Handbook of Dialysis

Handbook of Dialysis

Editor: Sean Eastwood

AMERICAN
MEDICAL PUBLISHERS
www.americanmedicalpublishers.com

AMERICAN
MEDICAL PUBLISHERS
www.americanmedicalpublishers.com

Cataloging-in-Publication Data

Handbook of dialysis / edited by Sean Eastwood.
p. cm.
Includes bibliographical references and index.
ISBN 978-1-63927-270-9
1. Dialysis. 2. Kidneys--Diseases. 3. Hemodialysis. 4. Nephrology. I. Eastwood, Sean.
RC903 .H36 2022
616.61--dc23

American Medical Publishers,
41 Flatbush Avenue,
1st Floor, New York,
NY 11217, USA

ISBN 978-1-63927-270-9 (Hardback)

Contents

Preface

The clinical process of removing excess solutes, toxins and water from the blood in patients with compromised kidney function is known as dialysis or renal replacement therapy. It is a common procedure in acute kidney disease or stage 5 chronic kidney disease. Dialysis is not a comprehensive therapy as it cannot heal the kidney. However it serves to replace its function through diffusion and ultrafiltration. Hemodialysis and peritoneal dialysis are two primary types of dialysis. In the former, blood is circulated outside the body through a dialyzer containing a semipermeable membrane and the wastes are removed, while in the latter, the peritoneum is used as a natural semipermeable membrane and the wastes are removed inside the body. Hemofiltration, intestinal dialysis and hemodiafiltration are some other dialysis techniques. This book outlines the techniques and applications of dialysis in detail. The various types of dialysis are glanced at and their practices and procedures are looked at in detail. This book will serve as a valuable source of reference for graduate and post graduate students.

Various studies have approached the subject by analyzing it with a single perspective, but the present book provides diverse methodologies and techniques to address this field. This book contains theories and applications needed for understanding the subject from different perspectives. The aim is to keep the readers informed about the progresses in the field; therefore, the contributions were carefully examined to compile novel researches by specialists from across the globe.

Indeed, the job of the editor is the most crucial and challenging in compiling all chapters into a single book. In the end, I would extend my sincere thanks to the chapter authors for their profound work. I am also thankful for the support provided by my family and colleagues during the compilation of this book.

Editor

1

Ankle-Brachial Index: A Simple Way to Predict Mortality among Patients on Hemodialysis

Zaida Noemy Cabrera Jimenez, Benedito Jorge Pereira, João Egidio Romão Jr, Sonia Cristina da Silva Makida, Hugo Abensur, Rosa Maria Affonso Moyses, Rosilene Motta Elias*

Renal Division, Internal Medicine, Hospital das Clínicas, University of São Paulo School of Medicine, São Paulo, Brazil

Abstract

Background: Ankle-brachial index (ABI) can access peripheral artery disease and predict mortality in prevalent patients on hemodialysis. However, ABI has not yet been tested in incident patients, who present significant mortality. Typically, ABI is measured by Doppler, which is not always available, limiting its use in most patients. We therefore hypothesized that ABI, evaluated by a simplified method, can predict mortality in an incident hemodialysis population.

Methodology/Principal Findings: We studied 119 patients with ESRD who had started hemodialysis three times weekly. ABI was calculated by using two oscillometric blood pressure devices simultaneously. Patients were followed until death or the end of the study. ABI was categorized in two groups normal (0.9–1.3) or abnormal (<0.9 and >1.3). There were 33 deaths during a median follow-up of 12 months (from 3 to 24 months). Age (1 year) (hazard of ratio, 1.026; $p = 0.014$) and ABI abnormal (hazard ratio, 3.664; $p = 0.001$) were independently related to mortality in a multiple regression analysis.

Conclusions: An easy and inexpensive technique to measure ABI was tested and showed to be significant in predicting mortality. Both low and high ABI were associated to mortality in incident patients on hemodialysis. This technique allows nephrologists to identify high-risk patients and gives the opportunity of early intervention that could alter the natural progression of this population.

Editor: Emmanuel A. Burdmann, University of Sao Paulo Medical School, Brazil

Funding: Zaida Noemy Cabrera Jimenez was supported by Conselho Nacional de Desenvolvimento Científico e Tecnológico (CNPQ), Brazil. The funders had no role in study design, data collection and analysis, decision to publish, or preparation of the manuscript.

Competing Interests: The authors have declared that no competing interests exist.

* E-mail: rosilenemotta@hotmail.com

Introduction

Despite significant technological advances, mortality among patients on hemodialysis remains inexcusably high, particularly in the first year of therapy [1].

One way to potentially reduce mortality is to alert medical staff to patients at increased risk of death in order to facilitate timely diagnostic and therapeutic interventions.

Hemodialysis patients are at an increased risk for atherosclerotic disorders, including peripheral arterial disease (PAD) [2]. PAD is a strong predictor for all-cause and cardiovascular mortality in hemodialysis patients [3,4].

Ankle-brachial index (ABI) is a simple, noninvasive, and reliable test for PAD screening. Usually ABI is classified as low (<0.9), normal (0.9–1.3) and high (>1.3). Both low and high ABI are correlated to high mortality in patients on hemodialysis [5]. Low ABI is related to PAD, and high ABI is caused by no compressible arteries and vascular calcification. Therefore, an abnormal ABI value is a significant predictor of mortality among patients on hemodialysis [4,6].

ABI was already identified as a predictor of mortality among prevalent patients on hemodialysis. Incident patients on hemodialysis are even at higher risk. The annual number of patients beginning dialysis has grown, mostly because of the growing prevalence of hypertension and diabetes, the main underlying cause of kidney disease [7,8]. Most analyses of survival on dialysis exclude the first 90-day period. There have been minimal improvements in mortality rate during the first year, over the past decade, even without including the initial 90 days [1,7]. ABI could be an easy way to identify patients at the highest risk.

We recently tested measuring ABI by using two oscillometric blood pressure devices simultaneously [9], simulating an ABI-form device.

The results demonstrated good reproducibility and low intra-observer variability. The ABI was extensively tested in three consecutive dialysis sessions, as well as pre and post dialysis. The question that remained was if this technique could be significant in predicting mortality.

We therefore tested the general hypothesis that ABI measured by two oscillometric blood pressure devices can predict mortality in an incident hemodialysis population.

Methods

Subjects

Patients were enrolled from January 2008 to January 2010. Inclusion criteria were patients with end-stage renal disease (ESRD) at least 18 years of age undergoing their first month of

Table 1. Characteristics of the study population.

Variables	N = 119
Age, years	53.1±18.8
Male, n (%)	82 (68.9)
Etiology of ESRD, n (%)	
Hypertension	35 (29.4)
Diabetes	44 (37.0)
Glomerulonephritis	18 (15.1)
Others	22 (18.5)
Hypertension, n (%)	118 (99.1)
Diabetes mellitus, n (%)	49 (47.2)
Family history of CV disease, n (%)	62 (52.1)
Smoking, ever vs. never, n (%)	36 (30.2)
Sedentary habits, n (%)	92 (77.3)
Ankle-brachial index	1.16±0.23
Systolic Blood Pressure, mmHg	149.4±23.8
Diastolic Blood Pressure, mmHg	85.9±17.2
Albumin level, g/dl	3.4±0.7
Phosphorus level, mg/dl	5.8±2.2
Calcium corrected, mg/dl	9.0±1.1
Calcium x Phosphorus, mg/dl	48.3±18.3
Total cholesterol, mg/dl	167.9±44.9
Hemoglobin, g/dl	9.3±1.7
C-reactive protein, mg/L	35.9±48.9
Parathyroid hormone, pg/ml	372.7±484.2

CV, cardiovascular; Calcium corrected = calcium + (4-albumin) ×0.8.
Values are expressed as mean ± SD or n (percentage).

conventional hemodialysis three times weekly in the University of Sao Paulo School of Medicine's Hospital das Clinicas. This was a prospective observational study.

We excluded anyone who had been treated for infection, had bilateral amputation, bilateral fistula or had atrial fibrillation. Prior to ABI measurement, demographic characteristics, and medical history were recorded. Biochemical data were measured within 2 weeks of ABI measurement and dialysis initiation.

ABI Measurement

The measurements were done by using two oscillometric devices (Omron Corp 705 CP Corp, Tokyo, Japan) simultaneously to measure blood pressure in the upper and lower extremities. The pre dialysis ABI was used in this new technique which was already intra-observer validated and described [9]. Briefly, measurements were done pre dialysis, with the patient at rest in the supine position, after 5 minutes of the beginning of the session. The protocol was performed by the same examiner in all situations. During the study, only raw blood pressure values were recorded, and stored on a database for later ABI calculation. Our technique showed that ABI can be measured by two oscillometric devices at the same time, with good reproductibility and low intra-observer variation.

Follow-up

The outcome of this study was all-cause mortality. Patients were censored in case of renal transplantation or recovery of renal function. Vital status was ascertained by telephone contact. The censor date was 31st January 2010. Date of death was verified by contacting relatives and/or the staff of the dialysis clinic. Survival time was defined as the time of the baseline (first day of ABI measurement) to the date of death or end of follow-up.

Ethic Statements

The protocol was approved by the Research Ethics Boards of the University of Sao Paulo School of Medicine, and all subjects provided written informed consent before participation.

Data Analysis

Differences between continuous variables and categorical variables were calculated using Student t test for normally distributed continuous variables and by Mann-Whitney U test for abnormally distributed variables. The $\chi 2$ or Fisher exact test was used to compare nominal variables. To compare the 3 groups according to ABI <0.9, from 0.9 to 1.3 and >1.3, one-way analysis of variance was applied, with Tukey post-hoc test.

Mortality was the outcome of the follow-up. The relation of ABI categories and all-cause mortality was analyzed by Kaplan-Meier survival plots and log-rank test. A stepwise multivariate cox regression was undertaken to identify the relative risk of all-cause mortality (entry threshold, $P<0.05$; removal threshold, $P<0.10$) with the significant candidate variables (age, diabetes, calcium x phosphorus product, parathyroid hormone and C-reactive protein). A lower level of the −2 log-likelihood indicates a better model fit. Data are presented as means ±SD unless indicated otherwise. A P-value <0.05 was considered significant. Analyses were performed with the use of SPSS 17.0.1 (SPSS Inc., Chicago, Ill).

Results

Subjects

Out of 123 consecutive ESRD patients, 4 lost the follow-up. Therefore, 119 patients were studied (82 men and 37 women), whose baseline characteristics were shown in Table 1. Diabetes, hypertension and glomerulonephritis accounted for 80% of the underlying causes of renal disease. The majority of the patients had a family history of cardiovascular disease (51.2%), 30.2% were smokers, 47.2% had diabetes, hypertension was found in almost 100% of the patients, and 77.3% presented sedentary behavior, which configure in a high cardiovascular risk population. Anemia, altered bone mineral metabolism, and inflammation (expressed by C-reactive protein) were also observed.

Characteristics of the study population regarding ABI categories (normal 0.9–1.3, low <0.9, and high >1.3 are presented in Table 2. Distribution of observed ABI at the baseline is shown in Figure 1. The significant differences between these 3 groups were age ($p = 0.011$), albumin ($p = 0.040$) and hemoglobin ($p = 0.010$). Cardiovascular risk factors observed at the baseline were well distributed among the three groups.

During the study there were 33 deaths on a median follow-up of 12 months (from 3 to 24 months). Table 3 shows the differences in basal characteristics between the group of patients who died and the group that survived. Patients who died were more likely to be older ($p = 0.003$), and with lower PTH ($p = 0.044$). Gender, diabetes, family history of cardiovascular disease, smoking and sedentary habitus, blood pressure, and biochemical variables did not distinguish survivors and non-survivors. The ABI as a continuous variable was virtually identical in survivors and non-survivors ($p = 0.998$). However, abnormal ABI was more frequent among patients who died than in patients who survived (63.6% vs. 13.9%, $p<0.0001$).

Preface

The clinical process of removing excess solutes, toxins and water from the blood in patients with compromised kidney function is known as dialysis or renal replacement therapy. It is a common procedure in acute kidney disease or stage 5 chronic kidney disease. Dialysis is not a comprehensive therapy as it cannot heal the kidney. However it serves to replace its function through diffusion and ultrafiltration. Hemodialysis and peritoneal dialysis are two primary types of dialysis. In the former, blood is circulated outside the body through a dialyzer containing a semipermeable membrane and the wastes are removed, while in the latter, the peritoneum is used as a natural semipermeable membrane and the wastes are removed inside the body. Hemofiltration, intestinal dialysis and hemodiafiltration are some other dialysis techniques. This book outlines the techniques and applications of dialysis in detail. The various types of dialysis are glanced at and their practices and procedures are looked at in detail. This book will serve as a valuable source of reference for graduate and post graduate students.

Various studies have approached the subject by analyzing it with a single perspective, but the present book provides diverse methodologies and techniques to address this field. This book contains theories and applications needed for understanding the subject from different perspectives. The aim is to keep the readers informed about the progresses in the field; therefore, the contributions were carefully examined to compile novel researches by specialists from across the globe.

Indeed, the job of the editor is the most crucial and challenging in compiling all chapters into a single book. In the end, I would extend my sincere thanks to the chapter authors for their profound work. I am also thankful for the support provided by my family and colleagues during the compilation of this book.

Editor

Table 2. Characteristics of the study population according to ABI.

Variable	ABI			
	<0.9 N = 12	0.9–1.3 N = 73	>1.3 N = 34	p
Age, years	68.8±16.6*	53.7±17.9	42.3±18.2	0.001
Male sex, n (%)	7 (58.3)	49 (67.1)	26 (76.5)	0.440
Diabetes mellitus, n (%)	5 (41.7)	29 (39.7)	15 (44.1)	0.911
Family history of CV disease, n (%)	6 (50)	41 (56.2)	15 (44.1)	0.503
Smoking, ever vs. never, n (%)	4 (33)	23 (31.5)	9 (26.5)	0.844
ABI	0.68±0.16*	1.13±0.11	1.40±0.08*	0.0001
Albumin level, g/dl	3.4±0.9	3.5±0.6	3.1±0.8*	0.040
Calcium x Phosphorus, mg^2/dl^2	47.7±22.0	49.7±18.6	45.6±16.6	0.564
Total cholesterol, mg/dl	162.4±36.8	168.3±46.9	169.1±43.9	0.903
Hemoglobin, g/dl	9.9±2,1	9.5±1.6	8.6±1.5*	0.010
C-reactive protein, mg/l	55.0±69.8	31.0±41.3	39.6±54.9	0.260
Parathyroid hormone, pg/ml	463.6±302.1	397.7±555.7	286.2±360.4	0.448

CV, cardiovascular; ABI, ankle-brachial index; Corrected Calcium = calcium + (4-albumin) ×0.8.
Values are expressed as Mean ± SD. *p<0.05 by post-test, comparing to ABI 0.9–1.3.

Figure 2 shows an unadjusted Kaplan-Meier survival curve analysis demonstrating that abnormal ABI was associated with greater all-cause mortality. The mean survival time and 95% confidence interval was 21.1±0.8 months (19.6–22.6) for normal ABI, and 16.2±1.2 months (13.8–18.7) for abnormal ABI; log-rank test p = 0.0001.

Upon multivariable Cox regression analyses of all-cause mortality by forward stepwise, the association between abnormal ABI and mortality remained. The HR associated with abnormal ABI was 3.664 times higher than normal ABI (p = 0.001, 95% CI, 1.708–7.861) (Table 4).

Discussion

Our study has given rise to important findings that provide novel possibilities into the diagnostic and interventions in an incident population on hemodialysis. We found that abnormal baseline ABI can predict mortality in hemodialysis patients. In addition, we accessed ABI by a simple and easy method. These findings suggest that ABI may be measured at patient's entry on hemodialysis therapy, even in centers without Doppler or an ABI-form device.

Our study population was representative of the total dialysis population in Brazil, according to the Brazilian Society of Nephrology [10,11] in terms of age, gender distribution and cause

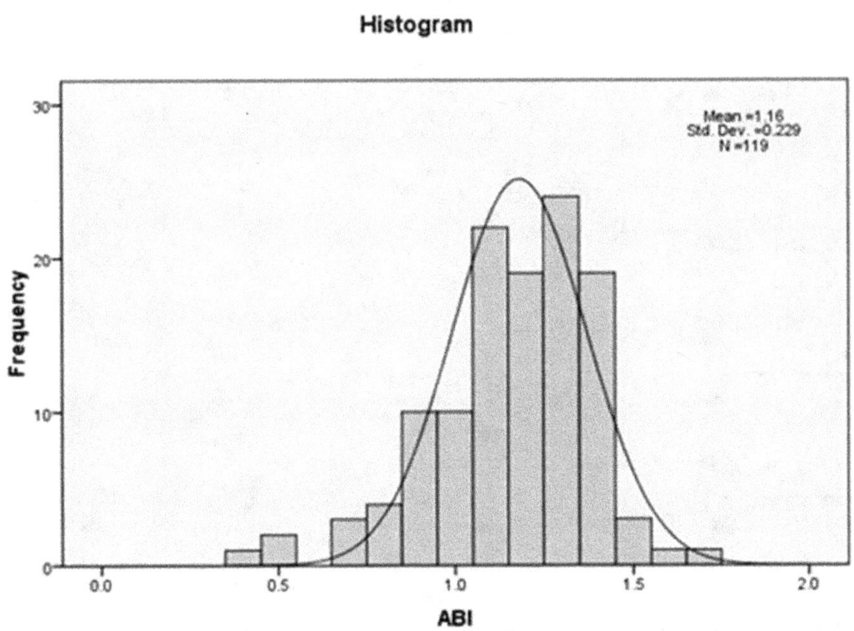

Figure 1. Frequency distribution of baseline ankle-brachial index (ABI).

Table 3. Survivors and non-survivors.

Variable	Survivors N = 86	Non-survivors N = 33	p
Age, years	50.0±18.3	61.2±17.8	0.003
Male sex, n (%)	58 (67.4)	27 (81.8)	0.671
Diabetes mellitus, n (%)	31 (36.0)	19 (57.6)	0.161
Family history of CV disease, n (%)	44 (51.2)	19 (57.6)	1
Smoking, ever vs. never, n (%)	26 (30.2)	10 (30.3)	0.830
Sedentary habitus, n (%)	68 (79.1)	26 (78.8)	0.355
ABI	1.16±0.18	1.15±0.32	0.998
Abnormal ABI, %	13.9	63.3	<0.0001
Systolic BP, mmHg	150.5±25.4	148.7±24.0	0.735
Diastolic BP, mmHg	86.9±19.9	81.0±16.9	0.146
Albumin level, g/dl	3.5±0.6	3.2±0.8	0.104
Calcium x Phosphorus, mg^2/dl^2	50.2±19.2	43.5±15.1	0.195
Total cholesterol, mg/dl	168.5±40.5	166.3±55.3	0.810
Hemoglobin, g/dl	9.2±1.8	9.4±13	0.612
C-reactive protein, mg/l	29.5±39.6	52.8±65.5	0.071
Parathyroid hormone, pg/ml	412.0±549.1	266.5±203.5	0.044

CV, cardiovascular disease; ABI, ankle-brachial index.
Values are expressed as Mean ± SD.

of ESRD. The prevalence of diabetes is also similar to the American and European reports [7,12,13]. However, all these data refer to the prevalent population and we studied an incident population. This specific population has an even higher risk of mortality. Some reported annual rate of mortality simply does not take into account the first 3 months of hemodialysis. The lack of information in the literature regarding diagnostic and possible therapeutic interventions in this selected population calls for new studies.

The incidence of patients in hemodialysis has increased in Brazil. The estimated number of patients starting treatment in 2010 was 18,972 (incidence rate: 99.5/million) [11].

We demonstrated that our sample size of incident patients on hemodialysis is at a high risk of mortality, with a family history of cardiovascular events, sedentary and smoking habits, presence almost universal of hypertension, diabetes and all dialysis-related biochemical abnormalities also associated to the high mortality risk. Indeed, we observed that 27.7% of the entire population had died after a 2-year period of follow-up.

The present data build on the previous findings showing that ABI is a good tool to detect high risk patients on hemodialysis. However, a mainly prevalent population on hemodialysis was studied, showing that both low and high ABI were associated to high overall and cardiovascular mortality [4,5,14,15].

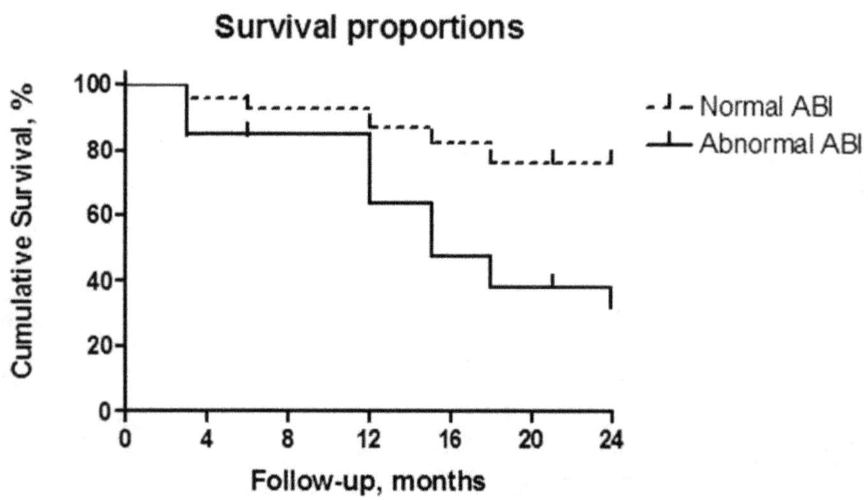

Figure 2. Kaplan-Meier survival curves according to ABI categories: normal (0.9–1.3) or abnormal (<0.9 and >1.3). A lower risk of mortality was observed for normal ABI [superior dashed line]; A higher risk of mortality was observed for abnormal ABI [continuous line]. Log-rank p = 0.0003;

Table 4. Cox regression Survival Analyses of All-cause Mortality, by Forward Stepwise (Likelihood ratio).

Variable	Hazard Ratio (95% Confidence interval)	P
Model 1		*0.001 (entire model)*
Abnormal ABI	3.564 (1.663–7.638)	0.001
Model 2		*0.0001 (entire model)*
Age (1 year)	1.026 (1.005–1.048)	0.014
Abnormal ABI	3.664 (1.708–7.861)	0.001

Initial Log Likelihood function −2 Log likelihood: 255.798.
Variables in the model: age, ABI as categorical (normal and abnormal), diabetes, C-reactive protein, albumin, hemoglobin, and PTH.

We could demonstrate similar results of previous studies by using a modified method in measuring ABI. It is important, however, to emphasize, that we had previously tested the intra-observer reproducibility. Based on this, we may suggest the use of this simple technique but we not guarantee applicability to other dialysis population. Different from previous studies, we accessed patients within their first month of dialysis. This approach allows us early recognition of patients at high risk of mortality.

The critical question is if the use of our simple technique in detecting abnormal ABI can eventually improve outcomes. There is no indication whether or not knowing the prognosis will improve outcomes. Possibly, we can at least alert medical staff to implement therapeutic interventions in those patients with abnormal ABI. Nevertheless, the clinical utility of our technique has to be studied rigorously in further studies. These studies should enrol larger sample sizes and evaluate different examiners measuring ABI.

Our study is subject to some limitations. First, it only shows associations between abnormal ABI and mortality in one selected dialysis population; this may not be applicable to all hemodialysis population. Second, the sample size was small. Third, we did not compare our technique to the gold-standard method, Doppler, in order to prove they can be interchangeable, although this was not an objective of the present data. Forth, we had no access to medication in use and dose of dialysis during the follow-up period. Finally, we could not distinguish between overall and cardiovascular cause of mortality, because the lack of accurate information relevant to the deaths of the patients within the study population.

However, our method was extensively tested and validated previously, and although we examined a small sample size, a direct relationship between abnormal ABI and mortality was found.

In conclusion, these data suggest that abnormal ABI was associated with increased mortality among incident patients on hemodialysis. The ABI could be measured by using at the same time two oscillometric blood pressure devices and then, making an easier and more largely applicable method in detecting patients with the highest risk of mortality. Our results also suggest the need for randomized trials to determine whether more aggressive interventions will change the outcomes.

Author Contributions

Conceived and designed the experiments: ZCNJ BJP SCSM JER RME. Performed the experiments: ZCNJ SCSM. Analyzed the data: ZCNJ SCSM BJP JER HA RMAM RME. Contributed reagents/materials/analysis tools: ZCNJ. Wrote the paper: ZCNJ BJP HA RMAM RME.

References

1. Himmelfarb J, Ikizler TA (2010) Hemodialysis. N Engl J Med 363: 1833–1845.
2. Cheung AK, Sarnak MJ, Yan G, Dwyer JT, Heyka RJ, et al. (2000) Atherosclerotic cardiovascular disease risks in chronic hemodialysis patients. Kidney Int 58: 353–362.
3. Newman AB, Shemanski L, Manolio TA, Cushman M, Mittelmark M, et al. (1999) Ankle-arm index as a predictor of cardiovascular disease and mortality in the Cardiovascular Health Study. The Cardiovascular Health Study Group. Arterioscler Thromb Vasc Biol 19: 538–545.
4. Ono K, Tsuchida A, Kawai H, Matsuo H, Wakamatsu R, et al. (2003) Ankle-brachial blood pressure index predicts all-cause and cardiovascular mortality in hemodialysis patients. J Am Soc Nephrol 14: 1591–1598.
5. Chen SC, Chang JM, Hwang SJ, Tsai JC, Liu WC, et al. (2010) Ankle brachial index as a predictor for mortality in patients with chronic kidney disease and undergoing haemodialysis. Nephrology (Carlton) 15: 294–299.
6. Kitahara T, Ono K, Tsuchida A, Kawai H, Shinohara M, et al. (2005) Impact of brachial-ankle pulse wave velocity and ankle-brachial blood pressure index on mortality in hemodialysis patients. Am J Kidney Dis 46: 688–696.
7. Collins AJ, Foley RN, Chavers B, Gilbertson D, Herzog C, et al. (2012) 'United States Renal Data System 2011 Annual Data Report: Atlas of chronic kidney disease & end-stage renal disease in the United States. Am J Kidney Dis 59: A7, e1–420.
8. Chan KE, Maddux FW, Tolkoff-Rubin N, Karumanchi SA, Thadhani R, et al. (2011) Early outcomes among those initiating chronic dialysis in the United States. Clin J Am Soc Nephrol 6: 2642–2649.
9. Jimenez ZN, de Castro I, Pereira BJ, de Oliveira RB, Romao JE, Jr., et al. (2012) When Is the Best Moment to Assess the Ankle Brachial Index: Pre- or Post-Hemodialysis? Kidney Blood Press Res 35: 242–246.
10. Censos Sociedade Brasileira de Nefrologia website. Available at http://www.sbn.org.br/leigos/index.php?censo Accessed 2011 Sep 10
11. Sesso RC, Lopes AA, Thome FS, Lugon JR, Santos DR (2011) 2010 report of the Brazilian dialysis census. J Bras Nefrol 33: 442–447.
12. Collins AJ, Foley RN, Herzog C, Chavers B, Gilbertson D, et al. (2009) United States Renal Data System 2008 Annual Data Report. Am J Kidney Dis 53: S1–374.
13. Zoccali C, Kramer A, Jager K (2009) The databases: renal replacement therapy since 1989–the European Renal Association and European Dialysis and Transplant Association (ERA-EDTA). Clin J Am Soc Nephrol 4 Suppl 1: S18–22.
14. Tanaka M, Ishii H, Aoyama T, Takahashi H, Toriyama T, et al. (2011) Ankle brachial pressure index but not brachial-ankle pulse wave velocity is a strong predictor of systemic atherosclerotic morbidity and mortality in patients on maintenance hemodialysis. Atherosclerosis 219: 643–647.
15. Adragao T, Pires A, Branco P, Castro R, Oliveira A, et al. (2012) Ankle–brachial index, vascular calcifications and mortality in dialysis patients. Nephrol Dial Transplant 27: 318–325.

2

Sympathetic Activation and Baroreflex Function during Intradialytic Hypertensive Episodes

Dvora Rubinger*, Rebecca Backenroth, Dan Sapoznikov

Nephrology and Hypertension Services, Department of Medicine, Hadassah University Medical Center, Jerusalem, Israel

Abstract

Background: The mechanisms of intradialytic increases in blood pressure are not well defined. The present study was undertaken to assess the role of autonomic nervous system activation during intradialytic hypertensive episodes.

Methodology/Principal Findings: Continuous interbeat intervals (IBI) and systolic blood pressure (SBP) were monitored during hemodialysis in 108 chronic patients. Intradialytic hypertensive episodes defined as a period of at least 10 mmHg increase in SBP between the beginning and the end of a dialysis session or hypertension resistant to ultrafiltration occurring during or immediately after the dialysis procedure, were detected in 62 out of 113 hemodialysis sessions. SBP variability, IBI variability and baroreceptor sensitivity (BRS) in the low (LF) and high (HF) frequency ranges were assessed using the complex demodulation technique (CDM). Intradialytic hypertensive episodes were associated with an *increased* (n = 45) or *decreased* (n = 17) heart rate. The maximal blood pressure was similar in both groups. In patients with *increased* heart rate the increase in blood pressure was associated with marked increases in SBP and IBI variability, with suppressed BRS indices and enhanced sympatho-vagal balance. In contrast, in those with *decreased* heart rate, there were no significant changes in the above parameters. End-of- dialysis blood pressure in all sessions associated with hypertensive episode was significantly higher than in those without such episodes. In logistic regression analysis, predialysis BRS in the low frequency range was found to be the main predictor of intradialytic hypertension.

Conclusion/Significance: Our data point to sympathetic overactivity with feed-forward blood pressure enhancement as an important mechanism of intradialytic hypertension in a significant proportion of patients. The triggers of increased sympathetic activity during hemodialysis remain to be determined. Intradialytic hypertensive episodes are associated with higher end-of- dialysis blood pressure, suggesting that intradialytic hypertension may play a role in generation of interdialytic hypertension.

Editor: Martin Gerbert Frasch, Université de Montréal, Canada

Funding: This study was self-funded by the investigators.

Competing Interests: The authors have declared that no competing interests exist.

* E-mail: rdvora@hadassah.org.il

Introduction

During hemodialysis treatment, blood pressure usually decreases with ultrafiltration and weight loss. In a significant proportion of patients, however, the blood pressure increases during or immediately after hemodialysis. Intradialytic hypertension has been recognized for many years, and it is believed to occur in at least 8–15% of patients [1]. There is no standard definition for intradialytic hypertension; some of the most common accepted criteria reviewed by Chazot and Jean [2] include a 15 mmHg increase of mean arterial pressure between the start and the end of a dialysis session [3], hypertension resistant to ultrafiltration occurring during or immediately after the dialysis procedure [4], or at least a 10 mmHg increase in the systolic blood pressure from pre-to post-dialysis [5]. Recent data have shown that intradialytic hypertension is associated with increased mortality and morbidity [5,6].

Several mechanisms are believed to lead to intradialytic increases in blood pressure. A positive sodium balance, resulting in extracellular fluid overload and hypertension in dialysis patients, is thought by many investigators to be the main cause of intradialytic increases in blood pressure [2,7]. Other popular hypotheses link intradialytic hypertension to variations in potassium or ionized calcium concentrations [8,9], antihypertensive drug removal during hemodialysis [10], hemoconcentration [11], recombinant erythropoietin administration, stimulation of the renin-angiotensin system during ultrafiltration [12], and to hemodynamic changes including increased cardiac output and vasoconstriction [13]. The latter is believed to be caused by endothelial dysfunction [14] and/or with increased endothelin secretion and altered nitric oxide/endothelin balance [13,15].

Sympathetic overactivity, believed to be generated by neurohormonal mechanisms arising within the diseased kidneys, is considered an important mechanism of hypertension in patients with chronic renal insufficiency [16–18]. Sympathetic nervous system activation during hemodialysis was proposed to be an important factor in the pathogenesis of intradialytic hypertension, via an increase in cardiac output and/or an increase in peripheral resistance. This hypothesis was supported by initial reports on increased plasma levels or increased turnover of cathecholamines in uremic patients and in experimental models of renal insufficiency [19–21]; no such changes, however, were found during hemodialysis treatment [22,23]. Furthermore, the baseline and intradialytic plasma levels of chatecholamines were reported to be similar in intradialytic hypertension-prone and in sex- matched control hemodialysis patients [15].

Sympathetic activity is best detected using microneurography (efferent post-ganglionic muscle sympathetic nerve activity, MSNA) and regional norepinephrine spillover technique [24]. Previous studies have shown that the basal MSNA firing was double in hypertensive hemodialysis patients as compared with age-matched healthy controls with normal blood pressure. Most studies, however, were performed in patients with residual renal function or in hemodialysis patients on a non-dialysis day [16,17,25]. To our knowledge, no such studies were performed in patients with intradialytic hypertension.

Since direct methods are not available or applicable in complex patients, sympathetic activity is assessed in many studies by non-invasive techniques. Heart rate variability (HRV), blood pressure variability (BPV) and baroreflex function (baroreceptor sensitivity, BRS) are the most frequently used methods to assess autonomic nervous system function and cardiovascular variability, a measure of the integrated control mechanisms of circulation [26]. In clinical settings, these measurements are usually computed from continuous beat to-beat recordings of heart rate and blood pressure oscillations [26–28]. Thus, the behavior of heart rate is considered an indirect index of adrenergic cardiovascular drive [29]. Spectral analysis of the heart rate oscillations allows the identification of low frequency (LF) component, believed to result from neural mechanisms related to sympathetic and vagal outflows, and a high frequency component (HF), related to respiration; the LF/HF ratio is frequently used as an index of sympatho-vagal interaction on the autonomic control of heart rate [26–28,30,31]. In humans, alterations of the low frequency band of blood pressure variability (LF SBP) were shown to be affected by sympathetic modulation of vascular tone as well as by myogenic vascular function [26–28,32].This relationship was well documented by studies measuring muscle sympathetic nerve activity in healthy volunteers, in whom sympathetic stimulation and nerve activity were associated with predominance of LF oscillations of blood pressure and of LF interbeat intervals [33,34]. In the recent years, in many studies, "spontaneous" BRS indices are also determined from continuous beat to beat surveys of blood pressure and heart rate, without pharmacological or external interventions. Both spontaneous and laboratory BRS indices correlate negatively with BPV and positively with HRV [26–28].

Complex demodulation is a newer method for assessing time dependent changes in signals around a specific frequency. The technique of complex demodulation (CDM) reveals instantaneous dynamic changes in heart rate and blood pressure that are not revealed by the standard spectral methods [35]. Therefore CDM may be particularly suitable to assess dynamic rapid changes in the autonomic nervous system during dialysis.

The present study was undertaken: 1. to detect increases in blood pressure during hemodialysis, and, 2. to assess the role of autonomic nervous system function during intradialytic hypertensive episodes. This is the first report of cardiovascular variability indices determined before and during intradialytic hypertensive episodes using the CDM methodology.

Methods

Continuous beat to beat blood pressure recordings were obtained during 113 routine midweek dialysis sessions in 108 chronic patients on maintenance hemodialysis. Patients with chronic atrial fibrillation or frequent ventricular premature beats, with debilitating illness and frequent hospital admissions, with permanent pacemakers or with severely decreased radial pulses following multiple vascular access surgical interventions were excluded from the study. Antihypertensive drugs were stopped 12–14 hr before the dialysis session. The study was approved by Hadassah Medical Organization Ethics Committee for Clinical Research. The patients signed an informed consent form before taking part in the study.

Demographic, clinical and laboratory data of all patients are shown in Tables 1 and 2. The patients were dialyzed 3.5 to 4 hours three to four times weekly, using the Gambro AK 200 delivery system and polyamide high flux dialyzers. The mean urea reduction rate (%URR) in all patients was 65–75%. Data on dialysate sodium concentration are given in Table 2; dialysate chloride, bicarbonate, potassium, dextrose and calcium concentrations were 108, 35, 2, 12 and 1.5 mmol/l, respectively.

The ultrafiltration rate during dialysis sessions never exceeded 1 liter/hour and was adjusted according to the presumed dry weight. The temperature of the dialysate was kept constant at 36°C.

All patients were treated with recombinant erythropoietin and phosphate binders (calcium carbonate, lanthanum carbonate and sevelamer hydrochloride) as needed.

Blood pressure signal acquisition

Blood pressure and inter-beat intervals were measured noninvasively by Finometer 1.10 (FMS, Finapres Medical Systems BV, Arnhem, The Netherlands). Continuous beat to beat recording of the finger arterial pressure waveform was performed as previously described [36] using the volume-clamp method of Penaz [37] and the Physiocal criteria of Wesseling [38]. In the volume-clamp method the diameter of the finger artery under the inflated cuff is kept constant. Changes in the arterial diameter, detected by a photo-plethysmographic method cause, via fast servo controller, pressure changes in an inflatable air bladder within the finger cuff. The Physiocal algorithm adjusts the correct diameter at which the finger artery is clamped. The transmural pressure is therefore zero all the time i.e., the finger cuff pressure equals the intra-arterial pressure. The finger cuff was wrapped on the middle phalanx of the middle finger. A height correction unit was attached to correct for finger height changes during the recording. An upper arm cuff unit was also attached and used to calibrate the systolic pressure for calculating the reconstructed brachial pressure from the finger pressure.

The data from Finometer were downloaded into a PC and analyzed by the BeatScope Software (TNO TPD Biomedical Instrumentation Amsterdam, The Netherlands) and our specifically designed programs. The BeatScope software performs beat to beat analysis of the finger arterial pressure and uses filtering and level correction to calculate reconstructed brachial pressures from finger pressures. The resulted data files containing beat to beat values of hemodynamic variables such as inter-beat intervals (IBI), systolic (SBP), diastolic (DBP) and mean blood pressures (MBP), were used for further processing. Data files included beat to beat values for the whole duration of hemodialysis. SBP and IBI signals were resampled at 1 Hz to obtain equidistant time series [35]. Aliasing was negligible as the Nyquist frequency is 0.5 Hz for this sampling rate and it was found to be above the frequency content of SBP and IBI signals. The recordings were scanned for hypertensive episodes. The *hypertensive episodes* were defined as: 1. a period of at least 10 mmHg increase in the systolic blood pressure (SBP) between the start and the end of a dialysis session, or, 2. hypertension occurring after significant ultrafiltration was

Table 1. Demographic and clinical data of all patients and of patients without and with hypertensive episodes.

	All Patients (n = 108)	Without hypertension (n = 51)	With hypertension (n = 57)	p[a]
Age (years)[b]	58 (15)	56 (16)	60 (15)	0.216
Males/females	69/39	32/19	37/20	0.815
Dialysis vintage (years)[b]	1.90 (3.02)	2.21 (3.51)	1.61 (2.49)	0.304
History of hypertension [n (%)]	98 (90.7)	45 (88.2)	53 (93.0)	0.396
Diabetes mellitus [n (%)]	38 (35.2)	18 (35.3)	20 (35.1)	0.982
History of ischemic heart disease [n (%)]	62 (57.4)	25 (49.0)	37 (64.9)	0.095
LV systolic dysfunction [n (%)][c]	28 (27.2)*	12 (23.5)	16 (30.8)	0.409
Diastolic dysfunction [n (%)]	37 (40.7)**	15 (34.1)	22 (46.8)	0.217
History of hyperlipidemia [n (%)]	79 (73.1)	37 (72.5)	42 (73.7)	0.894
History of frequent hypotensive episodes [n (%)]	53 (49.1)	23 (45.1)	30 (52.6)	0.434
Antihypertensive medication [n (%)]	80 (74.1)	36 (70.6)	44 (77.2)	0.578
Nitrates [n (%)]	20 (18.5)	5 (9.8)	15 (26.3)	0.027
Calcium blocking agents [n (%)]	40 (37.0)	15 (29.4)	25 (43.9)	0.121
Vasodilators[d] [n (%)]	20 (18.5)	3 (5.9)	17 (29.8)	0.001
ACE inhibitors [n (%)]	24 (22.2)	10 (19.6)	14 (24.6)	0.536
Angiotensin receptor blockers [n (%)]	10 (9.3)	4 (7.8)	6 (10.5)	0.631
Beta-blockers [n (%)]	55 (50.9)	25 (49.0)	30 (52.6)	0.708
Plasma Creatinine (μmol/l)[b,e]	728 (200)	757 (208)	702 (190)	0.154
Plasma calcium (mmol/l)[b, e]	2.22 (0.19)	2.24 (0.20)	2.21 (0.19)	0.434
Plasma phosphate (mmol/l)[b, e]	1.55 (0.36)	1.56 (0.37)	1.54 (0.36)	0.848
Hb (g/dl)[b, e]	11.1 (1.2)	11.1 (1.1)	11.2 (1.3)	0.751
Plasma albumin (g/l)[b, e]	38.0 (4.2)	38.7 (3.8)	37.4 (4.4)	0.112
PTH (pmol/l)[b, e]	49 (41)	51 (39)	48 (43)	0.684
CRP (mg/dl)[b, e]	3.36 (4.31)	2.85 (3.67)	3.82 (4.80)	0.254

[a]With vs. without hypertension.
[b]Mean (SD).
[c]Left ventricular ejection fraction (LVEF)<40%.
[d]Doxasozine or hydralazine.
[e]Predialysis values.
*Assessed in 103 patients, 52 with hypertensive episodes.
**Assessed in 91 patients, 47 with hypertensive episodes.
ACE, angiotensin-converting enzyme; CRP, C-reactive protein; Hb, hemoglobin; LV, left ventricle; PTH, parathyroid hormone.

achieved, i.e. during the second to the fourth hour of dialysis or immediately after the dialysis procedure [2,6]. During hemodialysis, blood pressure was also measured at 20 minute intervals using a digital oscillometric sphygmomanometer. During hypertensive episodes, blood pressure was double-checked by two different nurses or technicians every 5 minutes. The intradialytic episodes (n = 62) of increased blood pressure were further divided according to IBI changes into: a) *episodes with decreased IBI*, when the increase of at SBP was associated with a parallel increase in heart rate (n = 45) and, b) *episodes with increased IBI*, when the SBP increase was accompanied a decrease in heart rate (n = 17). Representative tracings of hypertensive episode associated with *increased* or *decreased* rate are depicted in Figure 1, left and mid panels. An episode with intradialytic hypotension and increased heart rate is depicted for comparison in the right panel.

Complex demodulation

Complex demodulation is a nonlinear time domain method of time series analysis. It is suited to the investigation of nonstationary oscillations and reveals instantaneous dynamic changes that are not revealed by the power spectrum methods. The analysis used in the present study was based on technique of Hayano et al [35]. In this analysis, signal X (t) is assumed to contain a frequency component which changes slowly around a specified center frequency, while Y(t) is the complex signal after shifting the frequency band around the frequency of interest to zero (see **Methods S1**).

Complex demodulation of SBP and IBI signals was performed at two frequency bands. The central frequencies (f_0) were 0.09 Hz for the low frequency (LF) and 0.30 Hz for the high frequency (HF) band. The result was then filtered by a low-pass 16th degree Butterworth filter with cut-off frequencies of 0.05 Hz and 0.16 Hz for the low and high frequencies range respectively. The signals were then smoothed by a 201 point least-square moving polynomial. Complex demodulation baroreflex (BRS) time series was computed as the ratio of the IBI and SBP time series instantaneous values in the two frequency ranges.

The amplitudes of SBP, IBI and BRS changes in the low (around center frequency of 0.09 Hz) and high (around center frequency of 0.30 Hz) frequency ranges were followed during the

Table 2. Dialysis data of all patients and of patients without and with hypertensive episodes.

	All Patients (n = 108)	Without hypertension (n = 51)	With hypertension (n = 57)	p[a]
Predialysis SBP (mmHg)*	134 (25)	135 (27)	133 (23)	0.694
Intradialytic weight loss (% of body weight)[b]	27.5 (15.3)**	28.1 (15.7)	26.9 (15.1)	0.714
Ultrafiltration rate (ml/min)[b]	9.29 (4.62)**	9.56 (4.67)	9.10 (4.57)	0.630
Dialysate Na concentration [n (%)] <140 mmol/l	2 (1.9)	1 (2.0)	1 (1.8)	0.663
140 mmol/l	98 (90.7)	45 (88.2)	53 (93.0)	
>140 mmol/l	8 (7.4)	5 (9.8)	3 (5.2)	
Predialysis plasma Na (mmol/l)[b]	139 (3)	139 (3)	139 (3)	0.340
Postdialysis plasma Na (mmol/l)[b]	140 (3)[c]	141 (4)[c]	140 (3)[d]	0.245
Gradient between dialysate and plasma Na (mmol/l)[b]	1.20 (3.52)	1.00 (3.70)	1.39 (3.38)	0.572
Increase in plasma Na after dialysis (mmol/l)[b]	1.37 (2.98)	1.45 (3.02)	1.30 (2.97)	0.792
Predialysis plasma K (mmol/l)[b]	4.97 (0.65)	5.10 (0.76)	4.85 (0.65)	0.065
Postdialysis plasma K (mmol/l)[b]	3.54 (0.43)[c]	3.63 (0.37)[c]	3.45 (0.47)[c]	0.030
Increase in plasma K after dialysis (mmol/l)[b]	1.43 (0.62)	1.47 (0.62)	1.40 (0.62)	0.537
Predialysis plasma osmolality (mosm/KgH_2O)[b]	318 (12)	319(10)	316 (12)	0.187
Postdialysis plasma osmolality (mosm/KgH_2O)[b]	305 (8)[c]	307 (8)[c]	303 (8)[c]	0.054

*Data given as median and interquartile range.
**Data available in 97 patients (53 with hypertensive episodes).
[a]With vs. without hypertension.
[b]Mean (SD).
p vs. predialysis values:
[c]<0.001;
[d]0.002.

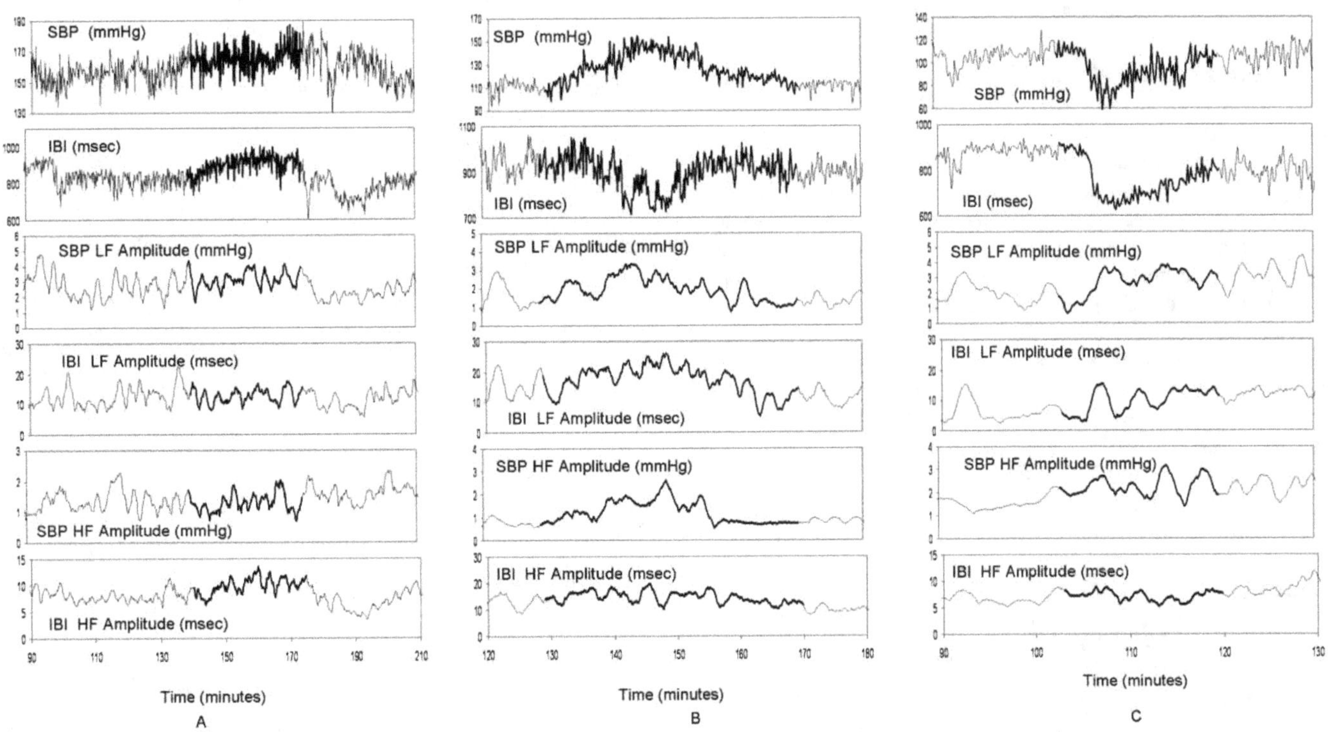

Figure 1. Representative tracings of continuous recordings of SBP and IBI oscillations and variability during intradialytic hypertension episodes with *decreased* (A) or *increased* heart rate (B). Tracings of a patient with marked intradialytic hypotension are depicted for comparison (C). The episodes associated with sudden changes in blood pressure are shown by the bolder parts of the tracings. LF, low frequency; HF, high frequency; IBI, interbeat interval.

whole dialysis session. Five minute averages of the LF and HF SBP, LF and HF IBI, LF IBI/HF IBI ratio (representative of sympatho-vagal balance) and BRS indices were calculated the following manually detected periods: 1) the first 20 minutes (beginning), 2) the last 20 minutes (end) of dialysis, 3) 20 minutes before, and, 4) during hypertensive episodes.

Statistics

Demographic and clinical categorical variables were compared by *chi*-square test. Age and laboratory data (mean and standard deviation) were compared using Student's *t* test. Blood pressure, inter-beat interval and baroreceptor variables are given as medians and inter-quartile ranges.

Wilcoxon signed-ranks test was used to compare paired differences at the beginning and the end of dialysis and to assess differences between the periods before and during hypertensive episodes. Mann-Whitney U-test was used to compare between sessions without and with hypertension, and between hypertensive episodes with increased and decreased heart rate.

Correlations of intradialytic changes in SBP with CDM indices and between different CDM variables were performed by Pearson correlation and linear regression analysis.

Logistic regression analysis

Logistic regression analysis (stepwise forward conditional procedure) was performed to select determinants of intradialytic hypertension. Age, gender, hemodialysis vintage (years), the presence of diabetes mellitus, history of hypertension, hyperlipidemia , ischemic heart disease and of intradialytic hypotensive episodes, administration of antihypertensive drugs, hypertensive medication, biochemical data and predialysis SBP, IBI and CDM measurements (LF IBI, HF IBI, LF SBP, HF SBP, LF BRS and HF BRS) were all included in the analysis.

Definitions of clinical variables

Ischemic heart disease was defined by: documentation of prior myocardial infarction or of coronary interventions, the presence of significantly abnormal Q waves on a 12-lead electrocardiogram, symptomatic angina pectoris or a thallium perfusion scan suggestive of myocardial ischemia. Left ventricular systolic dysfunction was defined as decreased left ventricular ejection fraction (LVEF) to less than 40% on echocardiography. Doppler interrogation of the mitral valve, pulmonary vein and mitral annulus was used to assess diastolic function. Severe diastolic dysfunction was defined as :a) pseudo-normalization of E (early filling wave) to A (late filling wave) ratio, suggesting an elevated left ventricular diastolic pressure, or, b) a restrictive pattern, suggesting reduced compliance, i.e. grade 2–4 diastolic dysfunction by echocardiographic criteria [39]. Patients with high triglyceride or/and high LDL cholesterol levels were considered to be hyperlipidemic.

Results

Clinical and laboratory data

One hundred and eight patients were examined during 113 hemodialysis sessions. Hypertensive episodes (n = 62) were detected in 57 patients. The timing of the occurrence of the hypertensive episode was different for each patient. Ten episodes occurred in the 1st, 22 in the 2nd ^{and} 24 in the 3rd hour, and 6 towards the end of hemodialysis session. The duration (mean ± SD) of the hypertensive episodes was 27±16 min (range 5–80 min). While many patients with intradialytic increases in blood pressure episodes complained of dizziness, palpitations or weakness, none developed syncope or loss of consciousness.

Patient clinical and biochemical data are listed in Table 1. Pre- and post dialysis SBP and other data related to the hemodialysis procedure are listed in Table 2. Age, sex distribution and dialysis vintage were similar in patients without and with intradialytic hypertensive episodes (Table 1). Diabetic nephropathy was the primary renal disease in 15 (29.4%) and in 18 (31.6%) patients without and with hypertensive episodes, respectively. Other causes of end stage renal failure in patients without and with intradialytic hypertension were glomerulonephritis (10 and 11), interstitial nephritis (5 and 5), familial nephropathy in 6 (6 and 3), nephrosclerosis and ischemic nephropathy (3 and 8), autosomal dominant polycystic kidney disease (1 and 3) and miscellaneous (11 and 9). A residual renal function was present in 44 patients, 17 without (mean creatinine clearance 5.87(4.12) ml/min) and 27 with intradialytic hypertension (mean creatinine clearance 5.29(3.65) ml/min, pNS). A history of essential or secondary hypertension was in the medical background of 45 (88.2%) and 53 (93%) patients without and with intradialytic hypertensive episodes, respectively (p NS). While the prevalence of diabetes mellitus, hyperlipidemia and the dialysis vintage was similar in both groups, that of ischemic heart disease was slightly increased in patients with hypertensive episodes (p = 0.095) . Fifty three (49.1%) patients, 23 patients with and 30 without hypertensive episodes (p NS) had a history of frequent hypotensive episodes during dialysis. The prevalence of patients receiving antihypertensive drugs was comparable in both groups, but the use of vasodilators and nitrates was more frequent in patients with intradialytic hypertensive episodes. There were no significant differences between groups with regard to cardiac function, biochemical data, dialysis prescription, intradialytic weight loss or ultrafiltration rate. While the decrease in plasma K^+ was similar in both groups, post dialysis K^+ level was lower in patients with hypertensive episodes (Table 2).

Effect of hemodialysis treatment on autonomic activity and on baroreceptor sensitivity in patients without and with intradialytic hypertensive episodes

Table 3 lists blood pressure, interbeat intervals and their variabilities, baroreflex sensitivity indices and LF IBI/HF IBI ratio during all screened hemodialysis sessions (n = 113), and sessions without (n = 51) and with (n = 62) hypertensive episodes. There was a significant decrease in SBP at the end of hemodialysis sessions without hypertensive episodes, while in those with hypertensive episodes, there were marked increases in SBP, DBP and MBP. A minimal decrease in LF SBP was noted, especially in session without hypertension, while HF SBP significantly increased at the end of dialysis in both groups. In both types of sessions, IBI was not significantly changed at the end of the dialysis. At the beginning of dialysis, LF BRS and HF BRS were higher in sessions associated with hypertensive episodes. Significant increases in LF IBI, HF IBI and LF BRS, and a decrease in LF IBI/HF IBI at the end of the treatment occurred only in the dialysis sessions without hypertension.

Blood pressure and interbeat interval variability, baroreflex sensitivity and sympatho-vagal balance during intradialytic hypertensive episodes

Forty-five (72.5%) intradialytic hypertensive episodes (mean duration 24±14 min) in 41 patients were associated with an *increase* in heart rate; the heart rate *decreased* during 17 (27.5%) episodes in 16 patients (lasting 34±19 min, p NS).The timing of occurrence of hypertension during dialysis was similar in the two

Table 3. Blood pressure variability, baroreflex sensitivity indices, interbeat intervals and low frequency/high frequency interbeat interval ratio at the beginning and at the end of hemodialysis*.

	All sessions (n = 113)**			Sessions without hypertension (n = 51)**			Sessions with hypertension (n = 62)**		
	Beginning	End	p	Beginning	End	p	Beginning	End	p
SBP (mmHg)	135 (31)	134 (36)	0.160	139 (42)	125 (34)	0.023	132 (30)	143 (36)[c]	0.001
DBP (mmHg)	67 (18)	73 (17)	0.001	69 (19)	71 (18)	0.056	67 (17)	76 (21)[d]	0.001
MBP(mmHg)	90 (20)	94 (22)	0.001	92 (25)	90 (16)	0.888	90 (17)	100 (17)[c]	0.001
IBI (msec)	827 (177)	862(216)	0.103	802 (196)	813(274)	0.606	850 (162)	878 (175)	0.089
LF SBP (mmHg)	1.92 (2.02)	1.90 (0.87)	0.726	1.98 (0.93)	1.95 (1.00)	0.051	1.92 (0.64)	1.88 (0.86)	0.188
HF SBP (mmHg)	1.40 (0.72)	1.69 (0.70)	0.001	1.54 (0.58)	1.89 (1.01)	0.003	1.21 (0.72)[b]	1.64 (0.52)	0.003
LF IBI (msec)	5.79 (4.74)	6.95 (6.38)	0.022	5.39 (4.49)	6.01 (6.80)	0.046	6.11 (4.92)	7.16 (5.49)	0.165
HF IBI (msec)	5.52 (3.28)	5.85 (4.07)	0.001	4.99 (2.45)	5.82 (5.32)	0.001	5.81 (3.39)	5.87 (2.77)	0.369
LF BRS (msec/mmHg)	3.48 (2.51)	3.60 (2.85)	0.003	3.03 (1.95)	3.21 (3.20)	0.001	3.62 (2.79)[a]	3.67 (2.67)	0.468
HF BRS (msec/mmHg)	3.87 (2.91)	3.69 (3.41)	0.783	3.29 (2.62)	3.42 (4.52)	0.376	4.39 (3.13)[b]	3.89 (2.54)	0.147
LF IBI/HF IBI	1.11 (0.59)	1.06 (0.50)	0.034	1.15 (0.64)	1.04 (0.58)	0.003	1.07 (0.57)	1.07 (0.60)	0.809

*Data given as median and interquartile range;
**Number of patients: all sessions-108; without hypertension-51; with hypertension-57. Beginning-the initial 20 minutes of the dialysis session; End-the last 20 minutes of the dialysis session. Comparison of sessions without and with hypotension-Beginning:
[a]p = 0.004;
[b]p = 0.008; End:
[c]p = 0.001;
[d]p = 0.035.

types of episodes. Five episodes were detected on repeated examinations; one patient was examined 3 times, and the remaining 3 patients were examined twice. Intradialytic hypertensive episodes with increased heart rate were detected during repeated examinations in 3 patients; in one remaining patient intradialytic increase in blood pressure with decreased heart rate was detected during two separate sessions.

During hypertensive episodes, the magnitude of the increase in blood pressure was similar in both subgroups. Maximal SBP, DBP and MBP [median (interquartile range)] were 158 (30), 80 (24) and 104 (19) mm Hg in patients with *increased* heart rate ($p<0.001$ vs. before) and 159 (25), 73 (17) and 102 (19) mm Hg in patients with *decreased* heart rate ($p<0.001$ vs. before). SBP, IBI and their variability before and during hypertensive episodes are depicted in Figure 2, while baroreceptor sensitivity indices and LF IBI/HF IBI during intradialytic hypertension are shown in Figure 3. At the initiation of hypertensive episodes (before), blood pressure and IBI were similar in all patients. LF SBP, HF SBP and LF IBI markedly increased during the hypertensive episodes in patients with *increased* heart rate (decreased IBI) , but did not significantly change in those in whom heart rate *decreased* (increased IBI, Figure 2). In *increased* heart rate episodes, the blood pressure elevation was associated with significantly diminished baroreflex indices (LF BRS and HF BRS) and enhanced LF/HF ratio (Figure 3). In *decreased* heart rate episodes, a tendency to increase in BRS indices was observed during hypertension; these changes, however, were not statistically significant.

Significant correlations between changes in heart rate variability with changes in blood pressure variability in both LF ($r = 0.526$) and HF ($r = 0.405$) bands ($p<0.001$) were found during hypertensive episodes, but only in those with *increased* heart rate (Figure 4). We found no correlations between the blood pressure increases during hypertensive episodes with changes in heart rate variability or blood pressure variability, with changes in baroreflex indices or LF IBI/HF IBI ratio. Likewise, there were no correlations between blood pressure increases and weight loss, ultrafiltration rate, the dialysate to predialysis plasma Na concentration gradient or the decrease in plasma potassium and in plasma osmolality during dialysis.

Comparisons of patients experiencing intradialytic hypertension with *increased* or *decreased* heart rate showed that age, medical history and comorbidities, the number of years in dialysis, dialysis prescription and the biochemical profile were similar for the two subgroups (not shown). A higher proportion of women, 9 of 16, was noted, however, in the subgroup of patients with decreased heart rate as compared with 11 of 41 in patients with increased heart rate during hypertensive episodes ($p = 0.036$). In addition, in the former subgroup, 8 (50%) patients were treated with an angiotensin converting enzyme inhibitor as compared with 6 (14.6%) patients in the latter ($p = 0.005$). Pre-and post-dialysis SBP, DBP, IBI and CDM measurements were similar in patients with increased or decreased heart rate during intradialytic hypertension episodes.

Predictors of intradialytic hypertension

Logistic regression analysis (stepwise forward conditional procedure) was performed to define independent predictors of intradialytic hypertension. Three different models were constructed including clinical, dialysis and laboratory data and CDM measurements (see **Methods**). The most significant predictors are listed in Table 4. Predialysis baroreflex sensitivity in the low frequency range (LF BRS) was found to be the most important predictor of intradialytic hypertension (1st and 2nd models, Odds Ratio 1.455 and 1.650, $p = 0.004$ and 0.001, respectively). Because of the strong correlation of baroreflex sensitivity with heart rate variability and the inverse correlation with blood pressure variability [28], these indices were analyzed in a different model (3rd model). In this model, a higher predialysis LF IBI (Odds ratio 1.228, $p = 0.006$) and a lower LF SBP (Odds ratio 0.223,

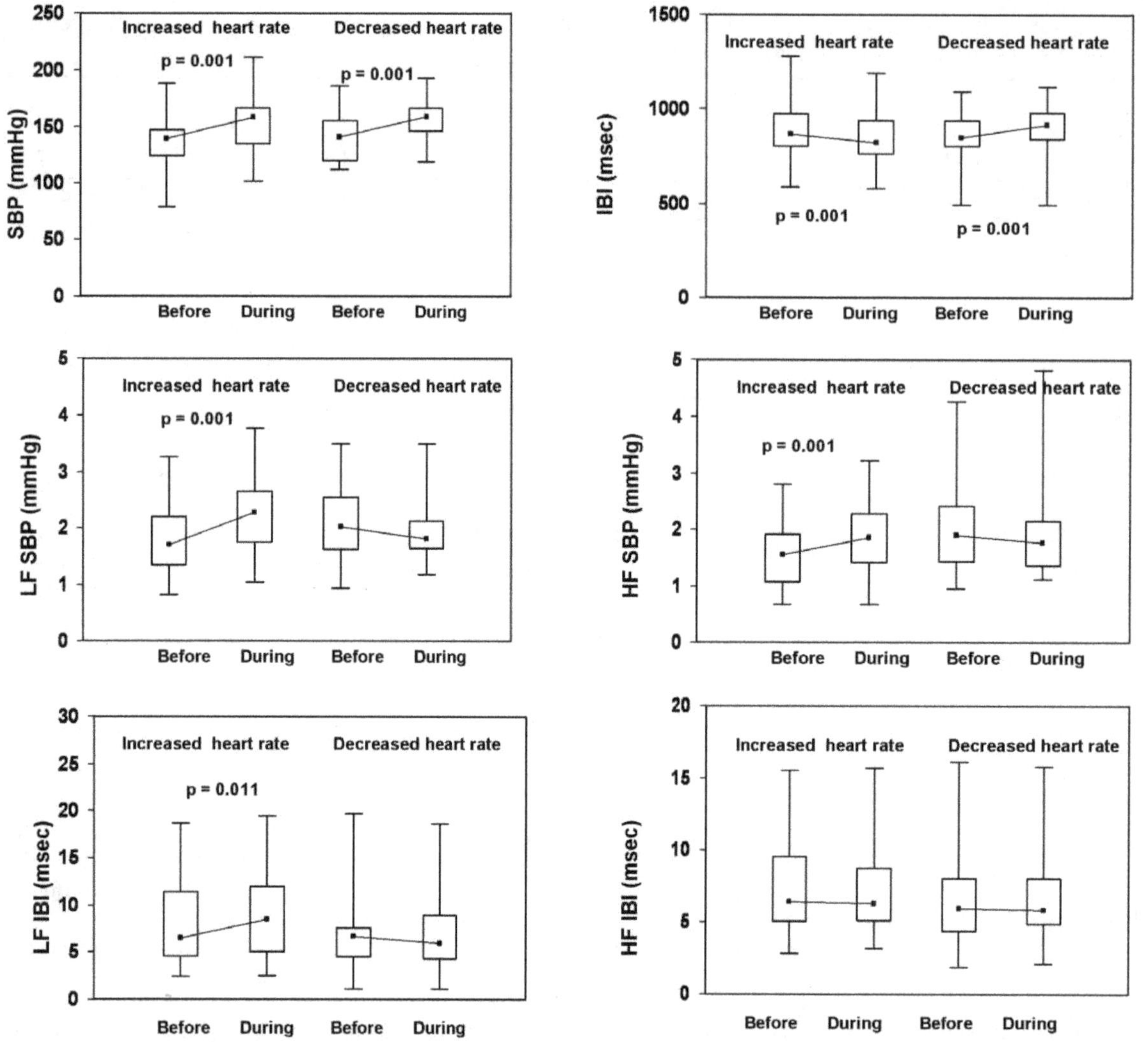

Figure 2. SBP and interbeat interval and their variability indices before and during intradialytic hypertensive episodes associated with *increased* (n = 45) or *decreased* (n = 17) heart rate. Data are presented as box plots. The box stretches from the 25th to the 75th percentile; the median is shown as a small black square in the box. The range (the upper and the lower extreme values) is indicated by whiskers. HF, high frequency; LF, low frequency, IBI, interbeat interval.

p = 0.001) were found to be significant predictors of hypertensive episodes.

Other significant predictors were lower serum albumin level (2nd and 3rd models, p = 0.020 and 0.037) and age (2nd model, p = 0.037).

Discussion

This study is the first, to our knowledge, to report on dynamic changes of SBP, IBI and baroreflex function during intradialytic hypertensive episodes. The principal new finding of this study is that a large proportion of hypertensive episodes are associated with increased heart rate, with marked increases in blood pressure variability (LF SBP and HF SBP), interbeat interval variability (LF IBI), decreased baroreceptor sensitivity (LF BRS and HF BRS) and enhanced sympatho-vagal balance (Figure 2 and 3).The above episodes, characterized by shortening of IBI intervals synchronous with SBP increase, are similar to those occurring during central autonomic activations [40]. These non- baroreceptor- related events are believed to be mediated by enhanced sympathetic outflow with feed-forward effects on blood pressure [41]. In contrast, during baroreceptor activation, increases or decreases in blood pressure are associated with feed-back mediated decreases or increases in heart rate (increased or decreased interbeat interval), respectively. In hemodialysis patients, baroreflex mechanisms were shown to be adequately activated during hypotensive episodes [36]. Our present findings suggest that sympathetic activation and feed–forward enhancement of blood pressure play an important role in the pathogenesis of intradialytic hypertension episodes.

Sympathetic activation during intradialytic hypertensive episodes

Sympathetic overactivity associated with chronic hypertension was detected by MSNA in patients with early or advanced chronic kidney disease and on maintenance hemodialysis [17,18,25,29,42]. In one single study, performed during dialysis, the sympathetic firing was shown to increase during the hemodialysis procedure, ultrafiltration and decrease in blood pressure [18].

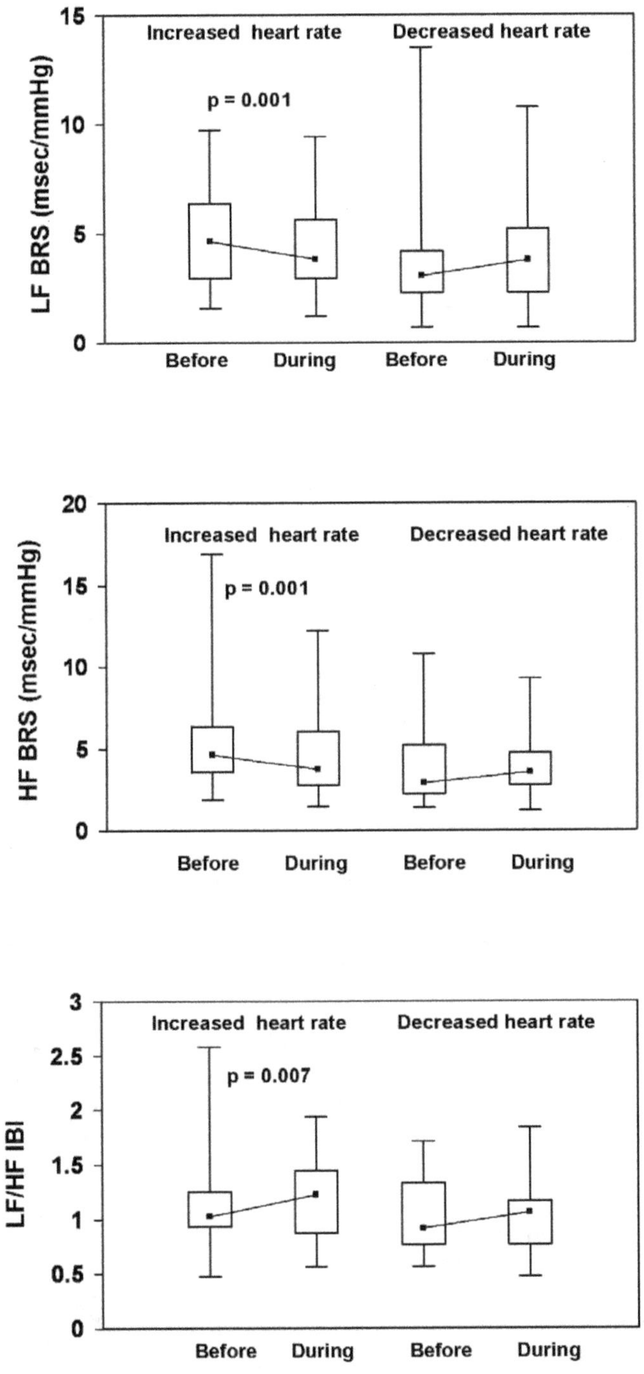

Figure 3. BRS indices and LF IBI/HF IBI ratio before and during intradialytic hypertensive episodes associated with *increased* (n = 45) or *decreased* (n = 17) heart rate. Data are presented as box plots. The box stretches from the 25th to the 75th percentile; the median is shown as a small black square in the box. The range (the upper and the lower extreme values) is indicated by whiskers. BRS, baroreceptor sensitivity; HF, high frequency; LF, low frequency, IBI, interbeat interval.

We have previously shown that in chronic dialysis patients, LF SBP was increased, while LF IBI and the baroreceptor sensitivity indices were markedly decreased as compared to normal individuals [43].These findings, similar to those reported in essential hypertension and congestive heart failure, were interpreted as evidence of background chronic sympathetic overactivity associated with end-stage kidney disease.

In the present study, the alterations noted during 45 (72.5%) of 62 intradialytic hypertensive episodes (Figures 2 and 3) are suggestive of acute bursts of sympathetic activity with feed forward enhancement of blood pressure. In the remaining 17 hypertensive episodes, similar increases in blood pressure were associated with decreased heart rate; no significant changes in interbeat interval variability, blood pressure variability or baroreflex indices were noted in these patients. One possible explanation for these findings may involve simultaneous co-activation of the parasympathetic system resulting in an elevated blood pressure without an increase in heart rate, as described in subjects under psychological stress [44]. The intradialytic elevation in blood pressure with no increase in heart rate might also be caused by mechanisms independent of autonomic nervous-system. Endothelial dysfunction was recently documented in patients with intradialytic hypertension [14,45]; in one study intradialytic hypertension was independently associated with both endothelial dysfunction and increased arterial stiffness [45]. Accordingly, a primary functional defect within the arterial wall may lead under special circumstances to an exaggerated pressure response due to increased endothelin and decreased nitric oxide (NO) availability and increased vascular resistance [14,15].

The mechanisms of acute intradialytic activation of the sympathetic nervous system are not well defined. Activation of RAS was suggested as a potential mechanism of both sympathetic stimulation and intradialytic hypertension. A recent study, however, did not show increases in plasma renin and aldosterone levels during hemodialysis in patients with intradialytic increases in blood pressure [15]. In our study, end-of dialysis plasma potassium level was lower in patients with hypertensive episodes. The lower plasma potassium in these patients could indeed have resulted from intradialytic activation of the renin-angiotensin system, leading to increased circulating angiotensin and aldosterone levels, with further activation of central nervous system mineralocorticoid and angiotensin type I receptors and enhanced sympathetic outflow [25,46]. In hemodialysis patients, an acute decrease in serum potassium was shown to be associated with increased blood pressure, presumably mediated by arteriolar constriction via sympathetic stimulation [8].

Another proposed mechanism extensively investigated in chronic kidney disease links between renal ischemia and hypoxia, activation of mechano- and chemo-receptors, secretion of adenosine and sympathetic activation [42]. The relevance of this mechanism, however, for hemodialysis-associated hypertension remains to be determined.

Tonic arterial chemoreceptor activation was also shown to be involved in sympathetic activation in patients with advanced renal failure [47]. Hypoxemic events during hemodialysis, initiated by intrapulmonary (ventilation-perfusion mismatching) and/or extra-pulmonary (ventilatory control) mechanisms [48] may elicit sympathetic activation [47]. Peripheral chemoreflex sensitivity is particularly enhanced in patients with obstructive sleep apnea, a common condition in chronic hemodialysis and frequently associated with hypertension. [49]. Studies in experimental animals have shown that prolonged blood flow reduction to carotid body enhances chemoreflex function and causes sympathetic activation [50]. Alterations of cerebral blood flow may occur in association with hemodynamic changes during hemodialysis [51].Taken together, these findings strongly support the hypothesis that sympathetic overactivity may be triggered by chemoreceptor dysregulation associated with fluid and electrolyte shifts during hemodialysis.

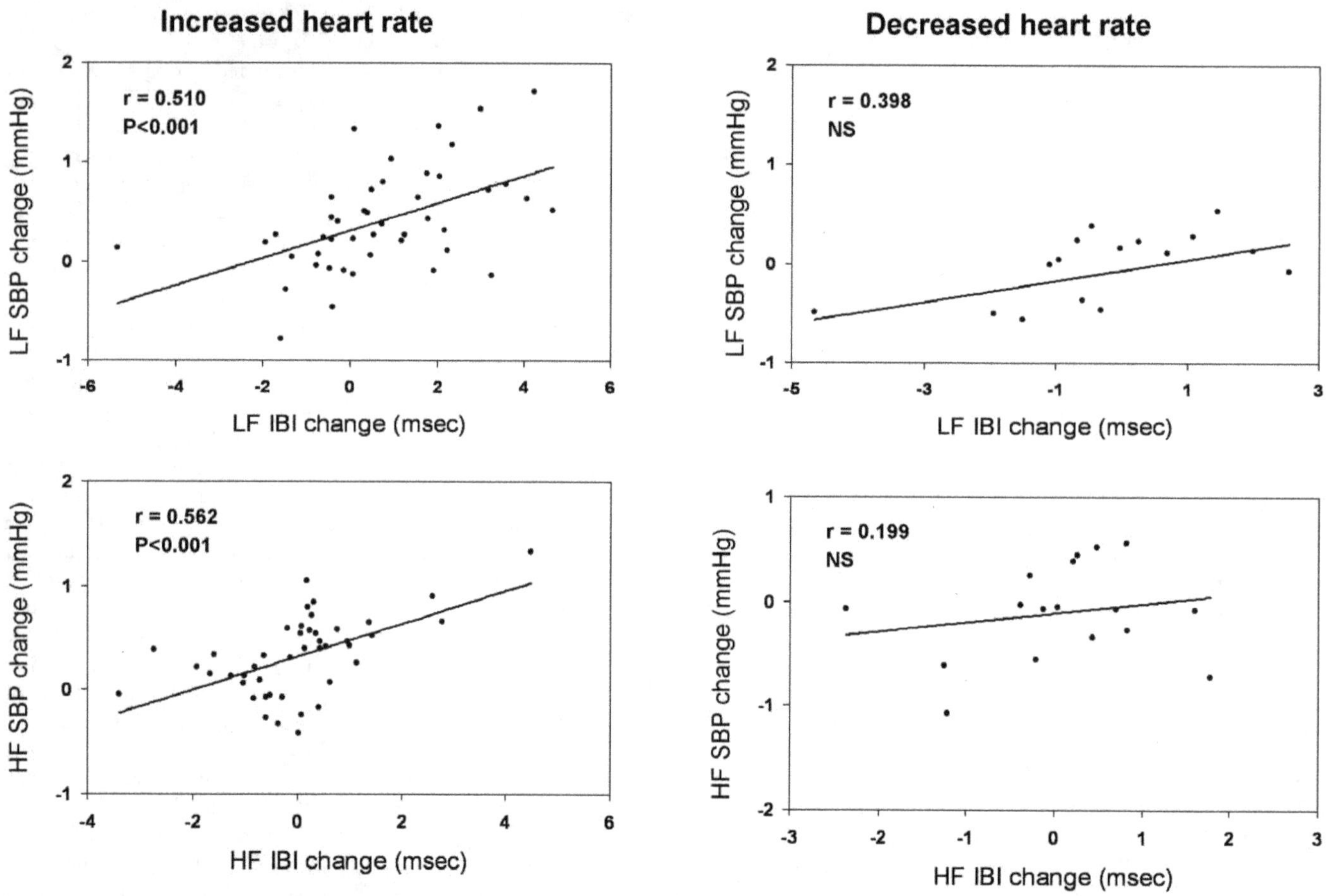

Figure 4. Correlations of changes in interbeat intervals with changes in SBP during intradialytic hypertensive episodes associated with *increased* (n = 45) or *decreased* (n = 17) heart rate. HF, high frequency; LF, low frequency, IBI, interbeat interval.

Other possible, non-mutually exclusive mechanism of intradialytic sympathetic activation may be related to a reduced vascular and hypothalamic availability of nitric oxide (NO) associated with alterations in sympathetic outflow and in vascular endothelial function [13,15,52]. Deficiency of the soluble monoamine oxidase renalase in end stage renal failure was also shown to be associated with increased sympathetic tone and with resistant hypertension [53]. The activation of the above mechanisms during intradialytic hypertensive episodes has yet to be explored.

Table 4. Predictors of intradialytic hypertension based on logistic regression analysis.

Variables	Predictors	Odds ratio	95% CI	b coefficient	p
1st **Model** (Clinical data, LF BRS and HF BRS)	LF BRS	1.455	1.130–1.875	0.375	0.004
2nd **Model** (Clinical and laboratory data, LF BRS and HF BRS)	Age	1.032	1.002–1.063	0.031	0.037
	Plasma albumin	0.875	0.781–0.979	−0.134	0.020
	LF BRS	1.650	1.222–2.228	0.501	0.001
3rd **Model** (Clinical and laboratory data, LF IBI, HF IBI, LF SBP, HF SBP)	Albumin	0.892	0.801–0.993	−0.114	0.037
	LF IBI	1.228	1. 061–1.422	0.206	0.006
	LF SBP	0.223	0.089–0.561	−1.499	0.001

CI: confidence interval.
Variables in logistic regression models:
Clinical data: age, gender, dialysis vintage, history of intradialytic hypotension, history of hypertension, diabetes, ischemic heart disease, hyperlipidemia, anti-hypertensive medication, pre-dialysis SBP and IBI.
Laboratory data: pre-dialysis creatinine, calcium, phosphate, potassium, albumin, hemoglobin and PTH concentrations and CRP levels.
CDM measurements: pre-dialysis LF IBI, HF IBI, LF SBP, HF SBP, LF BRS and HF BRS.

Insufficient sodium removal during hemodialysis and volume excess were proposed and are still believed by many investigators to be the main causes of intradialytic and interdialytic hypertension [2,7,54,55]. In experimental animals, excess salt may lead to hypertonic Na accumulation in skin, to endothelial activation and hypertension [56,57]. A central effect of excessive salt intake may occur via enhancement of the excitability of sympatho-regulatory circuits in the rostral ventro-lateral medulla and it was hypothesized that even small changes in plasma sodium may affect the responsiveness of these neurons [57]. Salt balance may also affect sympathetic activity via modulation of renalase expression [53]. Dialysis salt loading may occur with increased dialysate Na concentration and/or with increased dialysate to predialysis plasma Na gradient [55]. Indeed, a mild but significant increase in plasma sodium concentration was noted after dialysis in all our patients (Table 2). Pre-and post dialysis plasma Na and the dialysate to predialysis Na concentration gradient, however, were similar in patients without and with hypertension (Table 2), and in hypertensive patients with increased as compared with those with decreased heart rate (see **Results**). Furthermore, these indices did not predict the occurrence of hypertensive episodes in the logistic regression models (Table 4). Thus, while a positive salt balance might be present in many of our patients, it could not explain the sudden increase in blood pressure or spontaneous bursts of sympathetic activity occurring during dialysis.

Predictors of intradialytic hypertensive episodes

On logistic regression analysis, a higher predialysis BRS in the low frequency band (LF BRS) was found to be the main predictor of intradialytic hypertension (Table 4). Indeed, both LF BRS and HF BRS were higher at the beginning of dialysis sessions associated with intradialytic hypertension as compared with sessions without hypertensive episodes (Table 3). LF IBI was also higher, albeit not significantly at the beginning of hypertensive sessions. The increased *initial* BRS and LF IBI may suggest the presence of a more robust autonomic nervous system in patients with intradialytic hypertension and may be interpreted as resulting from the synergistic effect of enhanced sympathetic tone coupled with reflex vagal activation [58]. A recent paper underscores the dependency of the sympathetic baroreflex with the level of sympathetic activity at rest especially in young and old men and in postmenopausal women [59]. Extrapolation of these findings to our study, however, has to be done cautiously, in view of the different methodology and different study population. Genetic traits, including polymorphism of RAS genes [60] or of beta-adrenergic receptors [61] that affect autonomic activity and BRS were also not checked in the present study.

Comparisons of patients with and without hypertensive episodes (Table 1) shows a slightly higher ratio of ischemic heart disease and an increased proportion of patients treated with nitrates, calcium channel blockers and vasodilator drugs in the hypertensive group. These conditions, however, were reported to be most commonly associated with decreased or no significant changes in BRS [62–65]. The proportion of patients treated with beta blocker agents and with angiotensin receptors antagonists (ARB's) that may both increase BRS [66,67] was similar in patients with and in those without hypertension. When compared with patients with increased heart rate, a higher proportion of those with decreased heart rate were treated with ACE inhibitors. These agents were shown to enhance heart rate variability and increased baroreflex sensitivity [68]. Even though antihypertensive medication was stopped in all patients at least 12 hr before the study, a partial effect of drugs on CDM measurements can not be excluded.

Other predictors of intradialytic hypertension in the present study were lower plasma albumin and age. These factors may be suggestive of the link between autonomic imbalance and chronic inflammation in elderly individuals and in patients with end stage renal disease on maintenance hemodialysis [69,70]. The correlation of these markers with intradialytic hypertension has yet to be understood.

Intradialytic hypertension may contribute to interdialytic hypertension

The second important finding of this study is the markedly increased end-of-dialysis blood pressure in patients with intradialytic hypertensive episode (Table 3) as compared with the remaining patients, in which end-of dialysis blood pressure decreased. This finding confirms previous observations from other studies [54,71]; in one such study, intradialytic hypertension was associated with increased time-integrated blood pressure burden as measured by 44-hour ambulatory monitoring [71]. In our study, end-of dialysis blood pressure was similar in patients with hypertensive episodes with increased or decreased heart rate (not shown in tables). We did not find differences in ultrafiltration rates, intradialytic weight loss, pre-and post-dialysis plasma sodium concentration or dialysate sodium concentration between patients with and those without hypertensive episodes. Since blood volume monitoring techniques were not available, our patients' dry weight, however, was assessed by clinical criteria only. Thus, a residual volume and/or sodium excess in certain patients could not be ruled out, especially in the presence of a positive dialysate to plasma Na concentration gradient (Table 2). Chronic volume excess is thought to be the main cause of interdialytic hypertension. Within this regard our study corroborates the assumption that intradialytic hypertension may play a role in the generation of interdialytic hypertension [54].

Limitations

One main shortcoming of our study is the use of noninvasive methodology of assessment of autonomic nervous function, since more direct techniques as MNSA or pharmacological challenge were not applicable to our patient population. The study patient population included many elderly individuals with multiple comorbidities. These patients however, are most characteristic of the present day general hemodialysis population. Likewise, because of the methodology limitations, patients with arrhythmia or pacemakers were excluded from the study. Furthermore, blood volume and hemodynamic parameters were not assessed in parallel with the CMD determinations.

Perspectives

Our findings support the hypothesis that increased sympathetic activity mediates intradialytic hypertension. Intradialytic hypertensive episodes with elevated post-dialysis blood pressure may contribute to interdialytic hypertension. This association deserves further studies using hemodynamic monitoring, different dialysis protocols and pharmacological approaches. The prognostic impact of intradialytic sympathetic activation and hypertension on overall survival and cardiovascular morbidity of these patients remain to be further clarified.

Acknowledgments

We would like to thank Mr. Mordecai Bar-Ezer for his excellent technical assistance in the conduct of this study.

Author Contributions

Conceived and designed the experiments: DR DS. Analyzed the data: DS DR. Wrote the paper: DR DS. Surveyed the study: DR. Collected clinical data: DR RB. Designed the software used in the study: DS. Reviewed the manuscript: RB.

References

1. Inrig JK (2010) Intradialytic hypertension: a less-recognized cardiovascular complication of hemodialysis. Am J Kidney Dis 55: 580–589.
2. Chazot C, Jean G (2010) Intradialytic hypertension: it is time to act. Nephron Clin Pract 115: c182–c188.
3. Amerling R, Cu GA, Dubrow A, Levin NW, Osheroff RJ (1995) Complications during hemodialysis, in: Nissenson AR, Fine RN, Gentile DE, eds. Clinical Dialysis, 3rd ed. East Norwalk: Appleton & Lange. pp 235–267.
4. Chen J, Gul A, Sarnak MJ (2006) Management of intradialytic hypertension: the ongoing challenge. Semin Dialysis 19: 141–145.
5. Inrig JK, Patel UD, Toto RD, Szchzech LA (2009) Association of blood pressure increases during hemodialysis with 2-year mortality in incident hemodialysis patients: a secondary analysis of the Dialysis Morbidity and Mortality Wave 2 Study. Am J Kidney Dis 54: 881–890.
6. Inrig JK, Oddone EZ, Hasselblad V, Gillespie B, Patel UD, et al. (2007) Association of intradialytic blood pressure changes with hospitalization and mortality rates in prevalent ESRD patients. Kidney Int 71: 454–461.
7. Locatelli F, Covic A, Chazot C, Leunissen K, Luño J, et al. (2004) Hypertension and cardiovascular risk assessment in dialysis patients. Nephrol Dial Transplant 19: 1058–1068.
8. Dolson GM, Ellis KJ, Bernardo MV, Prakash R, Adrogué HJ (1995) Acute decreases in serum potassium augment blood pressure. Am J Kidney Dis 26: 321–326.
9. van Kujik WH, Mulder AW, Peels CH, Harff GA, Leunissen KM (1997) Influence of changes in ionized calcium on cardiovascular reactivity during hemodialysis. Clin Nephrol 47: 190–196.
10. Matzke GR, Aronoff GR, Atkinson AJ, Jr., Bennett WM, Decker BS, et al. (2011) Drug dosing consideration in patients with acute and chronic kidney disease- a clinical update from Kidney Disease: Improving Global Outcomes (KDIGO). Kidney Int 80: 1122–1137.
11. Boulager CM, Amabile N, Guérin AP, Pannier B, Leroyer AS, et al. (2007) In vivo shear stress determines circulating levels of endothelial microparticles in end-stage renal disease. Hypertension 49: 902–908.
12. Hörl MP, Hörl WH (2002) Hemodialysis –associated hypertension: pathophysiology and therapy. Am J Kidney Dis 39: 227–244.
13. Raj DS, Vincent B, Simpson K, Sato E, Jones KL, et al. (2002) Hemodynamic changes during hemodialysis: role of nitric oxide and endothelin. Kidney Int 61: 697–704.
14. Inrig JK, Van Buren P, Kim C, Vongpatanasin W, Povsic TJ, et al. (2011) Intradialytic hypertension and its association with endothelial cell dysfunction. Clin J Am Soc Nephrol 6: 2016–2024.
15. Chou KJ, Lee PT, Chen CL, Chiou CW, Hsu CY, et al. (2006) Physiological changes during hemodialysis in patients with intradialysis hypertension. Kidney Int 69: 1833–1838.
16. Augustyniak RA, Tuncel M, Zhang W, Toto RD, Victor RG (2002) Sympathetic overactivity as a cause of hypertension in chronic renal failure. J Hypertension 20: 3–9.
17. Converse RL, Jr., Jacobsen TN, Toto RD, Jost CM, Cosentino F, et al. (1992) Sympathetic overactivity in patients with chronic renal failure. New Engl J Med 327: 1912–1918.
18. Converse RL, Jr., Jacobsen TN, Jost CM, Toto RD, Grayburn PA, et al. (1992) Paradoxical withdrawal of reflex vasoconstriction as a cause of hemodialysis-induced hypotension. J Clin Invest 90: 1657–1665.
19. Bigazzi R, Kogosov E, Campese VM (1994) Altered norepinephrine turnover in the brown fat of rats with chronic renal failure. J Am Soc Nephrol 4: 1896–1900.
20. Bigazzi R, Kogosov E, Campese VM (1994) Altered norepinephrine turnover in the brain of rats with chronic renal failure. J Am Soc Nephrol 4: 1901–1907.
21. Eisenhofer G, Huysmans F, Pacak K, Walther MM, Sweep FC, et al. (2005) Plasma metanephrines in renal failure. Kidney Int 67: 668–677.
22. Hegbrant J, Thysell H, Mårtensson L, Ekman R, Boberg U (1993) Changes in plasma levels of vasoactive peptides during standard bicarbonate hemodialysis. Nephron 63: 303–308.
23. Katzarski KS, Randmaa I, Bergsrtöm J (1999) Influence of hemodialysis on intravascular volume and vasocative homones. Clin Nephrol 52: 304–311.
24. Grassi G (2009) Assessment of sympathetic cardiovascular drive in human hypertension; achievements and perspectives. Hypertension 54: 690–697.
25. Klein IH, Ligtenberg G, Neumann J, Oey PL, Koomans HA, et al. (2003) Sympathetic nerve activity is inappropriately increased in chronic renal disease. J Am Soc Nephrol, 14: 3239–3244.
26. Parati G, Saul JP, Di Rienzo M, Mancia G (1995) Spectral analysis of blood pressure and heart rate variability in evaluating cardiovascular regulation. A critical appraisal. Hypertension 25: 1276–1286.
27. Norton MR, Sloan RP, Bagiella E (2005) New approach to the statistical analysis of cardiovascular data. J Appl Physiol 98: 2298–303.
28. Parati G, Di Rienzo M, Mancia G (2000) How to measure baroreflex sensitivity: from the cardiovascular laboratory to daily life. J Hypertension 18: 7–19.
29. Grassi G, Quarti-Trevano F, Seravalle G, Arenare F, Volpe M, et al. (2011) Early sympathetic activation in the initial clinical stages of chronic renal failure. Hypertension 57: 846–51.
30. Elghozi JL, Julien C (2007) Sympathetic control of short-term heart rate variability and its pharmacological modulation. Fundam Clinical Pharmacology 21: 337–347.
31. Task Force of the European Society of Cardiology and the North American Society of Pacing and Electrophysiology (1996) Heart rate variability. Standards of measurement, physiological interpretation and clinical use. Circulation 93: 1043–1065.
32. Stauss HM (2007) Identification of blood pressure control mechanisms by power spectral analysis. Clin Exp Pharmacol Physiol 34: 362–368.
33. Pagani M, Montano N, Porta A, Malliani A, Abboud FM, et al. (1997) Relationship between spectral components of cardiovascular variabilities and direct measure of muscle sympathetic activity in humans. Circulation 18: 1441–1448.
34. Brychta RJ, Shiavi R, Robertson D, Biaggioni I, Diedrich A (2007) A simplified two –component model of blood pressure fluctuation. Am J Physiol Heart Circ Physiol 292: H1193–H1203.
35. Hayano J, Taylor JA, Mukai S, Okada A, Watanabe Y, et al. (1994) Assessment of frequency shifts in R-R interval variability and respiration with complex demodulation. J Appl Physiol 77: 2879–2888.
36. Sapoznikov D, Backenroth R, Rubinger D (2010) Baroreflex sensitivity and sympatho-vagal balance during intradialytic hypotensive episodes. J Hypertens 28: 314–324.
37. Penaz J (1973) Photoelectric measurement of blood pressure, volume and flow in the finger. Digest 10th Int Conf Med Biol Eng, Dresden. 104 p.
38. Wesseling KH, De Wit, van de Hoeven GMA, van Goudoever J, Settels J (1995) Physiocal, calibrating finger vascular physiology for Finapres. Homeostasis 36: 67–82.
39. Nagueh SF, Appleton CP, Gillebert TC, Marino PN, Oh JK, et al. (2009) Recommendations for the evaluation of the left ventricular diastolic function by echocardiography. J Am Soc Echocardiogr 22: 107–133.
40. Castiglioni P, DiRienzo M, Parati G (2011) How should the baroreflex sensitivity on the heart be estimated? J Electrocardiol 44: 391–392.
41. Legramante JM, Raimondi G, Massaro M, Cassarino S, Peruzzi G, et al. (1999) Investigating feed-forward neural regulation of circulation from analysis of spontaneous arterial pressure and heart rate fluctuations. Circulation 99: 1760–1766.
42. Schlaich MP, Socratous F, Hennebry S, Eikelis N, Lambert EA, et al. (2009) Sympathetic activation in chronic renal failure. J Am Soc Nephrol 20: 933–939.
43. Rubinger D, Backenroth R, Sapoznikov D (2009) Restoration of baroreflex function in patients with end-stage renal disease after renal transplantation. Nephrol Dial Transplant 24: 1305–13.
44. Berntson GG, Cacioppo JT, Quigley KS (1991) Autonomic determinism: the modes of autonomic control, the doctrine of autonomic space, and the laws of autonomic constraint. Psychol Rev 98: 459–487.
45. Dubin R, Owens C, Gasper W, Ganz P, Johansen K (2011) Associations of endothelial dysfunction with intradialytic hypotension and hypertension. Hemodial Int 15: 350–358.
46. Huang BS, Leenen FHH (2011) Mineralocorticoid actions in the brain and hypertension. Curr Hypertens Rep 13: 214–220.
47. Hering D, Zdrojewski Z, Król E, Kara T, Kucharska W, et al. (2007) Tonic chemoreflex activation contributes to the elevated muscle sympathetic nerve activity in patients with chronic renal failure. J Hypertension 25: 157–161.
48. Munger MA, Ateshkadi A, Cheung AK, Flaharty KF, Stoddard GJ, et al. (2000) Cardiopulmonary events during hemodialysis: effects of dialysis membranes and dialysate buffers. Am J Kidney Dis 36: 130–139.
49. Kara T, Narkiewicz K, Somers VK (2003) Chemoreflexes-physiology and clinical implications. Acta Physiol Scand 17: 377–384.
50. Ding Y, Li YL, Schultz HD (2011) Role of blood flow in carotid body chemoreflex function in heart failure. J Physiol 589.1: 245–258.
51. Prohovnik I, Post J, Uribarri J, Lee H, Sandu O, et al. (2007) Cerebrovascular effects of hemodialysis in chronic kidney disease. J Cereb Blood Flow Metab 27: 1861–1869.
52. Campese VM, Ye S, Zhong H (2002) Downregulation of neuronal nitric oxide synthase and interleukin 1beta mediates angiotensin II-dependent stimulation of sympathetic nerve activity. Hypertension 39: 519–524.
53. Desir GV (2011) Role of renalase in the regulation of blood pressure and the renal dopamine system. Curr Opin Nephrol Hypertension 20: 31–36.
54. Agarwal R, Light R (2010) Interdialytic hypertension is a marker of volume excess. Nephrol Dial Transplant 25: 3355–3361.

55. Flanigan M (2004) Dialysate composition and hemodialysis hypertension. Semin Dial 17: 279–283.
56. Machnik A, Neuhofer W, Jantch J, Dahlmann A, Tammela T, et al. (2009) Macrophages regulate salt-dependent volume and blood pressure by a vascular endothelial factor-C-dependent buffering mechanism. Nat Med 15: 545–552.
57. Stocker SD, Madden CJ, Sved AF (2010) Excess dietary salt intake alters the excitability of central sympathetic networks. Physiol Behav 100: 519–524.
58. La Rovere MT, Mortara A, Schwartz PJ (1995) Baroreflex sensitivity. J Cardiovasc Electrophysiol 6: 761–774.
59. Hart EC, Wallin BG, Curry TB, Joyner MJ, Karlson T, et al. (2011) Hysteresis in the sympathetic baroreflex: role of baseline nerve activity. J Physiol 589: 3395–3404.
60. Ylitalo A, Airaksinen KE, Hautanen A, Kupari M, Carson M, et al. (2000) Baroreflex sensitivity and variants of the renin angiotensin system genes. J Am Coll Cardiol 35: 194–200.
61. Mason DA, Moore JD, Green SA, Liggett SB (1999) A gain-of-function polymorphism in a G-protein coupling domain of the human β_1-adrenergic receptor. J Biol Chem 274: 12670–12674.
62. La Rovere MT, Bigger JT, Jr., Marcus FI, Mortara A, Schwartz PJ (1998) Baroreflex sensitivity and heart rate variability in prediction of total cardiac mortality after myocardial infarction. ATRAMI (Autonomic Tone and Reflexes after Myocardial Infarction) Investigators. Lancet 351: 478–484.
63. Gori T, Floras JS, Parker JD (2002) Effects of nitroglycerin treatment on baroreflex sensitivity and short-term rate variability in humans. J Am Coll Cardiol 40: 2000–2005.
64. Grassi G, Seravalle G, Turri C, Bolla G, Mancia G (2003) Short-versus long-term effects of different dihydropyridines on sympathetic and baroreflex function in hypertension. Hypertension 41: 558–562.
65. Eguchi K, Tomizawa H, Ishikawa J, Hoshide S, Fukuda T, et al. (2007) Effects of new calcium channel blocker, azelnidipine, and amlodipine on baroreflex sensitivity and ambulatory blood pressure. J Cardiovasc Pharmacol 49: 394–400.
66. Chern CM, Hsu HY, Hu HH, Chen YY, Hsu LC, et al. (2006) Effects of atenolol and losartan on baroreflex sensitivity and heart rate variability in uncomplicated essential hypertension. J Cardiovasc Pharmacol 47: 169–174.
67. Pitzalis MV, Mastropasqua F, Massari F, Passantino A, Totaro P, et al. (1998) Beta-blocker effects on respiratory sinus arrhythmia and baroreflex gain in normal subjects. Chest 114: 185–191.
68. Munakata M, Aihara A, Nunokawa T, Ito N, Imai Y, et al. (2003) The influence of one-year treatment by angiotensin converting enzyme inhibitor on baroreflex sensitivity and flow-mediated vasodilatation of the brachial artery in essential hypertension- comparison with calcium channel blockers. Clin Exp Hypertens 25: 169–181.
69. Sajadieh A, Nielsen OW, Rassmusen V, Hein HO, Abedini A, et al. (2004) Increased heart rate and reduced heart rate variability are associated with subclinical inflammation in middle-aged and elderly subjects with no apparent heart disease. Eur Heart J 25: 363–370.
70. Rubinger D, Backenroth R, Sapoznikov D (2008) Decreased baroreceptor sensitivity is an independent predictor of survival and cardiovascular morbidity in hemodialysis patients (Abs.). J Am Soc Nephrol 19: 725A. http://www.abstracts2view.com/asn08/authorindex.php. Available : www.asn-online.org/education_and_meeteings/kidneyweek/2008. Accessed 2012, May 1st.
71. Van Buren PN, Kim C, Toto R, Inrig JK (2011) Intradialytic hypertension and the association with interdialytic ambulatory blood pressure. Clin J Am Soc Nephrol 6: 1684–1691.

3

Hepcidin-25 in Chronic Hemodialysis Patients is Related to Residual Kidney Function and not to Treatment with Erythropoiesis Stimulating Agents

Neelke C. van der Weerd[1,2]*, Muriel P. C. Grooteman[1,3], Michiel L. Bots[4], Marinus A. van den Dorpel[5], Claire H. den Hoedt[5,6], Albert H. A. Mazairac[6], Menso J. Nubé[1,3], E. Lars Penne[1,6], Carlo A. Gaillard[1], Jack F. M. Wetzels[7], Erwin T. Wiegerinck[8,9], Dorine W. Swinkels[8,9], Peter J. Blankestijn[6], Piet M. ter Wee[1,3], CONTRAST investigators¶

1 Department of Nephrology, VU Medical Center, Amsterdam, The Netherlands, **2** Department of Nephrology, Academic Medical Center, University of Amsterdam, Amsterdam, The Netherlands, **3** Institute for Cardiovascular Research VU Medical Center (ICaR-VU), VU Medical Center, Amsterdam, The Netherlands, **4** Julius Center for Health Sciences and Primary Care, University Medical Center Utrecht, Utrecht, The Netherlands, **5** Department of Internal Medicine, Maasstad Hospital, Rotterdam, The Netherlands, **6** Department of Nephrology, University Medical Center Utrecht, Utrecht, The Netherlands, **7** Department of Nephrology, Radboud University Nijmegen Medical Center, Nijmegen, The Netherlands, **8** Department of Laboratory Medicine, Laboratory of Genetic, Endocrine and Metabolic Diseases, Radboud University Nijmegen Medical Center, Nijmegen, The Netherlands, **9** Hepcidinanalysis.com, Radboud University Nijmegen Medical Center, Nijmegen, The Netherlands

Abstract

Hepcidin-25, the bioactive form of hepcidin, is a key regulator of iron homeostasis as it induces internalization and degradation of ferroportin, a cellular iron exporter on enterocytes, macrophages and hepatocytes. Hepcidin levels are increased in chronic hemodialysis (HD) patients, but as of yet, limited information on factors associated with hepcidin-25 in these patients is available. In the current cross-sectional study, potential patient-, laboratory- and treatment-related determinants of serum hepcidin-20 and -25, were assessed in a large cohort of stable, prevalent HD patients. Baseline data from 405 patients (62% male; age 63.7±13.9 [mean SD]) enrolled in the CONvective TRAnsport STudy (CONTRAST; NCT00205556) were studied. Predialysis hepcidin concentrations were measured centrally with matrix-assisted laser desorption/ionization time-of-flight mass spectrometry. Patient-, laboratory- and treatment related characteristics were entered in a backward multivariable linear regression model. Hepcidin-25 levels were independently and positively associated with ferritin ($p<0.001$), hsCRP ($p<0.001$) and the presence of diabetes ($p=0.02$) and inversely with the estimated glomerular filtration rate ($p=0.01$), absolute reticulocyte count ($p=0.02$) and soluble transferrin receptor ($p<0.001$). Men had lower hepcidin-25 levels as compared to women ($p=0.03$). Hepcidin-25 was not associated with the maintenance dose of erythropoiesis stimulating agents (ESA) or iron therapy. In conclusion, in the currently studied cohort of chronic HD patients, hepcidin-25 was a marker for iron stores and erythropoiesis and was associated with inflammation. Furthermore, hepcidin-25 levels were influenced by residual kidney function. Hepcidin-25 did not reflect ESA or iron dose in chronic stable HD patients on maintenance therapy. These results suggest that hepcidin is involved in the pathophysiological pathway of renal anemia and iron availability in these patients, but challenges its function as a clinical parameter for ESA resistance.

Editor: Leighton R. James, University of Florida, United States of America

Funding: The Dutch CONvective TRAnsport STudy is financially supported by a grant from the Dutch Kidney Foundation (Nierstichting Nederland, grant C02.2019) and unrestricted grants from Fresenius Medical Care (The Netherlands) and Gambro Lundia AB (Sweden). Additional support for CONTRAST was received from the Dr. E.E. Twiss Fund, Roche Netherlands; the International Society of Nephrology/Baxter Extramural Grant Program; the Dutch Organization for Health Research and Development (ZonMW, grant 17088.2802); and for this particular study from Amgen BV Netherlands. The funders had no role in study design, data collection and analysis, decision to publish, or preparation of the manuscript.

Competing Interests: DWS is a co-founder and Medical Director of the "Hepcidinanalysis.com" initiative, which aims to serve the scientific and medical community with high-quality hepcidin-25 measurements (www.hepcidinanalysis.com). The other authors have declared that no competing interests exist. Furthermore, the main study was supported by funding from several commercial sources (Fresenius Medical Care, Gambro Lundia AB (Sweden), Roche Netherlands, Baxter Netherlands and Amgen BV Netherlands). This does not alter the authors adherence to all the PLoS ONE policies on sharing data and materials.

* E-mail: n.c.vanderweerd@amc.uva.nl

¶ Membership of the CONTRAST investigators is provided in the Acknowledgments.

Introduction

Hepcidin is a key regulator of iron homeostasis in humans. It induces internalization and degradation of ferroportin, which is a cellular iron exporter on enterocytes, macrophages and hepatocytes [1,2]. Hence, hepcidin reduces iron absorption from the gut and iron release from reticuloendothelial and hepatocyte stores. The bioactive form is hepcidin-25, a mainly protein-bound amino acid of 2.8 kD, whereas hepcidin-20 and hepcidin-22 are its isoforms with unknown biological function [2,3]. The expression of hepcidin is regulated in response to iron administration, erythropoietic demand, hypoxia and inflammatory signals [2,4].

Hepcidin is excreted with the urine. In patients with chronic kidney disease (CKD), serum levels of the active hepcidin-25 and its isoforms are increased [5,6]. In patients with end stage renal disease (ESRD) on dialysis, even higher levels of hepcidin have been observed [5,6]. Hepcidin is the intermediary between available iron stores on the one hand, and erythropoiesis on the other hand. Furthermore, it has been suggested that hepcidin is an important tool to predict the response to erythropoiesis stimulating agents (ESA) [7,8,9]. Therefore, hepcidin might be useful to assess the functional iron availability in patients with renal failure as high levels might indicate a blockade of iron release from its stores [10].

In several studies, patient-, laboratory- and treatment characteristics of CKD and ESRD patients have been related with hepcidin levels. Many studies have shown a relation between ferritin levels and hepcidin, both in CKD [5,6,9,11] and in hemodialysis (HD) patients [5,12,13,14,15]. Furthermore, studies in CKD and HD patients have shown associations with hepcidin and various other parameters such as residual kidney function (RKF) [6,11,16], ESA dose [11] and markers of inflammation including C-reactive protein (CRP), tumor necrosis factor α (TNF-α) and interleukin-6 (IL-6) [7,15]. In these studies, hepcidin has been measured with different techniques, mainly competitive immunoassays and mass spectrometry (MS) based methods, impeding direct comparisons [3,17,18]. Furthermore, most studies on hepcidin in HD patients included a limited number of patients, precluding multivariate statistics.

In the current study, patient-, laboratory- and treatment characteristics that are associated with hepcidin levels are evaluated with a state-of-the-art hepcidin assay in a prospective cohort of over 400 chronic HD patients, included in the CONvective TRAnsport STudy (CONTRAST).

Materials and Methods

Patients and Study Design

Baseline data from patients enrolled in the CONTRAST study (NCT00205556) were used. The rationale and the design of the CONTRAST study have been described before [19]. In short, prevalent HD patients were recruited from 2004 until 2010 and randomized to either continue treatment with low flux HD, or switch to treatment with post-dilution online hemodiafiltration, both with ultrapure dialysate, with a variable follow up until December 2010. Primary endpoint of the study is all cause mortality [20], and anemia management is a secondary endpoint. A total of 714 patients were recruited from 29 dialysis centers. In the design phase of CONTRAST, a protocol for blood sampling and storage was added, specifically for future studies on newly identified markers that would become potentially relevant and of interest. Hepcidin is an example of such a marker. In 17 of the 29 dialysis centers, in which blood sampling and storage was logistically feasible, predialysis blood samples from participating patients were drawn and stored at −80°C. The selection of centers participating in this sub-study was made prior to enrolment. The present analyses were based on a subset of patients from the main study, namely those participants (n = 405) from who additional blood samples were collected.

Patients were eligible for inclusion in the main study if they were treated two or three times per week with HD for at least two months. Exclusion criteria were age below 18 years, treatment with hemo(dia)filtration or high-flux HD in the six months prior to randomization, a life expectancy less than three months due to non-renal disease, participation in another clinical intervention trial evaluating cardiovascular outcomes and severe incompliance regarding frequency and/or duration of dialysis treatment.

The study was conducted in accordance with the Declaration of Helsinki and was approved by a central medical ethics committee and by all local medical ethics review boards. Written informed consent was obtained from all patients prior to enrolment (File S1). Patients provided informed consent for storage of blood samples for later analysis.

Treatment Protocol

Included patients were stable for at least two months with a minimum dialysis $spKt/V_{urea}$ of 1.2 per treatment and they were treated with either polysulfone (PS) or polyarylethersulfone (PAES) low-flux dialyzers with a UF coefficient varying between 10 and 21 ml/mmHg/h and a surface area from 1.3 to 2.2 m^2: F6HPS, F7HPS, F8HPS and F10HPS (Fresenius Medical Care, Bad Homburg, Germany) and Polyflux 14 L, 17 L and 21 L (Gambro Corporation AB, Lund, Sweden). Dialysis was performed with ultrapure dialysis fluids, containing less than 0.1 colony forming units per mL and less than 0.03 endotoxin units per mL.

Routine patient care and prescription of medication was practiced according to the opinion of the attending nephrologist and based on the Quality of Care Guidelines of the Dutch Federation of Nephrology. The Dutch Quality of Care Guideline on anemia management was derived from the European Best Practice Guidelines [21] and the KDOQI guidelines [22,23,24]. ESA and iron supplements were administered via the venous bloodline at the end of a dialysis session. Decisions on dose changes and the timing of these changes were made according to the opinion of the treating nephrologist.

Laboratory Protocol

Predialysis blood samples were drawn and routine laboratory assessments were analyzed in the local hospitals by standard laboratory techniques. The total iron-binding capacity (TIBC) was considered to represent serum transferrin level [25] and the transferrin saturation ratio (TSAT) was either provided by the local laboratory or calculated as serum iron divided by the TIBC. Hepcidin, soluble transferrin receptor (sTfR), hsCRP and IL-6 measurements were preformed centrally. For this purpose, predialysis blood samples were centrifuged at 1500 g and 4°C for 10 minutes and stored at −80°C.

Serum hepcidin-20 and -25 measurements were centrally performed by a validated combination of weak cation exchange (WCX) bead-based hepcidin enrichment followed by time-of-flight mass spectrometry (WCX-TOF-MS) [17]. For the quantification of hepcidin in serum, an internal standard (synthetic hepcidin-24, Peptide International Inc., Louisville, KY, USA) was used [26]. Peptide spectra were generated on a Microflex LT matrix-enhanced laser desorption/ionisation (MALDI-) TOF-MS platform (Bruker Daltonics GmbH, Bremen, Germany). Serum hepcidin-20 and -25 concentrations were expressed as nmol/L and the lower limit of detection of this method was 0.5 nmol/L. For hepcidin-25, the intra-assay coefficients of variation (CV) were 3.7% at 7.9 nmol/L, 2.3% at 13.4 nmol/L, and 2.2% at 3.1 nmol/L. The inter-assay CV were 9.1% at 7.8 nmol/L and 3.9% at 12.9 nmol/L [17]. This method enables the specific measurement of the hepcidin isoforms (hepcidin-25, hepcidin-22 and hepcidin-20) [17] and has been described before in CKD and HD patients [5]. It is an update of a previous method performed by the same laboratory [26,27]. sTfR (mg/L) was measured immunonephelometrically on a BN II System (Dade Behring Marburg GmbH, Marburg, Germany). hsCRP (mg/L) was measured with a particle-enhanced immunoturbidimetric assay on a Roche-Hitachi analyzer (Roche Diagnostics GmbH, Mannheim, Germany) with a lower quantification limit of 0.1 mg/L and

Table 1. Patient and treatment characteristics and laboratory parameters.[a]

	N = 405
Patient characteristics	
Male gender – no. (%)	252 (62)
Age (years)	63.7±13.9
Caucasian race – no. (%)	333 (82)
Dialysis vintage (years)	1.8 (0.9–3.6)
Cause of renal failure - no. (%)	
- vascular	131 (32)
- diabetes mellitus	63 (16)
- tubulointerstitial nephritis/glomerulo-nephritis/multisystem disease	96 (24)
- cystic disease	28 (7)
- other/unknown	87 (21)
Diabetes mellitus – no. (%)	85 (21)
History of cardiovascular disease – no. (%)	177 (44)
Current smoker – no. (%)	81 (20)
Body weight (kg)[b]	71.7±14.6
Systolic blood pressure (mmHg)[c]	142±18
Diastolic blood pressure (mmHg)[c]	73±11
BMI (kg/m^2)	25.0±4.8
Residual diuresis – no. (%)[d]	230 (57)
eGFR (ml/min/1.73 m^2)[e]	2.6 (1.2–5.1)
Treatment characteristics	
Treatment frequency 3x/week – no. (%)	375 (93)
Treatment time (min)	227±23
Bloodflow (mL/min)	298±39
Dialysis access – no. (%)	
- fistula	339 (84)
- graft	56 (14)
- central catheter	10 (2)
spKt/V (per dialysis)	1.39±0.20
Dialyzer – no. (%)	
- polysulfone	246 (61)
- polyarylethersulfone	147 (37)
- other	12 (3)
Prescription of ESA- no. (%)	364 (90)
Type of ESA – no. (%)	
- darbepoetin α	254 (70
- epoetin α/β	110 (30)
ESA dose (DDD/week)[f]	8.9 (6.0–15.4)
Use of iron replacement therapy – no. (%)	300 (74)
Irondose (mg/week)[g]	100 (50–100)
Prescription of RAS inhibitors – no. (%)	215 (53)
Prescription of statin – no. (%)	203 (50)
Laboratory parameters	
Hemoglobin (g/dL)	11.9±1.3
Hematocrit	0.36±0.04
MCV (fl)	94.9±6.2
Reticulocytes (x10^9/L)	65.3±30.5
Ferritin (ng/mL)	378 (211–631)
TSAT (%)	24.3±12.4
sTfR (mg/L)[h]	1.58 (1.24–2.11)
Cholesterol (mg/dL)	143.1±38.7
Albumin (g/dL)	3.6±0.5
hsCRP (mg/L)	3.95 (1.38–10.41)
Il-6 (pg/mL)	2.06 (1.21–3.82)
Hepcidin-20 (nM)	6.3 (3.9–9.3)
Hepcidin-25 (nM)[i]	13.8 (6.6–22.5)

[a]Values represent mean ± SD, median (interquartile range) or proportion (%).
[b]Weight after dialysis (dry weight) defined as the mean of three consecutive values.
[c]Mean of pre- and post-dialysis blood pressure of three consecutive dialysis sessions.
[d]Defined as >100 mL per day.
[e]eGFR (estimated glomerular filtration rate) calculated as mean of creatinine and urea clearance in 24 h urine collection adjusted for body surface area, exclusively in patients with residual diuresis.
[f]In patients on ESA therapy.
[g]In patients on iron therapy.
[h]Reference value: 0.76–1.76 mg/L (Dade Behring Marburg GmbH, Marburg, Germany).
[i]Reference value (median [95% range]): men 65–69 years 5.3 (<0.05–13.9); women 65–69 years 4.9 (<0.05–14.2) [29].
Conversion factors for units: hemoglobin in g/dL to mmol/L, x 0.62; cholesterol in mg/dL to mmol/L, x 0.026; albumin in g/dL to g/L, x 10; no conversion necessary for ferritin in ng/mL to μg/L.
BMI = body mass index; ESA = erythropoiesis stimulating agents; RAS = renin angiotensin system; TSAT = transferrin saturation ratio; sTfR = soluble transferrin receptor; PTH = parathyroid hormone; hsCRP = high sensitive c-reactive protein; IL-6 = interleukin-6.

an intra-assay variation of 1.9% at the level of 0.57 mg/L and 0.3% at the level of 3.00 mg/L. The inter-assay variation was 1.9% at the level of 0.67 mg/L and 1.2% at the level of 3.64 mg/L. IL-6 (pg/mL) was measured with an immunometric assay (Sanquin, Amsterdam, The Netherlands). The intra-assay variation was 12% at the level of 1 pg/mL and 8% at the level of 3 pg/mL. The inter-assay variation was 19% at the level of 0.35 pg/mL (which was the lower quantification limit) and 12% at the level of 2.3 pg/mL.

Data Collection

Data on demography, cause of renal failure, history of cardiovascular disease (CVD), diabetes mellitus (DM), type of vascular access, dialysis vintage and treatment parameters were collected, as well as medication use. ESA was prescribed as epoetin α or β (Eprex® or Neorecormon® respectively, IU) or darbepoetin α (Aranesp®, μg) and expressed as a dose per week. To compare the different types of ESA, prescribed dosages were converted to daily defined doses (DDD), using conversion factors as provided by the World Health Organization (WHO) Drug Classification (http://www.whocc.no/atc_ddd_index/). For darbepoetin α (ATC code B03XA02), DDD is 4.5 μg and for epoetin α and β (ATC code B03XA01), DDD is 1000 IU. All patients on iron therapy used iron sucrose (Venofer®, mg/week).

RKF was defined as a urine production of >100 mL/d. In patients with RKF, the eGFR (estimated glomerular filtration rate) was calculated as the mean of creatinine and urea clearance in a 24 h urine collection, adjusted for body surface area [28].

Statistical Analysis

Variables were reported as proportions or means ± standard deviation (SD), or medians with 25th–75th percentiles when appropriate. The relation between hepcidin-20 and hepcidin-25 was evaluated with a Spearman's correlation test. All patient characteristics, laboratory parameters and treatment characteristics listed in table 1, were considered as possible determinants of hepcidin-25. First, relations between these determinants and hepcidin-25 were studied using a backward multivariable linear regression model with a p-value <0.15 as a cut-off level. Subsequently, the determinants that were related with Hepcidin-25 (with a p-value <0.15) were entered in a second multivariable regression model. In this second regression model, a double sided p-value <0.05 was considered statistically significant. The natural logarithm of hepcidin-25 (ln-hepcidin-25) was applied as the dependent variable in all regression models since the distribution of hepcidin-25 was positively skewed. The regression coefficients (B) were retransformed into percentages of change in hepcidin-25 by using the formula $(e^{B}-1)\times100$, which means that for each increment in the determinant, hepcidin-25 changed with the specified percentage. Additionally, in a separate analysis, all regression models were adjusted for participating center to correct for local policies concerning anemia management and timing of ESA and iron administration and blood withdrawal.

To evaluate whether the relation between a determinant (e.g. hsCRP) and hepcidin-25 was modified by a second determinant (e.g. ferritin), the possibility of effect modification was explored by adding an interaction term (e.g. hsCRP x ferritin) to the multivariable regression model. If this interaction term turned out to be significant (p<0.05), the relation between the determinant and hepcidin-25 was analyzed separately in each stratum of the second determinant.

Statistical analyses were performed with PASW software (version 18.0, SPSS inc. Headquarters, Chicago, Illinois, US).

Results

Blood samples from 405 patients were available. All patient and treatment characteristics and laboratory parameters are listed in table 1 (baseline characteristics of the total CONTRAST cohort [n = 714] are listed in table S1). Mean (± SD) age of the patients was 63.7±13.9 years and 62% was male. Hepcidin-20 and hepcidin-25 were highly correlated (r = 0.76; p<0.001; figure 1). In this section, results for hepcidin-25 are presented. In analyses with hepcidin-20 as an outcome parameter, similar results were obtained (data not shown).

Multivariable Regression Analysis

In table 2, all determinants of hepcidin showing a p-value <0.15 in the backward multivariable linear regression model are listed. In the final model ($R2 = 0.49$), ferritin, hsCRP and the presence of diabetes mellitus showed a positive relation with hepcidin-25, whereas male gender, eGFR and sTfR had an inverse relation. Of note, no relation between hepcidin-25 and the weekly ESA dose and the administration of iron supplements was observed. Adjustment for participating center did not change the results (data not shown).

Interaction between Determinants

The relation between hsCRP and hepcidin-25 was modified by the ferritin level, as the interaction term (hsCRP x ferritin) was highly significant (p<0.001). This relation persisted after adjustment for other determinants of hepcidin-25. As depicted in figure 2, the relation between ferritin and hepcidin-25 was present

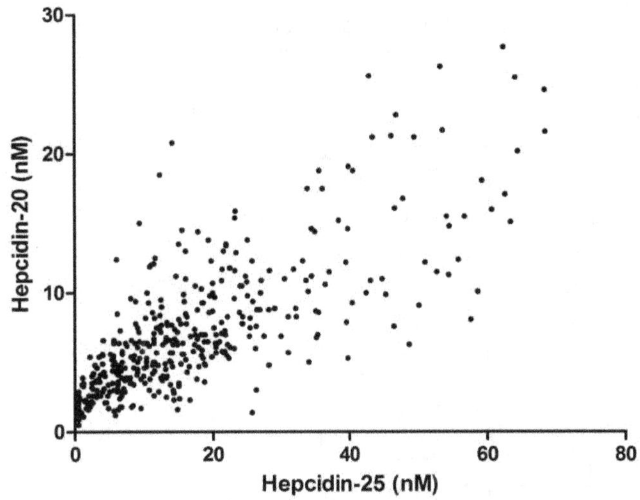

Figure 1. Correlation of Hepcidin-25 with its isoform hepcidin-20. Hepcidin-20 and -25 were measured with mass spectrometry (WCX-MALDI-TOF-MS, see section on laboratory protocol). r = 0.76; p-value <0.001.

irrespective of the level of inflammation (lowest hsCRP tertile: B = 0.020 per 10 ng/mL; 95%CI -0.015 to 0.026; p<0.001; middle hsCRP tertile: B = 0.014 per 10 ng/mL; 95%CI 0.010 to 0.018; p<0.001; highest hsCRP tertile: B = 0.015 per 10 ng/mL; 95%CI 0.010 to 0.020; p<0.001). In fact, the relation between hsCRP and hepcidin-25 was present in all three tertiles of ferritin (lowest tertile: B = 0.020 per mg/L; 95%CI −0.010 to 0.030; p<0.001; middle tertile: B = 0.009 per mg/L; 95%CI 0.000 to 0.018; p = 0.055; highest tertile: B = 0.007 per mg/L; 95%CI 0.001 to 0.013; p = 0.034).

No interaction between hemoglobin level and ESA dose on hepcidin-25 levels was observed as the interaction term (ESA dose X hemoglobin) was not statistically significant (p = 0.588). The absence of a relation between those parameters is readily apparent from figure 3.

Discussion

In this cross-sectional study in a cohort of stable prevalent HD patients, hepcidin-25 levels were shown to be independently and positively associated with iron stores (as reflected by ferritin levels), inflammation (hsCRP) and the presence of diabetes, and inversely with erythropoiesis (sTfR and reticulocyte count), residual kidney function (eGFR) and male gender. Of note, no relations between hepcidin-25 and either ESA dose or iron supplementation were observed.

In our study, ferritin was the strongest determinant of hepcidin, which has been well established before in healthy controls [29], CKD patients [5,6,9,11] and in patients with ESRD treated with HD and peritoneal dialysis [5,12,13,14,15]. Notably, the studies in HD patients included mostly low patient numbers. As can be seen from figure 2, the relation between hepcidin-25 and ferritin was present irrespective of the level of inflammation. However, whether hepcidin is upregulated in response to increased ferritin levels cannot be concluded from our study.

sTfR has proven to be a valuable tool to assess bone marrow erythropoietic activity and iron stores in HD patients treated with ESA [30,31]. However, it could not predict a response of intravenous iron administration on the hemoglobin level [32]. In our study, an inverse association between either sTfR and reticulocyte count, and hepcidin levels was observed, after

Table 2. Results from the multivariable regression analysis on hepcidin-25 levels.[a]

	Multivariable regression				
Determinant	**B[b]**	**95% CI[b]**	**% change[c]**	**95% CI[c]**	**P-value**
Gender (male)	−0.188	−0.361 to −0.016	−17.1	−30.3 to −1.6	0.032
Diabetes	0.246	0.034 to 0.458	27.9	3.5 to 58.1	0.023
Current smoker	−0.188	−0.390 to 0.014	−17.1	−32.3 to 1.4	0.067
Prescription of statins	−0.162	−0.332 to 0.009	−15.0	−28.3 to 0.9	0.063
Prescription of RAS inhibitors	0.113	−0.056 to 0.282	12.0	−5.4 to 28.7	0.053
eGFR (per mL/min/1.73 m^2)	−0.033	−0.057 to −0.008	−3.2	−5.5 to −0.5	0.008
Hemoglobin (per g/dL)	0.085	0.019 to 0.152	8.9	1.9 to 16.4	0.012
MCV	−0.011	−0.025 to 0.004	−1.1	−2.5 to 0.4	0.150
Reticulocytes (per 10 $*10^9$/L)	−0.034	−0.063 to −0.006	−3.3	−6.1 to −0.6	0.019
Ferritin (per 10 ng/mL)	0.016	0.013 to 0.018	1.6	1.3 to 1.8	<0.001
sTfR (per mg/L)	−0.409	−0.544 to −0.274	−33.6	−42.0 to −24.0	<0.001
hsCRP (per mg/L)	0.012	0.007 to 0.017	1.2	0.7 to 1.4	<0.001

[a]Regression analyses were performed with natural logarithm of hepcidin-25 as dependent variable. Potential determinants of hepcidin-25 were selected using a backward multivariable linear regression model with a p-value <0.15 used as a cut-off level in which all patient, treatment and laboratory characteristics as listed in table 1 were entered.
[b]The regression coefficient (B) denotes a natural logarithm. Positive values indicate an increase in hepcidin-25 and negative values a decrease with one unit increase of the determinant.
[c]Results of conversion of the regression coefficient (B) from natural logarithm to a percentage of change: for each increase in the determinant with one unit, hepcidin-25 changed with the percentage indicated in this column. Positive values indicate an increase in hepcidin-25 and negative values a decrease.
R^2 for multivariable regression model = 0.49. Further adjustment for participating center did not change the results (data not shown).

multivariable adjustments. Whether low hepcidin levels enhance erythropoiesis, or whether increased bone marrow erythropoietic activity suppresses expression of hepcidin, cannot be concluded from this cross-sectional study.

We showed a strong association between hepcidin-25 and hsCRP, but not with IL-6. Several studies have demonstrated a relation between CRP [5,7,15,33] or IL-6 [7,13] in small groups of chronic HD patients, whereas others did not [14]. The explana-

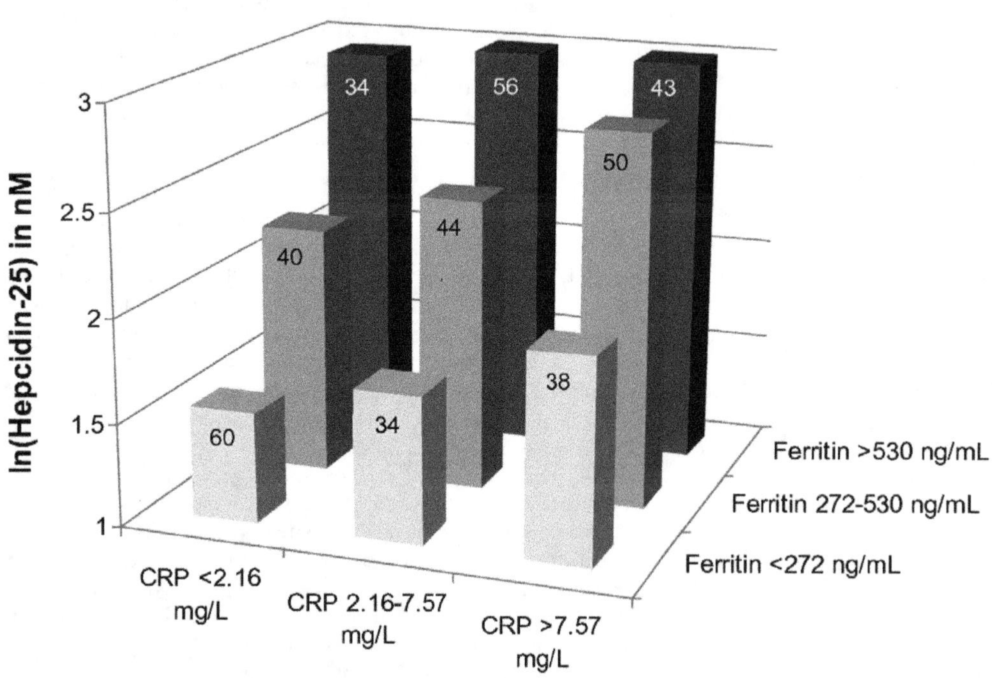

Figure 2. Relationship between ferritin, hsCRP and hepcidin-25. Hepcidin-25 was ln-transformed because of a positively skewed distribution. Values were adjusted for gender, diabetes, smoking status, prescription of statins and RAS inhibitors, eGFR, hemoglobin, MCV, absolute reticulocyte count and the level of soluble transferrin receptor. CRP and ferritin levels were divided in tertiles. Numbers in boxes represent number of patients per category. For 6 patients, ferritin and/or hsCRP levels were missing. P-value for interaction factor (hsCRP x ferritin) <0.001.

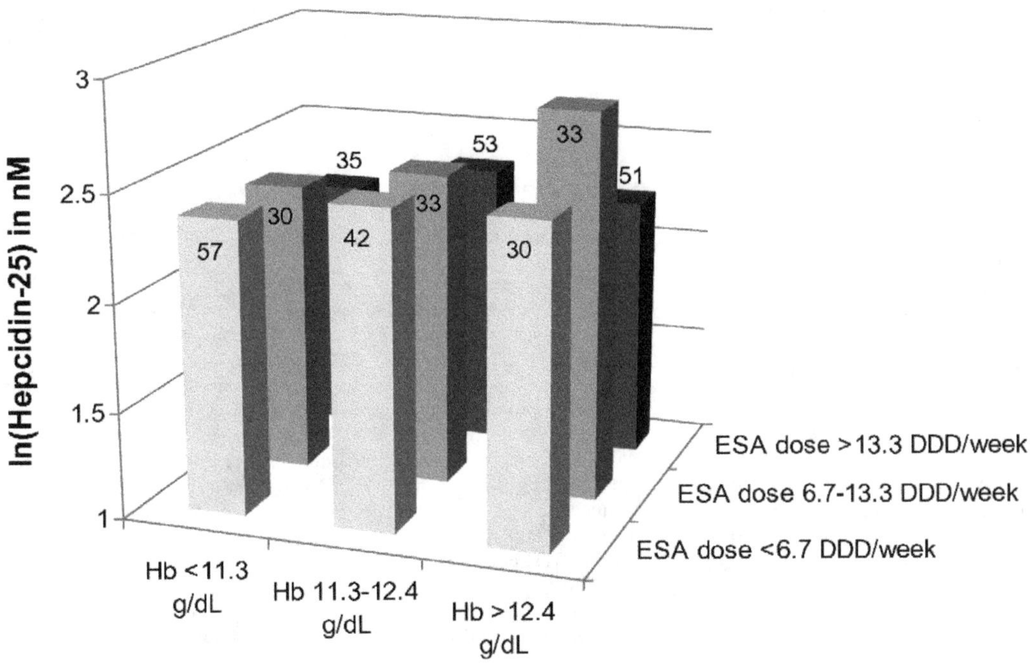

Figure 3. Relationship between ESA dose, hemoglobin and hepcidin-25. Hepcidin-25 was ln-transformed because of a positively skewed distribution. Values were adjusted for gender, diabetes, smoking status, prescription of statins RAS inhibitors, eGFR, MCV, absolute reticulocyte count, ferritin, hsCRP and soluble transferrin receptor. Only patients on ESA therapy are depicted (n = 364). Hemoglobin and ESA dose were divided in tertiles. Numbers in boxes represent number of patients per category. P-value for interaction factor (ESA dose x hemoglobin) NS.

tion for the association between hepcidin-25 and hsCRP, and not IL-6, is not readily apparent, especially as transcription of hepatic hepcidin is activated by binding of IL-6 to its receptor complex [1]. However, in a murine and human model investigating various factors associated with hepcidin expression, the role of IL-6 was limited [34]. Furthermore, the IL-6 assay used in our study showed a wide inter-assay variability, especially in the lower range. This could have resulted in less accurately measured values of IL-6 as compared to hsCRP, and hence less precision in the estimation.

We are the first to report an independent association between eGFR and both the active hepcidin-25 and the inactive isoform hepcidin-20 in HD patients. As we used a mass-spectrometry assay that specifically measures hepcidin-25, our results indicate that the observed association between eGFR and hepcidin-25 was not due to the concurrent measurement of inactive isoforms. To date, studies on the association between eGFR and hepcidin levels in CKD patients have been conflicting [5,6,11,35]. Low hepcidin levels (measured with a radioimmunoassay) were reported in HD and PD patients with residual diuresis [16], but RKF was not quantified in that study. Whether the high hepcidin levels in chronic HD patients were exclusively caused by decreased renal clearance, or whether other mechanisms are involved, cannot be concluded from our data.

In our study population, hepcidin-25 levels were significantly lower in men as compared to women. This can be explained by the fact that most women in our study will be post-menopausal, in whom higher hepcidin levels have been demonstrated [29]. Furthermore, we showed that diabetic patients had higher hepcidin levels. In one study, diabetic patients had higher levels of hepcidin than healthy age-matched controls, although this relation was not adjusted for possible confounders [36].

Interestingly, we did not observe an interaction between ESA dose and hemoglobin levels in relation to hepcidin-25 as has been demonstrated before by Ashby et al [11]. Therefore, it appears that hepcidin, measured with a mass spectrometric assay in chronic HD patients on maintenance therapy with ESA, is not a marker of ESA resistance. Whether hepcidin-25 can predict an ESA response, as has been shown in patients with the cardio-renal syndrome [9], cannot be concluded from our cross-sectional data. Nevertheless, in a study in 24 HD patients, hepcidin levels of ESA responsive patients did not differ from those who were ESA resistant [12], which is in accordance with our results.

Concerning iron supplementation in HD patients, various effects of iron loading on hepcidin levels have been reported [14,37,38]. We did not observe a relationship between hepcidin and iron supplementation, which can be explained by the fact that patients in our study received maintenance iron therapy instead of a (single) loading dose. Recently, it was shown that hepcidin-25 levels did not predict a response to the administration of intravenous iron supplementation in HD patients on ESA maintenance therapy [38]. Hence, it appears that hepcidin is more a marker of iron stores than a predictor of the effect of iron therapy.

A number of studies showed that hepcidin levels could be lowered over a single HD session [13,15,39], although concentrations were back to baseline only one hour after the treatment [13]. Lowering of hepcidin by HD can be partly explained by appearance of (low) levels of hepcidin in the ultrafiltrate [5,16]. In addition, it has been shown that hepcidin can attach to the membrane of the dialyzer [5], which can be explained by the amphipathic and protein-bound structure of hepcidin [2]. Prospective research is needed to draw any conclusions on the effect of different dialyzers on hepcidin-levels.

Limitations and Strengths

Our study is limited by its cross-sectional design, which impedes assessing causal relationships. Furthermore, a specific treatment protocol for ESA and iron administration and timing of blood sampling was not provided. We tried to compensate for this by adjusting the regression models for participating center in an additional analysis, as the intervals between ESA and/or iron administration and blood sample withdrawal are supposed to be similar within a single treatment center. Since this did not change our results, we conclude that the dosing schedule was not a major confounder in our study. Another potential limitation of our study is the patient selection, based on centers where blood sampling and storage was logistically feasible. This might have introduced a selection bias of which the magnitude and direction cannot be estimated. As selective participation or non-participation must have occurred based on a logistical aspect, which is most probable not related to factors associated with hepcidin or determinants of hepcidin, selection bias seems unlikely.

The strength of our study is the large sample size and the prospective data collection. As far as we know, our study comprises the largest cohort of HD patients in which hepcidin measurements were performed, currently published. The large sample size facilitates multivariable statistics, which is an important method when examining the complex regulation of hepcidin [40]. Moreover, hepcidin measurements have been performed with a validated mass spectrometric technique, enabling specific quantification of the bioactive hepcidin-25.

Conclusions

In this cohort of chronic, stable HD patients, hepcidin-25 levels were independently associated with iron stores (as reflected by ferritin levels), erythropoiesis (reticulocyte count and sTfR), inflammation (hsCRP), eGFR, the presence of diabetes and gender. Hepcidin-25 was strongly correlated with its bio-inactive isoform hepcidin-20, and similar associations with hepcidin-20 were identified. Of note, hepcidin-25 was not associated with the maintenance dose of ESA or iron therapy.

Our findings confirm the role of hepcidin as a biomarker of iron stores and erythropoiesis in chronic HD patients and indicate that hepcidin is not a biomarker of ESA resistance in patients on ESA maintenance therapy. Furthermore, it underscores the potential important role of (limited) RKF in HD patients. However, whether low hepcidin levels in HD patients are associated with a favorable outcome in terms of morbidity and mortality is not clear yet. Furthermore, whether hepcidin measurements in HD patients provide additional information concerning anemia management compared to current available markers such as ferritin is questionable.

Acknowledgments

The authors are grateful to patients and nursing staff participating in this project.

Local Investigators:

The Netherlands: Academic Medical Center, Amsterdam – MG Koopman; Dianet Dialysis Centers, Utrecht – M Kooistra and B van Jaarsveld; Gelderse Vallei Hospital, Ede – GW Feith; Haga Hospital, The Hague – M van Buren; Jeroen Bosch Hospital, 's Hertogenbosch – EK Hoogeveen; Maasstad Hospital, Rotterdam – PJ van de Ven; Martini Hospital, Groningen – TK Kremer Hovinga; Medical Center Alkmaar, Alkmaar – WA Bax; Onze Lieve Vrouwe Gasthuis, Amsterdam – JO Groeneveld; Rijnstate Hospital, Arnhem – LJM Reichert; Slingeland Hospital, Doetinchem – J Huussen; University Medical Center St Radboud, Nijmegen –HW van Hamersvelt; University Medical Center Utrecht, Utrecht – WH Boer; VieCuri Medical Center, Venlo – WH van Kuijk; VU University Medical Center, Amsterdam – MG Vervloet; Zeeuws-Vlaanderen Hospital, Terneuzen – IMPMJ Wauters.

Norway: Haukeland University Hospital, Bergen – I Sekse.

Author Contributions

Conceived and designed the experiments: NCW MPCG MLB MAD CHH AHAM MJN ELP CAG JFMW DWS PJB PMW. Performed the experiments: NCW MPCG MLB CHH AHAM MJN ELP ETW DWS. Analyzed the data: NCW MPCG MLB CAG JFMW PMW. Contributed reagents/materials/analysis tools: NCW MPCG CHH ETW DWS. Wrote the paper: NCW MPCG MLB MAD CHH MJN ELP JFMW DWS PJB PMW.

References

1. Babitt JL, Lin HY (2010) Molecular mechanisms of hepcidin regulation: implications for the anemia of CKD. AmJKidney Dis 55: 726–741.
2. KrootJJ, Tjalsma H, Fleming RE, Swinkels DW (2011) Hepcidin in human iron disorders: diagnostic implications. Clin Chem 57: 1650–1669.
3. Macdougall IC, Malyszko J, Hider RC, Bansal SS (2010) Current status of the measurement of blood hepcidin levels in chronic kidney disease. ClinJAmSocNephrol 5: 1681–1689.
4. Coyne DW (2011) Hepcidin: clinical utility as a diagnostic tool and therapeutic target. Kidney Int 80: 240–244.
5. Peters HPE, Laarakkers CMM, Swinkels DW, Wetzels JFM (2010) Serum hepcidin-25 levels in patients with chronic kidney disease are independent of glomerular filtration rate. NephrolDialTransplant 25: 848–853.
6. Zaritsky J, Young B, Wang HJ, Westerman M, Olbina G, et al. (2009) Hepcidin–a potential novel biomarker for iron status in chronic kidney disease. ClinJAmSocNephrol 4: 1051–1056.
7. Costa E, Swinkels DW, Laarakkers CM, Rocha-Pereira P, Rocha S, et al. (2009) Hepcidin serum levels and resistance to recombinant human erythropoietin therapy in haemodialysis patients. Acta Haematol 122: 226–229.
8. Swinkels DW, Wetzels JF (2008) Hepcidin: a new tool in the management of anaemia in patients with chronic kidney disease? NephrolDialTransplant 23: 2450–2453.
9. van der Putten K, Jie KE, van den Broek D, Kraaijenhagen RJ, Laarakkers C, et al. (2010) Hepcidin-25 is a marker of the response rather than resistance to exogenous erythropoietin in chronic kidney disease/chronic heart failure patients. EurJHeart Fail 12: 943–950.
10. Wish JB (2006) Assessing iron status: beyond serum ferritin and transferrin saturation. ClinJAmSocNephrol 1 Suppl 1: S4–S8.
11. Ashby DR, Gale DP, Busbridge M, Murphy KG, Duncan ND, et al. (2009) Plasma hepcidin levels are elevated but responsive to erythropoietin therapy in renal disease. Kidney Int 75: 976–981.
12. Kato A, Tsuji T, Luo J, Sakao Y, Yasuda H, et al. (2008) Association of prohepcidin and hepcidin-25 with erythropoietin response and ferritin in hemodialysis patients. AmJNephrol 28: 115–121.
13. Kuragano T, Shimonaka Y, Kida A, Furuta M, Nanami M, et al. (2010) Determinants of hepcidin in patients on maintenance hemodialysis: role of inflammation. AmJNephrol 31: 534–540.
14. Weiss G, Theurl I, Eder S, Koppelstaetter C, Kurz K, et al. (2009) Serum hepcidin concentration in chronic haemodialysis patients: associations and effects of dialysis, iron and erythropoietin therapy. EurJClinInvest 39: 883–890.
15. Zaritsky J, Young B, Gales B, Wang HJ, Rastogi A, et al. (2010) Reduction of serum hepcidin by hemodialysis in pediatric and adult patients. ClinJAmSocNephrol 5: 1010–1014.
16. Malyszko J, Malyszko JS, Kozminski P, Mysliwiec M (2009) Type of renal replacement therapy and residual renal function may affect prohepcidin and hepcidin. Ren Fail 31: 876–883.
17. Kroot JJ, Laarakkers CM, Geurts-Moespot AJ, Grebenchtchikov N, Pickkers P, et al. (2010) Immunochemical and mass-spectrometry-based serum hepcidin assays for iron metabolism disorders. Clin Chem 56: 1570–1579.
18. Kroot JJ, Kemna EH, Bansal SS, Busbridge M, Campostrini N, et al. (2009) Results of the first international round robin for the quantification of urinary and

plasma hepcidin assays: need for standardization. Haematologica 94: 1748–1752.

19. Penne EL, Blankestijn PJ, Bots ML, van den Dorpel MA, Grooteman MP, et al. (2005) Effect of increased convective clearance by on-line hemodiafiltration on all cause and cardiovascular mortality in chronic hemodialysis patients - the Dutch CONvective TRAnsport STudy (CONTRAST): rationale and design of a randomised controlled trial [ISRCTN38365125]. CurrControl Trials CardiovascMed 6: 8.
20. Grooteman MP, van den Dorpel MA, Bots ML, Penne EL, van der Weerd NC, et al. (2012) Effect of Online Hemodiafiltration on All-Cause Mortality and Cardiovascular Outcomes. J Am Soc Nephrol 23: 1087–1096.
21. Locatelli F, Aljama P, Barany P, Canaud B, Carrera F, et al. (2004) Revised European best practice guidelines for the management of anaemia in patients with chronic renal failure. NephrolDialTransplant 19 Suppl 2: ii1–47.
22. NKF-K/DOQI (2001) IV. NKF-K/DOQI Clinical Practice Guidelines for Anemia of Chronic Kidney Disease: update 2000. AmJKidney Dis 37: S182–S238.
23. NKF-K/DOQI (2006) KDOQI Clinical Practice Guidelines and Clinical Practice Recommendations for Anemia in Chronic Kidney Disease. AmJKidney Dis 47: S11–145.
24. NKF-K/DOQI (2007) KDOQI Clinical Practice Guideline and Clinical Practice Recommendations for anemia in chronic kidney disease: 2007 update of hemoglobin target. AmJKidney Dis 50: 471–530.
25. Gambino R, Desvarieux E, Orth M, Matan H, Ackattupathil T, et al. (1997) The relation between chemically measured total iron-binding capacity concentrations and immunologically measured transferrin concentrations in human serum. ClinChem 43: 2408–2412.
26. Swinkels DW, Girelli D, Laarakkers C, Kroot J, Campostrini N, et al. (2008) Advances in quantitative hepcidin measurements by time-of-flight mass spectrometry. PLoS One 3: e2706.
27. Kemna EH, Tjalsma H, Podust VN, Swinkels DW (2007) Mass spectrometry-based hepcidin measurements in serum and urine: analytical aspects and clinical implications. Clin Chem 53: 620–628.
28. Fouque D, Vennegoor M, ter WP, Wanner C, Basci A, et al. (2007) EBPG guideline on nutrition. NephrolDialTransplant 22 Suppl 2: ii45–ii87.
29. Galesloot TE, Vermeulen SH, Geurts-Moespot AJ, Klaver SM, Kroot JJ, et al. (2011) Serum hepcidin: reference ranges and biochemical correlates in the general population. Blood 117: e218–225.
30. Chiang WC, Tsai TJ, Chen YM, Lin SL, Hsieh BS (2002) Serum soluble transferrin receptor reflects erythropoiesis but not iron availability in erythropoietin-treated chronic hemodialysis patients. Clin Nephrol 58: 363–369.
31. Tarng DC, Huang TP (2002) Determinants of circulating soluble transferrin receptor level in chronic haemodialysis patients. Nephrol Dial Transplant 17: 1063–1069.
32. Singh AK, Coyne DW, Shapiro W, Rizkala AR (2007) Predictors of the response to treatment in anemic hemodialysis patients with high serum ferritin and low transferrin saturation. Kidney Int 71: 1163–1171.
33. Ford BA, Eby CS, Scott MG, Coyne DW (2010) Intra-individual variability in serum hepcidin precludes its use as a marker of iron status in hemodialysis patients. Kidney Int 78: 769–773.
34. Truksa J, Peng H, Lee P, Beutler E (2006) Bone morphogenetic proteins 2, 4, and 9 stimulate murine hepcidin 1 expression independently of Hfe, transferrin receptor 2 (Tfr2), and IL-6. Proc Natl Acad Sci U S A 103: 10289–10293.
35. Uehata T, Tomosugi N, Shoji T, Sakaguchi Y, Suzuki A, et al. (2012) Serum hepcidin-25 levels and anemia in non-dialysis chronic kidney disease patients: a cross-sectional study. Nephrol Dial Transplant 27: 1076–1083.
36. Jiang F, Sun ZZ, Tang YT, Xu C, Jiao XY (2011) Hepcidin expression and iron parameters change in Type 2 diabetic patients. Diabetes Res Clin Pract 93: 43–48.
37. Malyszko J, Malyszko JS, Mysliwiec M (2009) Serum prohepcidin and hepcidin in hemodialyzed patients undergoing iron therapy. Kidney Blood Press Res 32: 235–238.
38. Tessitore N, Girelli D, Campostrini N, Bedogna V, Pietro Solero G, et al. (2010) Hepcidin is not useful as a biomarker for iron needs in haemodialysis patients on maintenance erythropoiesis-stimulating agents. NephrolDialTransplant 25: 3996–4002.
39. Campostrini N, Castagna A, Zaninotto F, Bedogna V, Tessitore N, et al. (2010) Evaluation of hepcidin isoforms in hemodialysis patients by a proteomic approach based on SELDI-TOF MS. JBiomedBiotechnol 2010: 329646.
40. Zaritsky JJ, Young BY (2009) The utility of multivariate analysis in the study of hepcidin. Kidney Int 76: 912; author reply 912–913.

4

Plasma Protein Characteristics of Long-Term Hemodialysis Survivors

Yao-Ping Lin[1,2], Chih-Yu Yang[1,2], Chen-Chung Liao[3], Wen-Chung Yu[2], Chin-Wen Chi[4], Chao-Hsiung Lin[3,4,5,6]*

1 Institute of Clinical Medicine, School of Medicine, National Yang-Ming University, Taipei, Taiwan, **2** Department of Medicine, Taipei Veterans General Hospital, Taipei, Taiwan, **3** Proteomics Research Center, National Yang-Ming University, Taipei, Taiwan, **4** Department of Medical Research and Education, Taipei Veterans General Hospital, Taipei, Taiwan, **5** Department of Life Sciences and Institute of Genomic Sciences, National Yang-Ming University, Taipei, Taiwan, **6** Department of Education and Research, Taipei City Hospital, Taipei, Taiwan

Abstract

Hemodialysis (HD) patients are under recurrent circulatory stress, and hemodialysis has a high mortality rate. The characteristics of plasma proteomes in patients surviving long-term HD remain obscure, as well as the potential biomarkers in predicting prognoses. This study reports the proteome analyses of patient plasma from non-diabetic long-term HD (LHD, dialysis vintage 14.9±4.1 years, n = 6) and the age/sex/uremic etiology-comparable short-term HD (SHD, dialysis vintage 5.3±2.9 years, n = 6) using 2-DE and mass spectrometry. In addition, a 4-year longitudinal follow-up of 60 non-diabetic HD patients was subsequently conducted to analyze the baseline plasma proteins by ELISA in predicting prognosis. Compared to the SHD, the LHD survivors had increased plasma vitamin D binding proteins (DBP) and decreased clusterin, apolipoprotein A-IV, haptoglobin, hemopexin, complement factors B and H, and altered isoforms of α1-antitrypsin and fibrinogen gamma. During the 45.7±15 months for follow-up of the 60 HD patient cases, 16 patients died. Kaplan-Meier analysis demonstrated that HD patients with the lowest tertile of the baseline plasma DBP level have a significantly higher mortality rate. Multivariate Cox regression analysis further indicated that DBP is an independent predictor of mortality. In summary, the altered plasma proteins in LHD implicated accelerated atherosclerosis, defective antioxidative activity, increased inflammation/infection, and organ dysfunction. Furthermore, lower baseline plasma DBP in HD patients is related to mortality. The results suggest that the proteomic approach could help discover the potential biomarker in HD prognoses.

Editor: Christina Lynn Addison, Ottawa Hospital Research Institute, Canada

Funding: This work was supported in part by grants (NSC 93-2314-B-075-044, NSC96-2317-B-010-001, and NSC98-2311-B-010-003-MY3) from the National Science Council in Taiwan and grants (VGH 95DHA0100584, VGH 95DHA0100695,and VGHUST100-G7-5-1) from the Taipei Veterans General Hospital in Taiwan. No additional external funding was received for this study. The funders had no role in study design, data collection and analysis, decision to publish, or preparation of the manuscript.

Competing Interests: The authors have declared that no competing interests exist.

* E-mail: chlin2@ym.edu.tw

Introduction

A global incidence and prevalence of end-stage renal disease (ESRD) patients requiring maintenance dialysis has been on the rise [1]. Although hemodialysis (HD) is a major treatment modality to maintain their lives, these patients are under recurrent circulatory stress caused by intermittent dialysis sessions [2]. In addition, ESRD patients still have substantially reduced life expectancy, mostly because of cardiovascular disease [3].

For ease of obtaining research specimens, plasma has the advantage over cells or tissue because it can be collected in a relatively non-invasive manner. Moreover, all the protein components are readily accessible in a single compartment without requiring additional extraction procedures. Advances in proteomic techniques have facilitated the investigation of global changes in human plasma proteomes. Because of their pivotal clinical implications, intensive efforts and large-scale collaborative studies have been devoted to compiling human plasma proteomes for further integrated studies [4]. Applications of plasma proteome analysis are emerging in studies on cancer [5] and cardiovascular [6] and infectious diseases [7]. In HD patients, Chu et al. focused on the identification of toxins that accumulate in the uremic sera [8]. Langlois et al. aimed to clarify differences in the serum proteome between HD patients and healthy participants [9]. Weissinger et al. studied the effects of oral vitamin C supplementation on plasma polypeptide profiles in HD patients by CE-ESI-TOF MS [10]. Profiling plasma proteome in patients surviving long-term HD (LHD) and identifying potential biomarkers for prognoses is worthy of investigation.

The present study hypothesizes that plasma proteomes of LHD survivors might be different from those who received short-term HD (SHD). In addition, certain protective or beneficial markers might be evolved to reflect the dialysis-related circulatory stress. To address this issue, we conducted a 2-DE-based comparison of the plasma proteomes of ESRD patients receiving different maintenance HD vintage. Subsequently, the differentially expressed proteins were identified by MALDI-TOF mass spectrometry. Specifically, the plasma level of a potential protein marker, vitamin D binding protein (DBP), was measured using ELISA in another 60 HD patients to characterize the clinical significance of DBP during a 4-year prospective follow-up. Our study on plasma protein profiles in HD patients with different dialysis vintage might act as a reference for mining potential biomarkers for prognoses.

Materials and Methods

Human Subjects

Each patient gave written informed consent, and the study protocol was approved by the Institutional Review Board of Taipei Veterans General Hospital. Non-diabetic ESRD patients under maintenance HD were enrolled in the present study if they met the following criteria: (1) had undergone maintenance HD for more than 6 months, (2) had no recent cerebrovascular or cardiovascular events, and (3) had no symptoms or signs of concurrent infection, active autoimmune/collagen vascular disease, liver dysfunction, or malignancy. For a comparison of plasma proteomes, we enrolled long-term non-diabetic HD (dialysis vintage 14.9±4.1 years, n = 6) patients and the age/sex/uremic etiology comparable short-term HD (dialysis vintage 5.3±2.9 years, n = 6). To determine the clinical significance of our identified proteins, another 60 prevalent non-diabetic HD patients were further enrolled for prospective follow-up.

HD was prescribed as 4-h dialysis sessions 3× weekly using 1.8-m^2 surface area dialyzers with bicarbonate-based dialysate (HCO_3^- 39 mEq/L, Na^+140 mEq/L, K^+2.0 mEq/L, Ca^{2+}3 -mEq/L and Mg^{2+}1 mEq/L). All patients received subcutaneous

Table 1. Demographics and biochemistry of the studied HD population.

	Screening subjects		*P*
	Short-term hemodialysis n=6	**Long-term hemodialysis n=6**	**Short vs. Long-term hemodialysis**
Age, years	68.4±15.2	60.0±17.1	0.250
Gender, female/male	4/2	4/2	
Dialysis vintage, years	5.3±2.9	14.9±4.1	0.001
Etiology			
Chronic glomerulonephritis	3	3	
Chronci interstitial nephritis	3	3	
Body weight, kg	55.1±7.8	52.6±5.8	0.540
Height, cm	156.7±10.0	157.0±7.2	0.948
Body mass index, kg/m^2	21.6±2.9	20.3±1.8	0.359
Systolic blood pressure, mmHg	145.3±11.7	141.0±16.1	0.609
Diastolic blood pressure, mmHg	80.3±6.2	77.1±4.9	0.347
Blood chemistry			
Leukocyte count, ×10^3/μL	6.303±1.725	5.688±1.258	0.496
Hemoglobin, g/dL	11.1±2.1	10.1±1.9	0.425
Hematocrit, %	34.9±7.5	31.8±5.6	0.432
Albumin, g/dL	4.1±0.2	4.3±0.3	0.351
Blood urea nitrogen, mg/dL	84.2±10.3	92.9±6.8	0.113
Creatinine, mg/dL	10.8±1.9	12.1±1.3	0.202
Sodium, meq/dL	141.5±1.8	142.0±2.2	0.674
Potassium, meq/dL	5.1±0.6	5.0±0.8	0.875
Fasting blood sugar, mg/dL	99.7±6.6	98.1±16.3	0.827
Cholesterol, mg/dL	171.1±40.5	195.1±43.7	0.347
HDL-C, mg/dL	55.5±31.6	51.7±14.7	0.793
LDL-C, mg/dL	129.7±54.6	129.0±36.6	0.981
ApoB, mg/dL	106.3±41.9	104.3±24.3	0.922
Lp(a), mg/dL	8.1±4.3	12.3±8.8	0.594
Triglyceride, mg/dL	149.6±47.5	147.4±75.3	0.955
Uric acid, mg/dL	8.9±1.2	9.4±1.4	0.505
Alanine aminotransferase, U/L	19.1±5.7	23.3±5.0	0.200
γ-glutamyl transferase, U/L	31.1±29.5	14.6±5.2	0.207
Alkaline phosphatase, U/L	88.5±28.5	127.8±50.1	0.125
Calcium, mg/dL	9.5±0.9	9.6±0.8	0.675
Phosphate, mg/dL	5.3±0.7	5.6±1.4	0.643
Intact-parathyroid hormone, pg/mL	269.7±295.3	315.2±264.4	0.553
25(OH) Vitamin D, ng/mL	16.6±5.5	16.9±4.6	0.916
Kt/V	1.7±0.2	1.7±0.1	0.982

recombinant erythropoietin at a mean dosage of 20 000 units monthly to maintain a hematocrit level of 30%, according to the guidelines set by the National Health Insurance Bureau of Taiwan. Vitamin D supplements and statin were prescribed according to the Kidney Disease Outcome Quality Initiative (KDOQI) clinical practice guidelines. The efficacy (adequacy) of HD was indexed by the clearance index Kt/V [11]. Adherence to diet was assessed by serum K^+, $PO4^{3-}$, and albumin [12].

Preparation of Plasma Samples

All plasma samples were collected on a mid-week non-dialysis day to avoid possible acute generation or clearance of proteins by the dialysis procedure. The patients' blood was drawn in EDTA-tubes (BD, Franklin Lakes, NJ, USA) and immediately centrifuged at 3000 rpm at 4°C for 15 min. The plasma were thereafter divided into aliquots and stored at −80°C. Samples were centrifuged after thawing without visible fibrinogen precipitation, and subjected to subsequent 2D and ELISA analyses.

Two-dimensional Gel Electrophoresis (2-DE)

The 2-DE analyses of the collected plasma were performed individually. Before electrophoresis, all plasma samples were carefully inspected to ensure that no hemolysis was present, which might have affected the analysis results. Protein concentration was determined using the PlusOne 2-D Quant Kit (GE Healthcare, Piscataway, NJ, USA), according to the manufacturer's manual. To detect the less abundant proteins present in the plasma, Qproteome Albumin/IgG Depletion Kits (Qiagen, Hilden, Germany) were used as a prefractionation step to remove abundant human albumin and immunoglobulins with similar efficiency among samples. The 2-DE was performed using an IPGphor IEF system (GE Healthcare, Piscataway, NJ, USA) and a PROTEAN IIxi Cell electrophoresis unit (Bio-Rad, Hercules, CA, USA). Plasma protein was first dissolved in a lysis buffer containing 7 M urea, 2 M thiourea, 4% 3-[(3-cholamidopropyl)dimethylammonio]-1-propanesulfonate, and 2 mM triphenylphosphine. Thereafter, approximately 120 µg of protein was loaded into 18 cm, linear pH 3–10 Immobiline DryStrips (GE Health Care, Uppsala, Sweden) for in-gel rehydration. Isoelectric focusing was conducted using the following program: 0 V×3.5 h; 50 V×3.5 h; 200 V×1 h; 500 V×1 h; 1000 V×1 h. The gradient was raised from 1000 V to 8000 V within 30 min, and the focusing was terminated after 70 000 Vh. After isoelectric focusing, the IPG strips were equilibrated in an equilibrium buffer (50 mM Tris-HCl (pH 8.8), 6 M urea, 2% w/v SDS, 30% v/v glycerol, and 1% w/v dithiothreitol) for 15 min, and then soaked in the same buffer containing 2.5% w/v iodoacetamide for another 15 min. The strips were then placed on a 12% SDS-PAGE gel and immobilized with agarose sealing solution (0.5% w/v agarose, 25 mM Tris, 192 mM glycine, 0.1% w/v SDS, and a trace of bromophenol blue). SDS-PAGE was performed with this strip, and the resulting gel was subsequently fixed in the buffer (40% v/v methanol, 10% v/v acetic acid) for 30 min. The fixed gel was then incubated in 30% methanol for 15 min, washed by Milli-Q water, and placed in 0.05% w/v sodium thiosulfate for 2 min. After washing with Milli-Q water, gels were incubated in 0.2% silver nitrate for 25 min. The gels were then washed quickly and developed with 3% w/v sodium carbonate, 0.001% w/v sodium thiosulfate, and 0.02% formaldehyde, until the desired spot profiles were obtained. Development was stopped by 1.4% EDTA. Gel images were obtained using a flatbed scanner and were quantitatively analyzed by PDQuest v7.2 software (Bio-Rad, Hercules, CA, USA) for the MWs, pIs, and relative intensities of all protein spots.

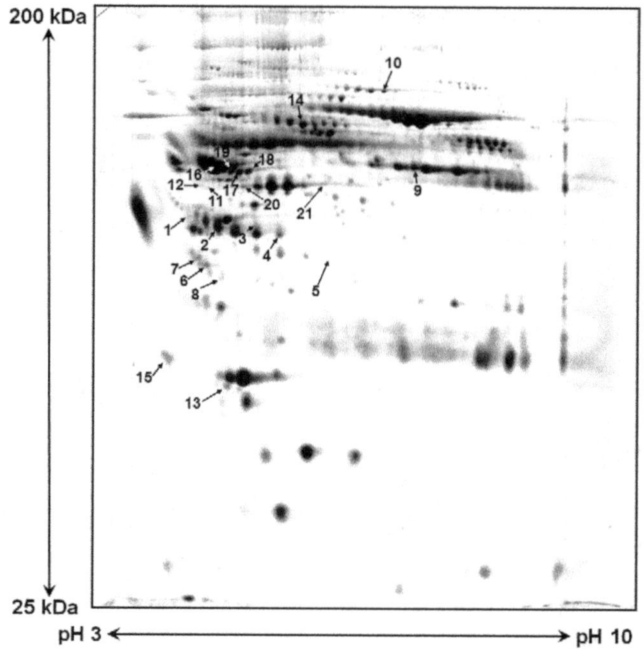

Figure 1. A representative 2D gel of plasma proteins from a long term HD patient. Plasma proteins were pre-treated with an albumin depletion kit and then separated according to their *pI* (IEF) and mass (SDS-PAGE). An average of 598 spots were detected per gel and further analyzed by MS or 2D database comparisons. The identified protein spots with differential expression related to HD duration were numbered and summarized in Table 2.

In-gel Digestion

Selected gel pieces were manually excised and placed into 1.5 mL Eppendorf tubes. For destaining, the gel pieces were washed 3× with 100 µL 25 mM NH_4HCO_3/50% (v/v) acetonitrile (ACN) for 15 min. The solution was removed and 100 µL of 100% ACN was added to dehydrate the gel pieces. Thereafter, 1.6 µL of 20 ng/µL sequencing grade trypsin (Promega, Madison, WI, USA) in 25 mM NH_4HCO_3 was added to the dried gel pellets, and the reaction was incubated at 4°C for 40 min. An extra 2 µL of 25 mM NH_4HCO_3 was added, and the tube was kept at 55°C for 1 h. Finally, the gel pieces were sonicated with 7 µL 1% formic acid for 15 min to release the peptides into the solution, and these final products were ready for protein identification by using the following mass-spectrometric analysis.

Mass Spectrometry

Protein identification by peptide mass fingerprinting was performed on an Ultraflex MALDI-TOF MS (Bruker Daltonics, Bremen, Germany). The tryptic peptides were mixed 1:1 with 2 mg/mL of α-cyano-4-hydroxycinnamic acid (CHCA) in a water/ACN/TFA (50:50:0.1 v/v) solution and deposited on an AnchorChip 600/384 (Brucker). A peptide mixture of Angiotensin II (MH^+1046.5418), Angiotensin I (MH^+1296.6848), Substance P (MH^+1347.7354), Bombesin (MH^+1619.8223), ACTH (1–17, MH^+2093.0862), and ACTH (18–39, MH^+2465.1983) was used as the external standard for molecular weight calibration. Peptide samples were analyzed over a detection range from 800 to 3500 m/z. The batch process for peak list analysis was conducted using flexAnalysis 2.0 (Bruker Daltonics, Bremen, Germany). During the batch process, the signal detection algorithm SNAP (Bruker Daltonics, Bremen, Germany) was used for peak detection, and

Table 2. Lists of differentially expressed proteins in the plasma of long-term HD compared to the short-term HD patients.

Spot No.	Protein names	Theoretical Mr (kDa)/pI	Observed Mr (kDa)/pI	Identification method[a]	Sequence coverage	MASCOT score	Fold changes
1	Haptoglobin	38/6.27	44/4.74	sequencing	37	617	↓ 2.6±0.8
2	Haptoglobin	38/6.27	43/5.04	pmf	22	79	↓ 4.3±1.4
3	Haptoglobin	38/6.27	42/5.32	sequencing	24	337	↓ 3.9±1.5
4	Haptoglobin	38/6.27	42/5.50	sequencing	27	349	↓ 2.0±0.5
5	Haptoglobin	38/6.27	38/5.90	pmf	17	47	↓ 2.9±0.4
6	Clusterin	52/6.06	37/4.92	sequencing	6	97	↓ 1.9±0.4
7	Clusterin	52/6.06	38/4.84	sequencing	6	86	↓ 1.8±0.3
8	Clusterin	52/6.06	35/5.08	sequencing	4	59	↓ 3.1±0.1
9	Complement factor H	51/6.77	60/6.32	sequencing	10	180	↓ 2.0±0.4
10	Complement factor B	85/6.55	102/6.17	sequencing	12	68	↓ 2.5±1.0
11	α1-antitrypsin	44/5.37	51/4.93	pmf	21	87	↓ 2.8±0.4
12	α1-antitrypsin	44/5.37	51/4.86	pmf	28	96	↓ 2.3±0.8
13	Apolipoprotein A-IV	28/5.39	22/5.11	pmf	41	130	↓ 3.2±0.8
14	Hemopexin precursor	51/6.55	80/5.69	pmf	18	69	↓ 2.2±0.1
15	α1-antitrypsin	44/5.37	25/4.56	pmf	17	56	↑ 3.6±1.4
16	α1-antitrypsin	44/5.37	59/5.02	pmf	35	89	↑ 2.6±0.8
17	Vitamin D binding protein	53/5.40	57/5.18	sequencing	19	313	↑ 2.8±1.0
18	Vitamin D binding protein	53/5.33	58/5.27	pmf	30	133	↑ 5.2±0.7
19	Vitamin D binding protein	53/5.33	57/5.25	pmf	47	140	↑ 2.3±0.5
20	Fibrinogen gamma chain	49/5.61	50/5.61	pmf	21	108	↑ 1.9±0.2
21	Fibrinogen gamma chain	52/5.37	50/5.61	pmf	36	134	↓ 2.1±0.4

[a]Protein identification was done by the peptide mass fingerprinting (pmf) using MALDI-TOF MS, or by sequencing amino acids using Q-TOF tandem MS, as shown in the supplementary materials including Figure S1 and Data S1.

the criterion for the signal-to-noise ratio was set to 4. Each recorded mass spectrum was further analyzed by the MASCOT program (http://www.matrixscience.com) by searching the NCBInr database with the following settings: digested enzyme, trypsin; missed cleavage site, one; variable modification: carbamidomethylation (Cysteine) and oxidation (Methionine, Histidine and Tryptophan); peptide tolerance, less than 150 ppm and mass values, MH^+, and monoisotopic. Only proteins with MOWSE scores above the significance level were considered identified.

For those spots that could not be identified by MALDI-TOF, further sequencing of peptide amino acids was performed using LC-MS/MS (QTOF-2 from Micromass, Manchester, UK). Briefly, tryptic peptides were separated on a reversed-phase C18 capillary column then delivered into to the electrospray source of mass spectrometer. The MS was operated in positive ion mode with source temperature at 80°C and cone voltage set to 45 V. A voltage of 3.2 kV was applied to the source capillary. Resulting MS/MS spectra were recorded in the data-dependent acquisition mode whereby the four most abundant doubly or triply-charged ions were selected for collision-induced dissociation of which collision energies were set to 10 and 30 V for MS and MS/MS scans respectively. Mass spectra were processed using the MassLynx 4.0 software (Micromass) and the protein identities were analyzed using the MS/MS peak lists generated from MassLynx. Protein identification was carried out by interpreting MS/MS data based on NCBInr gene database with the following parameters: taxonomy: Homo sapiens; digested enzyme: trypsin; missed cleavage site: one; variable modification: carbamidomethylation (cysteine) and oxidation (methionine); peptide mass tolerance: 1 Da; MS/MS tolerance: 0.6 Da; data format: micromass pkl file; monoisotopic mass and peptide charge of $2^+/3^+$ were chosen.

Enzyme Linked Immunosorbent Assay (ELISA)

The blood concentrations of human DBP and clusterin were measured using ELISA kits (Immun Diagnostik, Bensheim, Germany; BioVendor Laboratory Medicine Inc., Brno, Czech Republic), with a sensitivity of 0–60 ng/mL and 0–640 U, respectively. All reagents, samples, and working standards were prepared according to the manufacturer's instruction. Each measurement was performed in duplicate. In brief, a 100 μL assay dilution buffer was added to each well prior to the addition of the standard or sample in the capture antibody-coating microplate. Thereafter, 100 μL of samples, standard or control, were incubated at room temperature for 1 h with horizontal shaking. Unbound residue was washed off by a 350 μL wash buffer for 4 times; subsequently, 100 μL of HRP-conjugated antibody was added, and the mixture was incubated for 1 h. After 4 more washes with the buffer, a 100 μL premixed enhanced luminal and hydrogen peroxide substrate was added and incubated for 10 min to 20 min at ambient temperature. The relative light units of each sample reaction were then read within 30 min by an automated reader. Sample concentrations were calculated using the machine program by comparing with a best-fit 4-parameter logistic standard curve.

Statistics

SPSS 15.0 was used for statistical analysis. Continuous data were expressed as mean ± standard deviation (SD). Comparisons

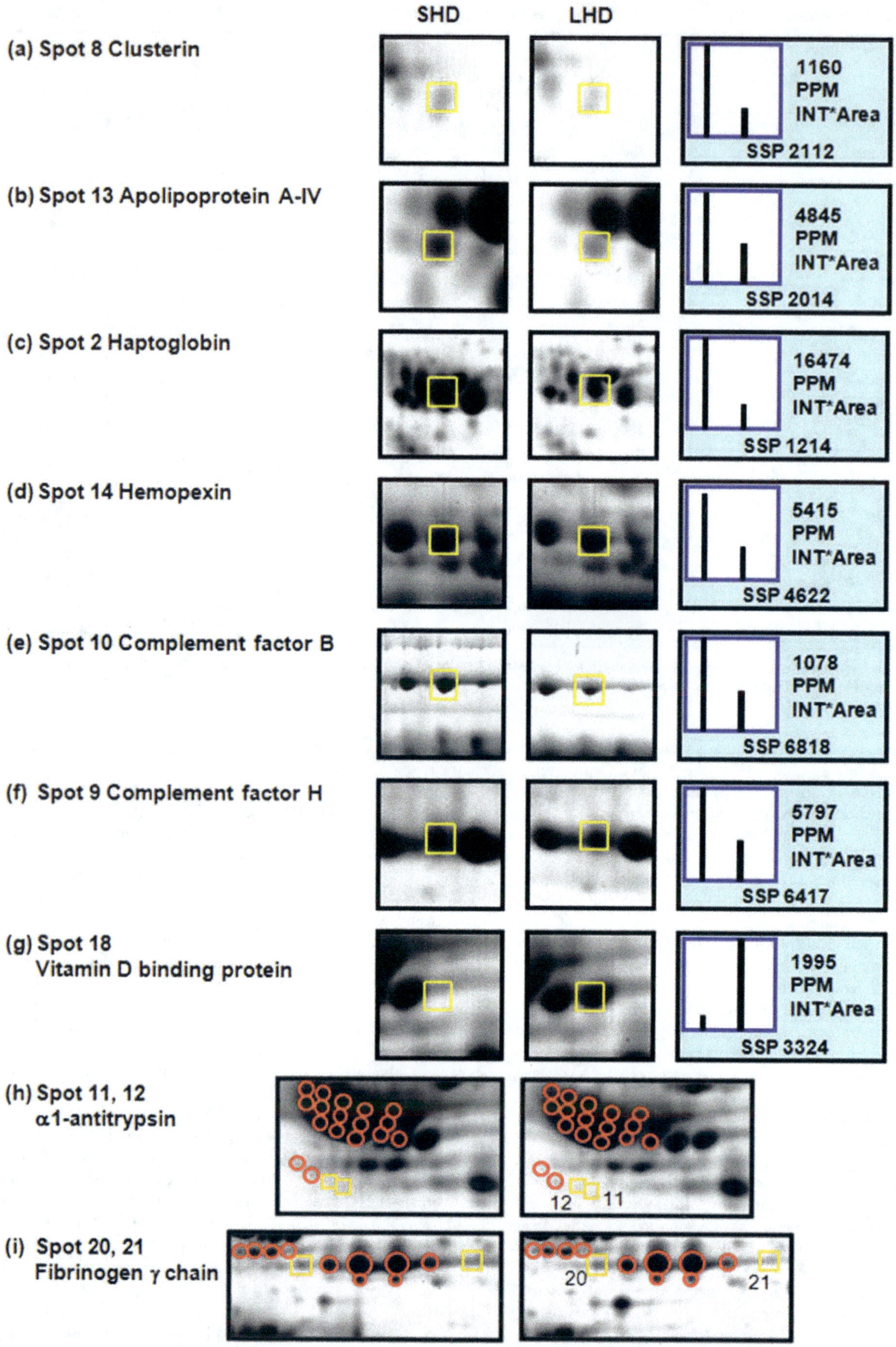
SHD
LHD
(a) Spot 8 Clusterin
1160
PPM
INT*Area
SSP 2112
(b) Spot 13 Apolipoprotein A-IV
4845
PPM
INT*Area
SSP 2014
(c) Spot 2 Haptoglobin
16474
PPM
INT*Area
SSP 1214
(d) Spot 14 Hemopexin
5415
PPM
INT*Area
SSP 4622
(e) Spot 10 Complement factor B
1078
PPM
INT*Area
SSP 6818
(f) Spot 9 Complement factor H
5797
PPM
INT*Area
SSP 6417
(g) Spot 18
Vitamin D binding protein
1995
PPM
INT*Area
SSP 3324
(h) Spot 11, 12
α1-antitrypsin
12
11
(i) Spot 20, 21
Fibrinogen γ chain
20
21

Figure 2. Representative gel sections of protein alterations related to HD duration. Each bar represents the intensity of the squared spot quantitatively analyzed by PDQuest software. Circles were used to indicate the α1-antitrypsin and fibrinogen γ chain respectively in (h) and (i) according to SWISS-2DPAGE (http://tw.expasy.org/ch2d/).

between different groups were analyzed by the Student's *t* test for continuous variables or $\chi 2$ test for categorical variables. Kaplan-Meier analysis was used to compare the mortality rate related to the tertile of the DBP protein level. The Cox proportional hazards model was used to investigate significant factors for determining mortality. Factors related to mortality under univariate Cox regression analysis with *p*-values less than 0.10 were entered for further multivariate Cox regression analysis. A *p*-value of less than 0.05 was considered statistically significant.

Results

The demographic and biochemical data of the participating HD patients are summarized in Table 1. Except for the dialysis vintage, the backgrounds of the SHD and LHD patients were similar for age, sex, and anthropometrical indices such as height, weight and body mass index, blood pressure, lipid profile, calcium, phosphate, and the dialysis adequacy index Kt/V.

Patient plasma samples were analyzed by 2-DE over a pH ranged between 3 and 10 to obtain optimal resolution and protein separation. An average of 598±116 spots in each silver-stained gel was visualized and subsequently quantified using PDQuest software (Bio-Rad). After deliberate inspection of each gel image and comparative analysis, a consistent trend of 2 increased spots (≥1.5 folds) and 19 decreased spots (≤1.5 folds) were observed in the LHD patients, compared to those of the other 6 age- and sex-comparable SHD counterparts. The locations of the differential spots are indicated with numbers in a representative gel of LHD patient plasma (Fig. 1).

Protein spots with greater than 1.5-fold intensity change upon HD duration were excised, trypsin-digested, and determined by mass spectrometry. Table 2 shows a summary of the protein identification results. The sequence coverage of the identified proteins ranges from 4% to 47%, depending on the protein size and quantity. The enlarged gel sections displayed in Fig. 2 show the expression patterns of plasma proteins, including clusterin, apolipoprotein A-IV, haptoglobin, hemopexin, complement factor B, complement factor H, DBP, α1-antitrypsin, and fibrinogen γ, in the representative SHD and LHD patients. In each bar representation, the intensities of the squared spots were quantitatively analyzed using PDQuest software (Fig. 2). In the plasma of LHD patients, we observed the presence of increased DBP protein, as well as downregulation of a number of proteins, including clusterin, apolipoprotein A-IV, haptoglobin, hemopexin, complement factor B, and complement factor H, compared with those of the SHD counterparts. In addition, the isoform profiles of α1-antitrypsin and fibrinogen γ were altered, as shown in Fig. 2.

Among the identified proteins, we further used ELISA to validate the plasma concentrations of DBP and clusterin in the same patients' plasma analyzed by 2-DE. Concordant with the 2-DE expression patterns, the LHD patients (n = 6, Group II in Table 1) have significantly higher DBP levels (204.5±63.9 mg/L vs 149.0±71.6 mg/L, $p = 0.036$) and lower clusterin (282.3±105.8 mg/L vs 438.5±174.2 mg/L, $p = 0.011$) than SHD patients (n = 6, Group I in Table 1) (Fig. 3).

To explore the clinical implication of plasma levels of DBP in HD patients, we followed up another 60 prevalent HD patient s based on their initial plasma DBP detected by ELISA. During the follow-up of 45.7±15.9 months, 16 patients died (10 acute coronary events and 6 heart failures). The baseline plasma ELISA data of the dead patients (n = 16) disclosed their lower DBP compared to the surviving patients (n = 44) (165.6±59.6 vs 214.7±60.8 mg/L, $p = 0.007$). No significant differences existed for HD duration, age, sex, anthropometrical indices, blood pressure, lipid profile, calcium, phosphate, and Kt/V between the dead and living patients (Table 3).

Kaplan-Meier analysis demonstrated that HD patients with the lowest tertile of baseline plasma DBP level have a significantly

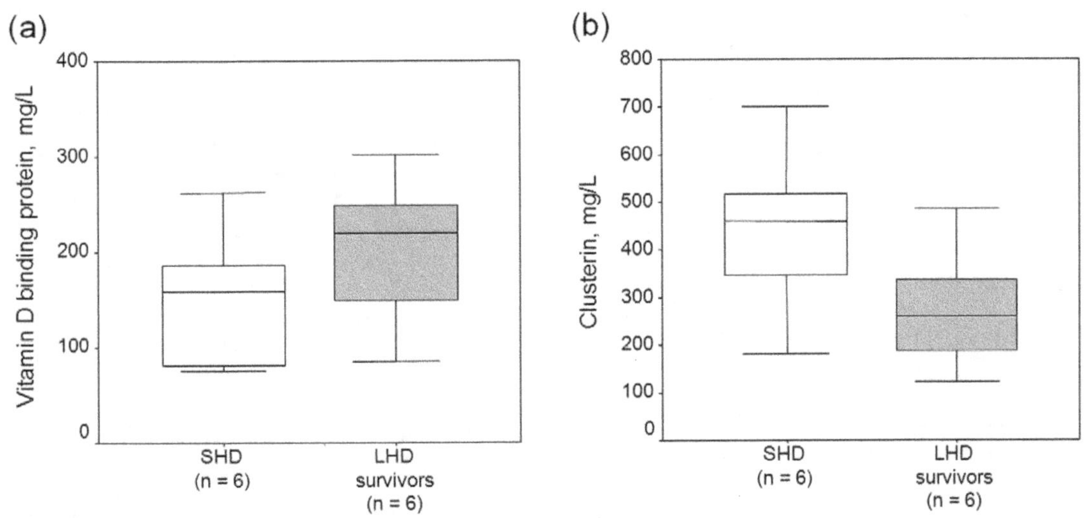

Figure 3. Box plots of plasma vitamin D binding protein and clusterin levels in HD patients. ELISA validation of vitamin D binding protein and clusterin concentration for patients' plasma originally analyzed by 2-DE. Long-term HD survivors have (a) higher vitamin D binding protein (204.5±63.9 mg/L vs. 149.0±71.6 mg/L, p = 0.036) and (b) lower clusterin (282.3±105.8 mg/L vs. 438.5±174.2 mg/L, p = 0.011) than the short-term HD patients, which are concordant with 2-DE expression pattern.

Table 3. Comparison between the surviving and deceased HD patients in a four-year follow-up.

	Survivors n = 44*	Deceased n = 16*	P
ELISA - Vitamin D binding protein, mg/L	214.7±60.8	165.6±59.6	0.007
Age, years	58.2±14.5	67.8±12.5	0.021
Gender, male %	35	44	0.530
Dialysis vintage, years	7.9±5.5	5.9±4.2	0.158
Etiology			0.981
Chronic glomerulonephritis	32	11	
Chronci interstitial nephritis	5	2	
Hypertensive nephrosclerosis	4	2	
Lupus nephritis	3	1	
Body weight, Kg	53.4±7.9	56.8±8.8	0.273
Height, cm	157.2±7.9	160.6±8.7	0.157
Body mass index, kg/m^2	21.2±2.8	21.9±2.9	0.365
Systolic blood pressure, mmHg	141.8±14.4	145.4±16.7	0.422
Diastolic blood pressure, mmHg	79.1±6.9	79.5±9.2	0.850
Laboratory data			
Leukocyte count, ×10^3/μL	6.231±1.345	5.696±1.180	0.163
Hemoglobin, g/dL	11.8±1.9	11.2±1.7	0.517
Hematocrit, %	31.8±3.2	31.8±5.9	0.994
Albumin, g/dL	4.2±0.2	4.1±0.3	0.113
Blood urea nitrogen, mg/dL	90.8±15.4	92.7±17.2	0.683
Creatinine, mg/dL	10.6±1.8	10.3±1.6	0.843
Sodium, meq/dL	140.6±2.4	140.6±2.2	0.983
Potassium, meq/dL	5.1±0.7	5.3±0.7	0.303
Fasting blood sugar, mg/dL	103.6±18.8	110.8±17.6	0.189
Cholesterol, mg/dL	177.3±36.4	173.5±35.6	0.717
HDL-C, mg/dL	54.8±20.9	55.4±16.1	0.921
LDL-C, mg/dL	125.1±45.5	109.5±54.8	0.309
ApoB, mg/dL	102.7±30.7	90.4±38.1	0.243
Lp(a), mg/dL	8.1±8.7	10.2±9.2	0.457
Triglyceride, mg/dL,	154.7±85.5	177.3±157	0.523
Uric acid, mg/dL	8.7±1.4	8.3±1.3	0.255
Alanine aminotransferase, U/L	19.5±14.4	23.2±11.1	0.360
γ-glutamyl transferase, U/L	26.6±24.2	26.5±22.3	0.992
Alkaline phosphatase, U/L	112.4±55.1	139.1±71.9	0.128
Calcium, mg/dL	9.4±0.9	9.2±0.8	0.153
Phosphate, mg/dL	5.5±1.3	5.8±1.3	0.458
Calcium × Phosphate product, mg^2/dL^2	53.2±12.2	53.6±14.5	0.932
Intact-parathyroid hormone, pg/mL	268.5±294.1	360.3±231.3	0.285
25(OH) Vitamin D, ng/mL	16.9±7.7	19.0±7.8	0.388
Kt/V	1.69±0.17	1.63±0.22	0.397

*Values are expressed as mean ± SD or percent unless otherwise listed.

higher mortality rate compared to patients with the top tertile level ($p = 0.030$; log-rank test) (Fig 4). In addition, initial univariate Cox regression analysis of factors significantly associated with mortality ($p<0.1$) disclosed that older age, lower plasma DBP, hypoalbuminemia, and decreased uremic solute clearance (as indexed by lower Kt/V) were at an increased of dying. Considering all these variables for multivariate Cox regression analysis, DBP remains an independent predictor of 4-year mortality in the current study's HD patients (Table 4).

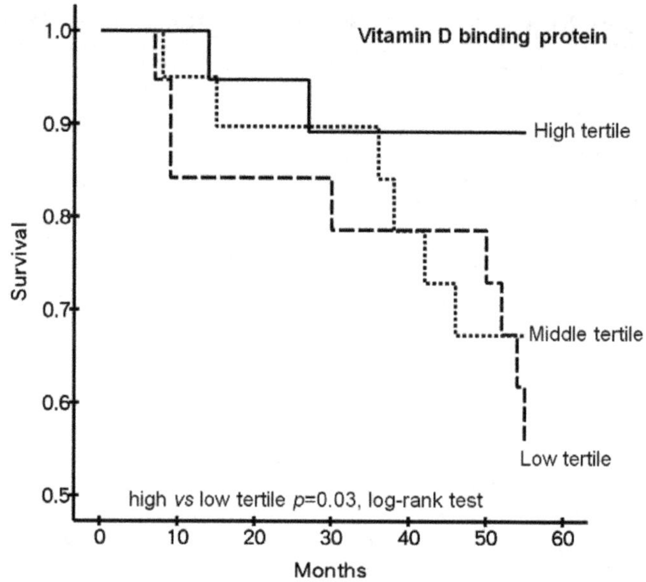

Figure 4. Kaplan-Meier analysis of plasma DBP level in HD patients. HD patients with the lowest plasma vitamin D binding protein level were at the highest risk for mortality than those with the top tertile plasma levels (p = 0.03; log-rank test).

Discussion

Chronic HD patients are under constant exposure to uremic toxins and hemodynamic stress caused by fluctuations in blood pressure and fluid status. HD patients who can survive long and remain in stable conditions might be likened to centenarians in the general population. We are curious as to whether their plasma proteomes are altered, or whether certain protective factors might exist to endure the prolonged deleterious uremic milieu. By harnessing the power of 2-DE-based comparative proteomic techniques, we profiled plasma protein changes in HD patients with different dialysis vintages and identified 9 differentially expressed proteins in the current study's LHD survivors. These protein profiles include increased DBP and decreased clusterin, apolipoprotein A-IV, haptoglobin, hemopexin, complement factors B and H, and altered isoform profiles of α1-antitrypsin and fibrinogen γ. We speculated that these protein changes might be related to intricate influences caused by adsorption [13] or elimination [14] of proteins by HD procedure, that is, altered catabolism resultant from deranged enzyme activities in the uremic state, and post-translational modifications by increased oxidative [15] and carbonyl stress [16] throughout the disease process.

By binding vitamin D, DBP is well recognized for regulating calcium-phosphate homeostasis [17] and exerting great impacts on cardiovascular calcifications [18]. It has been noted that, in addition to transporting vitamin D and its metabolites, DBP plays crucial roles in inflammation and immune reactions by mediating chemotaxis [19] and macrophage activation [20]. Moreover, DBP constitutes an important extracellular actin-scavenger system that eliminates actin released from cell lysis [21]. Without clearance, these accumulated extracellular actin filaments are extremely

Table 4. Cox proportional hazard model for prognosis of HD patients at a four-year follow-up.

Factor[b]	Univariate[a]				Multivariate[a]			
		95% CI[c]				95% CI		
	HR[d]	Lower	Upper	*p* Value	HR	Lower	Upper	*p* Value
ELISA - Vitamin D binding protein, 10 mg/L	0.895	0.817	0.980	0.013*	0.843	0.756	0.951	0.006
Age, year	1.045	1.003	1.089	0.037*	1.048	1.005	1.092	0.027
Male gender, %	1.445	0.538	3.883	0.465				
Dialysis vintage, years	0.900	0.800	1.013	0.080*				
Body weight, Kg	1.046	0.986	1.109	0.137				
Height, cm	1.048	0.987	1.113	0.129				
Body mass index, kg/m^2	1.040	0.889	1.217	0.620				
Systolic blood pressure, mmHg	1.011	0.978	1.045	0.514				
Diastolic blood pressure, mmHg	1.008	0.942	1.079	0.823				
Smoking index	1.167	0.795	1.712	0.430				
Medications								
ACE inhibitor/ARB, %	1.132	0.403	3.183	0.936				
Vitamin D_3, %	1.079	0.347	3.353	0.895				
Laboratory data								
Leukocyte count, $\times 10^3/\mu L$	1.000	0.999	1.000	0.117				
Hemoglobin, g/dL	1.011	0.684	1.495	0.954				
Hematocrit, %	1.012	0.887	1.154	0.863				
Albumin, g/dL	0.162	0.020	1.328	0.090*	0.064	0.008	0.574	0.012
Blood urea nitrogen, mg/dL	1.005	0.973	1.038	0.752				
Creatinine, mg/dL	1.134	0.648	1.983	0.660				
Sodium, meq/dL	1.023	0.835	1.254	0.826				
Potassium, meq/dL	1.464	0.721	2.973	0.291				
Fasting blood sugar, mg/dL	1.016	0.990	1.042	0.226				
Total cholesterol, mg/dL	0.998	0.985	1.012	0.777				
HDL-C, mg/dL	1.001	0.972	1.032	0.939				
LDL-C, mg/dL	0.992	0.980	1.004	0.210				
ApoB, mg/dL	0.985	0.966	1.005	0.147				
Lp(a), mg/dL	1.005	0.947	1.067	0.875				
Triglycerides, mg/dL	1.001	0.997	1.005	0.557				
Uric acid, mg/dL	0.821	0.576	1.170	0.275				
Alanine aminotransferase, U/L	1.008	0.982	1.036	0.542				
γ-glutamyl transferase, U/L	0.999	0.982	1.017	0.906				
Alkaline phosphatase, U/L	1.004	0.997	1.011	0.231				
Calcium, mg/dL	0.591	0.332	1.052	0.074*				
Phosphate, mg/dL	1.162	0.789	1.713	0.447				
Calcium $\times$ Phosphate product	1.003	0.964	1.044	0.876				
Intact-parathyroid hormone, pg/mL	1.001	1.000	1.003	0.157				
25(OH) Vitamin D, ng/mL	1.033	0.973	1.096	0.289				
Kt/V	0.026	0.002	0.545	0.124				

[a]Values are expressed as mean $\pm$ SD or percent.
[b]ACE, angiotensin converting enzyme; ARB, angiotensin receptor blocker.
[c]CI, confidence interval.
[d]HR, hazard ratio.
*$p<0.10$ in univariate Cox regression analysis.

detrimental because of microvasculature blockage, and consequently leads to organ dysfunction. Decreased plasma DBP has also been reported to affect patient prognoses in multiple organ failure [22], and to fulminant hepatic failure [23]. Because of our observations of higher DBP levels in long-term surviving HD patients, and because lower DBP is related to increased risk of

4-year mortality, we reasoned that DBP might exert protective effects on HD.

Clusterin is a highly conserved and ubiquitously expressed secretory glycoprotein that regulates lipid transport and local deposition. Augmented clusterin expression has been demonstrated in human atherosclerotic lesions [24] and in endothelial cell cultures exposed to laminar shear stress [25]. An elevated serum clusterin level was observed in patients with coronary artery disease and myocardial infarction [26]. Therefore, clusterin was proposed to be an index of underlying cardiovascular damage. Clusterin is also a senescence biomarker that is upregulated during replicative and stress-induced premature senescence [27]. It could interact with stress-induced extracellular amyloid aggregations [28]. Our observation of lower plasma clusterin expressed in LHD survivors implies that these specific patients might develop certain protective mechanisms to resist hemodynamics and uremic stress with less accumulated damages during the course of HD.

We found that the current study's LHD patients remained not refrained from injuries imposed by the uremic milieu. Their plasma revealed downregulation of certain cardiovascular-protective proteins such as apolipoprotein A-IV, haptoglobin, and hemopexin, which could explain the accelerated atherosclerosis process accompanying HD [29]. Apolipoprotein A-IV is an anti-atherogenic factor that participates in the reverse transport of cholesterol from peripheral cells to the liver and other steroidogenic organs, and acts as a potent inhibitor of lipid oxidation [30]. Decreased plasma apolipoprotein A-IV has also been demonstrated in patients with coronary artery disease [31]. Both haptoglobin and hemopexin are heme-binding glycoproteins that protect the body from hemoglobin-induced oxidative damage, nitric oxide toxicity, and pro-inflammatory effects induced by intravascular hemolysis. Haptoglobin also functions as a chaperone that inhibits oxidation-induced misfolding of extracellular proteins, and thus, exerts anti-inflammatory effects. In addition to binding heme, hemopexin could suppress neutrophil adhesion and phagocytosis. We believe that the downregulation of haptoglobin and hemopexin might reflect an exhausted antioxidant reserve in LHD patients while counteracting the persistent deranged redox state and inflammatory stresses.

Repetitive contact of blood with HD devices could activate the complement system and contribute to the lower level of complement factors B and H in the current study's LHD patients [32]. The complement system is the main mediator of innate immunity and contributes to the recognition, opsonization, and lysis of microorganisms. Therefore, HD patients with decreased factors B and H are immunocompromised, susceptible to bacterial infections, and in a state of chronic inflammation [33].

Altered isoform patterns of plasma α1-antitrypsin and fibrinogen γ were demonstrated in the study's HD patients with different dialysis vintages. α1-Antitrypsin is a potent inhibitor of several proteolytic enzymes that inhibit neutrophil superoxide production [34]. α1-Antitrypsin is related to the atherogenesis process, and different genotypes/phenotypes were related to diverse ischemic cerebrovascular and cardiovascular disease risks. Furthermore, serum α1-antitrypsin has been reported to be an important index of chronic inflammation in HD patients [35]. Exogenous administration of α1-antitrypsin could confer protection against ischemic/reperfusion injury [36]. Because HD is an ischemia-reperfusion process, α1-antitrypsin might serve as another therapeutic target.

Fibrinogen, the precursor of fibrin, is a 6-chain protein comprising 2 sets of the 3 polypeptide chains α, β, and γ. The γ chain interacts with other fibrin(ogen) molecules, coagulation factors, growth factors, and integrins. Therefore, fibrinogen γ prominently participates in platelet aggregation, coagulation, clot retraction, thrombosis, and inflammation [37]. The differential expression patterns of plasma α1-antitrypsin and fibrinogen γ chain isoforms have also been observed in other diseases. Mateos-Caceres et al. reported the differential expression of α1-antitrypsin and fibrinogen γ chain isoforms between the plasma of acute myocardial infarction and unstable angina patients [38]. We believe that these isoforms might reflect the disparate host responses to diverse pathological processes of HD and they merit further investigation.

High performance HD or more prolonged HD were expected to cause more efficient removal of uremic toxins. However, it might concurrently lead to the loss of plasma proteins as DBP [39]. To explore the impacts of dialysis efficiency on serum protein profiles, Hallbauer et al. [40] conducted a 10-week cross-over study of high- and low-flux dialysis treatments with the identical membrane material in 16 ESRD patients. The serum protein profiles were not altered by the increased pore size of HD membrane in the high performance HD. They reasoned that there might be no significant permeability differences in the dialysis and the clearance of proteins by HD might be compensated by de novo production. Complimentary to the proteomic researches, the clinical landmark study of HEMO neither obtained significant beneficial effects on patients' survival by increasing higher dialysis dose or adopting the high-flux dialysis membranes [41]. It is important to perform long-term studies by using more advanced proteomic techniques to elucidate the effects of HD procedure on plasma proteome.

In conclusion, we observed that several altered plasma proteins in LHD survivors were related to signaling moieties of accelerated atherosclerosis, defective antioxidative activity, increased inflammation/infection, and organ dysfunction. Specifically, lower plasma DBP levels might be a predictor of cardiovascular mortality in HD patients. Further large-scale studies are warranted to consolidate this protein as a biomarker in prognoses, and to elucidate their roles in salient uremic milieus.

Author Contributions

Conceived and designed the experiments: YPL CWC CHL. Performed the experiments: YPL CYY WCY. Analyzed the data: YPL CYY CCL WCY. Contributed reagents/materials/analysis tools: YPL CCL CWC CHL. Wrote the paper: YPL.

References

1. Collins AJ, Foley RN, Herzog C, Chavers B, Gilbertson D, et al. (2011) US Renal Data System 2010 Annual Data Report. American journal of kidney diseases : the official journal of the National Kidney Foundation 57: A8, e1–526.
2. McIntyre CW (2010) Recurrent circulatory stress: the dark side of dialysis. Seminars in dialysis 23: 449–451.
3. Himmelfarb J, Ikizler TA (2010) Hemodialysis. The New England journal of medicine 363: 1833–1845.
4. States DJ, Omenn GS, Blackwell TW, Fermin D, Eng J, et al. (2006) Challenges in deriving high-confidence protein identifications from data gathered by a HUPO plasma proteome collaborative study. Nature biotechnology 24: 333–338.

5. Pitteri SJ, Amon LM, Busald Buson T, Zhang Y, Johnson MM, et al. (2010) Detection of elevated plasma levels of epidermal growth factor receptor before breast cancer diagnosis among hormone therapy users. Cancer research 70: 8598–8606.
6. Kim CX, Bailey KR, Klee GG, Ellington AA, Liu G, et al. (2010) Sex and ethnic differences in 47 candidate proteomic markers of cardiovascular disease: the Mayo Clinic proteomic markers of arteriosclerosis study. PloS one 5: e9065.
7. Thongboonkerd V, Chiangjong W, Mares J, Moravec J, Tuma Z, et al. (2009) Altered plasma proteome during an early phase of peritonitis-induced sepsis. Clinical science 116: 721–730.
8. Chu J, Yuan Z, Liu X, Wu Q, Mi H, et al. (2001) Separation of six uremic middle molecular compounds by high performance liquid chromatography and analysis by matrix-assisted laser desorption/ionization time-of-flight mass spectrometry. Clinica chimica acta; international journal of clinical chemistry 311: 95–107.
9. Langlois RG, Trebes JE, Dalmasso EA, Ying Y, Davies RW, et al. (2004) Serum protein profile alterations in hemodialysis patients. American journal of nephrology 24: 268–274.
10. Weissinger EM, Nguyen-Khoa T, Fumeron C, Saltiel C, Walden M, et al. (2006) Effects of oral vitamin C supplementation in hemodialysis patients: a proteomic assessment. Proteomics 6: 993–1000.
11. Gotch FA (2000) Kt/V is the best dialysis dose parameter. Blood Purif 18: 276–285.
12. Unruh ML, Evans IV, Fink NE, Powe NR, Meyer KB (2005) Skipped treatments, markers of nutritional nonadherence, and survival among incident hemodialysis patients. American journal of kidney diseases : the official journal of the National Kidney Foundation 46: 1107–1116.
13. Mares J, Thongboonkerd V, Tuma Z, Moravec J, Matejovic M (2009) Specific adsorption of some complement activation proteins to polysulfone dialysis membranes during hemodialysis. Kidney international 76: 404–413.
14. Clark WR, Gao D (2002) Low-molecular weight proteins in end-stage renal disease: potential toxicity and dialytic removal mechanisms. Journal of the American Society of Nephrology : JASN 13 Suppl 1: S41–47.
15. Witko-Sarsat V, Gausson V, Nguyen AT, Touam M, Drueke T, et al. (2003) AOPP-induced activation of human neutrophil and monocyte oxidative metabolism: a potential target for N-acetylcysteine treatment in dialysis patients. Kidney international 64: 82–91.
16. Michelis R, Gery R, Sela S, Shurtz-Swirski R, Grinberg N, et al. (2003) Carbonyl stress induced by intravenous iron during haemodialysis. Nephrology, dialysis, transplantation : official publication of the European Dialysis and Transplant Association - European Renal Association 18: 924–930.
17. Silver J, Yalcindag C, Sela-Brown A, Kilav R, Naveh-Many T (1999) Regulation of the parathyroid hormone gene by vitamin D, calcium and phosphate. Kidney international Supplement 73: S2–7.
18. Johnson RC, Leopold JA, Loscalzo J (2006) Vascular calcification: pathobiological mechanisms and clinical implications. Circulation research 99: 1044–1059.
19. McVoy LA, Kew RR (2005) CD44 and annexin A2 mediate the C5a chemotactic cofactor function of the vitamin D binding protein. Journal of immunology 175: 4754–4760.
20. Yamamoto N, Naraparaju VR (1996) Role of vitamin D3-binding protein in activation of mouse macrophages. Journal of immunology 157: 1744–1749.
21. Lee WM, Galbraith RM (1992) The extracellular actin-scavenger system and actin toxicity. The New England journal of medicine 326: 1335–1341.
22. Dahl B, Schiodt FV, Ott P, Wians F, Lee WM, et al. (2003) Plasma concentration of Gc-globulin is associated with organ dysfunction and sepsis after injury. Critical care medicine 31: 152–156.
23. Schiodt FV, Bondesen S, Petersen I, Dalhoff K, Ott P, et al. (1996) Admission levels of serum Gc-globulin: predictive value in fulminant hepatic failure. Hepatology 23: 713–718.
24. Ishikawa Y, Ishii T, Akasaka Y, Masuda T, Strong JP, et al. (2001) Immunolocalization of apolipoproteins in aortic atherosclerosis in American youths and young adults: findings from the PDAY study. Atherosclerosis 158: 215–225.
25. Urbich C, Fritzenwanger M, Zeiher AM, Dimmeler S (2000) Laminar shear stress upregulates the complement-inhibitory protein clusterin : a novel potent defense mechanism against complement-induced endothelial cell activation. Circulation 101: 352–355.
26. Trougakos IP, Poulakou M, Stathatos M, Chalikia A, Melidonis A, et al. (2002) Serum levels of the senescence biomarker clusterin/apolipoprotein J increase significantly in diabetes type II and during development of coronary heart disease or at myocardial infarction. Experimental gerontology 37: 1175–1187.
27. Petropoulou C, Trougakos IP, Kolettas E, Toussaint O, Gonos ES (2001) Clusterin/apolipoprotein J is a novel biomarker of cellular senescence that does not affect the proliferative capacity of human diploid fibroblasts. FEBS letters 509: 287–297.
28. Hatters DM, Wilson MR, Easterbrook-Smith SB, Howlett GJ (2002) Suppression of apolipoprotein C-II amyloid formation by the extracellular chaperone, clusterin. European journal of biochemistry/FEBS 269: 2789–2794.
29. Lin YP, Chen CH, Yu WC, Hsu TL, Ding PY, et al. (2002) Left ventricular mass and hemodynamic overload in normotensive hemodialysis patients. Kidney international 62: 1828–1838.
30. Qin X, Swertfeger DK, Zheng S, Hui DY, Tso P (1998) Apolipoprotein AIV: a potent endogenous inhibitor of lipid oxidation. The American journal of physiology 274: H1836–1840.
31. Kronenberg F, Stuhlinger M, Trenkwalder E, Geethanjali FS, Pachinger O, et al. (2000) Low apolipoprotein A-IV plasma concentrations in men with coronary artery disease. Journal of the American College of Cardiology 36: 751–757.
32. Horl WH (2002) Hemodialysis membranes: interleukins, biocompatibility, and middle molecules. Journal of the American Society of Nephrology : JASN 13 Suppl 1: S62–71.
33. Jofre R, Rodriguez-Benitez P, Lopez-Gomez JM, Perez-Garcia R (2006) Inflammatory syndrome in patients on hemodialysis. Journal of the American Society of Nephrology : JASN 17: S274–280.
34. Sun Z, Yang P (2004) Role of imbalance between neutrophil elastase and alpha 1-antitrypsin in cancer development and progression. The lancet oncology 5: 182–190.
35. Borawski J, Naumnik B, Mysliwiec M (2003) Serum alpha1-antitrypsin but not complement C3 and C4 predicts chronic inflammation in hemodialysis patients. Renal failure 25: 589–593.
36. Daemen MA, Heemskerk VH, van't Veer C, Denecker G, Wolfs TG, et al. (2000) Functional protection by acute phase proteins alpha(1)-acid glycoprotein and alpha(1)-antitrypsin against ischemia/reperfusion injury by preventing apoptosis and inflammation. Circulation 102: 1420–1426.
37. Mosesson MW (2003) Fibrinogen gamma chain functions. Journal of thrombosis and haemostasis : JTH 1: 231–238.
38. Mateos-Caceres PJ, Garcia-Mendez A, Lopez Farre A, Macaya C, Nunez A, et al. (2004) Proteomic analysis of plasma from patients during an acute coronary syndrome. Journal of the American College of Cardiology 44: 1578–1583.
39. Dihazi H, Muller CA, Mattes H, Muller GA (2008) Proteomic analysis to improve adequacy of hemo- and peritoneal dialysis: Removal of small and high molecular weight proteins with high- and low-flux filters or a peritoneal membrane. Proteomics Clin Appl 2: 1167–1182.
40. Hallbauer J, Kreusch S, Klemm A, Wolf G, Rhode H (2010) Long-term serum proteomes are quite similar under high- and low-flux hemodialysis treatment. Proteomics Clin Appl 4: 953–961.
41. Eknoyan G, Beck GJ, Cheung AK, Daugirdas JT, Greene T, et al. (2002) Effect of dialysis dose and membrane flux in maintenance hemodialysis. The New England journal of medicine 347: 2010–2019.

5

Evidence of Increased Muscle Atrophy and Impaired Quality of Life Parameters in Patients with Uremic Restless Legs Syndrome

Christoforos D. Giannaki[1,6,8], Giorgos K. Sakkas[1,6]*, Christina Karatzaferi[5,6], Georgios M. Hadjigeorgiou[2,6], Eleftherios Lavdas[4], Vassilios Liakopoulos[1], Nikolaos Tsianas[7], Georgios N. Koukoulis[3], Yiannis Koutedakis[5,6], Ioannis Stefanidis[1,6]

1 Department of Nephrology, University of Thessaly, Larissa, Thessaly, Greece, **2** Department of Neurology, University of Thessaly, Larissa, Thessaly, Greece, **3** Department of Endocrinology, School of Medicine, University of Thessaly, Larissa, Thessaly, Greece, **4** Department of Medical Radiological Technologists, Technological Educational Institute of Athens, Athens, Attika, Greece, **5** Department of Sport Science, University of Thessaly, Trikala, Thessaly, Greece, **6** Centre for Research and Technology – Thessaly, Volos, Thessaly, Greece, **7** Department of Nephrology, General Hospital of Trikala, Trikala, Thessaly Greece, **8** Department of Life and Health Sciences, University of Nicosia, Nicosia, Cyprus

Abstract

Background: Restless Legs Syndrome is a very common disorder in hemodialysis patients. Restless Legs Syndrome negatively affects quality of life; however it is not clear whether this is due to mental or physical parameters and whether an association exists between the syndrome and parameters affecting survival.

Methodology/Principal Findings: Using the Restless Legs Syndrome criteria and the presence of Periodic Limb Movements in Sleep (PLMS/h >15), 70 clinically stable hemodialysis patients were assessed and divided into the RLS (n = 30) and non-RLS (n = 40) groups. Physical performance was evaluated by a battery of tests: body composition by dual energy X ray absorptiometry, muscle size and composition by computer tomography, while depression symptoms, perception of sleep quality and quality of life were assessed through validated questionnaires. In this cross sectional analysis, the RLS group showed evidence of thigh muscle atrophy compared to the non-RLS group. Sleep quality and depression score were found to be significantly impaired in the RLS group. The mental component of the quality of life questionnaire appeared significantly diminished in the RLS group, reducing thus the overall quality of life score. In contrast, there were no significant differences between groups in any of the physical performance tests, body and muscle composition.

Conclusions: The low level of quality of life reported by the HD patients with Restless Legs Syndrome seems to be due mainly to mental health and sleep related aspects. Increased evidence of muscle atrophy is also observed in the RLS group and possibly can be attributed to the lack of restorative sleep.

Editor: Ian Lanza, Mayo Clinic, United States of America

Funding: This study was supported by the 03ED375 research grant, implemented within the framework of the "Reinforcement Programme of Human Research Manpower" (ENTER) and co-financed by National and Community Funds (25% from the Greek Ministry of Development-General Secretariat of Research and Technology and 75% from E.U. European Social Fund). The funders had no role in study design, data collection and analysis, decision to publish, or preparation of the manuscript.

Competing Interests: The authors have declared that no competing interests exist.

* E-mail: gsakkas@med.uth.gr

Introduction

Restless Legs Syndrome (RLS) is a sensory-motor neurological disorder characterized by an irresistible urge to move one's extremities. This unpleasant sensation becomes worse during inactivity and especially at night [1]. RLS is a very common feature among patients receiving hemodialysis (HD) therapy [2–4] and in this case it is called uremic RLS. In uremic patients, RLS has been associated with poorer quality of life (QoL) compared to RLS free patients [5–8], however it is not clear whether the impaired QoL is due to physical or mental aspects of the QoL.

Reductions in physical performance and physical functioning, and increasing restraints to independent living are affecting QoL in HD population [9], whereas muscle wasting and low lean body mass are additionally associated to lower survival rates [10,11]. It has been reported that HD-RLS patients have a higher mortality rate compared to their non RLS counterparts [8,12]. However, it is still unknown whether HD patients with RLS experience any further declines in parameters directly affecting survival such as body composition, muscle quality and quantity, physical performance and functional capacity, compared to RLS free patients.

The possible effect of RLS on these parameters is ambiguous. On one hand, the discomfort that the syndrome induces to the patients, may lead to avoidance and lack of exercise. On the other hand, the repeated movement-relaxation cycle that the RLS patients experience in order to get relief from the symptoms could lead to a relatively increased physical activity. Nevertheless, both scenarios could affect body composition as well as the quality and quantity of muscle tissue, influencing thus the patients' mortality and morbidity rates.

Moreover, RLS, either in its idiopathic [13] or uremic [6] form, is well known to impair patients' sleep. Disturbed sleep is reported to be associated with reductions in circulating anabolic hormones [14,15] thus it could affect muscle metabolism. Indeed, some data indicates that the lack of sleep is associated with reduced muscle size in HD patients [16] and it is plausible that in HD patients with RLS the anabolic effect of sleep might be further reduced. Given that RLS disturbs sleep quality, we hypothesized that this could have a detrimental effect in the HD patient's muscle quantity and/or quality.

Given the high prevalence of undiagnosed RLS in HD patients,[5,17] and the fact that RLS by nature could influence aspects of physical performance, physical functioning and QoL, such as endurance, body composition and muscle size, it is conceivable to assume that research outcomes based on HD populations could have been confounded in the past.

The aims of the present study were to investigate whether HD patients with RLS, as compared to those without the syndrome, show evidence of further reduced quality of life and of overall physical performance and functional capacity, as well as further alterations in indices of body composition and muscle characteristics, parameters that could have a significant impact in the survival and quality of life in this patient- population.

Methods

Ethics Statement

The study was approved by the Ethics Committee of the University of Thessaly, and by the bioethics committee of the University General Hospital of Larissa, Greece and the bioethics committee of the General Hospital of Trikala, Greece. All patients gave their written informed consent prior to study participation.

Study Population

From September of 2006 to July of 2010, a total of eighty-five HD patients (the total number of patients receiving care in the study centers) were screened while seventy HD patients (51 male, 19 female, 54.1±16.9 years) were finally enrolled in the study (Figure 1). The patients were recruited from the HD units of the University Hospital of Larisa (UHL) and from the General Hospital of Trikala, Greece.

The inclusion criteria for the study were: dialysis for at least three months or more with adequate dialysis delivery and with stable clinical condition. In addition, none of the recruited patients should have been diagnosed with RLS prior to the study. Exclusion criteria included diagnosed neuropathies (n = 8, clinically examined by a neurologist) or reasons for being in a catabolic state (n = 4, including malignancies, opportunistic infections or active inflammation), within 3 months prior to the start of the study, or with abnormal C-Reactive Protein blood levels. In addition, another 3 patients refused to participate to the study for personal reasons.

Allocation

Patients were divided into two groups according to their RLS status: the RLS group (n = 30; 10 females, 55.4±13.4 years) and the non-RLS group (n = 40; 9 females, 53.1±19.3 years).

RLS diagnosis and severity assessment

RLS was diagnosed by a single RLS specialist neurologist, using the internationally recognised criteria of the IRLSSG [1], whereas the presence of Periodic Limb Movements in Sleep (PLMS) was derived from an overnight polysomnographic (PSG) study (Somnoscreen, Somnomedics GmbH, Randersacker, Germany). According the International RLS Study Group, the presence of PLMS is considered as a supportive and not conclusive clinical feature for the diagnosis of the syndrome and therefore it was used complementary to the IRLSSG criteria [1]. The assessment of PLMS was performed according to the official World Association of Sleep Medicine standards for recording and scoring of PLMS with a cut off threshold at >15 events per hour [18]. RLS patients were included in the study if they had at least one RLS episode per week excluding the episodes that took place during the dialysis session. Finally, RLS severity was assessed using the IRLSSG severity rating scale [19].

Study design

This is a cross sectional study. Patients screening for RLS took place prior to any measurements and the status of the patients was coded for blinding purposes. All investigators were blinded to the RLS status of the patients up to the completion of data analysis. Patients were studied in a single out-patients visit on a free dialysis day.

Body and muscle composition

A DEXA system (Lunar model DPX Madison, WI) was used to measure the patient's whole body fat and lean body mass [20]. *Post-hoc* regional analysis of the DEXA images was performed as described previously [21]. In addition, muscle size and composition of the right thigh was assessed by computed tomography (CT) (Philips Tomoscan SR5000) [22] with image analysis performed as previously described [16]. Waist to hip ratio (WHR) was calculated as waist circumference, at the midway between the iliac crest and the lowermost margins of the ribs, over the hip circumference at the maximum circumference of buttocks.

Physical performance assessment

Patients' physical performance was evaluated by a battery of tests. Briefly, we used the "North Staffordshire Royal Infirmary" walking test (NSRI), two gait speed tests (normal and fast walk tests) and two sit-to-stand tests (STS-5 and STS-60) as previously described [23–25].

Questionnaires

All questionnaires were completed with the interview method, by experienced personnel. The patient's subjective QoL outcomes were evaluated by using a Short Form-36 Health Survey (SF-36) version modified for patients receiving HD therapy [26]. Outcome scores can range from 0 to 100, with higher scores indicate better health status. The 8 multi-item scales of the SF-36 were summarized into two dimensions (mental and physical dimension respectively) and into a "total or overall SF-36 score" [26]. The patient's score in the physical health component was considered as the "physical functioning" score [27,28].

The patients' depression levels were evaluated by using a 20-item self-rating depression scale questionnaire developed by Zung [29], used successfully in the past in HD patients [16,30]. The cut-off point for the diagnosis of clinical depression is above 50.

The Epworth sleepiness scale (ESS) was used to assess the daily sleepiness level of the patients [31]. ESS consists of questions referring to eight situations. The patients are asked to rate on a scale of 0 up to 3 how likely they would be to doze off or fall asleep during the 8 situations. Outcome scores can range from 0 to 24. A score above 10 is considered to be pathological sleepiness.

A weekly sleep diary, adapted from the University of Massachusetts Medical School website (http://healthnet.umassmed.edu/

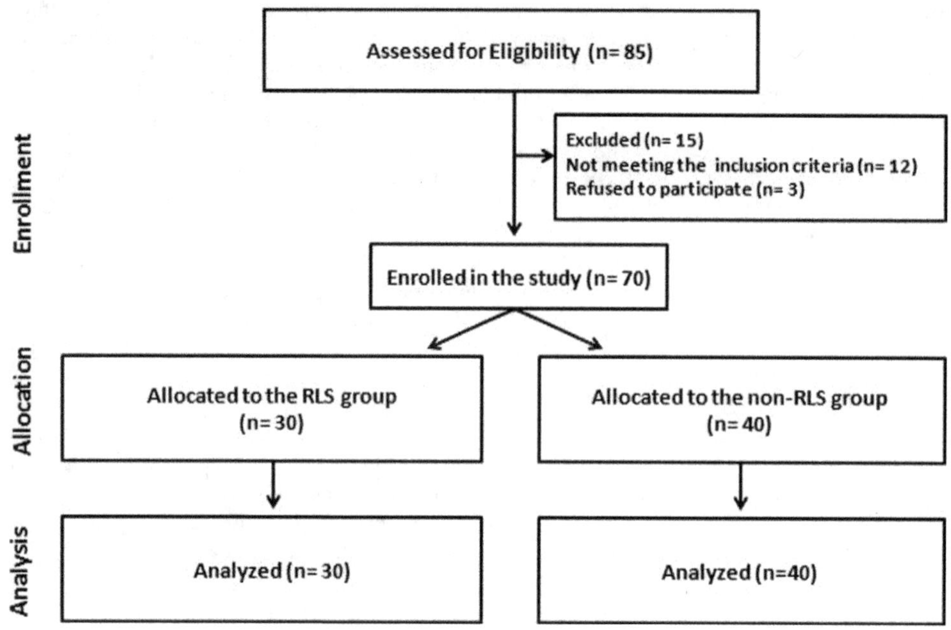

Figure 1. Patient recruitment flow diagram. Disposition of the patients into the two groups according to the RLS diagnosis as follows: the RLS group and the non-RLS group.

mhealth/WeeklySleepQuestionnaire.pdf), was used to evaluate the patient's quality of sleep. Briefly, the sleep diary contained questions regarding how often during the previous week HD patients experienced any of the following: (1) difficulties falling asleep, (2) number of nocturnal awakenings, (3) difficulties remaining asleep, (4) the sensation of waking-up tired and fatigued, (5) day time stress and (6) how often did they feel refreshed after the night's sleep. The sleep diary was scored as follows: 'never' (0 points), '1–2 times a week' (1 point), '3–5 times a week' (2 points), '6–7 times a week' (3 points). For question number 6 the scoring was reversed with 3 points for the answer 'never', and 0 points for the answer '6–7 times a week'. The sleep diary score was calculated as the sum of the total points with the minimum at zero points and the maximum score at 18.]

Nutritional assessment

The nutritional status of the patients was examined by the Subjective Global Assessment (SGA) method [32].

Biochemical assessment

Routine monthly laboratory results were recorded for HD subjects including ferritin, hematocrit, hemoglobin and dialysis efficiency parameters. A single-pool Kt/V was calculated from pre- and post-dialysis BUN measurements using the Daugirdas II equation [33]. The biochemical analysis was performed at the clinical lab of the UHL under standard hospital procedures.

Hemodialysis procedure

Patients underwent HD therapy (Fresenius 4008B, Oberursel, Germany) for at least 4 hours, 3 times/week, with hollow-fiber dialysers and bicarbonate buffer. Low molecular weight heparin (Enoxaparin, Clexane®, Sanofi-Aventis, Strasbourg, France) was applied for anticoagulation. Enoxaparin doses of 40–60 mg were administered intravenously before the beginning of HD treatment. EPO therapy was given after the completion of HD session in order to normalize hemoglobin within 11-12 (g/dL).

Statistical analysis

For the patients' characteristics (Table 1) an unpaired *t*-test were used to compare groups for continuous normally distributed variables; chi-square, for categorical variables; and Mann-Whitney *U* test, for non–normally distributed variables. Multivariate Analysis of covariance (MANCOVA) with "gender" as a covariance was used in order to control for possible differences between the examined variables (Tables 2–3). Spearman rank correlation test was used to assess the relationships between the examined variables, while for correlation between continuous and categorical variables a "Point Biserial Correlation Coefficient" test was used to assess this type of relationship. All analyses were carried out using the SPSS Statistical Package (SPSS 15.0, Chicago, Illinois). Data are presented as mean ± SD unless otherwise stated and the level for statistical significance was set at $P<0.05$.

Sample Size

Sample size calculations were conducted based in functional capacity [NSRI 73.5(30) vs 105(37)] and quality of life score [78.1(12.9) vs 63.7(20.2)] values in the hemodialysis patients from previous published articles [16,34]. The resulting minimum required sample size was an average of 30 for 2-sided type 1 and type 2 errors of 5%.

Results

In this cross sectional analysis, the prevalence of RLS within the HD population was approximately 42% (30 out of 70), whereas 57% of those (17 out of 30) co-experienced PLMS. The RLS patient's score in the IRLS severity scale was 24±9, which categorized them at the "severe" level of symptoms' intensity.

The prevalence of RLS was found to be higher in women compared to men (52% vs 39%), however no gender effect was observed in the current analysis ($P = 0.313$).

The patients' characteristics are presented in Table 1 and physical performance data are presented in Table 2. There were

Table 1. Patient's characteristics presented as pool data and divided in two groups according to RLS diagnosis.

Variables	Patients Pool Data	Non RLS	RLS	P values
N	70	40	30	-
Female / Male	19/51	9/31	10/20	0.313[¥]
Age (yr)	54.1±16.9	53.1±19.3	55.4±13.4	0.580
BMI (Kg/m^2)	25.5±4.2	25.2±4.5	25.8±3.9	0.580
Kt/V	1.24±0.4	1.25±0.5	1.22±0.4	0.802
Years in Hemodialysis	3.0±2.6	2.5±1.6	3.7±3.5	0.093
WHR	0.97±0.07	0.97±0.06	0.97±0.07	0.744
PLMS prevalence	26 (37%)	9 (22%)	17 (57%)	**0.008**[¥]
PLMS index (per hour)	20.4±29.3	10.3±20.2	31.5±33.7	**0.003**
IRLS score	-	-	23.7 ± 9.2	-
SGA (A/B/C)	31/9/1	22/7/1	9/2/0	0.820[¥]
Ferritin (ng/ml)	202.3±189.5	173.2±173.3	241.1±206.6	0.187
Hct	36.3±4.9	35.7±5.5	37.0±3.9	0.300
Hb (g/dL)	11.8±1.6	11.5±1.6	12.2±1.5	0.107

All data are mean ± SD. Abbreviations: BMI, body mass index; Kt/V, dialysis efficiency; WHR, waist to hip ratio; PLMS, Periodic Limb Movements in Sleep; IRLS, International Restless Legs Syndrome severity scale; SGA, subjective global assessment; Hct, hematocrit; Hb, hemoglobin.
[¥]For categorical data a chi-square test was performed.

Table 2. Physical performance, depression, daytime sleepiness and sleep quality data.

Variables	Patients Pool Data	Non RLS	RLS	P values
Physical Performance Tests				
STS- 5 (sec)	10.1±2.8	10.4±3.3	9.7±1.9	0.330
STS-60 (rep)	27.8±8.4	28.8±8.9	26.6±7.6	0.339
Normal Walk (sec)	5.9±1.4	5.9±1.5	5.8±1.2	0.572
Fast Walk (sec)	4.1±1.0	4.1±1.1	4.1±0.9	0.687
NSRI test (sec)	84.3±36.8	85.6±41.4	82.7±30.5	0.503
Questionnaires				
Sleep Diary	7.2±4.8	5.7±4.3	9.2±4.7	0.005
Epworth Sleepiness Scale	6.1±4.1	5.3±3.7	7.1±4.4	0.060
Zung Depression Scale	41.0±9.6	38.2±8.3	44.4±10.1	0.011

All data are mean ± SD. P values are adjusted for yrs in dialysis. Abbreviations: STS-5, sit-to- stand test 5-repetitions; STS-60, sit-to- stand test 60 seconds; NSRI, North Staffordshire royal infirmary test.

no significant differences between the two groups in all direct physical performance tests performed. In contrast, significant differences were found in the QoL assessment results (Figure 2), in the sleep diary [F (1,60) = 8.472, P = 0.005], in the severity of the Zung self-rating depression scale [F (1,60) = 6,922, P = 0.011] and a trend in the sleepiness scale [F (1,60) = 3,656, P = 0.060] (Table 2).

The severity of RLS symptoms 'score (IRLS) was correlated significantly with the score in sleep diary (r = 0.410, P = 0.030). The prevalence of RLS was correlated with sleep diary (r_{pb} = +0.31, P = 0.01), and Zung depression scale scores (r_{pb} = +0.29, P = 0.01), whereas significant negative correlations were found between the IRLS score and the overall score of the SF-36 (r = −.0423, P = 0.022).

Total body composition assessment did not show any differences between the two groups. The CT analysis showed that the thigh muscle total area, muscle cross sectional area (CSA) and the level of muscle fat infiltration (EMCL-extramyocellular lipids) were significantly reduced in the RLS group (Table 3). In addition, muscle CSA/total LBM ratio and EMCL CSA/total body fat ratio were found to be significantly increased in the non-RLS group [F (1,41) = 7.538, P = 0.009] and [F (1,41) = 4.130, P = 0.048] respectively, whereas, no significant differences were found in the percentage of muscle and EMCL between the two groups [F(1,41) = 2.207, P = 0.145].

Discussion

A 42 % of the examined patients were diagnosed with RLS in agreement with other recent studies [35]. To the best of our knowledge this is the first study assessing parameters that affect survival and quality of life in such detail in patients with uremic RLS. We found that the size of proximal muscles was significantly reduced in the RLS group, however, uremic RLS did not seem to have an additional detrimental impact on the already diminished physical performance, body and muscle composition and physical aspects of the quality of life in HD patients. The low level of QoL reported by the RLS- HD patients seems to be due mainly to mental health and sleep related aspects rather than the physical aspects.

It is well known that HD patients are characterized by low VO_2 peak,[9] reduced physical performance, high levels of weakness and exercise intolerance [36]. In the RLS population with normal kidney function, maximal oxygen uptake values [37] and physical fitness levels [38] have been found to be lower compared to non-RLS healthy individuals. It is, therefore, plausible to hypothesize that HD patients with RLS could have been affected in an additive or synergistic way by uremia and RLS, and that this combination would affect their functional capacity and physical performance. In the current study patients of both groups responded similarly in all physical performance tests, implying that there was no discernible effect of RLS on physical performance in patients receiving dialysis therapy. In agreement to our findings, a study that assessed elderly idiopathic RLS patients using the same methodology with us, found no significant differences in physical performance between sufferers and non-sufferers [39].

Moreover, it is known that HD patients are characterized by significant reductions in muscle size and increased muscle fat infiltration [40]. The analysis of CT images revealed among other that the total thigh area was reduced by 15%, the muscle CSA by 17% and the EMCL CSA area by 38% in the RLS-HD patients. This reduction of muscle mass is worrisome especially since muscle atrophy is usually prominent in HD patients and has been related to high mortality [11]. Independently from the increased levels of atrophy however, there were no visible changes in the muscle composition between groups and this could be speculated to be a positive counteracting effect induced by the increased muscle activity in which RLS patients involuntarily engage. The reduction of total thigh muscle area in the RLS group could be partially explained by the respective reductions in both EMCL and muscle CSAs that were found in that group and not by the amount of subcutaneous fat tissue as this appeared to be similar in both groups.

Table 3. Body composition data.

Variables	Patients Pool Data	Non RLS	RLS	P values
DEXA Body Composition Analysis				
Total Body Fat (%)	27.4±11.3	25.3±11.9	29.7±10.5	0.554
Trunk Fat (%)	27.9±11.3	26.1±12.3	29.9±9.7	0.559
% Legs Fat	27.4±11.2	25.0±12.2	30.0±11.9	0.515
% Arms Fat	24.4±12.6	22.3±12.7	26.6±12.3	0.744
Total LBM (Kg)	46.1±8.8	47.3±9.2	44.9±8.3	0.985
Legs LBM (kg)	14.5±3.1	15.2±3.4	13.8±3.7	0.333
Arms LBM (kg)	5.0±1.4	5.5±1.6	4.6±1.0	0.091
CT Thigh Analysis				
Thigh Total Area (cm^2)	112.1±25.5	119.4±28.9	104.3±18.8	**0.050**
EMCL CSA (cm^2)	17.4±8.7	20.1±8.6	14.5±8.0	**0.022**
EMCL CSA/Total Body Fat	1.1±1.2	1.6±1.7	0.7±0.4	**0.048**
EMCL (%)	15.7±7.4	17.2±6.8	14.1±7.7	0.089
Muscle CSA (cm^2)	94.5±25.2	101.4±28.8	87.1±18.4	0.066
Muscle CSA/Total LBM	2.1±0.4	2.2±0.4	1.9±0.3	**0.009**
Muscle (%)	82.7±6.9	82.4±6.8	83.1±7.2	0.187
Muscle (%)/EMCL (%)	7.4±5.3	6.3±3.1	8.4±6.7	0.145
SAT CSA (cm^2)	115.0±54.1	113.5±56.7	116.5±52.5	0.723

All data are mean ± SD. P values are adjusted for yrs in dialysis. Abbreviations: LBM, lean body mass; EMCL, extramyocellular lipids (fat infiltration); CSA, cross sectional area; SAT, subcutaneous adipose tissue.

The differences in the EMCL area in the RLS patients could be a result of an increased fat oxidation due to higher muscle activity, as it is observed in highly trained athletes [41] however this is only a hypothesis and it should be seen with caution. The fact that no-significant differences were observed in the nutritional status within the two groups, could indicate that the observed differences in the HD-RLS patient's muscle size were not caused by malnutrition. Overall, it seems that the observed changes in muscle size do not have the magnitude to worsen functionality and further reduce physical activity in HD patients with RLS.

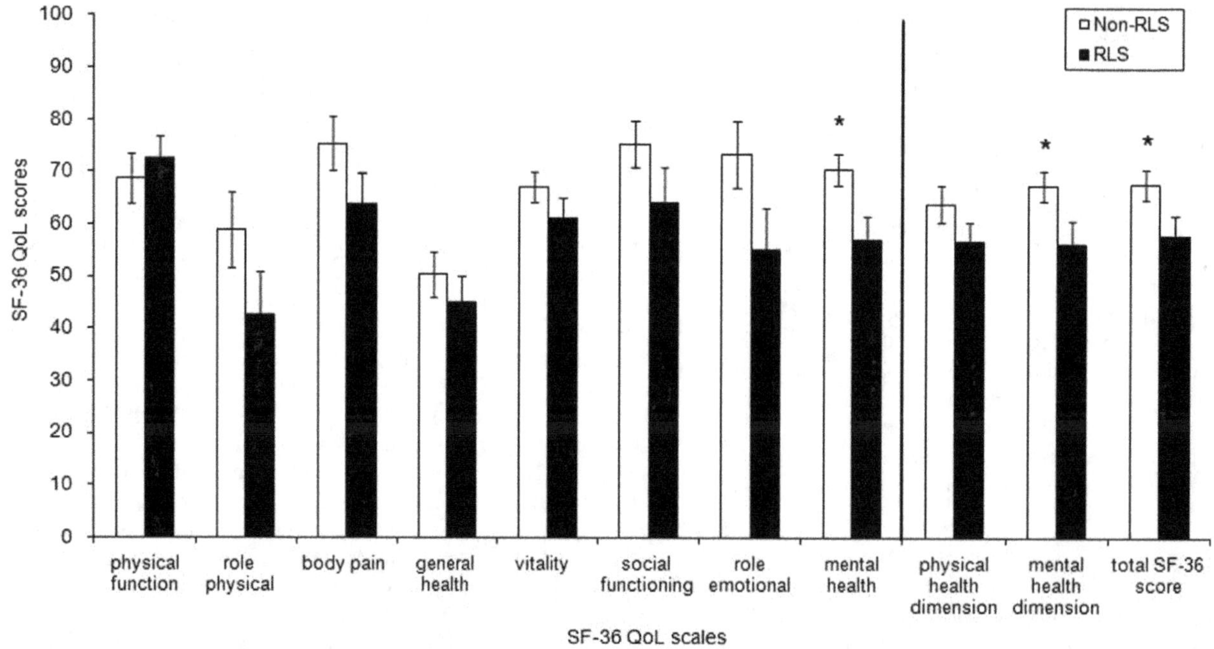

Figure 2. Health-related Quality of Life scores for the RLS (in black) and non-RLS (white bars) hemodialysis patients. Vertical line: The first two sets of bars on the right of the vertical bar are the summary physical and mental dimension score while the last set of bars at the far right is the total SF-36 score.

RLS has been blamed also for sleep deprivation [13] which in turn could evoke alterations in anabolic hormones secretion and circulation such as in growth hormone (GH) and insulin-like growth factor I (IGF-I) [14,15] eventually affecting the patient's anabolism and muscle mass. Subjective sleep quality was found reduced by 61% (sleep diary) reinforcing the hypothesis that the lack of restorative sleep could be one of the factors affecting muscle mass. The RLS-induced sleep deprivation is an important health issue that needs to be addressed further in order to reduce all the possible factors contributing to muscle atrophy and accelerated catabolism in HD patients.

Depression symptoms are common in patients receiving HD therapy [42,43]. It is plausible that HD patients with RLS might experience higher levels of depression as a result of their restless night, the related insomnia and the overall reduced QoL that RLS is associated with [44]. Indeed, the RLS group showed higher depression score than the non-RLS group confirming previous data [45,46], and the RLS status significantly correlated with the score in the Zung depression scale. Even thought depression score was elevated in both groups, none of them exceeded the threshold for the diagnosis of clinical depression (cut off<50). It is also known that low sleep quality exacerbates the severity of depression symptoms seen in HD patients [47] and this is in agreement with our findings. Given that the sleep quality in the HD patients with RLS is significantly impaired compared to the HD patients without the syndrome [5], this could explain in part the differences in depression symptoms severity score between the two groups. This also agrees with our PLMS results, as PLMS were two fold increased in the RLS HD patients affecting even more their sleeping pattern.

So far it was not clear whether the impaired QoL seen in RLS HD patients was due to physical or mental QoL components. A closer look at the questionnaires as well as the physical performance tests reveals that the differences between the two groups are better explained by their diminished mental rather than their physical aspects, confirming data derived from previous studies in RLS in HD patients [5,6]. To the best of our knowledge ours is the first study to carefully investigate, by using both indirect (surveys-questionnaires) and direct (physical performance tests) approaches, what quality of life aspects are the most affected in these patients. The revealed consequences seem to be common also for other symptomatic forms of the sleep disorder (e.g. RLS due to type 2 diabetes). In the past, Merlino et al. concluded that patients accustomed to severe physical dysfunctions (eg, uremia and diabetes) complain of RLS more as a mental distress than a physical one [48] without however providing measurable indices (e.g. functional tests) of the presence or lack of physical impairments. The current study reports a higher level of depression and even poorer sleep quality in the HD patients with RLS compared to their RLS-free counterparts.

RLS severity has been associated with lower survival [8] while PLMS severity is considered an independent predictor of mortality [49]. In the current study, the intensity of the syndrome in our RLS patients was categorized as "severe" [19] implying that those patients might be subjects to a higher CVD risk. However, such a claim will have to be further validated, as it was not straightforward substantiated by our findings.

Limitations

It has been reported that PLMS index can vary across nights in patients with idiopathic RLS [50] but it is not known if the same phenomenon exists in patients with secondary type of RLS. Thus, in that respect our data should be viewed with caution since the PLMS indices obtained by a single overnight PSG study may be not as reliable as if we had used an average of two or even three consecutive assessment nights.

In conclusion, hemodialysis patients with RLS reported lower quality of life and overall scored worse in mental rather than physical parameters compared to their RLS free counterparts. The size of proximal muscles was found to be significantly reduced in the RLS group, however, uremic RLS did not seem to have an additional detrimental impact on the already diminished physical performance, body and muscle composition and physical aspects of the quality of life in HD patients. It is possible that the potential negative impact of RLS on the above parameters could have been masked under the dominant impact of uremia and/or hemodialysis *per se*. Screening for RLS should be part of the routine general health assessment of the hemodialysis patients as it affects QoL and possibly overall health status.

Acknowledgments

We would like to thank all hemodialysis patients who volunteered for the purposes of this study, as well as the staff at the hemodialysis unit of the University Hospital of Larissa and General Hospital of Trikala, Greece, for their expert advice and valuable help.

Author Contributions

Conceived and designed the experiments: CDG GKS GMH YK IS. Performed the experiments: CDG GKS CK GMH EL YK NT GNK. Analyzed the data: CDG GKS CK GMH EL VL NT GNK. Contributed reagents/materials/analysis tools: CK EL VL IS. Wrote the paper: CDG GKS CK GMH EL VL YK IS.

References

1. Allen RP, Picchietti D, Hening WA, Trenkwalder C, Walters AS, et al. (2003) Restless legs syndrome: diagnostic criteria, special considerations, and epidemiology. A report from the restless legs syndrome diagnosis and epidemiology workshop at the National Institutes of Health. Sleep Med 4: 101–119.
2. Parker KP (2003) Sleep disturbances in dialysis patients. Sleep Med Rev 7: 131–143.
3. Merlino G, Piani A, Dolso P, Adorati M, Cancelli I, et al. (2006) Sleep disorders in patients with end-stage renal disease undergoing dialysis therapy. Nephrol Dial Transplant 21: 184–190.
4. Perl J, Unruh ML, Chan CT (2006) Sleep disorders in end-stage renal disease: 'Markers of inadequate dialysis'? Kidney Int 70: 1687–1693.
5. Mucsi I, Molnar MZ, Ambrus C, Szeifert L, Kovacs AZ, et al. (2005) Restless legs syndrome, insomnia and quality of life in patients on maintenance dialysis. Nephrol Dial Transplant 20: 571–577.
6. Kawauchi A, Inoue Y, Hashimoto T, Tachibana N, Shirakawa S, et al. (2006) Restless legs syndrome in hemodialysis patients: health-related quality of life and laboratory data analysis. Clin Nephrol 66: 440–446.
7. Rijsman RM, de Weerd AW, Stam CJ, Kerkhof GA, Rosman JB (2004) Periodic limb movement disorder and restless legs syndrome in dialysis patients. Nephrology (Carlton) 9: 353–361.
8. Unruh ML, Levey AS, D'Ambrosio C, Fink NE, Powe NR, et al. (2004) Restless legs symptoms among incident dialysis patients: association with lower quality of life and shorter survival. Am J Kidney Dis 43: 900–909.
9. Painter P (2005) Physical functioning in end-stage renal disease patients: update 2005. Hemodial Int 9: 218–235.
10. Kakiya R, Shoji T, Tsujimoto Y, Tatsumi N, Hatsuda S, et al. (2006) Body fat mass and lean mass as predictors of survival in hemodialysis patients. Kidney Int 70: 549–556.
11. Johansen KL (2009) Anabolic and catabolic mechanisms in end-stage renal disease. Adv Chronic Kidney Dis 16: 501–510.
12. La Manna G, Pizza F, Persici E, Baraldi O, Comai G, et al. (2011) Restless legs syndrome enhances cardiovascular risk and mortality in patients with end-stage kidney disease undergoing long-term haemodialysis treatment. Nephrol Dial Transplant 26(6): 1976–83.
13. Allen RP, Walters AS, Montplaisir J, Hening W, Myers A, et al. (2005) Restless legs syndrome prevalence and impact: REST general population study. Arch Intern Med 165: 1286–1292.
14. Everson CA, Crowley WR (2004) Reductions in circulating anabolic hormones induced by sustained sleep deprivation in rats. Am J Physiol Endocrinol Metab 286: E1060–1070.

15. Van Cauter E, Spiegel K, Tasali E, Leproult R (2008) Metabolic consequences of sleep and sleep loss. Sleep Med 9 Suppl 1: S23–28.
16. Sakkas GK, Gourgoulianis KI, Karatzaferi C, Liakopoulos V, Maridaki MD, et al. (2008) Haemodialysis patients with sleep apnoea syndrome experience increased central adiposity and altered muscular composition and functionality. Nephrol Dial Transplant 23: 336–344.
17. Kavanagh D, Siddiqui S, Geddes CC (2004) Restless legs syndrome in patients on dialysis. Am J Kidney Dis 43: 763–771.
18. Zucconi M, Ferri R, Allen R, Baier PC, Bruni O, et al. (2006) The official World Association of Sleep Medicine (WASM) standards for recording and scoring periodic leg movements in sleep (PLMS) and wakefulness (PLMW) developed in collaboration with a task force from the International Restless Legs Syndrome Study Group (IRLSSG). Sleep Med 7: 175–183.
19. Walters AS, LeBrocq C, Dhar A, Hening W, Rosen R, et al. (2003) Validation of the International Restless Legs Syndrome Study Group rating scale for restless legs syndrome. Sleep Med 4: 121–132.
20. Svendsen OL, Haarbo J, Hassager C, Christriansen C (1993) Accuracy of measurements of total-body soft-tissue composition by dual energy X-ray absorptiometry in vivo. Basic Life Sci 60: 381–383.
21. Lo JC, Mulligan K, Tai VW, Algren H, Schambelan M (1998) "Buffalo hump" in men with HIV-1 infection. Lancet 351: 867–870.
22. McIntyre CW, Selby NM, Sigrist M, Pearce LE, Mercer TH, et al. (2006) Patients receiving maintenance dialysis have more severe functionally significant skeletal muscle wasting than patients with dialysis-independent chronic kidney disease. Nephrol Dial Transplant 21: 2210–2216.
23. Johansen KL, Chertow GM, da Silva M, Carey S, Painter P (2001) Determinants of physical performance in ambulatory patients on hemodialysis. Kidney Int 60: 1586–1591.
24. Koufaki P, Mercer TH, Naish PF (2002) Effects of exercise training on aerobic and functional capacity of end-stage renal disease patients. Clin Physiol Funct Imaging 22: 115–124.
25. Mercer TH, Naish PF, Gleeson NP, Wilcock JE, Crawford C (1998) Development of a walking test for the assessment of functional capacity in non-anaemic maintenance dialysis patients. Nephrol Dial Transplant 13: 2023–2026.
26. Kalantar-Zadeh K, Kopple JD, Block G, Humphreys MH (2001) Association among SF36 quality of life measures and nutrition, hospitalization, and mortality in hemodialysis. J Am Soc Nephrol 12: 2797–2806.
27. Johansen KL, Kaysen GA, Young BS, Hung AM, da Silva M, et al. (2003) Longitudinal study of nutritional status, body composition, and physical function in hemodialysis patients. Am J Clin Nutr 77: 842–846.
28. Koufaki P, Mercer T (2009) Assessment and monitoring of physical function for people with CKD. Adv Chronic Kidney Dis 16: 410–419.
29. Zung WW (1965) A Self-Rating Depression Scale. Arch Gen Psychiatry 12: 63–70.
30. Suh MR, Jung HH, Kim SB, Park JS, Yang WS (2002) Effects of regular exercise on anxiety, depression, and quality of life in maintenance hemodialysis patients. Ren Fail 24: 337–345.
31. Johns MW (1991) A new method for measuring daytime sleepiness: the Epworth sleepiness scale. Sleep 14: 540–545.
32. Enia G, Sicuso C, Alati G, Zoccali C (1993) Subjective global assessment of nutrition in dialysis patients. Nephrol Dial Transplant 8: 1094–1098.
33. Daugirdas JT (1993) Second generation logarithmic estimates of single-pool variable volume Kt/V: an analysis of error. J Am Soc Nephrol 4: 1205–1213.
34. Sakkas GK, Karatzaferi C, Zintzaras E, Giannaki CD, Liakopoulos V, et al. (2008) Liver fat, visceral adiposity, and sleep disturbances contribute to the development of insulin resistance and glucose intolerance in nondiabetic dialysis patients. Am J Physiol Regul Integr Comp Physiol 295: R1721–1729.
35. Siddiqui S, Kavanagh D, Traynor J, Mak M, Deighan C, et al. (2005) Risk factors for restless legs syndrome in dialysis patients. Nephron Clin Pract 101: c155–160.
36. Johansen KL, Shubert T, Doyle J, Soher B, Sakkas GK, et al. (2003) Muscle atrophy in patients receiving hemodialysis: effects on muscle strength, muscle quality, and physical function. Kidney Int 63: 291–297.
37. Larsson BW, Kadi F, Ulfberg J, Aulin KP (2007) Skeletal muscle morphology in patients with restless legs syndrome. Eur Neurol 58: 133–137.
38. Schlesinger I, Erikh I, Avizohar O, Sprecher E, Yarnitsky D (2009) Cardiovascular risk factors in restless legs syndrome. Mov Disord 24: 1587–1592.
39. Rothdach AJ, Trenkwalder C, Haberstock J, Keil U, Berger K (2000) Prevalence and risk factors of RLS in an elderly population: the MEMO study. Memory and Morbidity in Augsburg Elderly. Neurology 54: 1064–1068.
40. Sakkas GK, Ball D, Mercer TH, Sargeant AJ, Tolfrey K, et al. (2003) Atrophy of non-locomotor muscle in patients with end-stage renal failure. Nephrol Dial Transplant 18: 2074–2081.
41. van Loon LJ (2004) Use of intramuscular triacylglycerol as a substrate source during exercise in humans. J Appl Physiol 97: 1170–1187.
42. Kimmel PL, Peterson RA (2006) Depression in patients with end-stage renal disease treated with dialysis: has the time to treat arrived? Clin J Am Soc Nephrol 1: 349–352.
43. Kimmel PL (2001) Psychosocial factors in dialysis patients. Kidney Int 59: 1599–1613.
44. Gigli GL, Adorati M, Dolso P, Piani A, Valente M, et al. (2004) Restless legs syndrome in end-stage renal disease. Sleep Med 5: 309–315.
45. Szentkiralyi A, Molnar MZ, Czira ME, Deak G, Lindner AV, et al. (2009) Association between restless legs syndrome and depression in patients with chronic kidney disease. J Psychosom Res 67: 173–180.
46. Tuncel D, Orhan FO, Sayarlioglu H, Isik IO, Utku U, et al. Restless legs syndrome in hemodialysis patients: ssociation with depression and quality of life. Sleep Breath.
47. Pai MF, Hsu SP, Yang SY, Ho TI, Lai CF, et al. (2007) Sleep disturbance in chronic hemodialysis patients: the impact of depression and anemia. Ren Fail 29: 673–677.
48. Merlino G, Valente M, Serafini A, Fratticci L, Del Giudice A, et al. (2010) Effects of restless legs syndrome on quality of life and psychological status in patients with type 2 diabetes. Diabetes Educ 36: 79–87.
49. Benz RL, Pressman MR, Hovick ET, Peterson DD (2000) Potential novel predictors of mortality in end-stage renal disease patients with sleep disorders. Am J Kidney Dis 35: 1052–1060.
50. Sforza E, Haba-Rubio J (2005) Night-to-night variability in periodic leg movements in patients with restless legs syndrome. Sleep Med 6: 259–267.

6

Sensitive Troponins – Which Suits Better for Hemodialysis Patients? Associated Factors and Prediction of Mortality

Ferruh Artunc[1]*, Christian Mueller[2], Tobias Breidthardt[2], Raphael Twerenbold[2], Andreas Peter[1], Claus Thamer[1], Peter Weyrich[1], Hans-Ulrich Haering[1], Bjoern Friedrich[1,3]

1 Department of Internal Medicine, Division of Endocrinology, Diabetology, Vascular Disease, Nephrology and Clinical Chemistry, University of Tuebingen, Germany, **2** Department of Internal Medicine, Division of Cardiology, University of Basel, Basel, Switzerland, **3** Dialysis Center, Leonberg, Germany

Abstract

Background: In hemodialysis patients, elevated plasma troponin concentrations are a common finding that has even increased with the advent of newly developed sensitive assays. However, the interpretation and relevance of this is still under debate.

Methods: In this cross-sectional study, we analyzed plasma concentrations of sensitive troponin I (TnI) and troponin T (TnT) in stable ambulatory hemodialysis patients (n = 239) and investigated their associations with clinical factors and mortality.

Results: In all of the enrolled patients, plasma TnI or TnT was detectable at a median concentration of 14 pg/ml (interquartile range: 7–29) using the Siemens TnI ultra assay and 49 pg/ml (31–74) using the Roche Elecsys high sensitive TnT assay. Markedly more patients exceeded the 99th percentile for TnT than for TnI (95% vs. 14%, $p<0.0001$). In a multivariate linear regression model, TnT was independently associated with age, gender, systolic dysfunction, time on dialysis, residual diuresis and systolic blood pressure, whereas TnI was independently associated with age, systolic dysfunction, pulse pressure, time on dialysis and duration of a HD session. During a follow-up period of nearly two years, TnT concentration above 38 pg/mL was associated with a 5-fold risk of death, whereas elevation of TnI had a gradual association to mortality.

Conclusion: In hemodialysis patients, elevations of plasma troponin concentrations are explained by cardiac function and dialysis-related parameters, which contribute to cardiac strain. Both are highly predictive of increased risk of death.

Editor: Wolf-Hagen Schunck, Max Delbrueck Center for Molecular Medicine, Germany

Funding: These authors have no support or funding to report.

Competing Interests: The authors have declared that no competing interests exist.

* E-mail: ferruh.artunc@med.uni-tuebingen.de

Introduction

Elevations of cardiac troponins in the plasma define are indicative of myocardial injury and necrosis [1]. According to the universal definition of myocardial infarction (MI) published in 2007, MI can be diagnosed based on a rise and fall in the plasma troponin concentrations above the 99th percentile when there is evidence of myocardial ischemia [2]. However, in patients with end-stage renal failure (ESRD), chronic elevations at the subclinical level have been shown to occur without signs of myocardial ischemia [3–5]. Several longitudinal studies have consistently shown that elevated troponin concentrations in ESRD patients add prognostic information and are associated with increased mortality [6–10]. A meta-analysis concluded that increases in plasma troponin T or troponin I concentrations conferred a 2.64 or 1.74-fold increase, respectively, in mortality risk in ESRD patients [11]. The current view is that an elevated troponin concentration reflects chronic myocardial strain and damage during the course of renal failure and ESRD [12] rather than reduced clearance [13] or cross-reactivity with troponins from skeletal muscle [14,15]. The cardiac work load of ESRD patients is greatly increased by several conditions, such as hypertension, shunt flow, chronic extracellular volume expansion, anemia or increased pulse pressure. These factors induce profound alterations in cardiac structure [16] and may lead to subsequent troponin release. In addition to a chronically increased cardiac work load, acute hemodialysis sessions induce cardiac stress due to circulatory alterations and may trigger myocardial stunning [17].

Typically, plasma troponin concentrations in ESRD patients are slightly elevated above the 99th percentile touching the lower detection limit of many troponin assays employed in routine diagnostics. At this point, the analytical precision of conventional troponin measurements is reduced, and the coefficient of variation (CV) can reach 10–20% [18]. To overcome this problem, sensitive assays with a CV of <10% at the 99th percentile have been developed and have shown improved accuracy in the diagnosis of MI [19]. Some of these tests can be designated as highly sensitive based on a high proportion (>50%) of subjects with measurable

Table 1. Patient characteristics of the cohort (n = 239).

median age		70 (61; 77) years (n = 239)
gender distribution		64% male (n = 153)/36% female (n = 86)
renal disease	diabetic nephropathy	26% (n = 63)
	hypertension	8% (n = 19)
	glomerulonephritis	30% (n = 71)
	polycystic disease	5% (n = 11)
	other/unknown	31% (n = 75)
cardiac comorbidities	coronary heart disease	31% (n = 74)
	revascularized	19% (n = 31)
	valvular heart disease	26% (n = 61)
	atrial fibrillation	23% (n = 55)
	pulmonary hypertension	7% (n = 16)
	AICD carrier	2% (n = 4)
other comorbidities	diabetes mellitus	38% (n = 90)
	peripheral vascular disease	33% (n = 80)
	stroke	16% (n = 38)
	vasculitis	3% (n = 8)
	malignoma	14% (n = 34)
	COPD	8% (n = 19)
length of time on dialysis		46 (19; 85) months (n = 239)
duration of dialysis session		4.0 (4.0; 4.5) hours (n = 239)
dialysis access	arteriovenous fistula	71% (n = 169)
	PTFE graft	13% (n = 31)
	tunneled catheter	16% (n = 38)
dialysis membrane	high-flux	92% (n = 219)
	low-flux	8% (n = 20)
residual diuresis		250 (0; 1000) mL/day (n = 239)
anuric patients		39% (n = 93)
interdialytic weight gain		1.85 (1.29; 2.47) kg (n = 239)
blood pump speed		300 (280; 340) mL/min (n = 239)
shunt flow		1080 (733; 1475) mL/min (n = 187)
blood pressure		134 (122; 144)/69 (63; 74) mm Hg (n = 239)
pulse pressure		65 (54; 74) mm Hg (n = 239)
singe pool Kt/V		1.55 (1.40; 1.73) (n = 239)
laboratory data	hemoglobin	11.5 (11.1; 12.0) g/dL (n = 239)
	C-reactive protein	8.6 (4.6; 15.0) mg/L (n = 239)
	albumin	37.1 (35.4; 39.3) g/L (n = 239)
	parathormone	204 (130; 348) pg/mL (n = 239)
	β2-microglobulin	23.4 (19.4; 25.4) mg/L (n = 239)
LV systolic function	normal	59% (n = 140)
	mildly reduced	13% (n = 32)
	moderately or severely reduced	12% (n = 29)
	unknown	16% (n = 38)

Values shown are the median and interquartile range. N indicates number of patients from which data were available.
abbreviations:
PTFE = polytetrafluorethylene, LV = left ventricle, AICD = automated implantable cardioverter-defibrillator.

values that fall below the 99th percentile [18,20]. Currently, only few clinically available assays, such as the Roche Elecsys high sensitive (hs) TnT, fulfill this criterion [18]. There are only a few studies that have applied sensitive troponin assays in ESRD patients [21–23]. In one study, sensitive troponin T was found to be the most powerful predictor of mortality in ESRD patients among other established cardiac biomarkers [22].

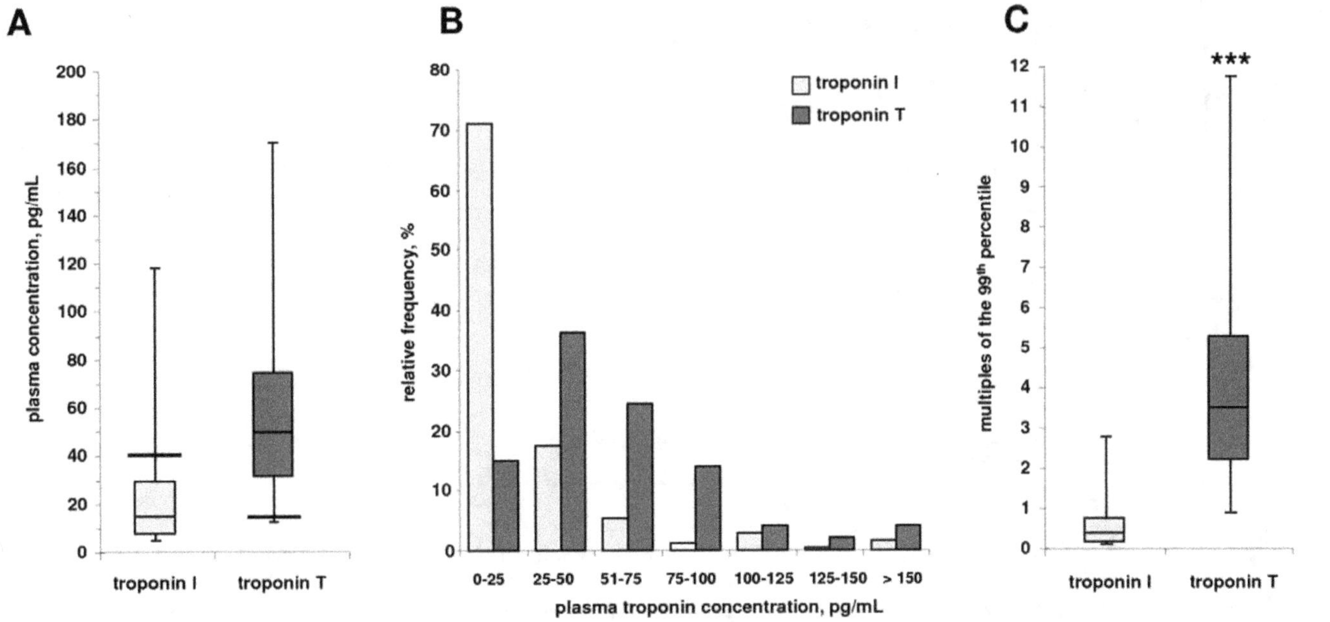

Figure 1. Depiction of the plasma troponin I and T concentrations in the cohort. A Box-and-Whiskers-Plot of the plasma troponin I and T concentrations indicating the median, interquartile range and the range between the 2.5^{th} and 97.5^{th} percentile. Solid lines represent the 99th percentile of the assay [19]. **B** Distribution of the plasma troponin I and T concentrations in the cohort (n = 239). **C** Box-and-Whiskers-Plot of the plasma troponin I and T concentrations expressed as multiples of the 99th percentile [19]. *** indicates a significant difference (p<0.0001) between the troponin T and troponin I concentrations.

With the advent of sensitive assays, cardiac troponins are now detected to a larger extent in hemodialysis patients raising questions about interpretation and relevance to nephrologists and cardiologists alike. The increased sensitivity and resolution of the assays, however, also improve the chance to identify factors that are associated with elevated plasma troponin concentrations, such as loss of residual renal function [24] or volume overload [25], both of which contribute to cardiac strain and are predictive of increased mortality. Since both troponins (I and T) can be measured with sensitive assays, results might also reflect different biochemical properties. Therefore, we measured both troponin I and T with sensitive assays in a comparative approach to investigate associated factors and to analyze the diagnostic performance in predicting death during a follow-up period of two years.

Methods

Patients and cohort

This cross-sectional, prospective multicenter study was conducted in stable, ambulatory hemodialysis patients from four dialysis centers in southwest Germany between September 2009 and April 2010. Patients without evidence of an acute illness and cardiac event or procedure within two months were included in the study after providing written informed consent. Patients with cardiac diseases leading to increased plasma troponin concentrations independent of ESRD, such as amyloidosis, were excluded. The study was approved by the local ethics committee of the University hospital Tuebingen.

Laboratory assays

Plasma concentrations of troponin I and troponin T were measured in three independent samples collected within two weeks. Each sample was collected prior to the start of a dialysis

Table 2. Univariate correlations (Pearson's r) of the plasma troponin concentration with general and dialysis-specific parameters (n = 210–239).

	troponin I, pg/ml	troponin T, pg/ml
age, y	0.32 ***	0.43 ***
systolic LVF, classes	0.44 ***	0.38 ***
time on dialysis, months	0.15 *	0.18 **
residual diuresis, ml/day	−0.13 *	−0.29 ***
interdialytic weight gain, kg	0.13 *	0.25 **
shunt flow, ml/min	−0.16 *	−0.14 #
systolic blood pressure, mm Hg	0.11 #	n.s.
diastolic blood pressure, mm Hg	−0.13 *	−0.19 **
pulse pressure, mm Hg	0.21 *	0.22 **
duration of a HD session	n.s.	n.s.
blood pump speed, ml/min	n.s.	0.15 *
Kt/V	n.s.	n.s.
hemoglobin, g/dL	n.s.	n.s.
plasma albumin, g/L	n.s.	n.s.
C-reactive protein, mg/L	n.s.	0.21 **
parathormone, pg/mL	0.16 *	0.14 *
β2-microglobulin, mg/dL	n.s	n.s

#p<0.10, * p<0.05, ** p<0.01, *** p<0.001, n.s. = not significant (p>0.10).

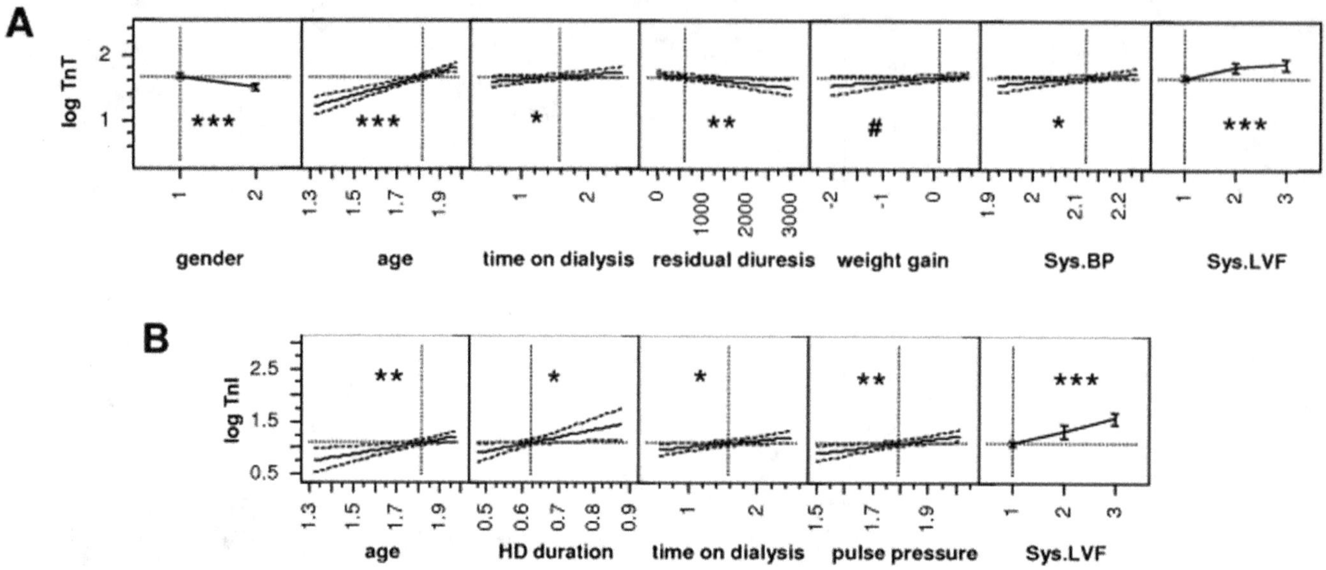

Figure 2. Plot showing the influence of single predictors in the multivariate model for troponin T (A) and troponin I (B). # p<0.10, * p<0.05, ** p<0.01, *** p<0.001.

session. Blood was collected in lithium-heparinized tubes (Sarstedt, Nuembrecht, Germany), cooled at 4°C, and centrifuged within 4 hours. The sera were stored at −80°C until further analysis. Plasma concentrations of troponin I were measured using the Troponin I Ultra assay on a Siemens ADVIA Centaur system (Siemens Healthcare Diagnostics, Eschborn, Germany) with a detection limit of 6 pg/ml, a 99th percentile at 40 pg/ml, and a CV of less than 10% at 30 pg/ml, as specified by the manufacturer. Plasma concentrations of troponin T were measured using an automated Roche assay on an Elecsys 2010 system with a detection limit of 2 pg/ml, a 99th percentile at 14 pg/ml, and a coefficient of variation of less than 10% at 13 pg/ml [19]. Plasma beta-2-microglobulin concentrations were measured using a turbidimetric assay (Randox Laboratories, Antrim, United Kingdom) on a Siemens ADVIA 1800 system with a measurable range between 0.56–20.9 mg/l and an upper reference concentration of 3 mg/l [26]. All other laboratory values (parathormone, hemoglobin, albumin and C-reactive protein) were extracted from the patients' medical records and represent an average of the available values from the previous year (4–12 values).

Clinical data

The following data were extracted from each patient: residual diuresis, as measured by 24 h urine collection: single pool Kt/V (mean of the most recent 4 values collected), interdialytic weight gain, predialytic systolic and diastolic blood pressure (mean of the most recent 12 values), dialysis access and membrane, length of

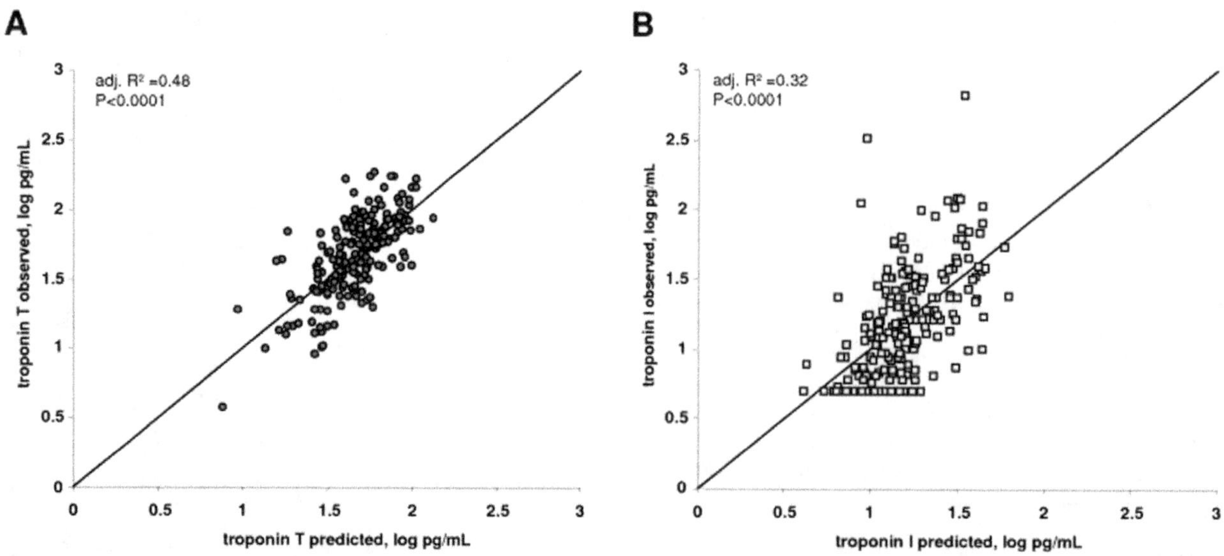

Figure 3. Agreement between predicted and observed log troponin I and T concentrations. Plot of the predicted and observed troponin values for troponin T (**A**) and troponin I (**B**) as a result of the models shown in table 4. The diagonal line represents the line of identity.

Table 3. Independent factors determining plasma troponin concentrations by multivariate linear modeling (n = 201).

	covariate	estimate ± SD	standardized estimate ± SD	p-value
troponin T, pg/ml	y-intercept	−1.25±0.61	1.59±0.02	0.0410
	age, y	0.84±0.14	0.27±0.05	<.0001
	systolic LVF, classes [2 vs. 1]	0.14±0.04	0.14±0.04	0.0016
	systolic blood pressure, mmHg	0.55±0.27	0.09±0.04	0.0432
	residual diuresis, ml/24 h	$-6\ 10^{-5}\pm2\ 10^{-5}$	-0.09±0.03	0.0050
	gender [1 = male]	0.08±0.02	0.08±0.02	<.0001
	interdialytic weight gain, kg	0.06±0.03	0.07±0.04	0.0688
	time on dialysis. months	0.08±0.04	0.07±0.04	0.0395
	systolic LVF, classes [3 vs. 2]	0.04±0.27	0.06±0.06	0.4715
	atrial fibrillatiom [1 = yes]	0.08±0.04	0.04±0.02	0.0324
troponin I, pg/ml	y-intercept	−2.32±0.69	1.10±0.03	0.0009
	duration of a HD session, h	1.30±0.58	0.26±0.12	0.0274
	systolic LVF, classes [3 vs. 2]	0.22±0.07	0.25±0.08	0.0042
	systolic LVF, classes [2 vs. 1]	0.25±0.08	0.22±0.07	0.0013
	age, y	0.62±0.24	0.20±0.08	0.0104
	pulse pressure, mm Hg	0.71±0.24	0.18±0.06	0.0032
	time on dialysis, months	0.11±0.06	0.11±0.05	0.0410
	valvular disease [1 = yes]	0.10±0.06	0.05±0.03	0.0767

time on dialysis, blood pump flow and shunt flow measured using a Transonic system (Ithaca, NY, USA). The left ventricular (LV) systolic function was classified from available echocardiography examinations in which class 1 indicated normal function, 2 was mildly reduced, and 3 was moderately or severely reduced. Determination of the LV systolic function was done at the discretion of the cardiologist and not standardized. Echocardiography was available in 84% of all patients within one year (plus-minus) relative to study enrollment.

Statistical analysis

Three samples were available in 87% of the patients and were averaged to calculate the arithmetic mean without excluding possible outliers. For further analysis, plasma troponin concentrations and continuous clinical data were log transformed to approximate normal distribution. The association of the plasma troponin concentrations with clinical or dialysis-related factors was analyzed by univariate parametric correlation. Multivariate linear regression analyses were performed to identify independent determinants of the plasma troponin concentrations. Selection of the variables entering the model were derived from forward, stepwise multiple linear regression, and all variables with a p-value <0.05 were included in the multivariate linear regression models. The residuals of each model were tested for normality. Averaged values of the deceased patients were compared to those from the surviving patients using t-Test or Wilcoxon's test. Kaplan-Meier curves were generated after stratification into tertiles of the variable according to its distribution. The follow-up period started on the first day of blood draw and was censored as of 31 December 2011. The diagnostic performance was analyzed using receiver-operator curves (ROC or c-index) and the best cut-off value was considered as the maximal difference of sensitivity and 1-specificity (Youden index). C-Index was calculated using Wessa, P. (2012), Free Statistics Software, Office for Research Development and Education, version 1.1.23-r7, http://www.wessa.net/. Univariate and multivariate proportional hazards were calculated to analyze the risk ratios of each predictor and the independence of the predictors. Data analysis was performed using the statistical software package JMP 10.0.1 (SAS Institute, Cary, NC).

Results

Patients

Of the n = 250 available patients that were treated in the participating centers, n = 239 were included in the study. The reasons for exclusion of the n = 11 patients were the following: patients declined to participate (n = 6), deaths occurred following the initial plasma collection (n = 2), cardiac amyloidosis (n = 2) and a recent enrollment in dialysis (n = 1). The characteristics of the study cohort are provided in table 1. Participants were primarily geriatric, with a median age of 70. They had been in a dialysis-dependent state for a median of 45 months and were dialyzed mainly using an arteriovenous (AV) fistula (71%) or a high flux membrane (95%). The dialysis sessions, which lasted 4 hours, had a Kt/V value above the recommended K/DOQI target value of 1.3. Median shunt flow was approximately 1 L/min. Residual diuresis was low (median of 250 ml/day), and 39% of the patients were anuric. The median plasma albumin concentration was slightly below the recommended KDOQI target of 40 g/L, although hemoglobin and parathormone levels were within the target range. Plasma β2-microglobulin concentrations were highly elevated (median concentration of 23.5 mg/L), indicating an accumulation due to reduced renal and low dialysis-driven clearance.

Cardiac comorbidities were present in a large proportion of the patients. Ischemic heart disease was the most frequent condition (31%). Systolic LV dysfunction was found in 26% of all of the patients (table 1).

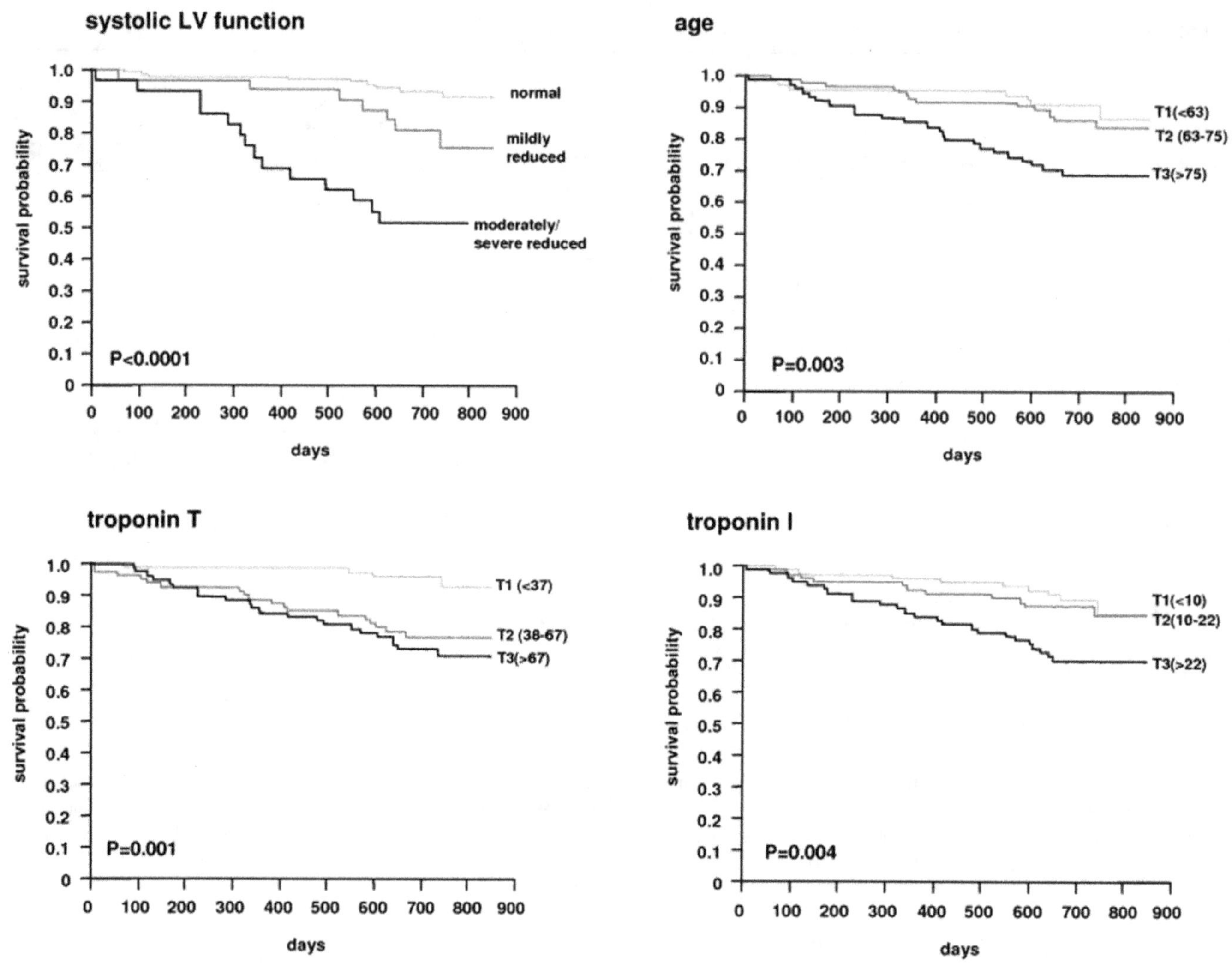

Figure 4. Survival curves of the cohort stratified according to classes of systolic LV function and tertiles of age, troponin T and troponin I.

Plasma troponin concentrations in the cohort

Plasma troponin I or T was detectable with the applied sensitive assays in all of the enrolled patients. The median TnT and TnI concentrations were 49 pg/ml and 14 pg/ml, with an interquartile range of 31 to 73 pg/ml and 7 to 28 pg/ml, respectively (Fig. 1A). The distributions of the plasma troponin concentrations are shown in Figure 1B. A large proportion of patients (95%) had a plasma TnT concentration above the 99th percentile at 14 pg/ml, while only 14% of the patients had a plasma TnI concentration above the 99th percentile at 40 pg/ml. Expressed as multiples of the 99th percentile, the TnT concentration was elevated 3.5 fold (interquartile range: 2.2 to 5.2) compared to 0.4 fold for TnI (interquartile range: 0.2 to 0.7; Figure 1C), which represented a highly significant difference ($p<0.0001$). Plasma troponin concentrations were moderately correlated with each other ($r=0.63$, $p<0.0001$). TnI had a greater variability within the three samples with a variation of 26±24% compared to 8±8% for TnT.

Univariate analyses

Table 2 lists the results of univariate correlation analyses of the plasma TnI and TnT concentrations with the collected parameters. Both troponins showed a significant positive correlation with age, degree of systolic dysfunction, interdialytic weight gain, pulse pressure and parathormone concentration. The troponins were negatively correlated with residual diuresis, diastolic blood pressure and shunt flow. TnT was positively correlated with blood pump speed and C-reactive protein concentrations. There was no correlation with the plasma β2-microglobulin concentration. Variations in TnT and TnI, expressed as the standard deviation of the three samples obtained from each patient, were not correlated to any of the parameters studied.

Multivariate analyses

To analyze independent determinants of the plasma TnI and TnT concentrations, multivariate linear regression modeling was performed. The parameters that entered the final model were selected using a stepwise forward approach with a p-value of <0.05. Table 3 and Figure 2 show the results of the multivariate linear regression models that were applied. Besides age and gender, the independent determinants of the plasma TnT concentration were systolic LV function, systolic blood pressure, time on dialysis and residual diuresis. The influence of interdialytic weight gain was close to reaching statistical significance ($p=0.0688$). Overall, the adjusted r^2 of the model was 0.48,

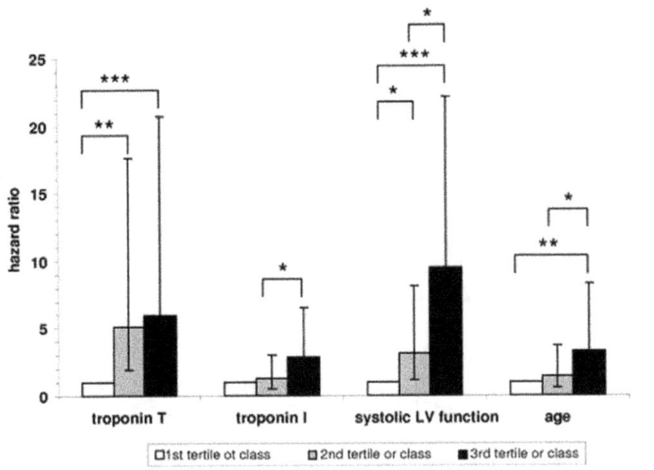

Figure 5. Hazard ratio of mortality according to tertiles of troponin T (<37; 38–67; >67 pg/ml), troponin I (<10; 10–22; >22 pg/ml), age (<63; 63–75; >75 years) and classes of systolic LV function (1 = normal, 2 = mildly reduced; 3 = moderately and severe reduced). Error bars represent lower and upper 95% confidence interval. The hazard ratio of the first tertile or class, respectively, was set to 1. ** p<0.01, *** p<0.001.

indicating that 48% of the variability in plasma TnT concentrations could be explained by these factors (Figure 3A). In contrast, the best model for TnI had an adjusted r^2 of 0.32, and age, systolic LV function, pulse pressure, length of time on dialysis and duration of a HD session were independent predictors (Figure 3B).

Prognostic value

After the initial blood draw, the cohort was followed for survival to analyze the prognostic value of elevated plasma troponin concentrations. During a median follow-up time of 710 days (679; 761), 44 patients died corresponding to an annual mortality rate of 9.2%. Compared to surviving patients, deceased patients were significantly older (77 years [68;82] vs. 69 [59; 76]; p<0.0001), were more likely to have LV dysfunction (68% vs. 24%; p<0.0001) and had lower diastolic blood pressure (65 mm Hg [59;72] vs. 69 [63; 74]; p = 0.0087). They had higher plasma CRP and parathormone concentrations (12.9 mg/L [8.8;20.1] vs. 7.7 [4.2; 13.6]; p<0.0001 and 240 pg/mL [169;431] vs. 203 [124; 326]; p = 0.0011, respectively). Plasma troponin T and I concentrations were also significantly (p<0.0001) higher in deceased patients (67 [46;87] pg/mL and 24 [11;46] pg/mL, respectively) compared to surviving patients (44 [29;70] pg/mL and 13 [7;24] pg/mL, respectively).

The survival curves stratified for tertiles of age, plasma troponin T and I concentrations as well as classes of systolic LV function are shown in Figure 4. The relative risk compared to the first tertile or class is shown in Figure 5. Systolic LV function was the strongest predictor of death during follow-up, followed by increased plasma troponin T concentration. When analyzing the diagnostic performance of plasma troponin T and I concentrations using contingency tables and receiver-operator curves (Table 4), both troponins showed similar AUC-values, however, plasma troponin T concentration had a higher sensitivity (91%) and negative predictive value (95%) compared to troponin I (61% and 77%, respectively). For each increase of the plasma troponin T or I concentration by 10 pg/ml, the risk ratio was increased by 13.9% and 5.2%, respectively. In a multivariate proportional hazards model with age, systolic function and troponin concentration, only systolic function and age remained independent predictors (data not shown).

Discussion

This study shows that plasma troponin T concentrations measured using a highly sensitive assay were elevated in the vast majority of the hemodialysis cohort studied and that both cardiac and dialysis-related parameters determined its concentrations. Compared to sensitive troponin I, TnT was elevated in more patients, reflected dialysis-related factors to a greater extent and tended to be a stronger predictor of mortality. This study is in agreement with previous studies of patients without ESRD that showed an association between increased plasma troponin concentrations and impaired systolic function [27,28]. In addition, plasma troponin concentrations were independently associated with dialysis-related parameters, such as time on dialysis, residual diuresis, interdialytic weight gain or duration of a HD session. These factors, which can be termed "dialysis heritage", are strongly interrelated to each other in that residual function was lost with an increasing time on dialysis, which favors volume overload. Residual function and interdialytic weight gain are both independent risk factors for increased mortality in ESRD patients [24,25]. The association between residual diuresis and plasma troponin concentration has been reported earlier [29].

Most of the studies evaluating plasma troponin concentrations in ESRD patients have investigated the prognostic value and association with mortality. However, only a few studies have addressed the determinants of plasma troponin concentration in ESRD patients. Several studies found that elevated troponin concentrations were associated with the extent of coronary disease [30,31], calcification [32] or left ventricular hypertrophy or dysfunction [33]. Interestingly, in our study shunt flow was negatively correlated with plasma troponin T or I concentrations and was an independent predictor with a borderline statistical significance in the multivariate analysis (p = 0.07). Despite the possible detrimental effects of a high shunt flow on the heart [16], our results suggest that a high shunt flow can be interpreted as a sign of better cardiac status as judged by a lower plasma troponin concentration. This also highlights the fact that association studies cannot distinguish between cause and consequence and can be influenced by phenomena such as reverse causation (i.e., a failing

Table 4. Prognostic performance of the plasma troponin concentration in predicting death during follow-up.

	AUC (c-index)	cut-off, pg/ml	Youden index	sensitivity, %	specificity, %	positive predictive value, %	negative predictive value, %
troponin T	0.684	38	0.32	91	41	26	95
troponin I	0.665	21	0.32	61	70	16	77

heart that leads to increased plasma troponin concentrations and low shunt flow).

In studies comparing troponin T to troponin I, ESRD patients were 2–3 times more likely to have elevated concentrations of troponin T than troponin I [34,35]. In this study, TnT was elevated in nearly all of the patients (95%) compared to TnI (14%). This is similar to the findings of Jacobs et al., who found elevations of TnT measured with the high sensitive Roche assay in all of the patients studied whereas TnI measured using a conventional assay was elevated in only 28% of the cases [21]. Using a sensitive troponin I assay and a cut-off point of 35 pg/ml, this proportion was increased to 37% [23]. This difference can be partially explained with our data, which showed a slight accumulation of troponin T during the course of ESRD in that residual diuresis and the length of time on dialysis were independent predictors of the plasma concentration of only TnT, but not TnI. The finding that plasma troponin I concentrations were not influenced by residual renal clearance is in agreement with a study in ESRD patients that showed no differences in the clearance of troponin I after an acute MI [36].

However, there should be caution when interpreting high troponin T values as mere accumulation [5,37]. Elevated troponin T and troponin I concentrations are both strong predictors of mortality. Accumulation of troponin T can only occur following release after myocyte damage and should be regarded as a pathologic finding in any ESRD patients. Furthermore, accumulation can only occur when residual renal function declines, which is a strong predictor of survival in hemodialysis patients [38]. Therefore, plasma troponin T concentrations provide information about cardiac release and dialysis heritage, which might explain the improved prognostic value of troponin T compared to troponin I, as seen in our study or in the study of Jacobs et al. [18,20].

A more meaningful cut-off point than the 99th percentile would be levels that are linked to an increased mortality risk. We found that a plasma troponin T concentration above 38 pg/mL which is roughly three-times the 99th percentile was associated with a 5-fold risk of death during 2 years of follow-up. In contrast, we could not find a clear cut-off for troponin I as the association with death was more gradual. So far, only one study reported the association of hs TnT with mortality and found reduced survival rates at levels above 24.15 pg/ml [22]. In our study, both troponins were not independent predictors of death such as age or systolic LV function and did not add prognostic information. However, they can be used as alternative markers to identify patients at risk when echocardiography or other cardiac workup is not available. Additional studies are needed to clarify the diagnostic value of sensitive TnT and sensitive TnI in terms of mortality and risk stratification in ESRD patients.

On average, patients in this cohort had a TnT value that was 3.5-fold greater than the 99th percentile. Given these elevated baseline values, acute MI can only be diagnosed or ruled out when one or more subsequent samples show a significant rise or fall. Sensitive troponin I offers advantages in this respect, as the plasma concentration of a minority of the patients (14%) was above the 99th percentile.

The study is limited by the paucity of cardiac parameters that were collected, which might have contributed to an unexplained variability of roughly 70% and 50% in plasma troponin I and troponin T concentrations during multivariate modeling. Survival analyses might be limited by the low mortality during the follow-up period. This study focused on nephrological parameters that are commonly available and accessible during hemodialysis treatment, such residual diuresis or shunt flow. Systolic left ventricular function served as a surrogate for cardiac status and showed a high correlation to the plasma troponin concentration. Other cardiac morbidities, such as valvular disease or atrial fibrillation were also contributors of the plasma troponin concentration. Again it should be emphasized that association studies cannot prove causality between the studied parameters and elevated troponin concentrations and cannot distinguish between cause and consequence.

In summary, elevations of plasma troponin concentrations in hemodialysis patients measured with sensitive assays are influenced by cardiac function and dialysis-related parameters. Both are strong predictors of mortality in the short-term and are useful markers to identify patients at risk, however, troponin T is more retained during ESRD compared to troponin I.

Acknowledgments

We thank Andrea Janessa, Claudia Stelzig, Boris Huegle, MD & M.Sc. and Aline Naumann for their valuable assistance during the study.

Author Contributions

Conceived and designed the experiments: FA BF. Analyzed the data: HUH TB RT CT PW. Contributed reagents/materials/analysis tools: AP. Wrote the paper: FA BF CM.

References

1. Wu AH, Ford L (1999) Release of cardiac troponin in acute coronary syndromes: ischemia or necrosis? Clin Chim Acta 284: 161–174.
2. Thygesen K, Alpert JS, White HD (2007) Universal definition of myocardial infarction. Eur Heart J 28: 2525–2538.
3. Freda BJ, Tang WH, Van Lente F, Peacock WF, Francis GS (2002) Cardiac troponins in renal insufficiency: review and clinical implications. J Am Coll Cardiol 40: 2065–2071.
4. Artunc F, Haap M, Heyne N, Weyrich P, Wolf S (2010) [Interpretation of elevated serum troponin levels in end stage renal disease – case 2/2010]. Dtsch Med Wochenschr 135: 240.
5. Katus HA, Haller C, Muller-Bardorff M, Scheffold T, Remppis A (1995) Cardiac troponin T in end-stage renal disease patients undergoing chronic maintenance hemodialysis. Clin Chem 41: 1201–1203.
6. Porter GA, Norton T, Bennett WB (1998) Troponin T, a predictor of death in chronic haemodialysis patients. Eur Heart J 19 Suppl N: N34–N37.
7. Stolear JC, Georges B, Shita A, Verbeelen D (1999) The predictive value of cardiac troponin T measurements in subjects on regular haemodialysis. Nephrol Dial Transplant 14: 1961–1967.
8. Dierkes J, Domrose U, Westphal S, Ambrosch A, Bosselmann HP, et al. (2000) Cardiac troponin T predicts mortality in patients with end-stage renal disease. Circulation 102: 1964–1969.
9. Apple FS, Murakami MM, Pearce LA, Herzog CA (2002) Predictive value of cardiac troponin I and T for subsequent death in end-stage renal disease. Circulation 106: 2941–2945.
10. Mallamaci F, Zoccali C, Parlongo S, Tripepi G, Benedetto FA, et al. (2002) Troponin is related to left ventricular mass and predicts all-cause and cardiovascular mortality in hemodialysis patients. Am J Kidney Dis 40: 68–75.
11. Khan NA, Hemmelgarn BR, Tonelli M, Thompson CR, Levin A (2005) Prognostic value of troponin T and I among asymptomatic patients with end-stage renal disease: a meta-analysis. Circulation 112: 3088–3096.
12. Wang AY, Lai KN (2008) Use of cardiac biomarkers in end-stage renal disease. J Am Soc Nephrol 19: 1643–1652.
13. Diris JH, Hackeng CM, Kooman JP, Pinto YM, Hermens WT, et al. (2004) Impaired renal clearance explains elevated troponin T fragments in hemodialysis patients. Circulation 109: 23–25.
14. Bodor GS, Survant L, Voss EM, Smith S, Porterfield D, et al. (1997) Cardiac troponin T composition in normal and regenerating human skeletal muscle. Clin Chem 43: 476–484.
15. Zumrutdal A, Bakinen O, Ucan H, Atalay HV, Bodur H (2000) Relationship between uremic myopathy and false-positive cardiac troponin T test. Nephron 86: 522–523.
16. London GM (2002) Left ventricular alterations and end-stage renal disease. Nephrol Dial Transplant 17 Suppl 1: 29–36.

17. Breidthardt T, McIntyre CW (2011) Dialysis-induced myocardial stunning: the other side of the cardiorenal syndrome. Rev Cardiovasc Med 12: 13–20.
18. Apple FS (2009) A new season for cardiac troponin assays: it's time to keep a scorecard. Clin Chem 55: 1303–1306.
19. Reichlin T, Hochholzer W, Bassetti S, Steuer S, Stelzig C, et al. (2009) Early diagnosis of myocardial infarction with sensitive cardiac troponin assays. N Engl J Med 361: 858–867.
20. Keller T, Munzel T, Blankenberg S (2011) Making it more sensitive: the new era of troponin use. Circulation 123: 1361–1363.
21. Jacobs LH, van de KJ, Mingels AM, Kleijnen VW, van der Sande FM, et al. (2009) Haemodialysis patients longitudinally assessed by highly sensitive cardiac troponin T and commercial cardiac troponin T and cardiac troponin I assays. Ann Clin Biochem 46: 283–290.
22. McGill D, Talaulikar G, Potter JM, Koerbin G, Hickman PE (2010) Over time, high-sensitivity TnT replaces NT-proBNP as the most powerful predictor of death in patients with dialysis-dependent chronic renal failure. Clin Chim Acta 411: 936–939.
23. Kumar N, Michelis MF, DeVita MV, Panagopoulos G, Rosenstock JL (2011) Troponin I levels in asymptomatic patients on haemodialysis using a high-sensitivity assay. Nephrol Dial Transplant 26: 665–670.
24. van der Wal WM, Noordzij M, Dekker FW, Boeschoten EW, Krediet RT, et al. (2011) Full loss of residual renal function causes higher mortality in dialysis patients; findings from a marginal structural model. Nephrol Dial Transplant.
25. Kalantar-Zadeh K, Regidor DL, Kovesdy CP, Van Wyck D, Bunnapradist S, et al. (2009) Fluid retention is associated with cardiovascular mortality in patients undergoing long-term hemodialysis. Circulation 119: 671–679.
26. Evrin PE, Wibell L (1972) The serum levels and urinary excretion of 2 -microglobulin in apparently healthy subjects. Scand J Clin Lab Invest 29: 69–74.
27. Peacock WF, De Marco T, Fonarow GC, Diercks D, Wynne J, et al. (2008) Cardiac troponin and outcome in acute heart failure. N Engl J Med 358: 2117–2126.
28. Horwich TB, Patel J, MacLellan WR, Fonarow GC (2003) Cardiac troponin I is associated with impaired hemodynamics, progressive left ventricular dysfunction, and increased mortality rates in advanced heart failure. Circulation 108: 833–838.
29. Fernandez-Reyes MJ, Mon C, Heras M, Guevara P, Garcia MC, et al. (2004) Predictive value of troponin T levels for ischemic heart disease and mortality in patients on hemodialysis. J Nephrol 17: 721–727.
30. deFilippi C, Wasserman S, Rosanio S, Tiblier E, Sperger H, et al. (2003) Cardiac troponin T and C-reactive protein for predicting prognosis, coronary atherosclerosis, and cardiomyopathy in patients undergoing long-term hemodialysis. JAMA 290: 353–359.
31. Hayashi T, Obi Y, Kimura T, Iio K, Sumitsuji S, et al. (2008) Cardiac troponin T predicts occult coronary artery stenosis in patients with chronic kidney disease at the start of renal replacement therapy. Nephrol Dial Transplant 23: 2936–2942.
32. Jung HH, Ma KR, Han H (2004) Elevated concentrations of cardiac troponins are associated with severe coronary artery calcification in asymptomatic haemodialysis patients. Nephrol Dial Transplant 19: 3117–3123.
33. Mallamaci F, Zoccali C, Parlongo S, Tripepi G, Benedetto FA, et al. (2002) Diagnostic value of troponin T for alterations in left ventricular mass and function in dialysis patients. Kidney Int 62: 1884–1890.
34. Kanderian AS, Francis GS (2006) Cardiac troponins and chronic kidney disease. Kidney Int 69: 1112–1114.
35. Hickman PE, Koerbin G, Southcott E, Tate J, Dimeski G, et al. (2007) Newer cardiac troponin I assays have similar performance to troponin T in patients with end-stage renal disease. Ann Clin Biochem 44: 285–289.
36. Ellis K, Dreisbach AW, Lertora JL (2001) Plasma elimination of cardiac troponin I in end-stage renal disease. South Med J 94: 993–996.
37. Giannitsis E, Katus HA (2004) Troponin T release in hemodialysis patients. Circulation 110: e25–e26.
38. Termorshuizen F, Dekker FW, van Manen JG, Korevaar JC, Boeschoten EW, et al. (2004) Relative contribution of residual renal function and different measures of adequacy to survival in hemodialysis patients: an analysis of the Netherlands Cooperative Study on the Adequacy of Dialysis (NECOSAD)-2. J Am Soc Nephrol 15: 1061–1070.

7

Endotoxaemia in Haemodialysis: A Novel Factor in Erythropoetin Resistance?

Laura E. A. Harrison[1], James O. Burton[1], Cheuk-Chun Szeto[2], Philip K. T. Li[2], Christopher W. McIntyre[1,3]*

1 Department of Renal Medicine, Royal Derby Hospital, Derby, United Kingdom, **2** Department of Medicine and Therapeutics, Chinese University of Hong Kong, Hong Kong, China, **3** School of Graduate Entry Medicine and Health, University of Nottingham, Derby, United Kingdom

Abstract

Background/Objectives: Translocated endotoxin derived from intestinal bacteria is a driver of systemic inflammation and oxidative stress. Severe endotoxaemia is an underappreciated, but characteristic finding in haemodialysis (HD) patients, and appears to be driven by acute repetitive dialysis induced circulatory stress. Resistance to erythropoietin (EPO) has been identified as a predictor of mortality risk, and associated with inflammation and malnutrition. This study aims to explore the potential link between previously unrecognised endotoxaemia and EPO Resistance Index (ERI) in HD patients.

Methodology/Principal Findings: 50 established HD patients were studied at a routine dialysis session. Data collection included weight, BMI, ultrafiltration volume, weekly EPO dose, and blood sampling pre and post HD. ERI was calculated as ratio of total weekly EPO dose to body weight (U/kg) to haemoglobin level (g/dL). Mean haemoglobin (Hb) was 11.3±1.3 g/dL with a median EPO dose of 10,000 [IQR 7,500–20,000] u/wk and ERI of 13.7 [IQR 6.9–23.3] ((U/Kg)/(g/dL)). Mean pre-HD serum ET levels were significantly elevated at 0.69±0.30 EU/ml. Natural logarithm (Ln) of ERI correlated to predialysis ET levels ($r = 0.324$, $p = 0.03$) with a trend towards association with hsCRP ($r = 0.280$, $p = 0.07$). Ln ERI correlated with ultrafiltration volume, a driver of circulatory stress ($r = 0.295$, $p = 0.046$), previously identified to be associated with increased intradialytic endotoxin translocation. Both serum ET and ultrafiltration volume corrected for body weight were independently associated with Ln ERI in multivariable analysis.

Conclusions: This study suggests that endotoxaemia is a significant factor in setting levels of EPO requirement. It raises the possibility that elevated EPO doses may in part merely be identifying patients subjected to significant circulatory stress and suffering the myriad of negative biological consequences arising from sustained systemic exposure to endotoxin.

Editor: Martin Gerbert Frasch, Université de Montréal, Canada

Funding: No external funding was received for this study.

Competing Interests: The authors have declared that no competing interests exist.

* E-mail: chris.mcintyre@nottingham.ac.uk

Introduction

Anaemia commonly occurs in patients with chronic kidney disease (CKD), as a result of insufficient production of erythropoietin (EPO) by the kidneys. Effective treatment of anaemia has been possible since the introduction of recombinant Human Erythropoetin therapy in 1986 [1].

Initial observational studies of EPO in CKD suggested a reduced risk of mortality with increasing haemoglobin levels, associated with improved quality of life [2,3,4]. However, several clinical trials in recent years have raised significant concerns regarding the optimum haemoglobin targets and erythropoietin stimulating agent (ESA) doses [5,6,7]. The randomised trials of Normal Haematocrit Cardiac Trial [8] and TREAT, comparing lower to higher haemoglobin (Hb) targets on composite endpoints, have demonstrated an increased risk of cardiovascular (CV) events. These include stroke and vascular access thrombosis and a potential increased risk of death and provide no clear signal concerning improved patient quality of life.

There remains controversy over whether the poorer outcomes are due to higher absolute levels of haemoglobin or elevated EPO dose, particularly in those patients who fail to achieve target haemoglobin [9]. Patients who do not achieve Hb targets despite elevated doses of EPO, or who require higher doses to maintain their Hb are considered to be Erythropoietin Resistant or Hyporesponsive [10,11].

Resistance to EPO, previously identified as a predictor of mortality risk [12], is widespread. Iron deficiency is recognised as a significant factor affecting ESA response, and is usually treated alongside erythropoietin replacement as part of co-ordinated anaemia management in the CKD population. Other important factors modulating the individual's response and potentially increasing ESA resistance include infection, hyperparathyroidism, inadequate dialysis, malnutrition and chronic inflammation [13,14].

Despite attempts to identify and treat known risk factors, ESA resistance cannot always be explained, suggesting that there may be alternative causes driving the condition. The drivers of systemic inflammation are often obscure. In order to more fully understand the complex relationship between EPO dose, Hb, clinical condition and the dialysis process itself, we identified circulating endotoxin as a potential factor influencing EPO response.

Endotoxin (without sepsis) was initially proposed as a stimulus for immune activation in the pro-inflammatory state of congestive heart failure (CHF) [15]. Endotoxin is released by bacterial cell wall breakdown, within and beyond the gut lumen, from effective host defence mechanisms and by autolysis. Endotoxin enters the circulation via bacterial translocation, passage of intact bacteria and macro-molecules such as endotoxin across the intestinal barrier [16].

Exposure to endotoxin, a profoundly pro-inflammatory stimulus, results in release of a wide variety of pro-inflammatory cytokines, and has been implicated in a broad range of other pathophysiological responses, including oxidative stress, endothelial dysfunction and impaired circulatory autoregulation [17,18]. We have recently reported significant incremental endotoxaemia with worsening renal function across the range of CKD, with levels roughly tripling after initiation of dialysis [19]. In HD patients the severity of endotoxaemia was associated with both the drivers (ultrafiltration volume and rate) and the consequences (dialysis induced myocardial injury) of dialysis induced circulatory stress.

We hypothesised that there was a potential link between endotoxaemia and EPO resistance in HD patients, and aimed to describe the relative contribution of circulating endotoxin levels to EPO resistance in HD patients.

Methods

Objectives

This study aims to explore the potential link between previously unrecognised endotoxaemia and EPO resistance in HD patients.

Ethics Statement

Ethical approval for the study was granted by Derbyshire Local Research Ethics Committee. Written informed consent was received from all participants.

Participants

Fifty prevalent HD patients were recruited from a single hospital-based haemodialysis unit. All patients were haemodialysed thrice weekly via native arterio-venous fistulae. Exclusion criteria comprised; change in target weight in the preceding six weeks, clinical evidence of blood loss, active infection or malignancy, bone marrow disease or haemoglobinopathy, or pre-existing severe LV systolic dysfunction (NYHA IV).

Methodology: Description of Procedures or Investigations Undertaken

Haemodialysis details. Dialysis was performed using Hospal Integra monitors (Hospal, Mirandola, Italy). Dialysate fluid contained sodium, 138 mmol/L; potassium, 1 mmol/L; calcium 1.25 mmol/L; magnesium, 0.5 mmol/L; bicarbonate, 32 mmol/L; glucose, 5.6 mmol/L; and acetate, 3 mmol/L. Dual pass water treatment was used with undetectable levels of endotoxin throughout study duration.

All studies were conducted after a 2 day interdialytic period. Anticoagulation was with unfractionated heparin. Dialysate flow was 500 mL/min, and dialysate temperature was set at 37°C. Net fluid removal was set on an individual basis according to ideal dry weight. Patients were permitted to eat during HD if this was their usual preference.

Ultrafiltration rate. The rate of volume removal at dialysis, expressed in ml/h/kg BW, measured by the weight change per duration of HD treatment using the post HD weight as denominator.

Data collection. The following basic demographic information was obtained: age (years), sex, dialytic vintage (months), cardiovascular comorbidities, diabetes mellitus, body weight (BW; kg), body mass index (BMI; kg/m^2). The following factors were collected during the dialysis session: interdialytic weight gain (IDWG, kg), ultrafiltration volume (l), ultrafiltration rate (UFR: ml/h/kg body weight), pre-HD systolic and diastolic blood pressure, mean arterial blood pressure (MAP; mmHg), dialysis dose (Kt/V).

Erythropoietin dose. In order to normalize the amount of EPO required depending on the severity of anaemia, we calculated an EPO resistance (responsiveness) index (ERI), as described in previous studies [20], defined as the weekly EPO dose divided by Hb level (g/dl). Both the EPO dose and ERI were divided by target body weight to indicate the required EPO dose per kilogram of dry body weight.

Blood samples. All blood samples were taken before and after a dialysis session with rapid separation of serum and storage at −85°C before endotoxin measurement. Patients were not fasted prior to blood sampling. Haemoglobin (Hb), ferritin, reticulocytes, serum sodium, potassium, urea, creatinine, albumin, corrected calcium, albumin, and intact parathyroid hormone (PTH) were analyzed using standard autoanalyzer techniques (Roche diagnostics modular IIP®). Commercially available enzyme-linked immunosorbent assay (ELISA) kits (DRG instruments, Germany) were used to assess high-sensitivity C-reactive protein (hsCRP) and Interleukin-6 (IL-6), according to the manufacturer's protocol.

Circulating endotoxin level measurement. The method of lipopolysaccharide (LPS) quantification has been described previously [21]. Briefly, serum samples were diluted to 20% with endotoxin-free water and then heated to 70°C for 10 minutes to inactivate plasma proteins. Serum LPS was then quantified with a commercially available Limulus Amebocyte assay (Cambrex, Verviers, Belgium), according to the manufacturer's protocol. The detection limit of this assay was 0.01 EU/ml. Samples with LPS level below the detection limit were taken as 0.01 EU/ml. All samples were run in duplicate and background subtracted.

Statistical analysis. Results are presented as mean ± standard deviation (SD) or the median and interquartile range (IQR) unless otherwise stated. All data were tested for normality. Categorical data were compared using Chi-square test, continuous data using paired or unpaired Students t-test or one-way ANOVA with Tukey's correction as appropriate. Correlation between continuous variables was examined by Pearson's or Spearman's rank correlation coefficient. Factors associated with ERI/circulating endotoxin levels were further explored by a multivariable linear regression model. Analysis was performed using SPSS v16.0 (SPSS Inc, Chicago, IL). P value of less than 0.05 was considered significant. All probabilities were two-tailed.

Results

The patient characteristics and blood results are summarized in **Table 1**. Mean Hb was 11.3±1.3 g/dL with a median weekly EPO dose 169 IU/wk/kg [IQR 85–257]. EPO Resistance Index for the whole population was 13.7 IU/kg/wk/gm per dl [IQR 6.9–23.9]. Mean pre-HD serum endotoxin levels were appreciably elevated at 0.69±0.30 EU/ml, significantly higher than those of non-CKD patients (0.04±0.01 EU/ml, $p<0.001$) [22].

Predialysis endotoxin levels correlated to both EPO dose and natural logarithm (Ln) of ERI ($r=0.318$, $p=0.03$ and $r=0.324$, $p=0.03$ respectively). EPO dose and Ln ERI demonstrated a stronger relationship with ET than with traditional markers of inflammation, including high sensitivity C-Reactive Protein (hsCRP), Interleukin-6 (IL-6) and albumin. Endotoxin demonstrated a trend towards correlation with haemodynamic instability,

Table 1. Patient demographics, clinical characteristics and laboratory parameter results.

Parameter	Results
Age (yrs)	62.2±14.7
Gender (Male : Female)	36:14
Dialysis vintage (months; median [IQR])	38 [18,70]
Ethnicity (%)	
Caucasian	94
Asian	6
Cause of end-stage renal disease (%)	
Diabetic nephropathy	28
Glomerular disease	22
Adult polycystic kidney disease	12
Urological	10
Multiple myeloma	4
Tubulointerstitial nephritis	4
Unknown	10
Other	10
Diabetes Mellitus (%)	38
Cardiovascular Comorbidities (%)	42
EPO dose (IU/week)	10,000 [7,500–20,000]
ERI (IU/kg/wk/g/dl)	13.7 [6.9–23.9]
Weight (kg)	78.9±17
Body Mass Index (kg/m^2)	27±5.5
Kt/V $_{urea}$	1.3±0.2
Ultrafiltration volume (Litres)	1.97±0.76
Predialysis systolic BP (mmHg)	144±22
Predialysis diastolic BP (mmHg)	76±14
Haemoglobin (g/dl)	11.3±1.3 g
Haematocrit (%)	36±4
Ferritin (ug/L)	307 [213–454]
Phosphate (mmol/L)	1.45±0.39
Adjusted Calcium (mmol/L)	2.4±0.13
Albumin (g/L)	36±3.8
Parathyroid Hormone (ng/L)	240 [96–342]
hsCRP (mg/L)	1.32 [0.82–2.23]
IL-6 (pg/ml)	0.099 [0.086–0.115]

Data are mean±SD or median [IQR].
ERI, EPO Resistance Index, BP, Blood pressure; hsCRP, high sensitivity C Reactive Protein; IL-6, Interleukin 6.

assessed by maximum drop in systolic blood pressure over the HD treatment ($r = -0.270$, $p = 0.063$), as did ultrafiltration volume ($r = -0.270$, $p = 0.058$). Endotoxin levels were not significantly affected by the presence of diabetes mellitus ($p = 0.61$) or aspirin use ($p = 0.56$).

Ln ERI correlated significantly with ultrafiltration (UF) volume ($r = 0.332$, $p = 0.026$), a known driver of circulatory stress previously identified to be associated with increased intradialytic endotoxin translocation. Adjusting UF volume for body weight (L/kg), further strengthened this relationship ($r = 0.419$, $p = 0.004$). Ln ERI demonstrated a trend towards correlation with hsCRP ($r = 0.281$, $p = 0.075$) and inversely with BMI ($r = -0.259$, $p = 0.082$).

Ln ERI was not significantly affected by the presence of cardiovascular comorbidities ($p = 0.28$), diabetes mellitus ($p = 0.78$), or RAAS blockade ($p = 0.41$). EPO dose and Ln ERI did not demonstrate significant correlations with other parameters previously identified as linked to erythropoietin resistance, including ferritin, parathyroid hormone levels, ktV and serum albumin. This patient group were characterised by being well dialysed, iron replete with well controlled hyperparathyroidism. Univariable analysis is summarised in **Table 2**.

Multivariable analysis of factors contributing to EPO resistance revealed that serum endotoxin and ultrafiltration volume corrected for weight were independent variables associated with the natural logarithm of EPO resistance index in models adjusted for age, albumin, ferritin, PTH and Kt/V (see **Table 3**). In stepwise linear regression, the model predicting ln ERI comprised ultrafiltration volume corrected for body weight ($\beta = 0.472$, $p = 0.001$) and hsCRP ($\beta = 0.301$, $p = 0.033$) with a model fit of $R^2 = 0.297$ (Adjusted $R^2 = 0.260$).

Discussion

In this study, we demonstrated for the first time endotoxin as an independent determinant of EPO resistance. Significant endotoxaemia has been identified and described in the severe CKD and dialysis population [19,23] and these data confirm previous findings. Endotoxin levels seen in HD patients are extremely high, comparable with those reported in severe liver disease [24], post gut irradiation [25] and in severe decompensated congestive heart failure (CHF) [15]. Previous work in patients with acute heart failure showed ET to be systemically elevated, with higher levels in the hepatic vein compared to the left ventricle [26], identifying the gut as the source of ET. In CHF, bowel oedema and hypoperfusion have been identified as the two main factors influencing bowel wall permeability [27], and therefore ET translocation.

Factors involved in EPO resistance that can be modulated include iron deficiency, hyperparathyroidism, inadequate dialysis and malnutrition. Chronic inflammation, a common finding in CKD and dialysis patients, is strongly associated with EPO resistance [20]. Elevated circulating pro-inflammatory cytokines (PIC) including hsCRP, IL-6, and TNF-α demonstrate significant correlation with increasing levels of EPO hyporesponsiveness in

Table 2. Univariable associates of clinical and laboratory parameters with natural logarithm of EPO Resistance Index.

Parameter	R value	P value
Serum endotoxin (EU/ml)	0.311	0.04
Ultrafiltration volume (L)	0.332	0.026
UF volume/body weight (L/kg)	0.470	0.001
Age (years)	0.057	0.711
Body Mass Index (kg/m^2)	−0.259	0.082
Ferritin (ug/L)	0.08	0.6
Parathyroid Hormone (ng/L)	0.19	0.25
Kt/V$_{urea}$	−0.18	0.26
Albumin (g/L)	−0.70	0.67
hsCRP (mg/L)	0.280	0.07
IL-6 (ng/ml)	0.16	0.32

UF, ultrafiltration; hsCRP, high sensitivity C Reactive Protein; IL-6, Interleukin 6.

Table 3. Multivariable analysis model for natural logarithm of EPO Resistance Index (adjusted for age, albumin, ferritin, PTH and Kt/V).

	R^2	Adjusted R^2	Beta	SE	P value
UF volume/body weight (L/kg)	0.325	0.202	40.3	12.2	0.002
Serum endotoxin (EU/ml)	0.214	0.071	1.06	0.49	0.037

the dialysis population [20,28]. A variety of factors have been postulated as drivers of chronic inflammation in CKD, and endotoxin is a potential unifying feature of the interlinked malnutrition, inflammation and CV disease state in dialysis patients.

In this patient group, hsCRP demonstrated a trend towards correlation with ln ERI. This may be attributable to the narrow range of hsCRP values in this patient group, differences in immunoreactivity or insufficient patient numbers to achieve significance. Tachyphylactic response to endotoxin has been previously described, where further contact with, or incremental exposure to endotoxin can result in a diminishing physiological response. The use of native AV fistulae, ultrapure dialysis solution and absence of active intercurrent clinical events such as infection or vascular access issues will affect levels of inflammatory markers in the patient group. The complexities of the uraemic environment, dialysis related and patient specific factors will contribute towards variability in the individual's inflammatory response.

Exposure to ET results in release of a wide variety of PICs and binding via CD14 to systemic immune competent cells. Mechanisms of cytokine related anaemia include reduction of renal EPO production, inhibition of the proliferation and differentiation of erythroid progenitor cells in the bone marrow, impaired iron absorption and reduced iron delivery [29,30]. In animal models, induced endotoxaemia has been demonstrated to suppress ESA ability to stimulate erythropoiesis [31].

Endotoxin contamination of dialysis water has long been recognised as a cause of low grade inflammatory response and CV instability during dialysis [32]. Endotoxin exposure in sub-optimally prepared dialysis water has been linked to increased EPO resistance [33], whereas transition to ultrapure dialysate can reduce systemic inflammation and EPO dose requirements [34]. Circulating serum ET levels of 0.69 EU/ml in our patient group were greatly elevated, above even the maximum current permitted levels of endotoxin in dialysate fluid of 0.25 EU/ml. Dialysis water in this study had undetectable levels of endotoxin during the study period, following dual pass water treatment. Circulating ET in these patients therefore originates from an alternate source, namely the gastrointestinal tract.

HD itself appears to be responsible for increasing exposure to translocated intestinal endotoxin, as evidenced by a large difference between patients with very severe CKD stage 5, but not yet started on dialysis, and those receiving dialysis [19]. HD, in combination with ultrafiltration, results in significant systemic haemodynamic perturbation and clinically significant reduction of regional perfusion in critical organs such as the heart and brain [35]. HD is well described as being capable of inducing recurrent cardiac ischaemic injury, associated with long term myocardial damage and increased mortality [36]. Previous work has demonstrated significant correlation between endotoxin and severity of HD-induced cardiac stunning and relative hypotension [19].

Patients on long-term maintenance haemodialysis have evidence of mucosal ischaemia [37] and ultrafiltration causes a reduction in splanchnic blood volume [38] despite preserved blood pressure [39]. Mesenteric ischaemia results in disrupted gut mucosal structure and function, with increased gut permeability [40]. HD may result in recurrent regional hypoperfusion, particularly in the splanchnic vasculature. This can result in subclinical mesenteric ischaemia and injury, leading to altered membrane permeability and increased translocation of endotoxin.

Increasing ERI is associated with higher volumes of fluid removal during dialysis, and unsurprisingly this association increases when UF volume is corrected for body weight. Previous work has demonstrated significant correlation between endotoxaemia and dialysis induced haemodynamic stress, including severity of HD-induced cardiac stunning, markers of cardiac injury and relative hypotension [19]. Ultrafiltration volume is potentially a driver of both myocardial and splanchnic hypoperfusion, with end-organ injury resulting in system specific short-term injury and long-term damage, as well as a generalised inflammatory response.

Adding endotoxin into a simple linear regression model for ln ERI containing UF volume/weight and hsCRP strengthened the R^2 of the model (0.307), but both ET and hsCRP were no longer independent predictors within it. This is not unexpected, given the underlying pathophysiological processes linking these factors. The relationships between potential causes and consequences of endotoxaemia, may, in turn, influence EPO resistance. Multivariable analysis confirmed the independent association of serum endotoxin and of ultrafiltration volume corrected for weight with the natural logarithm of EPO resistance index, when adjusted for factors previously identified as influencing the response to EPO.

In terms of potential intervention, extended dialysis schedules are associated with marked reductions in UF requirements and intradialytic hypotension, lessening the haemodynamic insult [19], as well as improving Hb and lowering EPO requirements [41].

This study has potential limitations. Although this observational study was able to demonstrate a relationship between endotoxaemia and EPO resistance in HD patients, the sample size is inadequate to fully resolve factors relating to the degree of endotoxaemia or EPO hypo-responsiveness. Patients were not prevented from eating during HD, which could potentially influence gut perfusion and permeability, however the relatively high fibre and low fat meals provided are likely to have only limited impact on ET translocation. Areas of further work include longitudinal studies on ET, inflammatory response and EPO requirements, exploration of the effects of reduced endotoxin exposure on EPO requirements, and comparison of ET and ERI between different dialysis modalities.

Summary

This study suggests that endotoxaemia, either by direct interaction, or through its well documented effects on systemic inflammation, is a significant and potentially dominant factor in setting levels of EPO requirement. It raises the possibility that elevated EPO doses may in part merely be identifying patients subjected to significant haemodynamic perturbation, and suffering the myriad of negative biological consequences arising from sustained systemic exposure to endotoxin.

A greater understanding of the mechanism and factors influencing endotoxin translocation in the dialysis population is required. In addition, turning our attention to the dialysis procedure itself may yield additional benefits, both in terms of

EPO requirements, but also alleviating the haemodynamic impact of HD to improve long-term patient outcomes.

Acknowledgments

The authors gratefully acknowledge the time and commitment of patients and staff at Royal Derby Hospital.

Author Contributions

Conceived and designed the experiments: CWM JOB. Performed the experiments: JOB CCS PKT. Analyzed the data: LEAH JOB CCS PKT CWM. Contributed reagents/materials/analysis tools: LEAH JOB CCS PKL. Wrote the paper: LEAH JOB CCS PKL CWM.

References

1. Winearls CG, Oliver DO, Pippard MJ, Reid C, Downing MR, et al. (1986) Effect of human erythropoietin derived from recombinant DNA on the anaemia of patients maintained by chronic haemodialysis. Lancet 2: 1175–1178.
2. Ofsthun N, Labrecque J, Lacson E, Keen M, Lazarus JM (2003) The effects of higher hemoglobin levels on mortality and hospitalization in hemodialysis patients. Kidney Int 63: 1908–1914.
3. Macdougall IC, Tomson CR, Steenkamp M, Ansell D (2010) Relative risk of death in UK haemodialysis patients in relation to achieved haemoglobin from 1999 to 2005: an observational study using UK Renal Registry data incorporating 30,040 patient-years of follow-up. Nephrol Dial Transplant 25: 914–919.
4. Perlman RL, Finkelstein FO, Liu L, Roys E, Kiser M, et al. (2005) Quality of life in chronic kidney disease (CKD): a cross-sectional analysis in the Renal Research Institute-CKD study. Am J Kidney Dis 45: 658–666.
5. Pfeffer MA, Burdmann EA, Chen CY, Cooper ME, de Zeeuw D, et al. (2009) A trial of darbepoetin alfa in type 2 diabetes and chronic kidney disease. N Engl J Med 361: 2019–2032.
6. Singh AK, Szczech L, Tang KL, Barnhart H, Sapp S, et al. (2006) Correction of anemia with epoetin alfa in chronic kidney disease. N Engl J Med 355: 2085–2098.
7. Drueke TB, Locatelli F, Clyne N, Eckardt KU, Macdougall IC, et al. (2006) Normalization of hemoglobin level in patients with chronic kidney disease and anemia. N Engl J Med 355: 2071–2084.
8. Besarab A, Bolton WK, Browne JK, Egrie JC, Nissenson AR, et al. (1998) The effects of normal as compared with low hematocrit values in patients with cardiac disease who are receiving hemodialysis and epoetin. N Engl J Med 339: 584–590.
9. Badve SV, Hawley CM, Johnson DW (2011) Is the problem with the vehicle or the destination? Does high-dose ESA or high haemoglobin contribute to poor outcomes in CKD? Nephrology (Carlton) 16: 144–153.
10. Stivelman JC (1989) Resistance to recombinant human erythropoietin therapy: a real clinical entity? Semin Nephrol 9: 8–11.
11. Locatelli F, Aljama P, Barany P, Canaud B, Carrera F, et al. (2004) Revised European best practice guidelines for the management of anaemia in patients with chronic renal failure. Nephrol Dial Transplant 19 Suppl 2: ii1–47.
12. Regidor DL, Kopple JD, Kovesdy CP, Kilpatrick RD, McAllister CJ, et al. (2006) Associations between changes in hemoglobin and administered erythropoiesis-stimulating agent and survival in hemodialysis patients. J Am Soc Nephrol 17: 1181–1191.
13. Drueke T (2001) Hyporesponsiveness to recombinant human erythropoietin. Nephrol Dial Transplant 16 Suppl 7: 25–28.
14. Richardson D (2002) Clinical factors influencing sensitivity and response to epoetin. Nephrol Dial Transplant 17 Suppl 1: 53–59.
15. Anker SD, Egerer KR, Volk HD, Kox WJ, Poole-Wilson PA, et al. (1997) Elevated soluble CD14 receptors and altered cytokines in chronic heart failure. Am J Cardiol 79: 1426–1430.
16. Kotanko P, Carter M, Levin NW (2006) Intestinal bacterial microflora– a potential source of chronic inflammation in patients with chronic kidney disease. Nephrol Dial Transplant 21: 2057–2060.
17. Charalambous BM, Stephens RC, Feavers IM, Montgomery HE (2007) Role of bacterial endotoxin in chronic heart failure: the gut of the matter. Shock 28: 15–23.
18. Feng SY, Samarasinghe T, Phillips DJ, Alexiou T, Hollis JH, et al. (2010) Acute and chronic effects of endotoxin on cerebral circulation in lambs. Am J Physiol Regul Integr Comp Physiol 298: R760–766.
19. McIntyre CW, Harrison LE, Eldehni MT, Jefferies HJ, Szeto CC, et al. (2011) Circulating endotoxemia: a novel factor in systemic inflammation and cardiovascular disease in chronic kidney disease. Clin J Am Soc Nephrol 6: 133–141.
20. Gunnell J, Yeun JY, Depner TA, Kaysen GA (1999) Acute-phase response predicts erythropoietin resistance in hemodialysis and peritoneal dialysis patients. Am J Kidney Dis 33: 63–72.
21. Brenchley JM, Price DA, Schacker TW, Asher TE, Silvestri G, et al. (2006) Microbial translocation is a cause of systemic immune activation in chronic HIV infection. Nat Med 12: 1365–1371.
22. John SG, Owen PJ, Harrison LE, Szeto CC, Lai KB, et al. (2010) The impact of antihypertensive drug therapy on endotoxemia in elderly patients with chronic kidney disease. Clin J Am Soc Nephrol 6: 2389–2394.
23. Szeto CC, Kwan BC, Chow KM, Lai KB, Chung KY, et al. (2008) Endotoxemia is related to systemic inflammation and atherosclerosis in peritoneal dialysis patients. Clin J Am Soc Nephrol 3: 431–436.
24. Lumsden AB, Henderson JM, Kutner MH (1988) Endotoxin levels measured by a chromogenic assay in portal, hepatic and peripheral venous blood in patients with cirrhosis. Hepatology 8: 232–236.
25. Maxwell A, Gaffin SL, Wells MT (1986) Radiotherapy, endotoxaemia, and nausea. Lancet 1: 1148–1149.
26. Peschel T, Schonauer M, Thiele H, Anker SD, Schuler G, et al. (2003) Invasive assessment of bacterial endotoxin and inflammatory cytokines in patients with acute heart failure. Eur J Heart Fail 5: 609–614.
27. Krack A, Sharma R, Figulla HR, Anker SD (2005) The importance of the gastrointestinal system in the pathogenesis of heart failure. Eur Heart J 26: 2368–2374.
28. Kalantar-Zadeh K, McAllister CJ, Lehn RS, Lee GH, Nissenson AR, et al. (2003) Effect of malnutrition-inflammation complex syndrome on EPO hyporesponsiveness in maintenance hemodialysis patients. Am J Kidney Dis 42: 761–773.
29. Carrero JJ, Stenvinkel P (2010) Inflammation in end-stage renal disease–what have we learned in 10 years? Semin Dial 23: 498–509.
30. Weiss G, Goodnough LT (2005) Anemia of chronic disease. N Engl J Med 352: 1011–1023.
31. Brendt P, Horwat A, Schafer ST, Dreyer SC, Gothert J, et al. (2009) Lipopolysaccharide evokes resistance to erythropoiesis induced by the long-acting erythropoietin analogue darbepoetin alfa in rats. Anesth Analg 109: 705–711.
32. Raij L, Shapiro FL, Michael AF (1973) Endotoxemia in febrile reactions during hemodialysis. Kidney Int 4: 57–60.
33. Molina M, Navarro MJ, Palacios ME, de Gracia MC, Garcia Hernandez MA, et al. (2007) [Importance of ultrapure dialysis liquid in response to the treatment of renal anaemia with darbepoetin in patients receiving haemodialysis]. Nefrologia 27: 196–201.
34. Go AS, Chertow GM, Fan D, McCulloch CE, Hsu CY (2004) Chronic kidney disease and the risks of death, cardiovascular events, and hospitalization. N Engl J Med 351: 1296–1305.
35. McIntyre CW, Burton JO, Selby NM, Leccisotti L, Korsheed S, et al. (2008) Hemodialysis-induced cardiac dysfunction is associated with an acute reduction in global and segmental myocardial blood flow. Clin J Am Soc Nephrol 3: 19–26.
36. Burton JO, Jefferies HJ, Selby NM, McIntyre CW (2009) Hemodialysis-induced cardiac injury: determinants and associated outcomes. Clin J Am Soc Nephrol 4: 914–920.
37. Diebel L, Kozol R, Wilson RF, Mahajan S, Abu-Hamdan D, et al. (1993) Gastric intramucosal acidosis in patients with chronic kidney failure. Surgery 113: 520–526.
38. Mann JF, Gerstein HC, Pogue J, Bosch J, Yusuf S (2001) Renal insufficiency as a predictor of cardiovascular outcomes and the impact of ramipril: the HOPE randomized trial. Ann Intern Med 134: 629–636.
39. Jakob SM, Ruokonen E, Vuolteenaho O, Lampainen E, Takala J (2001) Splanchnic perfusion during hemodialysis: evidence for marginal tissue perfusion. Crit Care Med 29: 1393–1398.
40. Khanna A, Rossman JE, Fung HL, Caty MG (2001) Intestinal and hemodynamic impairment following mesenteric ischemia/reperfusion. J Surg Res 99: 114–119.
41. Chan CT, Floras JS, Miller JA, Richardson RM, Pierratos A (2002) Regression of left ventricular hypertrophy after conversion to nocturnal hemodialysis. Kidney Int 61: 2235–2239.

8

Intravenous Ferric Chloride Hexahydrate Supplementation Induced Endothelial Dysfunction and Increased Cardiovascular Risk among Hemodialysis Patients

Ko-Lin Kuo[1,4,5], Szu-Chun Hung[4,5], Yao-Ping Lin[7], Ching-Fang Tang[7], Tzong-Shyuan Lee[1], Chih-Pei Lin[3,6]*, Der-Cherng Tarng[1,2,7]*

1 Department and Institute of Physiology, National Yang-Ming University, Taipei, Taiwan, **2** Institute of Clinical Medicine, National Yang-Ming University, Taipei, Taiwan, **3** Department of Biotechnology and Laboratory Science in Medicine and Institute of Biotechnology in Medicine, National Yang-Ming University, Taipei, Taiwan, **4** School of Medicine, Tzu Chi University, Hualien, Taiwan, **5** Division of Nephrology, Buddhist Tzu Chi General Hospital, Taipei Branch, Taipei, Taiwan, **6** Division of General Laboratory, Department of Pathology and Laboratory Medicine, Taipei Veterans General Hospital, Taipei, Taiwan, **7** Division of Nephrology, Department of Medicine and Immunology Centre, Taipei Veterans General Hospital, Taipei, Taiwan

Abstract

Background: The association between intravenous (IV) iron administration and outcomes in hemodialysis (HD) patients is still debated. Therefore, this study was aimed to assess the relationship between the IV administration of ferric chloride hexahydrate (Atofen®) and cardiovascular (CV) outcome and the interaction between iron-induced oxidative stress and endothelial dysfunction in chronic HD patients.

Methodology/Principal Findings: A cohort of 1239 chronic HD patients was recruited. In a follow-up of 12 months, Kaplan-Meier survival curves showed that higher doses of IV Atofen associated with higher risks for CV events and deaths in HD patients. In multivariate Cox models, compared to no iron supplementation, IV Atofen administration was an independent predictor for CV events and overall mortality. However, the nature of the observational cohort study possibly bears selection bias. We further found that IV Atofen enhanced the superoxide production of mononuclear cells (MNCs), the levels of circulating soluble adhesion molecules, and the adhesion of MNCs to human aortic endothelial cells (HAECs). *In vitro* experiments showed that Atofen increased the expression of intracellular cell adhesion molecule-1 and vascular cell adhesion molecule-1 in HAECs and aggravated the endothelial adhesiveness in a dose-dependent manner. These iron-induced changes were significantly attenuated by the co-treatment of HAECs with N-acetylcysteine and inhibitors of NADPH oxidase, nuclear factor κB, and activator protein-1.

Conclusion: A cumulative dose of IV Atofen >800 mg within 6 months was associated with an adverse CV outcome and a higher mortality among chronic HD patients. The detrimental effects of IV iron supplementation were partly due to the increased oxidative stress and induction of MNC adhesion to endothelial cells, a pivotal index of early atherogenesis.

Editor: Thomas Thum, Integrated Research Centre, Germany

Funding: This work was supported by grants from the National Science Council (NSC 96-2628-B-010-001-MY3 and NSC 99-2314-B-303-002-MY3), Taipei Veterans General Hospital (V100C-143 and V100E4-003), Ministry of Education's Aim for the Top University Plan, and Taipei Tzu Chi General Hospital (TCRD-TPE-97-15). The funders had no role in study design, data collection and analysis, decision to publish, or preparation of the manuscript.

Competing Interests: The authors have declared that no competing interests exist.

* E-mail: cplin@vghtpe.gov.tw (C-PL); dctarng@vghtpe.gov.tw (D-CT)

Introduction

Anemia is associated with cardiovascular (CV) and global outcomes in patients with chronic kidney disease (CKD) [1]. The correction of anemia requires erythropoiesis-stimulating agents (ESAs) in most instances. The potential role of intravenous (IV) iron therapy in enhancing the efficacy of ESAs in CKD patients has received increasing attention in recent years [2]. IV iron therapy is valuable because it helps to reduce ESA requirements, allows dialysis patients to achieve increased hemoglobin levels, and increases the cost-effectiveness of ESA treatment [3,4]. However, iron is a transition metal and potent pro-oxidant that is capable of redox cycling. Acute high IV iron dose administration may provoke the generation of bioactive iron (non-transferrin-binding iron), subsequently elevate reactive oxygen species (ROS) in plasma and reduce the forearm flow-mediated dilatation in healthy individuals [5]. Drueke *et al.* [6] disclosed an interrelation of the annual IV iron dose administered with the common carotid artery intima-media thickness and with the generation of advanced oxidation products from proteins in hemodialysis (HD) patients. It is speculated that the chronic cumulative administration of IV iron might exaggerate oxidative stress and potentially increase the CV risk in CKD patients.

Table 1. Baseline characteristics of hemodialysis patients after receiving 6-month of IV administration of ferric chloride hexahydrate or not.

Parameters	Non-IV Iron group (n = 583)	IV Iron group (n = 656)	*P* value
Age, years	58±14	59±14	0.078[a]
Male sex, n (%)	271 (46)	308 (47)	0.830[b]
Diabetes mellitus, n (%)	167 (29)	165 (25)	0.176[b]
Hypertension, n (%)	244 (42)	256 (39)	0.332[b]
Prior cardiovascular disease, n (%)	87 (15)	93 (14)	0.667[b]
Causes for chronic renal failure			
Glomerulonephritis, n (%)	280 (48)	302 (46)	0.636[b]
Interstitial nephritis, n (%)	47 (8)	66 (10)	0.361[b]
Diabetic nephropathy, n (%)	157 (27)	164 (25)	0.511[b]
Nephrosclerosis, n (%)	41 (7)	39 (6)	0.336[b]
Others, n (%)	58 (10)	85 (13)	0.419[b]
Statin, n (%)	98 (17)	123 (19)	0.473[b]
ACEI and/or ARB, n (%)	232 (40)	250 (38)	0.744[b]
Other antihypertensives, n (%)	167 (27)	183 (28)	0.608[b]
Hemodialysis vintage, months	56±44	60±50	0.134[a]
Albumin, g/dL	4.0±0.4	4.0±0.40	0.189[a]
Total cholesterol, mg/dL	182±48	182±44	0.888[a]
Triglyceride, mg/dL	171±131	163±117	0.259[a]
Fasting glucose, mg/dL	139±74	131±68	0.063[a]
C-reactive protein, mg/L	5.21 [0.40, 9.82]	4.8 [0.30, 9.65]	0.103[c]
Hemoglobin, g/dL	10.4±1.5	10.2±1.7	0.062[a]
Erythropoietin dose, U/kg/week	70.3±41.1	70.6±34.9	0.888[a]
IV Iron dose, mg/6months	0 [0, 0]	320 [160, 1000]	
0 mg, n (%)	583 (100)	0 (0)	
40 to 800 mg, n (%)		451 (67)	
840 to 1600 mg, n (%)		111 (20)	
1640 to 2400 mg, n (%)		94 (13)	

Abbreviations: ACEI, angiotensin converting enzyme inhibitor; ARB, angiotensin II receptor blockade; IV, intravenous; nPCR, normalized protein catabolic rate; PTH, parathyroid hormone.
Other antihypertensives consisted of calcium channel blockers, β blockers, α blockers and diuretics.
Values of C-reactive protein, and IV iron dose are reported as medians with interquartile ranges; other continuous variables are reported as means ± SD.
Comparisons between two groups by [a]Student's t test;
[b]Person's chi-square test, and [c]Mann-Whitney U test.

So far, there is no definitive safe upper limit of the cumulative dose of IV iron. Three observational studies in large study cohorts did not provide definitive conclusions. Feldman *et al.* first showed a significantly increased mortality in 5833 HD patients receiving an IV iron dose >1000 mg over a 6-month period [7]. In contrast, in a different cohort of 32,566 HD patients, Feldman *et al.* failed to identify a statistically significant association between iron administration and mortality [8]. Kalantar-Zadeh *et al.* analyzed data from a cohort of 58,038 HD patients and found, after appropriate adjustments, that patients receiving a monthly IV iron dose >400 mg had significantly increased global and CV deaths compared with those who received no IV iron [9]. Accordingly, the adverse effects of iron supplementation on CV outcomes in CKD patients remain a matter of debate. Today, evidence from experimental studies to support the toxicity of iron to cells or tissues is still fragmentary and contradictory.

In the early stage of atherosclerosis, adhesion molecules, such as vascular cell adhesion molecule-1 (VCAM-1), intracellular cell adhesion molecule-1 (ICAM-1), and endothelial cell selectin (E-selectin), are expressed on the endothelial cell surface to facilitate the adhesion of circulating mononuclear cells (MNCs) to endothelial cells and their subsequent migration to the subendothelial space. ROS serve as common intracellular messengers for the redox-sensitive pathways and induce the expression of adhesion molecules in vascular endothelial cells [10,11]. Iron provokes ROS production *in vivo* [6,12]. Therefore, it seems rational to postulate that IV iron can promote early atherogenesis by increasing the expression of adhesion molecules and the adhesion of MNCs to endothelial cells. This speculation deserves further clinical studies as well as *in vitro* experiments.

Therefore, first, we conducted a prospective observational study to validate the association of the cumulative 6-month dose of IV ferric chloride hexahydrate (Atofen®; Uji pharmaceutical Co. Ltd., Japan) with CV events or overall mortality among 1239 patients receiving chronic HD in a follow-up period of 12 months. Second, another HD cohort was recruited to assess the *in vivo* pro-oxidant effects of IV Atofen by measuring the intracellular production of ROS in circulating MNCs and soluble adhesion molecule levels in

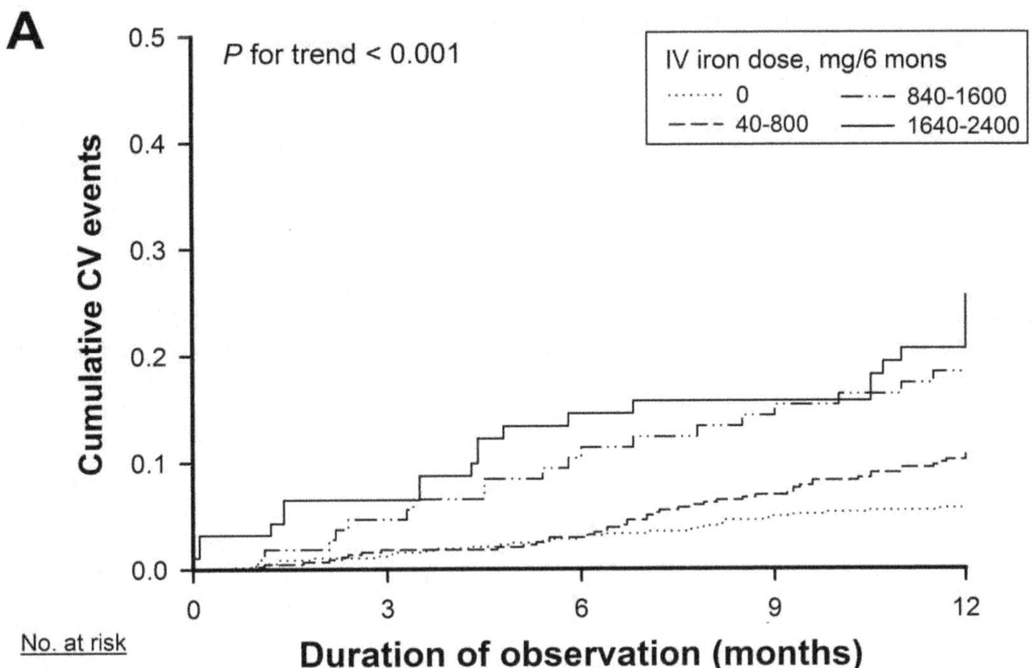

No. at risk

IV iron dose, mg/6 mons					
0	583	566	549	533	517
40-800	451	431	421	396	376
840-1600	111	102	91	85	78
1640-2400	94	84	73	70	60

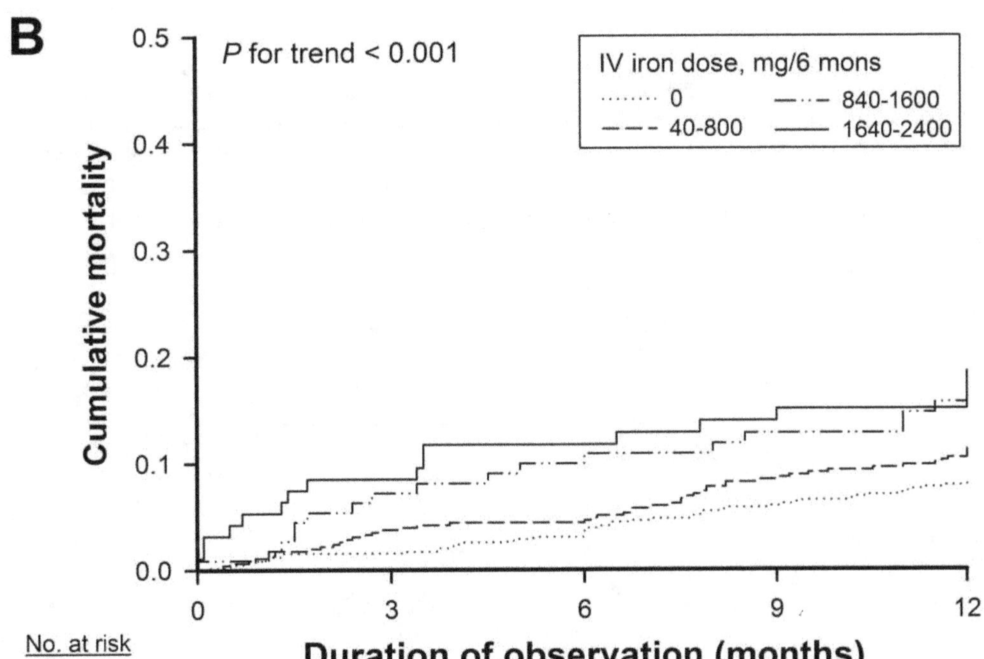

No. at risk

IV iron dose, mg/6 mons					
0	583	574	559	547	531
40-800	451	433	428	409	397
840-1600	111	103	96	92	87
1640-2400	94	86	80	75	70

Figure 1. IV iron was associated with CV events and overall mortality. Kaplan-Meier curves demonstrated cumulative CV events (A) and overall mortality (B) among 1239 hemodialysis patients. All patients were stratified into 4 groups according to the cumulative dose of IV iron within the 6 months prior to the enrollment.

plasma, as well as the *ex vivo* cell adhesion between cultured human aortic endothelial cells (HAECs) and circulating MNCs following IV Atofen therapy. Finally, we carried out *in vitro* experiments to assess the effects of iron on early atherogenesis by examining the expression of ICAM-1 and VCAM-1 in HAECs treated with Atofen and the subsequent endothelial cell adhesiveness to circulating MNCs. Our study suggests a novel role of IV-administered Atofen in initiating atherosclerosis and affecting CV outcome in HD patients.

Materials and Methods

Patients and Study Protocol

This prospective cohort study was carried out at the dialysis facility of Excelsior Renal Service Co., Ltd., Taiwan, to assess the safety of IV Atofen iron supplementation in terms of CV outcome and all-cause mortality among chronic HD patients. The study subjects were recruited between January 1 and June 30, 2004. Initially, 1911 patients undergoing chronic HD were screened, and 1687 clinically stable patients older than 20 years of age with a HD vintage of more than 6 months before the study and with a life expectancy of more than 6 months were included. The medical history of each patient was reviewed and confirmed by checking patient records; one physician (H. S.-C.) did this to minimize interobserver variations. The exclusion criteria were: dialysis for less than 12 h per week; inadequacy of dialysis, defined as a Kt/V urea <1.2; malignancy, infectious disease, sepsis, hepatobiliary disease, or hospitalization within 3 months before study; and those who were unable to give informed consent. Ultimately, our study population was comprised of 1239 patients (579 men and 660 women; mean age of 59±14 years). The baseline demographic, comorbidity, and laboratory measurements were recorded at enrollment. The study subjects were followed up from July 1, 2004 to June 30, 2005. All of the patients were subjected to a standard bicarbonate dialysis session. HD was performed three times weekly using single-use dialyzers with a membrane surface area of 1.6–1.7 m^2. Dialysis machines were sterilized daily, and water treatment circuits and tanks were sterilized weekly.

All patients were divided into two groups: with (n = 656) and without (n = 583) IV administration of Atofen 6 months prior to enrollment. Iron-treated patients were further stratified into 3 subgroups according to the cumulative 6-month iron dose: 40 to 800 mg (Group I, n = 451), 840 to 1600 mg (Group II, n = 111) and 1640 to 2400 mg (Group III, n = 94), respectively. The group without IV iron treatment was defined as the reference. In a follow-up of 12 months, fatal and non-fatal CV events and all-cause deaths were recorded. In all patients, a thorough medical history was taken at the time of study enrollment. The presence of CV disease was defined with a medical history and clinical findings of congestive heart failure (CHF), coronary artery disease, or cerebrovascular and/or peripheral vascular disease (PVD). Diabetes mellitus was diagnosed according to the American Diabetes Association criteria or if the patients were taking oral hypoglycemic agents or receiving insulin injection therapy at the time of enrollment. No major modifications were made in the dialysis treatments or schedules during the follow-up period. The primary outcome measures were CV events and all-cause mortality from the time of inclusion in the study. CV events included myocardial infarction, stroke, CHF, complicated PVD, and sudden death. CHF was ascertained by the dyspnea plus two of the followings: raised jugular venous pressure, bibasilar crackles, pulmonary venous hypertension or interstitial edema on chest X-ray. Complicated PVD is defined if patients with PVD requires the hospital-based interventions, including non-traumatic amputation, percutaneous transluminal angioplasty or bypass surgery. All clinical events were confirmed by hospital records.

Table 2. Multivariate Cox proportional hazards analysis for relative risk of cardiovascular events and overall mortality calculated for intravenous iron groups in a follow-up of 12 months.

	Intravenous iron administered dose, mg/6 months				
	0	40 to 800	840 to 1600	1640 to 2400	
	Hazard Ratio (95% CI)				*P* for trend
Cardiovascular events					
Crude	1	1.8 (1.1–2.9)	3.4 (1.9–6.0)	4.8 (2.9–8.4)	<0.001
Adjusted[a]	1	1.7 (1.0–2.7)	3.5 (1.9–6.1)	5.1 (3.0–9.7)	<0.001
Fatal and nonfatal MI and stroke, and sudden death					
Crude	1	1.4 (0.8–1.8)	1.9 (1.1–3.2)	2.5 (2.0–6.3)	0.009
Adjusted[a]	1	1.2 (0.9–1.9)	2.4 (1.2–4.7)	3.0 (1.5–5.6)	<0.001
All-cause mortality					
Crude	1	1.3 (0.9–2.0)	2.0 (1.1–3.4)	2.4 (1.3–4.1)	0.004
Adjusted[a]	1	1.3 (0.9–2.0)	3.1 (1.6–6.3)	3.7 (1.8–7.7)	<0.001

Hazard ratios and 95% confidence intervals (CIs) were derived from Cox regression analysis with intravenous iron dose taken into account as a time-dependent covariate.

[a]The multivariate model included variables for age, sex, diabetes, hypertension, prior cardiovascular disease, hemodialysis duration, serum albumin, hemoglobin, and C-reactive protein.

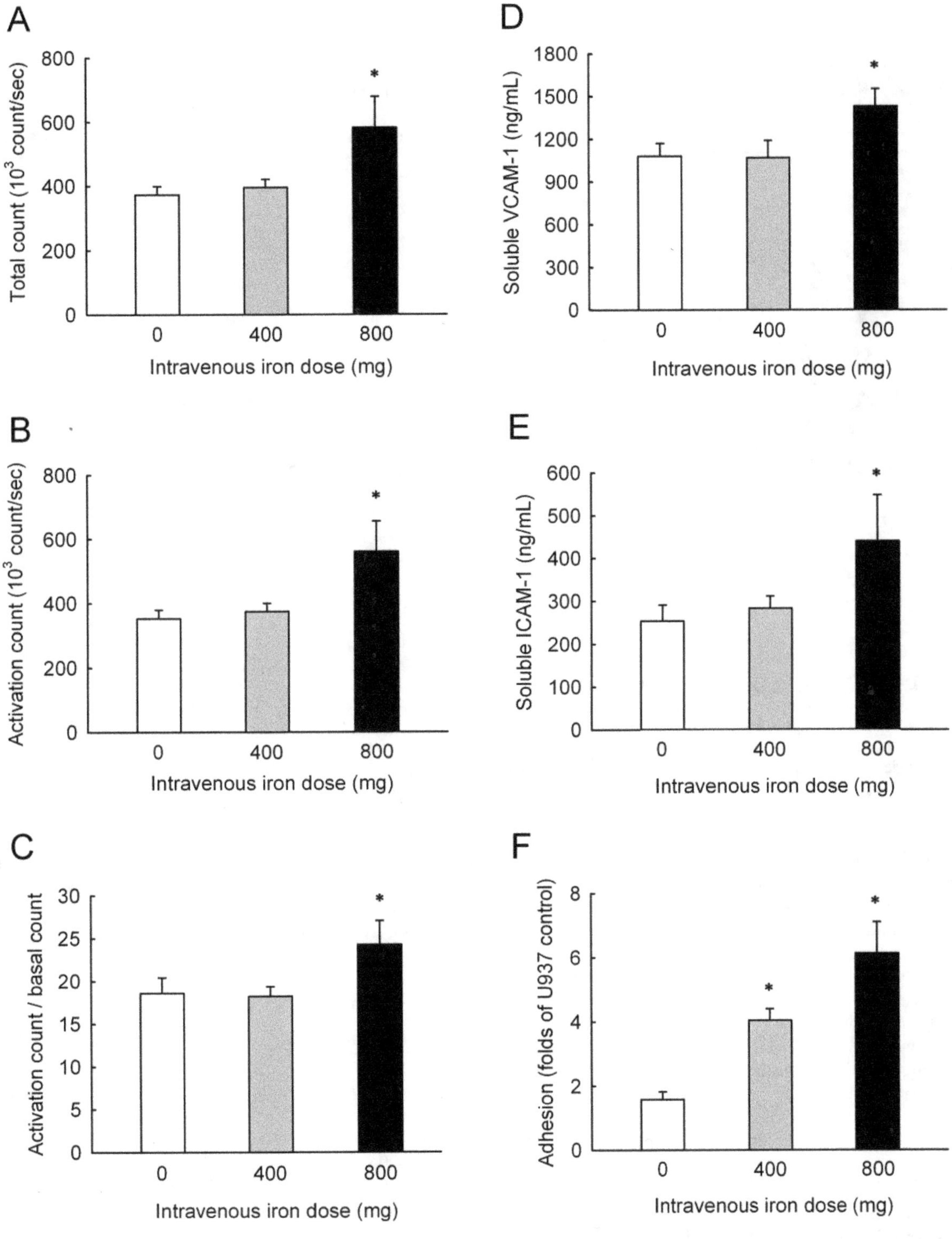

Figure 2. IV iron significantly increased superoxide production and endothelial damage *in vivo.* Total (A) and activated (B) intracellular production of superoxide, the ratio of activated to total superoxide (C) in circulating MNCs, plasma levels of VCAM-1 (D) and ICAM-1 (E), and endothelial adhesiveness of circulating MNCs (F) in hemodialysis patients. All patients were randomly allocated into 3 groups according to the IV Atofen iron doses of 0 mg (n = 20), 400 mg (n = 20), and 800 mg (n = 20). *$P<0.05$ compared with patients not receiving IV iron therapy. Abbreviations: ICAM-1, intracellular cell adhesion molecule-1; VCAM-1, vascular cell adhesion molecule-1.

To assess the possible molecular mechanisms of IV iron in CV disease, a second cohort of 60 patients (30 men and 30 women; mean age of 65±12 years) on maintenance HD for more than 6 months was recruited for superoxide production of MNCs, circulating levels of soluble adhesion molecules, and mononuclear-endothelial cell adhesion assays, which served as an index of early atherogenesis *ex vivo* [13–16]. Patients who had a malignancy, infectious disease, or sepsis, or hepatobiliary disease were

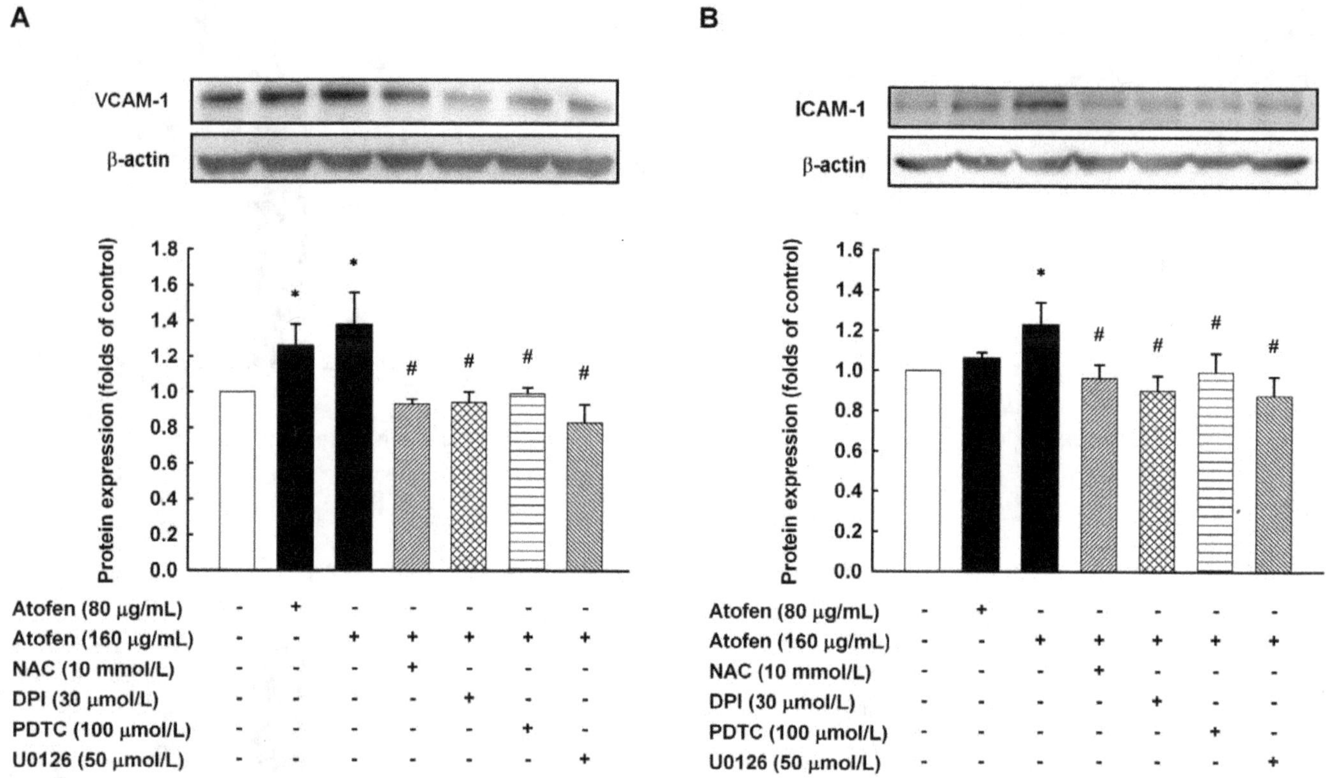

Figure 3. Iron upregulated the expressions of VCAM-1 and ICAM-1 in HAECs. The expressions of VCAM-1 (A) and ICAM-1 (B) in iron-stimulated HAECs were determined by Western blotting. HAECs were treated with ferric chloride hexahydrate (Atofen) with or without NAC (100 mmol/L), DPI (30 μmol/L), PDTC (100 μmol/L), and U0126 (50 μmol/L) for 4 hours. Data (mean ± SEM) are shown as a bar graph of densitometry data from 3 separate experiments. *$P<0.05$ compared with baseline without any treatment. #$P<0.05$ compared with 160 μg/mL ferric chloride hexahydrate for 4 h. Abbreviations: DPI, diphenyleneiodonium; HAECs, human aortic endothelial cells; ICAM-1, intracellular cell adhesion molecule-1; NAC, N-acetylcysteine; PDTC, pyrrolidine dithiocarbamate; VCAM-1, vascular cell adhesion molecule-1.

excluded from this study. Initially, all patients were randomly allocated to three groups receiving IV supplementation of Atofen iron or normal saline. IV supplementation with Atofen (40 mg and 80 mg elemental iron diluted in 250 mL of 0.9% saline) or 250 mL of 0.9% saline (control) was administered intravenously for 60 minutes postdialysis once a week for 10 weeks. Blood samples were taken two weeks after administration the last iron dose. All study subjects fasted for 12 hours immediately before the blood samples were taken. Any ongoing medications were continued without changes in dosage during the study. Both the observational and international studies were approved by the Committee on Human Research at Taipei Tzu Chi General Hospital. Written informed consent was obtained from each of the study subjects before study entry.

Isolation of Peripheral Blood Mononuclear Cells

Circulating MNCs from iron-treated HD patients and healthy subjects were isolated and extracted by density ultracentrifugation. In brief, 10 mL peripheral venous blood was drawn into a VACUTAINER® CPT™ Tube with 0.1 M sodium citrate at room temperature at bedside after 30 min of bed rest, with the study subjects in a supine position. The tubes were inverted 10 times gently. The blood was centrifuged and washed with EDTA/Hanks' balanced salt solution (HBSS) as per the operational instructions [17]. The isolated circulating MNCs were then resuspended with serum-free RPMI 1640 medium for labeling. All samples used in these experiments had at least 95% viability of the isolated MNCs assessed using trypan blue exclusion. The isolation procedures were carried out at room temperature within 2 h of blood collection. After density ultracentrifugation, the separated plasma was frozen to −20°C and stored at that temperature until the analysis of the circulating levels of adhesion molecules.

Assessment of Superoxide Generated by Mononuclear Cells

Using ultra-weak and luminol-enhanced chemiluminescence, superoxide generation of circulating MNCs was measured [18]. Briefly, after blood sampling, MNCs were immediately isolated by centrifuging (1500×*g*) whole blood in CPT tubes. The MNC suspension was then adjusted to 10^6 cells/mL (average lymphocytes: monocytes, 93:7) determined using a Coulter Counter (STKS, Coulter Electronics, Hialeah, FL). After adding 1 mL of 0.25 mm lucigenin to 100 μL of cell suspension, the photon emission at 200–750 nm was measured as the basal photon counts using the BJL-Ultra-Weak Chemiluminescence Analyzer (American Biologics, Chula Vista, CA; sensitivity 1.85×10^{-17} W/cm^2 count), which were recorded as the basal superoxide generated by MNCs. MNCs (suspended at 1×10^6/mL) were then activated by adding phorbol-12-myristate-13-acetate molecule (1 μg/mL), and the activated photon counts were recorded for 30 min. The total count of superoxide free radicals was a summation of the basal and the activated counts.

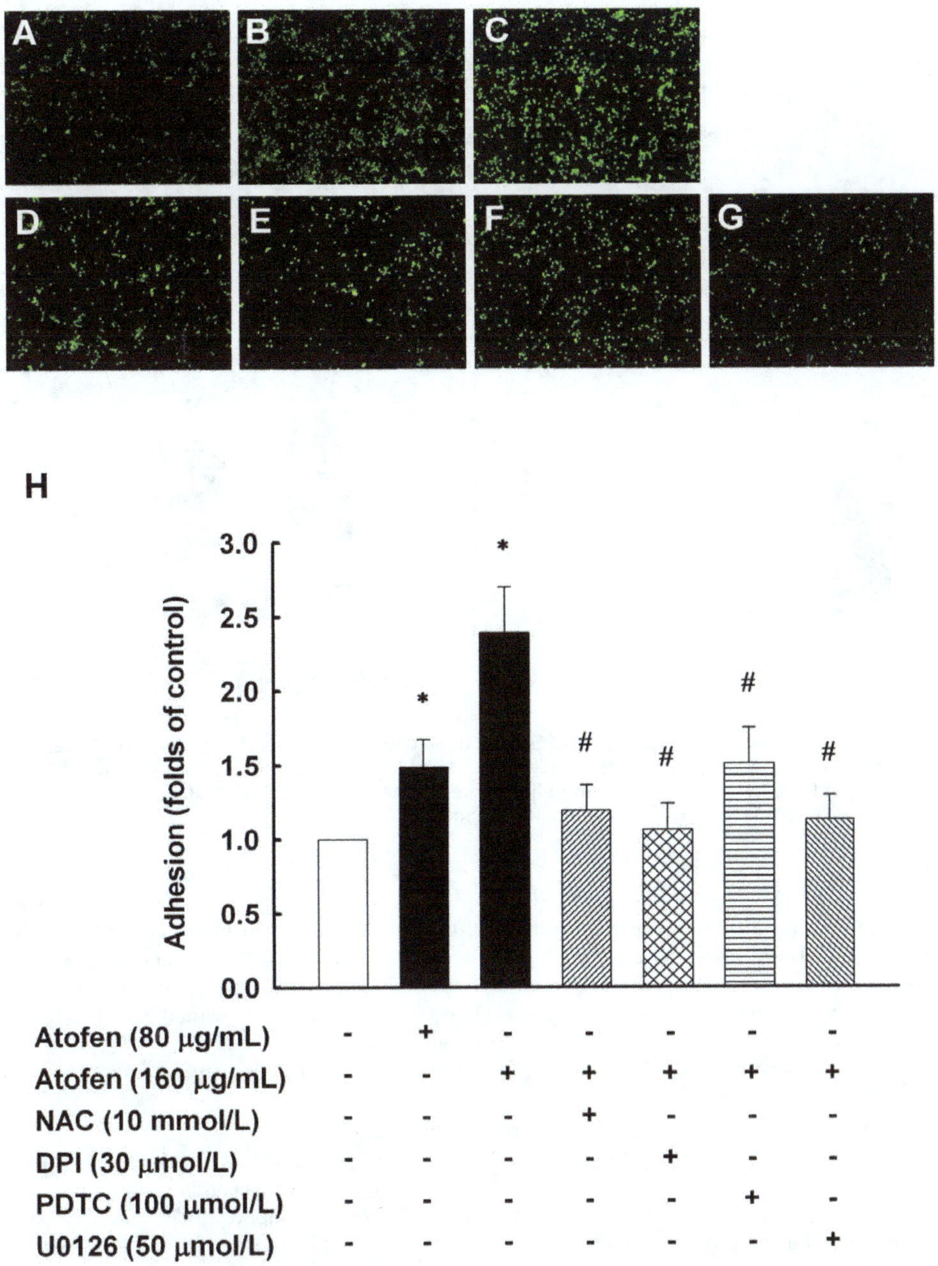

Figure 4. Iron enhanced adhesiveness of human MNCs to HAECs. HAECs were treated with ferric chloride hexahydrate (Atofen) with or without NAC (100 mmol/L), DPI (30 µmol/L), PDTC (100 µmol/L), and U0126 (50 µmol/L) for 4 hours. In upper panel, HAECs were unstimulated (control) (A), or stimulated by 80 µg/mL of Atofen alone (B), by 160 µg/mL of Atofen alone (C), and by co-treatment with 160 µg/mL of Atofen and NAC (D), DPI (E), PDTC (F), U0126 (G), respectively. Cell adherence was expressed as the fold difference over the untreated control. Values are expressed as mean ± SEM. *$P<0.05$ compared with baseline. #$P<0.05$ compared with 160 µg/mL Atofen for 4 h. Abbreviations: DPI, diphenyleneiodonium; HAECs, human aortic endothelial cells; NAC, N-acetylcysteine; PDTC, pyrrolidine dithiocarbamate.

Measurement of Plasma Levels of Soluble Adhesion Molecules

Plasma levels of human soluble VCAM-1 and ICAM-1 were determined by enzyme-linked immunosorbent assay with commercial kits (BioSource, Camarillo, CA). The procedures were carried out according to the instructions of the manufacturer.

Cell Culture of Human Aortic Endothelial Cells

Human aortic endothelial cells (Cascade Biologics, Portland, OR) were grown in Medium 200 (Cascade Biologics) supplemented with low-serum growth supplement (Cascade Biologics) in an atmosphere of 95% air and 5% CO_2 at 37°C in plastic flasks. At confluence, the cells were subcultured at a 1:3 ratio and used at passage numbers three through eight in this experiment.

Mononuclear-endothelial Cell Adhesion Assay

The adhesion assay was performed as previously described [13–16], with minor modifications. Before the adhesion assay, human MNCs were labeled with 10 µmol/L of 2′,7′-bis(2-carboxyethyl)-5(6)-carboxyfluorescein acetoxymethyl ester (BCECF-AM; Molec-

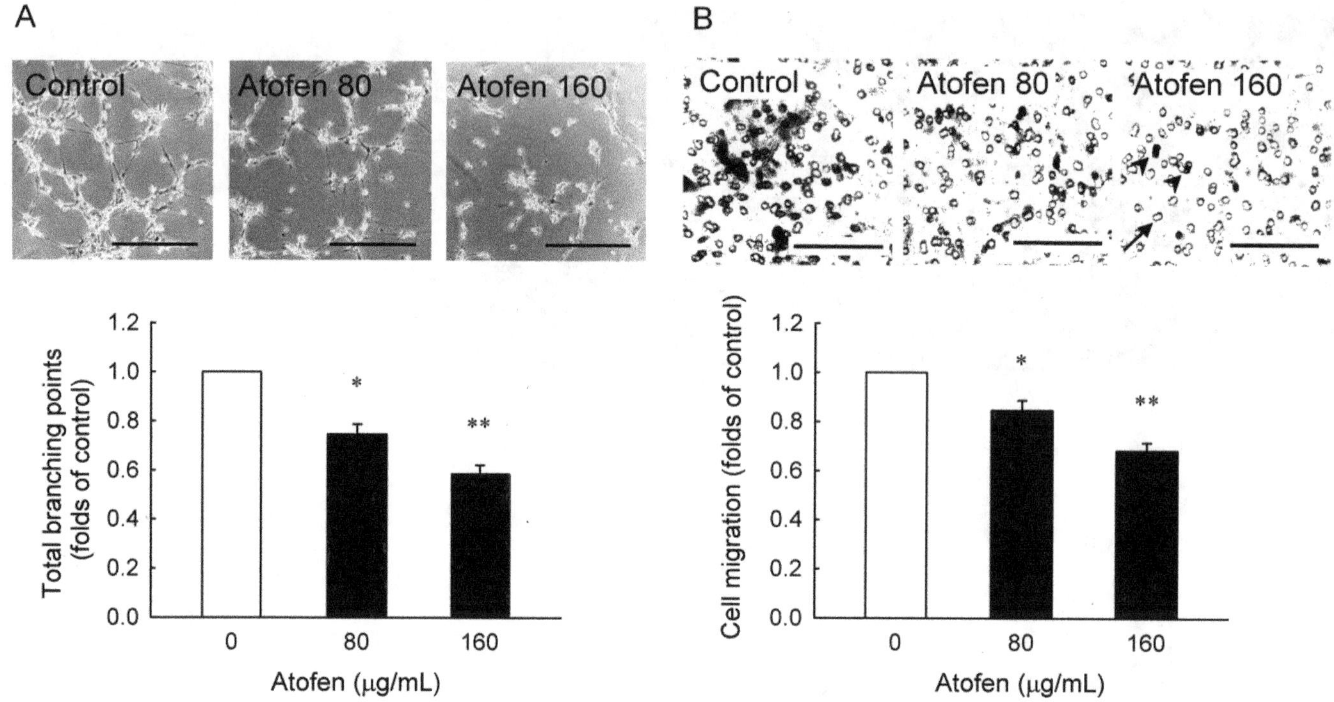

Figure 5. Iron inhibited tube formation and migratory capacity in HAECs. HAECs were treated with ferric chloride hexahydrate (Atofen) for 4 hours in tube formation (A) and 12 hours in cell migration (B). Values are expressed as mean ± SEM. Scale bar represents 50 μm in Figure 5A and 30 μm in Figure 5B. The arrowheads indicate migrated endothelial cells and the arrow indicates membrane pore. *$P<0.05$, **$P<0.001$ compared with baseline without Atofen treatment, $n=3$ in each group. Abbreviations: HAECs, human aortic endothelial cells.

ular Probes) in serum-free RPMI 1640 medium for 45 minutes at 37°C in darkness, and the surplus was washed with HBSS. Labeled MNCs (1×10^6) were then added to each well of control or Atofen-treated HAECs that were confluent in 24-well plates. After incubation at 37°C for 1 hour, non-adherent cells were removed with gentle HBSS washing for 3 times. MNC adhesion to HAECs was counted by an automated fluorometer at an emission of 530 nm and an absorption of 435 nm after cells were lysed with DMSO. The data were expressed as the fold difference over the untreated control in each experiment.

Western Blot

Confluent HAECs were stimulated with 80 or 160 μg/mL of Atofen with or without N-acetylcysteine (NAC, 10 mmol/L), diphenyleneiodonium (DPI; NADPH oxidase inhibitor, 30 μmol/L), pyrrolidine dithiocarbamate [PDTC; Nuclear factor κB (NF-κB) inhibitor, 100 μmol/L] and U0126 [activator protein-1 (AP-1) inhibitor, 50 μmol/L] for 4 hours. Protein extracts were prepared as previously described [17]. Total protein was quantified by the Bio-Rad protein assay, and processed for Western blot using primary goat antibodies for VCAM-1 and ICAM-1. Afterward, species-directed secondary goat HRP-conjugated monoclonal antibodies were used. Anti-β-actin antibody was used as a loading control. Densitometric analysis using ImageQuant software was conducted to semiquantify the data.

Tube Formation Assay

Tube formation assay was performed as previously described [19], with minor modifications. Angiogenesis μ-slides (Ibidi Gmbh, Germany) were coated with 10-μl growth factor-containing gel (ECMatrix; Millipore, Billerica, MA) and incubated at 37°C for 1 hour in CO_2 incubator according to the manufacturer's instructions. HAECs were plated on the coated plates at 5×10^3 cells/well in the presence of 0, 80 and 160 μg/ml of Atofen, respectively. After 4 hours of incubation in a 5% CO_2-humidified atmosphere at 37°C, tube-like formation in the center field was observed by an inverted photomicroscope and captured with a CCD camera. Total branching points were analyzed by WimTube Quantitative Image Analysis (Wimasis, https://mywim.wimasis.com).

Cell Migration Assay

Cell migration assay was performed as previously described [19], with minor modifications. Assay was conducted using 8.0-μm pore size 24-well Millicell insert (Millipore, Billerica, MA). Nine hundred μl medium with 10% FBS and 0, 80 or 160 μg/ml of Atofen were placed in the lower wells. Cell suspensions (200 μl; 2×10^4 cells/well) in the presence of different concentrations (0, 80 and 160 μg/ml) of Atofen were added to the upper well, respectively, and cultured at 37°C for 12 hours. Migrated cells on the lower surface of the membrane were fixed in 10% PFA and stained with Hematoxylin. Five random microscopic fields (200X) per well were quantified by ImageJ software.

Statistical Analysis

All variables are expressed as percentages for categorical data and the mean ± SD (normally distributed data) or medians with interquartile ranges (IQR) (non-normally distributed data). Comparisons between two groups were assessed by Student's *t* test, Pearson's chi-square test, or the Mann-Whitney *U* test, as appropriate. Potential differences among the 3 patient groups with different IV iron doses were assessed by multivariate analysis of variance (ANOVA). The Kaplan-Meier method was used to describe survival curves. Cox proportional hazards regression analysis was used to examine the associations of the cumulative dose of IV Atofen with CV events and all-cause mortality. The assumption of proportional hazards was confirmed by a log minus log plot and was met in the Cox models. Univariate and multivariate Cox regression analyses are presented as hazard ratios (HRs) and 95% confidence intervals (CIs). Adjustments for age and gender were initially performed to calculate the adjusted HRs. The multivariate regression analysis was further adjusted for age, sex, the presence of diabetes, hypertension, prior CV disease, hemodialysis duration, serum albumin, hemoglobin and CRP. The *in vitro* results are expressed as the mean ± SEM, and these data were analyzed using one-way ANOVA followed by the LSD test. A *P* value less than 0.05 was considered statistically significant. All statistical analyses were performed using the Statistical Package for the Social Sciences (SPSS), version 16.0 (SPSS Inc., Chicago, IL).

Results

IV Atofen Iron Associated with CV Events and All-cause Mortality

Among 1239 HD patients, 332 (27%) had diabetes mellitus and 180 (15%) had a previous history of CV disease. All patients were stratified into two groups with (n = 656) and without (n = 583) supplementation of IV Atofen during 6 months prior to enrollment (Table 1). The patients in the two groups did not differ significantly from each other. The baseline ferritin levels were 566 [IQR: 352, 594] μg/L in non-iron group and 354 [188, 518] μg/L in iron-treated group. The difference between two groups might be due to that the lower the ferritin level, the more the need of IV iron. The follow-up ferritin and hemoglobin levels were 480 [302, 819] μg/L and 10.3±1.8 g/dL at 6 months and 497 [307, 818] μg/L and 10.2±1.7 g/dL at 12 months in non-iron group; and were 392 [254, 583] μg/L and 10.4±1.4 g/dL at 6 months and 400 [228, 583] μg/L and 10.4±1.4 g/dL at 12 months in iron-treated group, respectively. No significant differences in ferritin and hemoglobin levels between the two groups were found during the follow-up.

During a follow-up period of 12 months, 154 patients died, and 83 (53.8%) died of CV-related causes and 71 (46.2%) died of non-CV causes including infection, sepsis, malignancy, gastrointestinal bleeding, chronic obstructive lung disease, and cachexia. There were 207 fatal and non-fatal CV events, i.e. 61 myocardial infarction, 50 stroke, 54 CHF, 15 PVD and 27 sudden death. Figure 1 shows the Kaplan-Meier survival curves for the endpoints of first CV event and the all-cause mortality among the 4 subgroups stratified by the cumulative iron dose within 6 months prior to the study: 0 mg (reference group, n = 583), 40 to 800 mg (Group I, n = 451), 840 to 1600 mg (Group II, n = 111), and 1640 to 2400 mg (Group III, n = 94). The survival analysis showed that higher IV iron doses were significantly associated with a higher risk for CV events (Figure 1A) and a lower probability of survival (Figure 1B) in HD patients.

Cox proportional hazards models (Table 2) corroborated the finding that compared to the reference group, the crude HR was 3.4 (95% CI, 1.9 to 6.0) in Group II and 4.8 (95% CI, 2.9 to 8.4) in Group III for CV events (*P* for trend <0.001), as well as 2.0 (95% CI, 1.1 to 3.4) in Group II and 2.4 (95% CI, 1.3 to 4.1) in Group III for all-cause mortality (*P* for trend = 0.004). After adjustment for potential confounders, including age, gender, dialysis vintage, comorbidities, and baseline traditional and uremic factors, the adjusted HR was 3.5 (95% CI, 1.9 to 6.1) in Group II and 5.1 (95% CI, 3.0 to 9.9) in Group III for CV events (*P* for trend <0.001), as well as 3.1 (95% CI, 1.6 to 6.3) in Group II and 3.7 (95% CI, 1.8 to 7.7) in Group III for mortality (*P* for trend <0.001). When CV events were confined to the fatal and nonfatal myocardial infarction, stroke and sudden cardiac death, the crude and adjusted HRs showed the similar results (Table 2). In general, a cumulative dose of IV Atofen >800 mg during the 6 months significantly increased the risks for CV events and overall mortality in HD patients.

Pro-oxidant Effects of IV Atofen Iron *in vivo*

HD patients were randomly assigned the treatment with normal saline (n = 20), and IV Atofen 400 mg (n = 20) and 800 mg (n = 20), respectively. The patients in the three groups did not differ significantly from each other in age, gender, comorbidities, HD vintage, weekly dose of ESA, hemoglobin, serum albumin, and ferritin. The intracellular superoxide production of circulating MNCs was measured in HD patients 2 weeks after a course of IV iron supplementation. As compared to the subjects not receiving IV iron, those receiving IV iron dose of 800 mg significantly had higher total (373±27 *vs.* 582±96×10^3 count/sec, P = 0.003; Figure 2A) and activated counts of superoxide (353±27 *vs.* 560±95×10^3 count/sec, P = 0.003; Figure 2B) and the ratio of the activated count to the basal count (18.6±1.9 *vs.* 24.3±2.8, P = 0.049; Figure 2C). Similarly, they had higher plasma levels of soluble VCAM-1 (1081±89 *vs.* 1429±123 ng/mL, P = 0.046; Figure 2D) and ICAM-1 (254±37 *vs.* 439±108 ng/mL, P = 0.028; Figure 2E) than those not receiving IV iron did. Trends of increased superoxide production and plasma adhesion molecules were noted in patients receiving IV iron of 400 mg, but not reach statistical significance. Using the *ex vivo* assay of MNC-endothelial cell adhesion, a significant increase of MNC adhesion to HAECs in a dose-dependent manner was observed in HD patients (1.6±0.2, 4.0±0.4, and 6.1±1.0 folds of U937 control in patients receiving 0 mg, 400 mg and 800 mg, respectively, P<0.001; Figure 2F).

Atofen Iron Upregulated the Expression of VACM-1 and ICAM-1 in HAECs

We examined the *in vitro* effects of Atofen on the expression of endothelial adhesion molecules in HAECs using Western blotting. In the following experiments, the non-cytotoxic Atofen concentrations of ≤160 μg/mL were used based on the MTT cell viability assay (Figure S1) and the report by Zager *et al.* [20]. Atofen at concentrations of 80 and 160 μg/mL significantly upregulated VCAM-1 expression in HAECs at 4 hours (P = 0.045 versus control; Figure 3A). Similarly, Atofen at 160 μg/mL significantly enhanced ICAM-1 expression in HAECs (P = 0.046 versus control; Figure 3B). Co-treatment of HAECs with NAC (10 mmol/L), DPI (30 μmol/L), PDTC (100 μmol/L) and U0126 (50 μmol/L) significantly suppressed the iron-induced expression of VCAM-1 (P = 0.007, 0.006, 0.008 and <0.001 versus Atofen at 160 μg/mL; Figure 3A) and ICAM-1 (P = 0.023, 0.006, 0.041 and 0.004 versus Atofen at 160 μg/mL; Figure 3B), respectively.

Atofen Iron Enhanced Endothelial Adhesiveness of Circulating MNCs in HAECs

Atofen's effects in endothelial adhesiveness were further examined, and BCECF-AM–labeled human MNCs and Atofen-treated HAECs were submitted to adhesiveness assays for 4 hours (Figure 4). Atofen induced a dose-dependent increase of endothelial adhesiveness in HAECs at concentrations of 80 to 160 μg/mL (1.48±0.49 and 2.39±0.30 folds of control, P = 0.018 and <0.001; Figure 4). Co-treatment of HAECs with NAC (10 mmol/L), DPI (30 μmol/L), PDTC (100 μmol/L) and U0126 (50 μmol/

L) attenuated the iron-induced endothelial adhesiveness (P = 0.003, 0.001, 0.035 and 0.002 versus Atofen at 160 μg/mL; Figure 4), respectively. Accordingly, iron-induced ROS generation via the activation of NAPDH oxidase and the downstream redox-sensitive transcription factors may in part lead to endothelial dysfunction.

Atofen Iron Inhibited Tube Formation and Migratory Capacity in HAECs

To further examine the Atofen's effects in angiogenesis and migratory capacity of HAECs, Atofen-treated HAECs were submitted to tube formation assay for 4 hours and Boyden chamber assay for 12 hours, respectively. The quantitative analysis of branching points showed that Atofen induced a dose-dependent decrease of tube formation in HAECs at concentrations of 80 and 160 μg/mL (0.75±0.04 and 0.58±0.04 folds of control, P = 0.011 and <0.001, respectively, Figure 5A). Similarly, Atofen inhibited the migration of HAECs at concentrations of 80 and 160 μg/mL in the Boyden chamber assay (0.85±0.04 and 0.68±0.03 folds of control, P = 0.001 and <0.001, respectively, Figure 5B).

Discussion

Iron is a cellular transition element, and its ionic forms are prone to participate in one-electron transfer reactions. However, this property also allows iron to generate ROS. In the presence of iron, reactive hydroxyl radicals can be formed via the Fenton reaction and the iron-catalyzed Haber-Weiss reaction [21,22]. The generated ROS subsequently initiate various types of damage to the human body. In 1981, Sullivan [23] suggested that iron depletion may protect against ischemic heart disease in humans. This "iron hypothesis" has been verified by many epidemiological studies. Bodily iron stores, as measured by the serum ferritin concentration, are positively correlated with the incidence of CV disease [24,25]. Subsequent cohort studies have found that higher body iron storage may increase the risk for CV disease [26,27]. In addition, several lines of evidence have indicated an increased iron level in human atherosclerotic plaques [28,29]. This observation was further supported by Lee *et al.* [30], who found that iron deposition was closely associated with the progression of atherosclerosis in ApoE-deficient mice. Restrictions in dietary iron intake led to a significant reduction of atherosclerotic lesion formation in ApoE-deficient mice. However, the contention that iron participates in vascular inflammation and the subsequent atherosclerosis still remains to be confirmed.

Iron therapy has positive and negative impacts in the clinical outcome of CKD patients. First, anemia can promote left ventricular hypertrophy and augment CV disease in CKD patients. Iron supplementation can improve the efficacy of ESA therapy and increase hemoglobin concentration [3,4]. Second, over-treatment with iron may increase the risk of CV disease and infection [31,32]. Third, iron can enhance ROS generation, exaggerate uremia-associated oxidative stress, and subsequently promote atherosclerosis via the oxidation of low-density lipoprotein (LDL) and endothelial dysfunction [33,34]. Accordingly, the optimal dosage of iron supplementation in CKD patients is still debatable. The main reasons for this are the absence of large clinical, especially randomized controlled, trials, as well as insufficient *in vivo* and *in vitro* experimental evidence.

Atofen is a new iron preparation for parenteral administration to treat anemia and iron deficiency in CKD patients. To our knowledge, this is the first study to assess whether IV Atofen supplementation had detrimental effects on CV events and mortality in HD patients. In this prospective cohort study, compared with those who did not receive IV iron, there were significant dose-dependent risks for fatal and non-fatal CV events and overall mortality among 1239 HD patients. We further observed that supplementation with Atofen of >800 mg over 6 months was significantly associated with poor CV outcome and increased mortality in chronic HD patients. Kalantar-Zadeh *et al.* [9] have observed a J-shaped association between iron dose and outcome, which is different from our observations. Because both were observational studies, the reasons for this discrepancy are mainly due to differences in iron regimens, patient selection, ethnicity, and statistical methodology. In the randomized study, we further found significant increases in ROS production and endothelial adhesion by circulating MNCs from HD patients receiving IV Atofen compared to those without IV iron therapy (Figure 2). Our observations are in line with the finding by Yin *et al.* [13] that the *ex vivo* MNC-endothelial cell adhesion assay can predict the clinical outcome in patients with chronic heart failure.

The molecular mechanisms of the association of iron administration with tissue oxidation or atherosclerosis have not been fully clarified. Zager *et al.* [35] first demonstrated that iron sucrose inhibits aortic endothelial cell proliferation *in vitro*. Carlini *et al.* [36] also found that the inhibitory effect of iron sucrose on endothelial cell proliferation probably results from the overexpression of proteins related to the cell-cycle arrest and apoptosis stress pathways. In rats with a remnant kidney, the IV administration of iron dextran can induce oxidant stress in CV tissues but has no impact on atherosclerotic lesions [37]. Our previous data together with those of others reveal that the activation of NF-κB [14,38] and AP-1 [39,40], two major redox-sensitive eukaryotic transcription factors, regulates genes relevant to the expression of adhesion molecules on endothelial cell surface. Furthermore, the activation of these genes can be diminished by various antioxidants [38–40]. Intriguingly, our *in vitro* experiments showed that the Atofen-induced expression of adhesion molecules and endothelial adhesiveness were attenuated by the co-treatment of HAECs with NAC and inhibitors of NADPH oxidase, NF-κB, and AP-1 (Figure 3 and 4). Endothelial adhesiveness to MNCs *in vitro* is a reliable cell model for early stages of atherogenesis [14–16,41], indicating that intracellular ROS production by iron therapy may play a central role in atherogenesis. In addition, we also demonstrated that iron can attenuate angiogenesis and inhibit migratory capacity *in vitro*. Taken collectively, the data indicate that IV iron acts as an *in vivo* pro-oxidant to provoke intracellular ROS production, which may induce redox-sensitive transcription pathway activation and adhesion molecule expression, promote the development of atherosclerosis, and even restrain angiogenesis.

Several points from our studies deserve discussion. First, the iron concentrations used (80 and 160 μg/mL) fall within a clinically achievable range of plasma iron concentrations (e.g., ~150 μg/mL following ~500 mg IV iron infusion) [20]. Our data provide insight into the molecular mechanisms of iron-related endothelial damage in normal physiologic situations, and an increase in iron levels from a high iron dosage (>800 mg IV infusion) may predispose to more endothelial dysfunction and exacerbate the risk of atherosclerosis in CKD. Second, in the process of MNC-endothelial cell adhesion, arrest and firm adhesion of the MNCs on activated endothelial cell surfaces also depends on the expression of the integrins very late antigen (VLA-4) and lymphocyte function-associated antigen-1 (LFA-1). Kartikasari *et al.* [42] found that VLA-4 and LFA-1 were upregulated on monocytes after 1 hour of 10 μmol/L Fe(III) citrate treatment, suggesting that iron may also enhance monocyte activation. Third, NADPH oxidase-derived ROS, in particular, superoxide radicals and their dismutation product, hydrogen peroxide, have been implicated in the development of human atherosclerotic lesions [43]. Clinically, there is a close relationship between cellular iron status and NADPH oxidase activity. Kurtoglu *et al.* [44] reported that the activity of NADPH oxidase was significantly lower in patients with iron-deficient anemia, and iron supplementation increased NADPH oxidase activity. Li *et al.* [45] found that iron increased endothelial NADPH oxidase activity by increasing $p22^{phox}$ gene transcription. These results support the findings in our study. We demonstrated that IV iron can significantly enhance the total and activated superoxide production of circulating MNCs isolated from HD patients. Our *in vitro* study further demonstrated that the co-treatment of iron-stimulated HAECs with an NADPH oxidase inhibitor ameliorated the iron-enhanced expression of adhesion molecules and endothelial adhesiveness. It implies that antioxidants may potentially protect against iron-mediated endothelial dysfunction in clinical practice.

Some limitations of this study should be acknowledged. There was no random allocation of treatment in our study on CV outcome and mortality. The nature of the observational cohort study might bear the possibility of selection bias. Nevertheless, the two groups of patients, those receiving and not receiving IV iron, did not differ significantly from each other in the baseline demographic and laboratory data. Furthermore, in analyzing the association of iron dosage with the end points, we used multivariate Cox hazards models to adjust for the likelihood of potential confounders. Unlike the previous studies [7–9], the single IV iron regimens applied in our cohort reduced the potential discrepancy that can result from the use of various IV iron medications and minimized the confounders in some associations. Finally, the type of vascular access, native arteriovenous fistula, arteriovenous graft or temporary catheter might represent an additional confounding variable. Despite the above-mentioned limitations, our data from the randomized controlled study and *in vitro* experiments still provide a causal interrelation among iron supplementation, ROS production and endothelial dysfunction, and provided the pathomechanism of IV iron-induced arthergenesis in HD patients.

In summary, our prospective cohort study demonstrates that high cumulative IV iron supplementation significantly increased the risks for fatal and non-fatal CV events and all-cause mortality in chronic HD patients, especially in those receiving Atofen >800 mg over 6 months. In addition, IV-administered iron acts as a pro-oxidant *in vivo* to enhance superoxide production of circulating MNCs, soluble adhesion molecule levels in the plasma, and the endothelial adhesion of circulating MNCs in chronic HD patients. Furthermore, our *in vitro* experiments showed that Atofen increased adhesion molecule expression and aggravated MNC-endothelial cell adhesion in cultured HAECs. Our findings may indicate a novel role of Atofen iron in exacerbating atherosclerosis in HD patients. From a clinical point of view, to confront the enhanced oxidant stress and subsequent vascular injury caused by IV-administered Atofen, long-term, randomized controlled studies of IV Atofen are needed to better define the clinically safe dose, if any, of this therapy.

Acknowledgments

The authors are extremely grateful to Ms. P.C. Lee for her expert secretarial assistance and graphic design.

Author Contributions

Conceived and designed the experiments: K-LK D-CT. Performed the experiments: K-LK S-CH Y-PL C-FT D-CT. Analyzed the data: K-LK D-CT Y-PL. Contributed reagents/materials/analysis tools: Y-PL C-FT T-SL C-PL. Wrote the paper: K-LK S-CH. Reviewed and edited the manuscript: D-CT.

References

1. Parfrey PS, Foley RN, Wittreich BH, Sullivan DJ, Zagari MJ, et al. (2005) Double-blind comparison of full and partial anemia correction in incident hemodialysis patients without symptomatic heart disease. J Am Soc Nephrol 16: 2180–2189.
2. Hörl WH (2007) Clinical aspects of iron use in the anemia of kidney disease. J Am Soc Nephrol 18: 382–393.
3. Besarab A, Amin N, Ahsan M, Vogel SE, Zazuwa G, et al. (2000) Optimization of epoetin therapy with intravenous iron therapy in hemodialysis patients. J Am Soc Nephrol 11: 530–538.
4. Sunder-Plassmann G, Hörl WH (1995) Importance of iron supply for erythropoietin therapy. Nephrol Dial Transplant 10: 2070–2076.
5. Rooyakkers TM, Stroes ES, Kooistra MP, van Faassen EE, Hider RC, et al. (2002) Ferric saccharate induces oxygen radical stress and endothelial dysfunction in vivo. Eur J Clin Invest 32: 9–16.
6. Drüeke T, Witko-Sarsat V, Massy Z, Descamps-Latscha B, Guerin AP, et al. (2002) Iron therapy, advanced oxidation protein products, and carotid artery intima-media thickness in end-stage renal disease. Circulation 106: 2212–2217.
7. Feldman HI, Santanna J, Guo W, Furst H, Franklin E, et al. (2002) Iron administration and clinical outcomes in hemodialysis patients. J Am Soc Nephrol 13: 734–744.
8. Feldman HI, Joffe M, Robinson B, Knauss J, Cizman B, et al. (2004) Administration of parenteral iron and mortality among hemodialysis patients. J Am Soc Nephrol 15: 1623–1632.
9. Kalantar-Zadeh K, Regidor DL, McAllister CJ, Michael B, Warnock DG (2005) Time-dependent associations between iron and mortality in hemodialysis patients. J Am Soc Nephrol 16: 3070–3080.
10. Griendling KK, Sorescu D, Lassègue B, Ushio-Fukai M (2000) Modulation of protein kinase activity and gene expression by reactive oxygen species and their role in vascular physiology and pathophysiology. Arterioscler Thromb Vasc Biol 20: 2175–2183.
11. Ross R (1999) Atherosclerosis: an inflammatory disease. N Engl J Med 340: 115–126.
12. Kuo KL, Hung SC, Wei YH, Tarng DC (2008) Intravenous iron exacerbates oxidative DNA damage in peripheral blood lymphocytes in chronic hemodialysis patients. J Am Soc Nephrol 19: 1817–1826.
13. Yin WH, Chen JW, Young MS, Lin SJ (2007) Increased endothelial monocyte adhesiveness is related to clinical outcomes in chronic heart failure. Int J Cardiol 121: 276–283, 2007.
14. Lin CP, Chen YH, Chen JW, Leu HB, Liu TZ, et al. (2008) Cholestin (Monascus purpureus rice) inhibits homocysteine-induced reactive oxygen species generation, nuclear factor-kappaB activation, and vascular cell adhesion molecule-1 expression in human aortic endothelial cells. J Biomed Sci 15: 183–196.
15. Chen JW, Chen YH, Lin FY, Chen YL, Lin SJ (2003) Ginkgo biloba extract inhibits tumor necrosis factor-alpha-induced reactive oxygen species generation, transcription factor activation, and cell adhesion molecule expression in human aortic endothelial cells. Arterioscler Thromb Vasc Biol 23: 1559–1566.
16. Chen JW, Lin FY, Chen YH, Wu TC, Chen YL, et al. (2004) Carvedilol inhibits tumor necrosis factor-alpha-induced endothelial transcription factor activation, adhesion molecule expression, and adhesiveness to human mononuclear cells. Arterioscler Thromb Vasc Biol 24: 2075–2081.
17. Lin CP, Chen YH, Lin WT, Leu HB, Liu TZ, et al. (2008) Direct effect of statins on homocysteine-induced endothelial adhesiveness: potential impact to human atherosclerosis. Eur J Clin Invest 38: 106–116.
18. Leu HB, Lin CP, Lin WT, Wu TC, Lin SJ, et al. (2006) Circulating mononuclear superoxide production and inflammatory markers for long-term

prognosis in patients with cardiac syndrome X. Free Radic Biol Med 40: 983–991.
19. Ikeda Y, Tajima S, Yoshida S, Yamano N, Kihira Y, et al. (2011) Deferoxamine promotes angiogenesis via the activation of vascular endothelial cellfunction. Atherosclerosis 215: 339–47.
20. Zager RA, Johnson AC, Hanson SY (2004) Parentral nephrotoxity: potential mechanisms and consequences. Kidney Int 66: 144–156.
21. Henle ES, Luo Y, Gassmann W, Linn S (1996) Oxidative damage to DNA constituents by iron-mediated fenton reactions. The deoxyguanosine family. J Biol Chem 271: 21177–21186.
22. Luo Y, Henle ES, Linn S (1996) Oxidative damage to DNA constituents by iron-mediated fenton reactions. The deoxycytidine family. J Biol Chem 271: 21167–21176.
23. Sullivan JL (1981) Iron and the sex difference in heart disease risk. Lancet 1: 1293–1294.
24. Salonen JT, Nyyssönen K, Korpela H, Tuomilehto J, Seppänen R, et al. (1992) High stored iron levels are associated with excess risk of myocardial infarction in eastern Finnish men. Circulation 86: 803–811.
25. Tuomainen TP, Punnonen K, Nyyssönen K, Salonen JT (1998) Association between body iron stores and the risk of acute myocardial infarction in men. Circulation 97: 1461–1466.
26. Kiechl S, Willeit J, Egger G, Poewe W, Oberhollenzer F (1997) Body iron stores and the risk of carotid atherosclerosis: prospective results from the Bruneck study. Circulation 96: 3300–3307.
27. Klipstein-Grobusch K, Koster JF, Grobbee DE, Lindemans J, Boeing H, et al. (1999) Serum ferritin and risk of myocardial infarction in the elderly: the Rotterdam Study. Am J Clin Nutr 69: 1231–1236.
28. Evans PJ, Smith C, Mitchinson MJ, Halliwell B (1995) Metal ion release from mechanically-disrupted human arterial wall. Implications for the development of atherosclerosis. Free Radic Res 23: 465–469.
29. Stadler N, Lindner RA, Davies MJ (2004) Direct detection and quantification of transition metal ions in human atherosclerotic plaques: evidence for the presence of elevated levels of iron and copper. Arterioscler Thromb Vasc Biol. 24: 949–954.
30. Lee TS, Shiao MS, Pan CC, Chau LY (1999) Iron-deficient diet reduces atherosclerotic lesions in apoE-deficient mice. Circulation 99: 1222–1229.
31. Hoen B, Paul-Dauphin A, Hestin D, Kessler M (1998) EPIBACDIAL: a multicenter prospective study of risk factors for bacteremia in chronic hemodialysis patients. J Am Soc Nephrol 9: 869–876.
32. Sengoelge G, Kletzmayr J, Ferrara I, Perschl A, Hörl WH, et al. (2003) Impairment of transendothelial leukocyte migration by iron complexes. J Am Soc Nephrol 14: 2639–2344.
33. Heinecke JW, Rosen H, Chait A (1984) Iron and copper promote modification of low density lipoprotein by human arterial smooth muscle cells in culture. J Clin Invest 74: 1890–1894.
34. Smith C, Mitchinson MJ, Aruoma OI, Halliwell B (1992) Stimulation of lipid peroxidation and hydroxyl-radical generation by the contents of human atherosclerotic lesions. Biochem J 286: 901–905.
35. Zager RA, Johnson AC, Hanson SY, Wasse H (2002) Parenteral iron formulations: A comparative toxicologic analysis and mechanisms of cell injury. Am J Kidney Dis 40: 90–103.
36. Carlini RG, Alonzo E, Bellorin-Font E, Weisinger JR (2006) Apoptotic stress pathway activation mediated by iron on endothelial cells in vitro. Nephrol Dial Transplant 21: 3055–3061.
37. Lim CS, Vaziri ND (2004) The effects of iron dextran on the oxidative stress in cardiovascular tissues of rats with chronic renal failure. Kidney Int 65: 1802–1809.
38. DiDonato JA, Hayakawa M, Rothwarf DM, Zandi E, Karin M (1997) A cytokine-responsive IkappaB kinase that activates the transcription factor NF-kappaB. Nature 388: 548–554.
39. Martin T, Cardarelli PM, Parry GC, Felts KA, Cobb RR (1997) Cytokine induction of monocyte chemoattractant protein-1 gene expression in human endothelial cells depends on the cooperative action of NF-kappa B and AP-1. Eur J Immunol 27: 1091–1097.
40. Zhu Y, Lin JH, Liao HL, Friedli O Jr, Verna L, et al. (1998) LDL induces transcription factor activator protein-1 in human endothelial cells. Arterioscler Thromb Vasc Biol 18: 473–480.
41. Lin CP, Lin WT, Leu HB, Wu TC, Chen JW (2003) Differential mononuclear cell activity and endothelial inflammation in coronary artery disease and cardiac syndrome X. Int J Cardiol 89: 53–62.
42. Kartikasari AE, Georgiou NA, Visseren FL, van Kats-Renaud H, van Asbeck BS, et al. (2004) Intracellular labile iron modulates adhesion of human monocytes to human endothelial cells. Arterioscler Thromb Vasc Biol 24: 2257–2262.
43. Griendling KK, Harrison DG (2004) Out, damned dot: studies of the NADPH oxidase in atherosclerosis. J Clin Invest 108: 1423–1424.
44. Kurtoglu E, Ugur A, Baltaci AK, Mogolkoc R, Undar L (2003) Activity of neutrophil NADPH oxidase in iron-deficient anemia. Biol Trace Elem Res 96: 109–115.
45. Li L, Frei B (2009) Prolonged exposure to LPS increases iron, heme, and p22phox levels and NADPH oxidase activity in human aortic endothelial cells: inhibition by desferrioxamine. Arterioscler Thromb Vasc Biol 29: 732–738.

Circulating MicroRNAs are not Eliminated by Hemodialysis

Filippo Martino[1]☯, Johan Lorenzen[1,2]☯, Julius Schmidt[2], Mascha Schmidt[1], Michael Broll[2], Yvonne Görzig[1], Jan T. Kielstein[2]¶, Thomas Thum[1,3]*¶

1 Institute for Molecular and Translational Treatment Strategies (IMTTS), Hannover Medical School, Hannover, Germany, 2 Department of Medicine, Division of Nephrology and Hypertension, Hannover Medical School, Hannover, Germany, 3 Centre of Clinical and Basic Research, IRCCS San Raffaele, Rome, Italy

Abstract

Background: Circulating microRNAs are stably detectable in serum/plasma and other body fluids. In patients with acute kidney injury on dialysis therapy changes of miRNA patterns had been detected. It remains unclear if and how the dialysis procedure itself affects circulating microRNA level.

Methods: We quantified miR-21 and miR-210 by quantitative RT-PCR in plasma of patients with acute kidney injury requiring dialysis and measured pre- and post-dialyser miRNA levels as well as their amount in the collected spent dialysate. Single treatments using the following filters were studied: F60 S (1.3 m^2, Molecular Weight Cut Off (MWCO): 30 kDa, $n = 8$), AV 1000 S (1.8 m^2, MWCO: 30 kDa, $n = 6$) and EMiC 2 (1.8 m^2, MWCO: 40 kDa, $n = 6$).

Results: Circulating levels of miR-21 or -210 do not differ between pre- and post-dialyzer blood samples independently of the used filter surface and pore size: miR-21: F60S: $p = 0.35$, AV 1000 S $p = 1.0$, EMiC2 $p = 1.0$; miR-210: F60S: $p = 0.91$, AV 1000 S $p = 0.09$, EMiC2 $p = 0.31$. Correspondingly, only traces of both miRNAs could be found in the collected spent dialysate and ultrafiltrate.

Conclusions: In patients with acute kidney injury circulating microRNAs are not removed by dialysis. As only traces of miR-21 and -210 are detected in dialysate and ultrafiltrate, microRNAs in the circulation are likely to be transported by larger structures such as proteins and/or microvesicles. As miRNAs are not affected by dialysis they might be more robust biomarkers of acute kidney injury.

Editor: Emmanuel A. Burdmann, University of Sao Paulo Medical School, Brazil

Funding: This work was supported by a grant from the German Federal Ministry of Education and Research (IFB-Tx: 01EO0802 to T.T.) and by Deutsche Forschungsgemeinschaft (DFG 903/7-2 to T.T.) as well as by an unrestricted grant of Fresenius Medical Care to JTK. The funders had no role in study design, data collection and analysis, decision to publish, or preparation of the manuscript.

Competing Interests: The authors have read the journal's policy and have the following conflicts: JL, JTK and TT filed a patent regarding diagnostic applications of miRNA in acute kidney injury. Patent name and number is EP12152245.2 "Device and method for analysis of kidney failure" (submitted to European patent office). The study was supported by an unrestricted grant of Fresenius Medical Care to JTK. This does not alter the authors' adherence to all the PLoS ONE policies on sharing data and materials.

* E-mail: Thum.Thomas@mh-hannover.de

☯ These authors contributed equally to this work.

¶ These authors also contributed equally to this work.

Introduction

MicroRNAs (miRNAs) are a class of endogenous small noncoding RNAs. The single-stranded molecules have a length of 19–23 nt [1]. Gain and loss of function studies revealed that miRNAs play a critical role in the regulation of basically all biological cell functions such as proliferation, differentiation and apoptosis [2–8]. MiRNAs are also involved in pathologic pathways of many disease models [6,9]. Recent studies discovered that miRNAs are detectable in extracellular human body fluids such as blood or urine in a rather stable form [10–12].

A potential reason that circulating miRNAs are not degraded by RNAses, is that they are partly included in microvesicles, such as exosomes or bound to protein complexes such as argonaute protein 2 (Ago 2) [13]. Especially in the intensive care unit there is a wide range of filters used for hemodialysis of patients with acute kidney injury. Dialysis membranes do usually not allow passage of larger molecules (>30–40 kDa). However, the dialysis procedure itself might influence the amount of circulating miRNAs. In the present study we therefore analyzed the effect of hemodialysis on circulating miRNA levels in blood and collected spent dialysate in order to investigate, whether the procedure removes miRNAs from circulation. Dialysis membranes of varying pore sizes (degree of molecular weight cut off) were compared.

Materials and Methods

Patients and Dialysis unit

The study protocol was approved by the Hannover Medical School Ethics Committee and conducted in accordance with the

German Federal Guidelines and the Declaration of Helsinki. Part of this represents a secondary analysis of samples collected for a study published elsewere [14]. Fourteen patients with acute kidney injury (AKI) treated by slow extended daily dialysis (SLEDD) were included (see table 1), using the GENIUS^{TM} dialysis system (Fresenius Medical Care, Bad Homburg, Germany). Its technical details are described elsewhere [15]. In brief, sterile bicarbonate dialysate is filled into a 75- or 90-L tank and is then circulated in a closed loop circuit. During dialysis, fresh dialysate is taken from the top of the tank, whereas the spent dialysate flows back to the bottom. Eight patients of the collective were treated only with the regularly used filter system (polysulfone high-flux dialyzer (F60S), 1.3 m^2 effective surface area, inner lumen 200 μm, wall thickness 40 μm, Fresenius Medical Care, Molecular weight cut off (MWCO): 30 kDa). Two of them received a second dialysis session at a later point in time which let us classify these results as an independent event. For further validation we recruited six more patients that received a dialysis session with two other different filter systems. The EmiC 2 (1.8 m^2 effective surface area, inner lumen 220 μm, wall thickness 35 μm, polysulfone, Fresenius Medical Care) has an enhanced middle molecule clearance and therefore among other things a higher MWCO of 40 kDa. We tested whether a larger pore size might result in depletion of circulating miRNAs. The AV 1000 S dialysis filter system (Fresenius Medical Care) effective surface area 1.8 m^2, inner lumen 220 μm, wall thickness 35 μm; allowing elimination of substances with a molecular weight of up to 30 kDa. The dialysate and countercurrent blood flow ranged between 150 to 165 mL/min in all dialysis sessions. Samples from pre-dialyser and post-dialyser blood line directly before and after the dialysis filter were collected 30 minutes after starting the dialysis session. Spent dialysate and ultrafiltrate samples were collected after the end of treatment (Duration: 490 min (480 min to 630 min)). The system, dialyser and sampling ports are described in figure 1.

RNA Isolation

RNA isolation was performed with plasma, ultrafiltrate and dialysate samples by using the MasterPure RNA Purification kit (Epicenter Technologies) according to the instructions of the manufacturer. In addition, we supplemented the samples with 1 μL of 3 fmol/μL *Caenorhabditis elegans* miR-39 (cel_miR-39) to normalize results.

Detection and Quantification of miRNAs

Isolated RNA was reverse transcribed with hsa_mir-21, hsa_miR-210 and cel_miR-39 primers using the TaqMan microRNA Reverse Transcription kit (Applied Biosystems, Foster City, CA) according to the manufacturers advices. Then both miRNAs were detected and validated by quantitative real-time PCR (qRT-PCR) via TaqMan MicroRNA Assays (Applied Biosystems). Levels of circulating miRNA were normalized to cel_miR-39 which was spiked in as external control.

Statistical Analysis

All statistics were performed with Graph Pad Prism 4. A nonparametric two-tailed Mann-Whitney test was used for statistical analysis of two groups. Data are represented as median and lower and upper quartile, if not described differently.

Results

Patients with acute kidney injury undergoing SLEDD using a F60S filter, we did not identify any effect of the dialysis procedure on circulating miRNA-21 and -210 levels comparing pre-dialyser and post-dialyser blood samples (miR-21: $p=0.35$; miR-210: $p=0.91$ (Figure 2A)). In line with this only traces of miR-21 and miRNA-210 could be found in both, dialysate and ultrafiltrate (miR-21: Dialysate: 1.6×10^{-6} (3.0×10^{-7} to 2.8×10^{-6}), ultrafiltrate: 1.3×10^{-6} (3.4×10^{-7} to 2.4×10^{-6}); miR-210: dialysate: 1.0×10^{-7} (2.8×10^{-8} to 4.5×10^{-7}), ultrafiltrate: 8.3×10^{-8} (3.0×10^{-8} to 2.1×10^{-7})). Also there was no difference between dialysate and ultrafiltrate (miR-21: $p=0.80$; miR-210: $p=0.74$ (Figure 2A)). As shown in Figure 2B miRNA values in blood within the F60S system for miR-21 and miR-210 were significantly higher than in dialysate/ultrafiltrate ($p<0.0001$) suggesting only minimal passage of miRNAs throughout the dialyser membrane.

Also dialysers with a larger surface area and pore size (Fresenius AV 1000 S 1.8 m^2 (MWCO: 30 kDa), EMiC 2 1.8 m^2 (MWCO: 40 kDa)) had no significant effect on circulating miRNA levels (miR-21: AV1000S pre-dialyser vs. EMiC 2 pre-dialyser $p=0.59$, post-dialyser $p=0.70$, dialysate $p=0.94$, ultrafiltrate $p=0.39$; miR-210: pre-dialyser $p=0.02$, post-dialyser $p=0.82$, dialysate $p=0.59$, ultrafiltrate $p=0.31$) (figure 3). The significant difference between the pre-dialyser line of AV 1000 S versus EMiC2 in miRNA-210 levels cannot be caused by different filter properties and is therefore not relevant for our main conclusion.

Also, the difference of miRNA-21 and -210 levels in blood versus spent dialysate levels using the EmiC 2 or AV 1000 S filter showed similar results for both miRNAs as previously shown for the F60S dialyser ($p<0.0001$; data not shown). Difference in miR-21 and -210 depletion ratios between the predialyser blood line and spent dialysate for AV 1000 S (miR-21: 2.2×10^{-3} (3.6×10^{-4}

Table 1. Demographic and clinical patient characteristics.

	Total	F60S	EMiC 2/Ultraflux AV 1000 S	p-value
Number of Patients: **Male (n; %)** **Female (n; %)**	14 8; 57.1% 6; 42.9%	8 4; 50.0% 4; 50.0%	6 4; 66.7% 2; 33.3%	0.8
Age (years)	49 (36 to 59)	53 (41 to 59)	40 (32 to 62)	0.7
BMI	25.7 (20.8 to 29.2)	24.6 (20.8 to 25.7)	31.5 (23.0 to 30.9)	0.4
Residual renal function (ml/d)	0 (0 to 0)	0 (0 to 0)	28 (22 to 33)	0.8
Urea (mmol/l)	15.4 (8.5 to 23.7)	13.4 (7.8 to 29.7)	18.6 (9.9 to 23.9)	0.7
APACHE II Score	23 (20 to 28)	22 (21 to 26)	27 (16 to 29)	0.9

BMI, Body mass index; APACHE II, Acute Physiology and Chronic Health Evaluation.

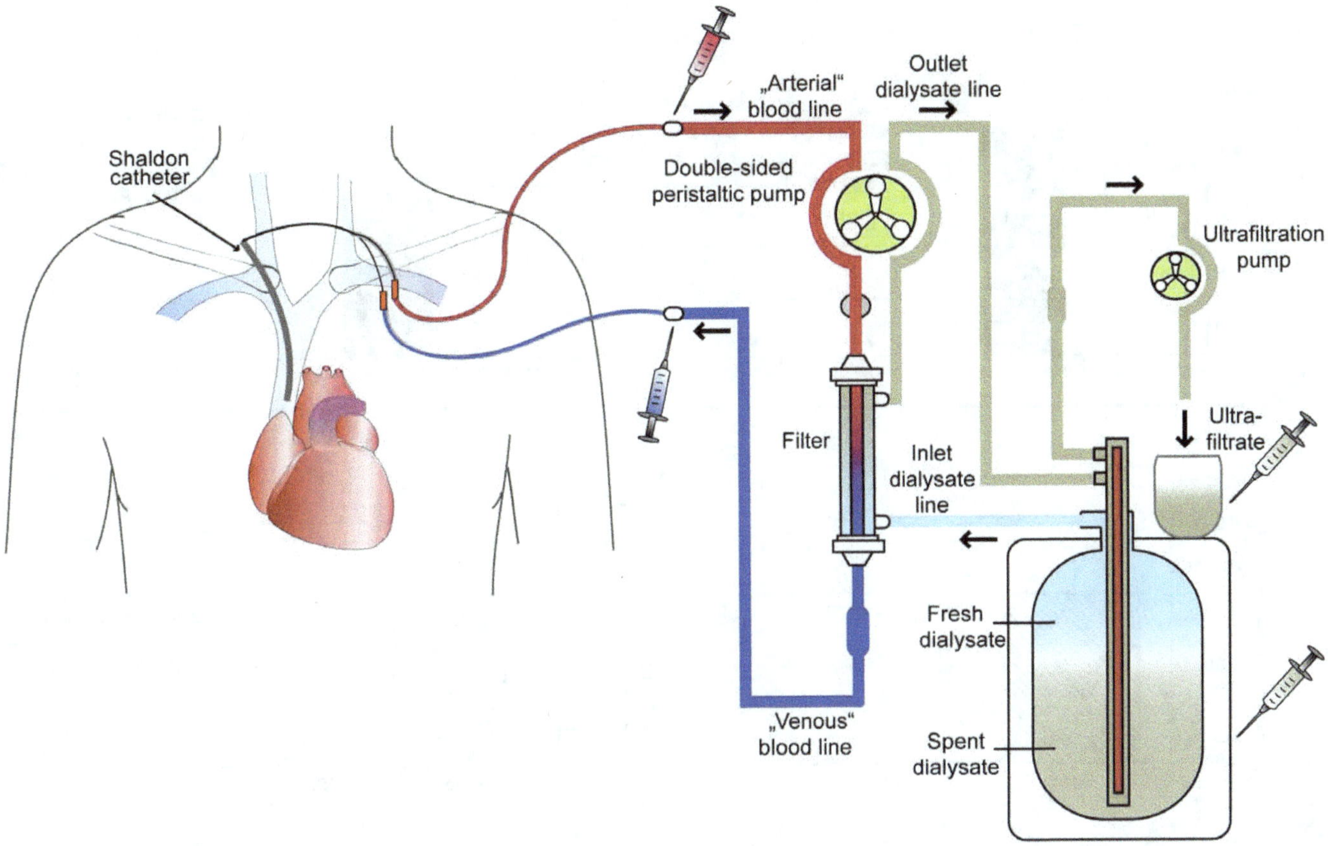

Figure 1. Structure and function of the Genius 75/90 Dialysis System and sample collection. Patient's blood runs countercurrent to dialysate and enters the dialysis circuit from a Shaldon catheter. The "arterial", i.e. predialyser blood line (red) passes the filter and blood flows back to the patient via the "venous", i.e. post-dialyser blood line (blue). Fresh dialysate is prepared individually for every patient's conditions and stored in a 75 or 90 liter tank. A tube leads the fresh dialysate (light-blue) to the dialysis filter. Exchange of substances and filtration is mediated by an osmotic and pressure gradient and is supported by counter-flow principle. Spent dialysate (grey) flows through the outlet dialysate line back into the tank. Phase formation prevents the mixture of fresh and spent dialysate. An ultrafiltration pump transports the excess filtrate and maintains the pressure gradient of the system. Samples are taken at the marked locations.

to 7.9×10^{-2}); miR-210: 7.3×10^{-3} (3.0×10^{-3} to 3.3×10^{-1})) and EMiC 2 (miR-21: 1.2×10^{-2} (5.9×10^{-4} to 1.1×10^{-1}); miR-210: 4.2×10^{-3} (8.3×10^{-4} to 1.1×10^{-2})) were not different (miR-21: $p=0.70$; miR-210: $p=0.31$ (data not shown)). This implicates that the different filter properties does not significantly alter circulating levels of at least miRNA-21 and -210.

Anticoagulation with heparin had no effect on the detectable miRNA levels in this study. Neither miR-21 (non-heparin treated pre-dialyser vs. heparin treated pre-dialyser $p=0.49$, post-dialyser $p=1.00$) nor miR-210 (non-heparin treated pre-dialyser vs. heparin treated pre-dialyser $p=0.19$, post-dialyser $p=0.98$) showed a significant difference in the entire patient collective between heparin treated and non heparin treated group.

Discussion

This is the first study, which describes the influence of hemodialysis therapy on circulating miRNA levels in patients with AKI. The salient finding is that miRNA, although only small in size, are not removed by various dialyser membranes, even those designed to remove middle-sized molecules.

MiRNAs interfere with a variety of pathologic pathways [6,16,17]. MiRNA-21 is a crucial player in various disease models such as cancer, heart failure or fibrosis in heart, lung or kidney [8,18–23]. Furthermore published evidence implicates that miR-21 is important in immune cell development and function [24,25]. Patient number 6 showed relatively high values of circulating miRNAs. Interestingly, this patient was involved in complex disease processes such as hepatitis B and C co-infection which led to liver transplantation. It is possible that these circumstances induced high levels of circulating miR-21. In fact there is a growing body of evidence that this miRNA is elevated in the circulation of patients with hepatitis C and therefore might be a potential biomarker [26]. MiR-210 has beenshown to be involved in kidney disease such as T-cell mediated rejection or clear cell carcinoma [16,27]. Furthermore it is a strong predictor of survival in critically ill patients with acute kidney injury in plasma [9,16].

Recent studies suggest that circulating miRNAs in general might have biosignaling functions and are transported by microvesicles and/or proteins [12,28,29]. Therefore we hypothesized that a dialysis procedure could remove miRNAs at least partially from blood, which lead to altered circulating levels of these small ribonucleotides of the circulation. This might have biological consequences. Surprisingly, we could not find a significant alteration of miRNAs in plasma after passing the dialysis filters. This leads to the conclusion that dialysis therapy does not deplete patient's blood of possibly biologically active miRNAs in the circulation. However, small amounts of miRNAs were detectable in the ultrafiltrate as well as in spent dialysate

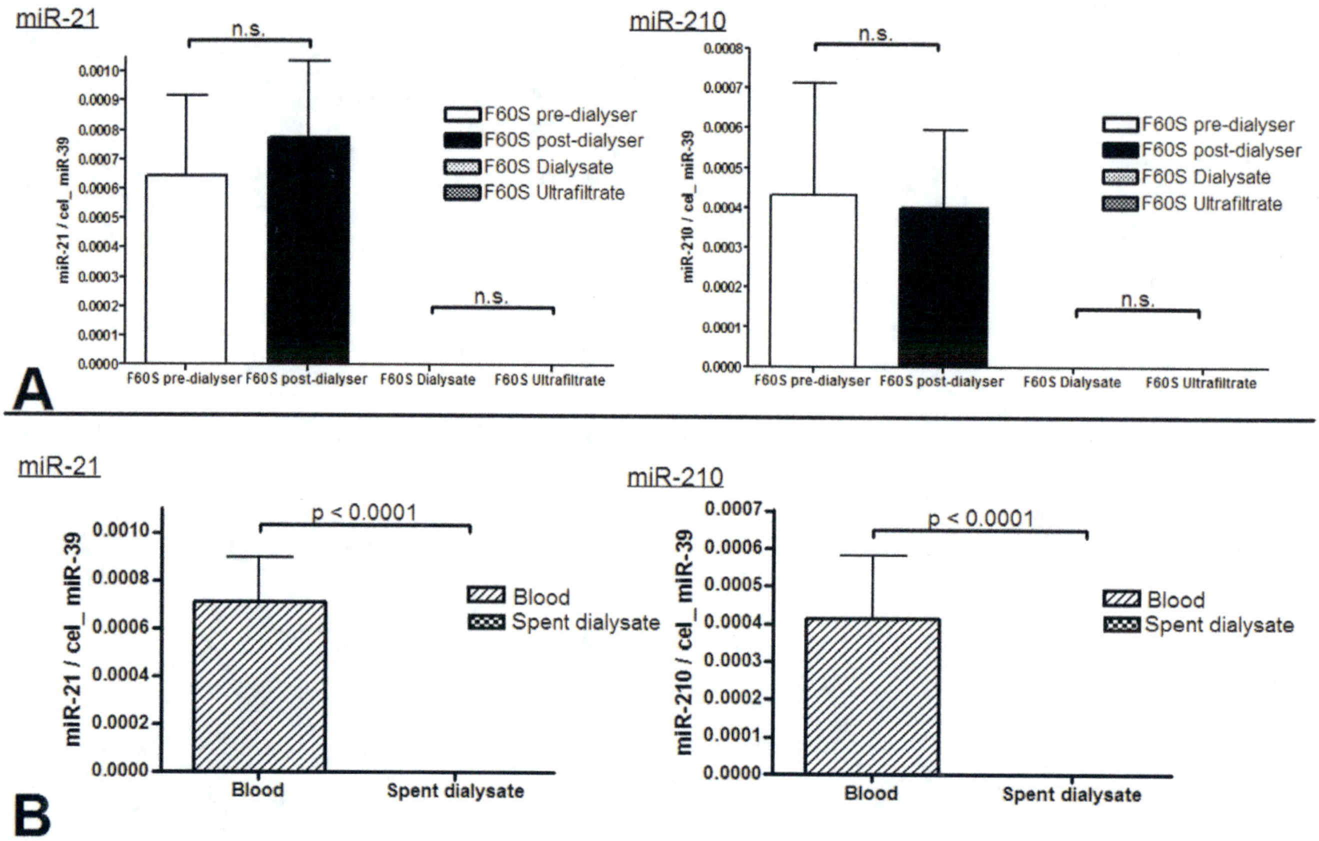

Figure 2. Levels of circulating miR-21 and -210 in different sample types with the F60S dialysate filter. Ten independent dialysis sessions in eight different patients were analyzed for the F60S filter system. MiR-21 and miR-210 levels are not significantly different between pre-dialyser and corresponding post-dialyser blood lines (miR-21: $p = 0.35$; miR-210: $p = 0.91$). Also the difference between spent dialysate and ultrafiltrate is not of statistical significance (miR-21: $p = 0.80$; miR-210: $p = 0.74$). However, averaged values of blood side versus spent dialysate reached high statistical significance for both microRNAs with p-values of <0.0001. Data are represented as mean and standard error of the mean.

suggesting that a small portion of miRNAs in the blood is transported by very small structures or as a free unbound form.

There are several possibilities of stabilizing circulating miRNAs in the blood; two main transporter systems have been identified. MiRNAs are transported in microvesicles and/or exosomes, apoptotic bodies and other microparticles [30]. In addition miRNAs are transported by non-vesicle associated protein and lipoprotein complexes [13]. Turchinovich et al. showed that the majority of circulating miRNAs are bound to a molecular family called argonaute proteins [31]. Especially Ago 2, a 97 kDa member of the RNA-induced silencing complex (RISC), is the most frequent miRNA carrier [32]. Furthermore, this group suggests that other transport forms such as exosomes may play only a minor role and more than 97% of the miRNAs are not exosome-associated [31]. However our study only permits the conclusion that miRNAs must be mainly transported by RNA-binding proteins (>30–40 kDa), microvesicles and/or other structures larger than 30–40 kDa.

Previous studies demonstrated unbound/naked miRNAs not to be protected against the endogenous RNAses in the extracellular fluids and may therefore be very unstable [13]. That makes it implausible that the detectable traces of miR-21 and -210 in ultrafiltrate and dialysate are not accompanied by stabilizing factors. Recent investigations describe two RNA-binding proteins that possibly could be candidates for this passage, namely nucleophosmin 1 (NPM 1) and dead end 1 (Dnd 1) [33]. As shown in figure 4 NPM 1 and Dnd 1 are the only known miRNA-carriers which are small enough to permeate at least the EMiC2 filter. Here it should be noted that filter-characteristics depend on pressure differences between the blood and effluent circuit. Because of this slight pressure dependent shift of the sieving coefficient curves towards a little higher molecular weight cut offs, it could be possible that very small exosomes might pass the dialyser as well. All other known transport forms such as Low and High density protein (LDL/HDL), microvesicles or even Ago 2 are too large to penetrate the membrane effectively. Thus, these structures are likely the major transporters of miRNAs. A recent study in chronic hemodialysis patients suggested that levels of miR-499 are in fact eliminated by hemodialysis [34]. This finding thus runs contradictory to the results presented here. In order for miRNAs to be eliminated by hemodialysis they have to be either bound to very small molecules or circulate unbound in blood. The study by Mitchell and coworkers suggests that "naked" (i.e. unbound) miRNAs are degraded within less than 2 minutes after addition to human plasma [11]. In addition, as figure 4 suggests only Dndl or NPMl are able to pass the EMIC2 filter system. Based on this we do not believe that circulating miRNAs can be altered by the hemodialysis procedure. Thus, an alteration of miR-499 levels in chronic hemodialyis patients might rather be due to other factors (i.e. degradation). However, different miRNAs have been shown to be transported by varying means [35]. The mirRNA let-7a was shown to be mainly detected in microvesicles,

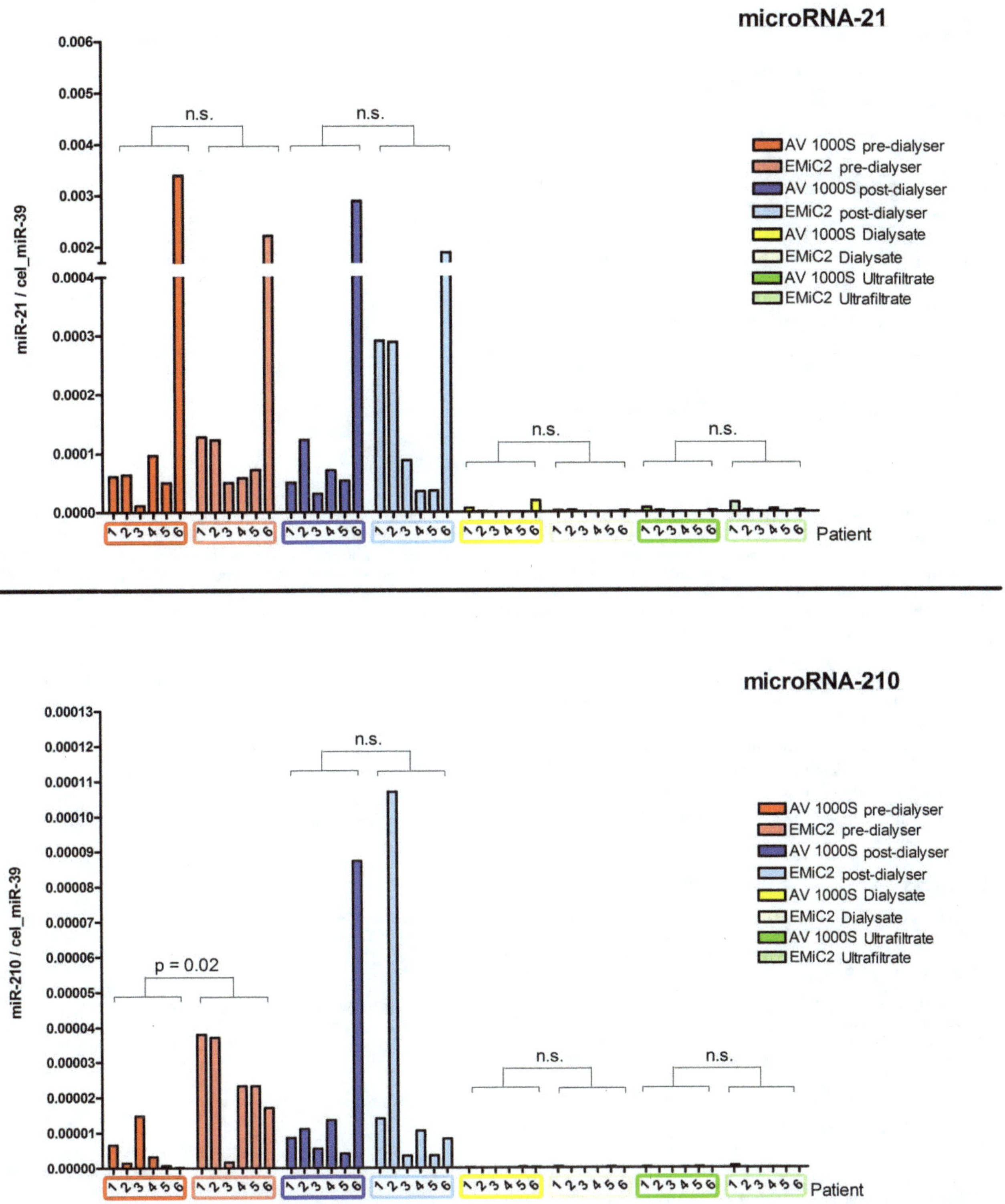

Figure 3. Comparison of influence of two different filter properties on circulating microRNA levels. Six patients received at least one dialysis session with each of the two filter systems AV 1000 S and EMiC 2. Circulating levels of miR-21 and -210 were not differently altered by the two different dialyser properties. (miR-21: AV1000S pre-dialyser vs. EMiC 2 predialyser $p = 0.59$, post-dialyser $p = 0.70$, dialysate $p = 0.94$, ultrafiltrate $p = 0.39$; miR-210: pre-dialyser $p = 0.02$, post-dialyser $p = 0.82$, dialysate $p = 0.59$, ultrafiltrate $p = 0.31$) Only pre-dialyser line showed a significant alteration, which is not of relevance for our main conclusion. Data are represented as mean and standard error of the mean.

while others were associated with Ago2 (e.g. miR-16 and miR-92a) [35]. Thus, miRNA packaging into microvesicles or RNA binding proteins likely follows a cell type-specific expression and/or release pattern. It is therefore conceivable that miR-499 is subjected to different kinetics. In pre-dialysis patients with chronic kidney disease the levels of circulating miRNAs have been shown to be

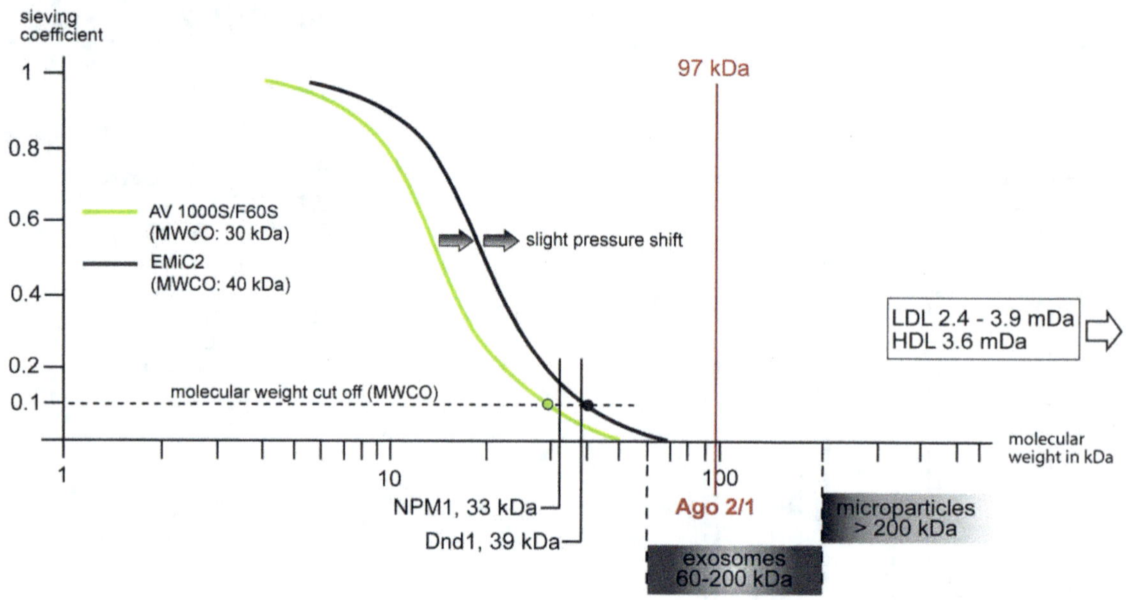

Figure 4. Filter-characteristics and potential microRNA carriers. The figure shows the filter properties characterized by their sieving coefficients depending on the molecular weight of the possibly passing molecules. Sieving coefficient is the ratio between passing and retained mass of molecules of a defined molecular weight. Molecular weight cut off (MWCO) is a special indicator to describe filter-characteristic. It characterizes the weight of molecules which are ~ 90% retained and therefore negligibly passing the filter. A slight pressure dependent shift towards higher MWCOs is possible. Furthermore there are marked various known microRNA carriers with their molecular weight. NPM1, Nucleophosmin 1; Dnd1, Dead end 1; Ago2/1, Argonaute protein 2/1; LDL, Low density protein; HDL, High density protein.

reduced suggesting altered miRNAs kinetics depending on renal function [36]. However, our results suggest that the hemodialysis technique as such does not influence levels of circulating miRNAs.

Based on our results we concluded, that: (I) miRNAs are likely to be carried and stabilized by larger structures (e.g. RNA-binding proteins and or microvesicles) (II) These structures must have a molecular weight not less than 30 respectively 40 kDa and (III) a small but detectable amount of miRNAs is carried in smaller structures with a kDa of less than 30 or is freely available in the blood.

Author Contributions

Conceived and designed the experiments: FM JL JTK TT. Performed the experiments: FM JL JS MS MB. Analyzed the data: FM JL JTK TT. Contributed reagents/materials/analysis tools: YG. Wrote the paper: FM JL JTK TT.

References

1. Bartel DP. (2004) MicroRNAs: Genomics, biogenesis, mechanism, and function. Cell 116(2): 281–297.
2. Delaloy C, Liu L, Lee JA, Su H, Shen F, et al. (2010) MicroRNA-9 coordinates proliferation and migration of human embryonic stem cell-derived neural progenitors. Cell Stem Cell 6(4): 323–335.
3. Zhao X, He X, Han X, Yu Y, Ye F, et al. (2010) MicroRNA-mediated control of oligodendrocyte differentiation. Neuron 65(5): 612–626.
4. Xiong Y, Fang JH, Yun JP, Yang J, Zhang Y, et al. (2010) Effects of microRNA-29 on apoptosis, tumorigenicity, and prognosis of hepatocellular carcinoma. Hepatology 51(3): 836–845.
5. Sayed D, Abdellatif M. (2011) MicroRNAs in development and disease. Physiol Rev 91(3): 827–887.
6. Thum T, Galuppo P, Wolf C, Fiedler J, Kneitz S, et al. (2007) MicroRNAs in the human heart: A clue to fetal gene reprogramming in heart failure. Circulation 116(3): 258–267.
7. van Rooij E, Sutherland LB, Thatcher JE, DiMaio JM, Naseem RH, et al. (2008) Dysregulation of microRNAs after myocardial infarction reveals a role of miR-29 in cardiac fibrosis. Proc Natl Acad Sci U S A 105(35): 13027–13032.
8. Thum T, Gross C, Fiedler J, Fischer T, Kissler S, et al. (2008) MicroRNA-21 contributes to myocardial disease by stimulating MAP kinase signalling in fibroblasts. Nature 456(7224): 980–984.
9. Lorenzen JM, Kielstein JT, Hafer C, Gupta SK, Kumpers P, et al. (2011) Circulating miR-210 predicts survival in critically ill patients with acute kidney injury. Clin J Am Soc Nephrol 6(7): 1540–1546.
10. Volinia S, Galasso M, Costinean S, Tagliavini L, Gamberoni G, et al. (2010) Reprogramming of miRNA networks in cancer and leukemia. Genome Res 20(5): 589–599.
11. Mitchell PS, Parkin RK, Kroh EM, Fritz BR, Wyman SK, et al. (2008) Circulating microRNAs as stable blood-based markers for cancer detection. Proc Natl Acad Sci U S A 105(30): 10513–10518.
12. Zampetaki A, Kiechl S, Drozdov I, Willeit P, Mayr U, et al. (2010) Plasma microRNA profiling reveals loss of endothelial miR-126 and other microRNAs in type 2 diabetes. Circ Res 107(6): 810–817.
13. Zampetaki A, Willeit P, Drozdov I, Kiechl S, Mayr M. (2011) PROFILING OF CIRCULATING MICRORNAs: FROM SINGLE BIOMARKERS TO RE-WIRED NETWORKS. Cardiovasc Res Nov 9.; Epub ahead of print.
14. Lorenzen JM, Broll M, Kaever V, Burhenne H, Hafer C, et al. (2012) Pharmacokinetics of Ampicillin/Sulbactam in critically ill patients with acute kidney injury undergoing extended dialysis. Clin J Am Soc Nephrol 7(3): 385–390.
15. Fliser D, Kielstein JT (2006) Technology insight: Treatment of renal failure in the intensive care unit with extended dialysis. Nat Clin Pract Nephrol 2(1): 32–39.
16. Lorenzen JM, Volkmann I, Fiedler J, Schmidt M, Scheffner I, et al. (2011) Urinary miR-210 as a mediator of acute T-cell mediated rejection in renal allograft recipients. Am J Transplant 11(10): 2221–2227.
17. Nana-Sinkam SP, Croce CM (2011) Non-coding RNAs in cancer initiation and progression and as novel biomarkers. Mol Oncol 5(6): 483–491.
18. Kumarswamy R, Volkmann I, Thum T (2011) Regulation and function of miRNA-21 in health and disease. RNA Biol 8(5).
19. Shen J, Todd NW, Zhang H, Yu L, Lingxiao X, et al. (2011) Plasma microRNAs as potential biomarkers for non-small-cell lung cancer. Lab Invest 91(4): 579–587.
20. Zaman MS, Shahryari V, Deng G, Thamminana S, Saini S, et al. (2012) Up-regulation of MicroRNA-21 correlates with lower kidney cancer survival. PLoS One 7(2): e31060.
21. Liu G, Friggeri A, Yang Y, Milosevic J, Ding Q, et al. (2010) miR-21 mediates fibrogenic activation of pulmonary fibroblasts and lung fibrosis. J Exp Med 207(8): 1589–1597.

22. Chau BN, Xin C, Hartner J, Ren S, Castano AP, et al. (2012) MicroRNA-21 promotes fibrosis of the kidney by silencing metabolic pathways. Sci Transl Med 4(121): 121ra18.
23. Zarjou A, Yang S, Abraham E, Agarwal A, Liu G (2011) Identification of a microRNA signature in renal fibrosis: Role of miR-21. Am J Physiol Renal Physiol 301(4): F793–801.
24. Wu H, Neilson JR, Kumar P, Manocha M, Shankar P, et al. (2007) miRNA profiling of naive, effector and memory CD8 T cells. PLoS One 2(10): e1020.
25. van der Fits L, van Kester MS, Qin Y, Out-Luiting JJ, Smit F, et al. (2011) MicroRNA-21 expression in CD4+ T cells is regulated by STAT3 and is pathologically involved in sezary syndrome. J Invest Dermatol 131(3): 762–768.
26. Bihrer V, Waidmann O, Friedrich-Rust M, Forestier N, Susser S, et al. (2011) Serum microRNA-21 as marker for necroinflammation in hepatitis C patients with and without hepatocellular carcinoma. PLoS One 6(10): e26971.
27. Valera VA, Walter BA, Linehan WM, Merino MJ. (2011) Regulatory effects of microRNA-92 (miR-92) on VHL gene expression and the hypoxic activation of miR-210 in clear cell renal cell carcinoma. J Cancer 2: 515–526.
28. Taylor DD, Zacharias W, Gercel-Taylor C. (2011) Exosome isolation for proteomic analyses and RNA profiling. Methods Mol Biol 728: 235–246.
29. Bhattacharyya SN, Habermacher R, Martine U, Closs EI, Filipowicz W (2006) Relief of microRNA-mediated translational repression in human cells subjected to stress. Cell 125(6): 1111–1124.
30. Gupta SK, Bang C, Thum T. (2010) Circulating microRNAs as biomarkers and potential paracrine mediators of cardiovascular disease. Circ Cardiovasc Genet 3(5): 484–488.
31. Turchinovich A, Weiz L, Langheinz A, Burwinkel B (2011) Characterization of extracellular circulating microRNA. Nucleic Acids Res 39(16): 7223–7233.
32. Arroyo JD, Chevillet JR, Kroh EM, Ruf IK, Pritchard CC, et al. (2011) Argonaute2 complexes carry a population of circulating microRNAs independent of vesicles in human plasma. Proc Natl Acad Sci U S A 108(12): 5003–5008.
33. McDonald JS, Milosevic D, Reddi HV, Grebe SK, Algeciras-Schimnich A (2011) Analysis of circulating microRNA: Preanalytical and analytical challenges. Clin Chem 57(6): 833–840.
34. Emilian C, Goretti E, Prospert F, Pouthier D, Duhoux P, et al. (2012) MicroRNAs in Patients on Chronic Hemodialysis (MINOS Study). Clin J Am Soc Nephrol. 7(4): 619–23.
35. Lorenzen JM, Thum T (2012) Circulating and urinary microRNAs in kidney disease. Clin J Am Soc Nephrol. in press.
36. Neal CS, Michael MZ, Pimlott LK, Yong TY, Li JY, et al. (2011) Circulating microRNA expression is reduced in chronic kidney disease. Nephrol Dial Transplant. 26(11): 3794–802.

10

Novel Evolved Immunoglobulin (Ig)-Binding Molecules Enhance the Detection of IgM against Hepatitis C Virus

Jie Cao[1], Qiuli Chen[1], Huaqun Zhang[1], Peipei Qi[1], Chao Liu[1], Xufang Yang[1], Niansong Wang[2,3], Baohua Qian[4], Jinhong Wang[1], Shaohua Jiang[1,5], Hua Yang[1,6], Shuhan Sun[7], Wei Pan[1]*

1 Department of Microbiology, Shanghai Key Laboratory of Medical Biodefense, Second Military Medical University, Shanghai, China, **2** Department of Nephrology, Zhongshan Hospital, Fudan University, Shanghai, China, **3** Department of Nephrology, Shanghai Sixth People's Hospital, Shanghai Jiao Tong University, Shanghai, China, **4** Department of Blood Transfusion, Changhai Hospital, Second Military Medical University, Shanghai, China, **5** Department of Cardiothoracic Surgery, The Military General Hospital of Tibet PLA, Lasa, China, **6** Shanghai Key Laboratory of Tuberculosis, Shanghai Pulmonary Hospital, Tongji University School of Medicine, Shanghai, China, **7** Department of Medical Genetics, Second Military Medical University, Shanghai, China

Abstract

Detection of specific antibodies against hepatitis C virus (HCV) is the most widely available test for viral diagnosis and monitoring of HCV infections. However, narrowing the serologic window of anti-HCV detection by enhancing anti-HCV IgM detection has remained to be a problem. Herein, we used LD5, a novel evolved immunoglobulin-binding molecule (NEIBM) with a high affinity for IgM, to develop a new anti-HCV enzyme-linked immunosorbent assay (ELISA) using horseradish peroxidase-labeled LD5 (HRP-LD5) as the conjugated enzyme complex. The HRP-LD5 assay showed detection efficacy that is comparable with two kinds of domestic diagnostic kits and the Abbott 3.0 kit when tested against the national reference panel. Moreover, the HRP-LD5 assay showed a higher detection rate (55.9%, 95% confidence intervals (95% CI) 0.489, 0.629) than that of a domestic diagnostic ELISA kit (Chang Zheng) (53.3%, 95% CI 0.463, 0.603) in 195 hemodialysis patient serum samples. Five serum samples that were positive using the HRP-LD5 assay and negative with the conventional anti-HCV diagnostic ELISA kits were all positive for HCV RNA, and 4 of them had detectable antibodies when tested with the established anti-HCV IgM assay. An IgM confirmation study revealed the IgM reaction nature of these five serum samples. These results demonstrate that HRP-LD5 improved anti-HCV detection by enhancing the detection of anti-HCV IgM, which may have potential value for the early diagnosis and screening of hepatitis C and other infectious diseases.

Editor: John E. Tavis, Saint Louis University, United States of America

Funding: This study was funded by the National Natural Science Foundation of China (NSFC) [Grant numbers 30872405, 30872246, 30972632 and 30972799], Shanghai Committee of Science and Technology [05dz19317], National High Biotechnology Development Program of China [2006AA02A238], the Chinese National Key Special Project for the Prevention and Control of Major Infectious Diseases [2009ZX10004-105] and the Chinese National Key Special Project for Major New Drug Discovery [2011ZX09506-001]. The funders had no role in study design, data collection and analysis, decision to publish, or preparation of the manuscript.

Competing Interests: The authors have declared that no competing interests exist.

* E-mail: pwpanwei@yahoo.com.cn

Introduction

Serologic determination of specific antibodies against hepatitis C virus (HCV) and detection of viral RNA are the most widely available tests for viral diagnosis and monitoring of HCV infection. Since the cloning of HCV in 1989 [1], several generations of anti-HCV enzyme immunoassay (EIA) have been developed [2–4]. The sensitivity of the third-generation EIA was greater than 98%, a significant improvement over the approximately 80% sensitivity of the first-generation EIA, and the average seroconversion period of 10 to 16 weeks using first-generation EIA was shortened to approximately 8 weeks [3–7]. This improvement was mostly attributed to the addition of HCV coating antigens, core proteins (c22–3), NS3 (c33c) and NS5 to the NS4 protein (c100–3) used in the first-generation EIA.

However, this 8 weeks serologic window of anti-HCV detection remains to be a problem for early viral diagnosis and efficient screening of blood donors. It is difficult to narrow the serologic window significantly by adding new HCV coating antigens. In an individual's response against virus infection, immunoglobulin M (IgM) antibodies appear first within the first week. Therefore, it should be possible to narrow the serologic window of anti-HCV detection by enhancing the anti-HCV IgM detection.

Novel evolved immunoglobulin-binding molecules (NEIBMs), characterized by MDPL-MDPA (MDPL, mono-domain of protein L; MDPA, mono-domain of protein A), have been generated by *in vitro* molecular evolution [8,9]. These proteins have been shown to simultaneously bind to κ light chains and V_H3 heavy chains of immunoglobulin and have shown high affinity for IgM in addition to IgG. In this study, we developed a new anti-HCV enzyme-linked immunosorbent assay (ELISA) by using horseradish peroxidase-labeled LD5 (HRP-LD5), a NEIBM, as the conjugated enzyme complex. Comparison studies using Chinese hemodialysis samples demonstrated that HRP-LD5 based assay can improve anti-HCV detection because of its enhanced anti-HCV IgM detection efficacy.

Materials and Methods

Ethics statement

All aspects of the study were approved by the Shanghai Society of Medical Ethics, China and the Changhai Hospital Ethics

Committee affiliated to the Second Military Medical University, China. Written informed consent was obtained from all participants in the study.

Serum samples

A total of 195 hemodialysis patient serum samples were obtained from the hemodialysis room of Zhongshan Hospital of Fudan University (Shanghai, China; 1997). All samples were aliquoted upon receipt and stored at −20°C. The national reference panel for anti-HCV (Lot No. 0501) was from the National Institute for the Pharmaceutical and Biological Products of China and consists of 30 anti-HCV-positive human plasma samples and 30 HCV-negative serum samples that have been solvent-detergent treated. Two hundred serum specimens from healthy blood donors (Changhai Hospital, Second Military Medical University, Shanghai, China) were used to establish a cut-off value for the new diagnostic method.

Novel evolved immunoglobulin-binding molecule

The novel evolved immunoglobulin-binding molecule (NEIBM) LD5 (B3-D-B3-D-B3) was previously generated with the characteristic structure of alternately arranged *Finegoldia magna* protein L B3 domains (B3) and staphylococcal protein A (SpA) D domains (D). LD5 showed substantially higher affinity for IgG-F(ab')2, IgM, and IgA than did either 4L (B3-B3-B3-B3) or SpA, which creates synergistic double-site binding sites to the V_H3 and V_k regions of the fragment of antigen binding [8].

Diagnostic ELISA kits and reagents

Anti-HCV diagnostic ELISA kits were purchased from Shanghai Chang Zheng Co. (China), Shanghai Ke Hua Bio-engineering Co., Ltd. (China) and Abbott Diagnostics (Abbott anti-HCV 3.0 kits, Chicago, IL, USA). Human IgG (hIgG), human IgM (hIgM), human IgA (hIgA), goat anti-human IgG, horseradish peroxidase (HRP), HRP-conjugated streptavidin, HRP-conjugated goat anti-human polyclonal polyvalent immunoglobulins (G, A, M) (HRP-goat anti-human PcAb), HRP-conjugated anti-hIgG and HRP-conjugated anti-hIgM were obtained from Sigma (St. Louis, MO, USA). hIgG, hIgM and hIgA antibodies were biotinylated using biotinyl-N-hydroxy-succinimide (Pierce, Rockford, IL, USA) in our lab (data not shown). β-mercaptoethanol (BME) was from Janssen Chimica (Geel, Belgium). Prokaryotic expressed SpA (Genbank: P02976) was kindly provided by Shanghai Fudan-Zhangjiang Bio-Pharmaceutical Co. Ltd. (Shanghai, China). HCV Nucleocapsid/NS3/NS4/NS5 recombinant proteins were from GenWay Biotech Inc. (CA, USA).

Biosensor analyses of LD5

The binding properties of LD5 to hIgG/hIgM/hIgA were studied by surface plasmon resonance (SPR) using a Biacore 3000 instrument (Biacore, Uppsala, Sweden). Briefly, 1 mg/ml hIgG, hIgM, or hIgA resuspended in 10 mM sodium acetate (1:5 diluted), pH 5.0, 4.5, or 4.0, was coupled to CM-5 sensor chips using amine-coupling chemistry. The association and dissociation were measured at a flow rate of 40 μl/min using NaCl/HEPES supplemented with 0.005% surfactant P20 as flow buffer. The sensor-chip surfaces were regenerated with 100 mM alanine-HCl (pH 2.5).

HRP labeling

HRP-labeled LD5 (HRP-LD5) was prepared by using sodium periodate according to the following procedure. Five milligrams of HRP was dissolved in 1 ml distilled water, and then 200 μl of a freshly prepared solution of 0.1 M sodium periodate was added. After stirring for 20 min in the dark, the above solution was dialyzed overnight against a 1 mM sodium acetate buffer (pH 4.4) at 4°C, then 1 ml of a 5 mg/ml LD5 in a phosphate-buffered saline (PBS) (pH 7.2) was added immediately after adding a 20 μl of a 0.2 M carbonate buffer (pH 9.5). After stirring gently for 2 h in the dark, 100 μl of a 4 mg/ml sodium borohydride solution was added, and the mixture was reacted for 3 h at 4°C. At the end of the reaction, the HRP-LD5 was dialyzed overnight against 0.15 M PBS (pH 7.4) at 4°C and stored at −40°C.

Detection of HRP-LD5 binding to Ig molecules by ELISA

hIgG, hIgM and hIgA molecules were diluted in a coating buffer (0.1 M $NaHCO_3$, pH 9.6) to make a 10 μg/ml solution and then coated onto a sterile 96-well microtiter plates at 37°C for 3 h. After blocking the plates with blocking buffer (10% degreased milk powder, 0.1% Tween 20 and 0.2% mercurothiolate in 0.01 M PBS) for at least 2 h, 100 μl of 1:2 serial dilutions of 1 mg/ml HRP-LD5 or HRP-goat anti-human PcAb were added to each well and incubated for 45 min at 37°C. Plates were developed by addition of 3, 3', 5, 5'-tetramethylbenzidine (TMB) (Sigma, St. Louis, MO, USA), and read at 450 nm with an ELISA Reader (Bio Rad).

Detection of anti-HCV antibody

For detection of anti-HCV using HRP-LD5, the immunoassay strips (Nunc, Rochester, NY, USA) were coated with 1.2 μg of each HCV Nucleocapsid/NS3/NS4/NS5 recombinant proteins diluted in carbonate buffer (pH 9.6). The strips were maintained at 37°C for 3 h and washed four times with a solution of PBS-Tween 20 (PBST) and blocked with blocking buffer as above. The strips were dried under reduced pressure for 2.5 h, and wrapped individually with aluminum foil under vacuumed conditions, which enable the precoated strips to be stored until use. Whenever a serum specimen was received and ready for the diagnostic test, a strip was removed from its wrapper and washed four times with PBST. Then 100 μl of a 10-fold dilution of the serum specimen, a blank, a positive and a negative reference serum sample were each added to a separate well. The strip was then placed in a 37°C incubator for 1 h. After washing four times with PBST, 100 μl of a 1,000-fold dilution of HRP-LD5 (1 mg/ml) was added to the strip and incubated for 45 min at 37°C. The strips were developed by addition of TMB and read at 450 nm in an ELISA Reader. The procedure for detection of anti-HCV IgG antibody was the same as above except for the addition of HRP-conjugated anti-hIgG instead of HRP-LD5. For anti-HCV IgM detection, goat anti-human IgG (1:10) was added to the serum and the detection was performed using HRP-conjugated anti-hIgM instead of HRP-LD5. The anti-HCV detection by the three ELISA kits (Abbott 3.0 from Chicago, USA and both Ke Hua and Chang Zheng from Shanghai, China) was performed according to the manufacturers' instructions.

Confirmation of anti-HCV IgM

100 μl of the serum samples (diluted 1:10 in PBS) were treated without or with β-mercaptoethanol (BME) at the concentration of 50 mM at 37°C for 30 min and then anti-HCV detection was performed as above using HRP-LD5 assay, anti-HCV IgM assay and Chang Zheng anti-HCV diagnostic ELISA kit.

Qualitative detection of HCV RNA

Reverse-transcriptase nested polymerase chain reaction (RT-PCR) was performed for HCV RNA qualitative detection [10].

The HCV RNA was extracted from serum as described previously [11]. The first-strand cDNA of the highly conserved 5'-end noncoding region [12] was synthesized by RT with an antisense primer (5'-CCGGTCGTCCTGGCAATTCCGG-3') and amplified by PCR with the same antisense primer and another sense primer (5'-GGCGACACTCCACCATAGATCAC-3'). All oligonucleotides were obtained from Shanghai Sangon Biological Engineering Technology & Services Co., Ltd. (China). The PCR conditions for 35 thermal cycles were 1 min at 94°C, 2 min at 42°C, and 2 min at 72°C, followed by a 5 min extension at 72°C (Perkin Elmer Applied Biosystems, Foster City, CA, USA). PCR products were analyzed by electrophoresis in a 1.2% agarose gel and detected by staining with ethidium bromide.

Statistical analyses

Statistical analysis between the detection rates by different diagnostic ELISA kits was performed by chi-square test. 95% confidence intervals (95% CI) are presented for the detection rates. A value of $P<0.05$ was considered statistically significant.

Results

NEIBM LD5 has significantly enhanced affinity for IgM

Our previous ELISA results had shown that LD5 molecules had much stronger binding to human immunoglobulins (Igs) than SpA [8]. In this study, binding properties of LD5 for human IgM, IgA and IgG were further detected by SPR (Table 1). LD5 showed high affinity for hIgG with an equilibrium dissociation constant (K_D) of 0.89 nM. Moreover, the affinity of LD5 binding to hIgM, with a K_D of 0.31 nM, was higher than that binding to hIgG and reached the level of the binding of SpA with the hIgG. LD5 also showed weak binding to hIgA (Table 1).

Binding properties of HRP-LD5 to human Igs

The LD5 conjugate HRP-LD5 was produced to compare its human Igs binding properties with the binding of HRP-goat anti-human PcAb, which is routinely used in most commercial anti-HCV diagnostic ELISA kits. ELISA results showed that HRP-LD5 had a much stronger binding reaction with hIgM and hIgA than did HRP-goat anti-human PcAb, and had similar binding to hIgG compared with HRP-goat anti-human PcAb (Fig. 1).

Table 1. Kinetic constants of the LD5 and SpA binding to three types of human Igs[1].

Analyte	Constant	Ligand		
		hIgG	**hIgM**	**hIgA**
LD5	$k_a(M^{-1}s^{-1})$	$(1.22\pm0.06)\times10^5$	$(7.23\pm0.07)\times10^4$	$(3.24\pm0.04)\times10^4$
	$k_d(s^{-1})$	$(1.08\pm0.05)\times10^{-4}$	$(2.21\pm0.05)\times10^{-5}$	$(9.44\pm0.11)\times10^{-5}$
	K_D(nM)	0.89 ± 0.003	0.31 ± 0.01	2.91 ± 0.07
SpA	$k_a(M^{-1}s^{-1})$	$(1.54\pm0.12)\times10^5$	$(1.15\pm0.13)\times10^5$	$(4.16\pm0.23)\times10^5$
	$k_d(s^{-1})$	$(4.40\pm0.31)\times10^{-5}$	$(8.17\pm0.13)\times10^{-4}$	$(2.92\pm0.08)\times10^{-3}$
	K_D(nM)	0.29 ± 0.01	7.15 ± 0.67	7.03 ± 0.22

[1]Binding experiments were performed by surface plasmon resonance with serial 1:2 dilutions of LD5 and SpA from 1.25 and 0.8 μM for binding to hIgA, hIgG and hIgM. k_a, association rate constants; k_d, dissociation rate constants; K_D, equilibrium dissociation constants. Data shown are averages ± standard deviation of three independent experiments.

HRP-LD5 based EIA enhance the detection of anti-HCV IgM

An anti-HCV ELISA assay was established using HRP-LD5 as conjugate and 200 serum specimens from healthy blood donors were tested to establish a cut-off value for this assay. The A_{450} values ranged from 0.017 to 0.093 (0.062±0.023). Therefore, 0.200, the average plus 6-fold of the standard deviation value, was chosen to distinguish positive from negative tests. This assay was compared with two kinds of domestic diagnostic kits (Chang Zheng and Ke Hua) and the Abbott 3.0 kit against the national reference panel (Lot No. 0501) (Table 2). All 30 HCV-positive reference serum samples were detected as positive with the HRP-LD5 assay and with the Abbott 3.0 kit, whereas one was not positive, according to the two domestic kit assays. All 30 HCV-negative reference serum samples were negative in the domestic kit assays, whereas one was detected as positive in Abbott 3.0 kit and HRP-LD5 assays (Table 2). The relative sensitivity and specificity of detection of the HRP-LD5 based assay and the domestic diagnostic kits and Abbott 3.0 kit were above 96%, which is the national standard for batch production quality control.

To test the detection efficacy of the HRP-LD5 based assay, we did a comparison study in an HCV high-risk population, hemodialysis patients. We also established an anti-HCV IgG assay and an anti-HCV IgM assay as reference tests. The cut-off value of the anti-HCV IgG and anti-HCV IgM ELISA were determined as above, and were 0.015 and 0.200 respectively. Serum samples from 195 hemodialysis patients were measured using the HRP-LD5 based assay, anti-HCV diagnostic ELISA kit (Chang Zheng), the established anti-HCV IgG assay and anti-HCV IgM assay (Fig. 2, Table 3). The results showed that the HRP-LD5 assay had a statistically higher positive detection rate (55.9% (109/195), 95% CI 0.489, 0.629) than that of a domestic diagnostic ELISA kit (Chang Zheng) (53.3% (104/195), 95% CI 0.463, 0.603) (P-value<0.05), and 108 were positive according to the anti-HCV IgG assay or the anti-HCV IgM assay. Interestingly, 104 samples that were positive using the anti-HCV IgG assay were scored as being positive by both the HRP-LD5-based assay and the Chang Zheng kit, and 33 were positive based on the anti-HCV IgM assay. The five serum samples which were positive by HRP-LD5 based assay and negative by Chang Zheng kit were also not detectable by the Abbott 3.0 kit (data not shown). All of the five positive for HRP-LD5 were positive for HCV RNA by RT-PCR (data not shown). However, only four of the samples that produced a false negative by the Chang Zheng kit were positive in the established anti-HCV IgM assay. The serum samples of the five patients that were false negative by the Chang Zheng kit were collected again 3 weeks later and were positive according to the Chang Zheng kit (Table 4) and the Abbott 3.0 kit (data not shown).

To further verify that these five serum samples positive in the HRP-LD5 based assay were due to specific anti-HCV IgM, the IgM confirmation test for these samples and the samples from the same patients three weeks later were performed. The A_{450} values of all five original samples were negative when the samples were treated with BME to destroy IgM (Table 4). The A_{450} values of second set of samples dramatically decreased when measured with both the HRP-LD5-based assay and the Chang Zheng kit when the samples were treated with BME, and these decreases corresponded well to the destruction of IgM as demonstrated by IgM detection assay (Table 4). These results demonstrated that the higher anti-HCV sensitivity of the HRP-LD5 based assay was due to enhanced IgM detection.

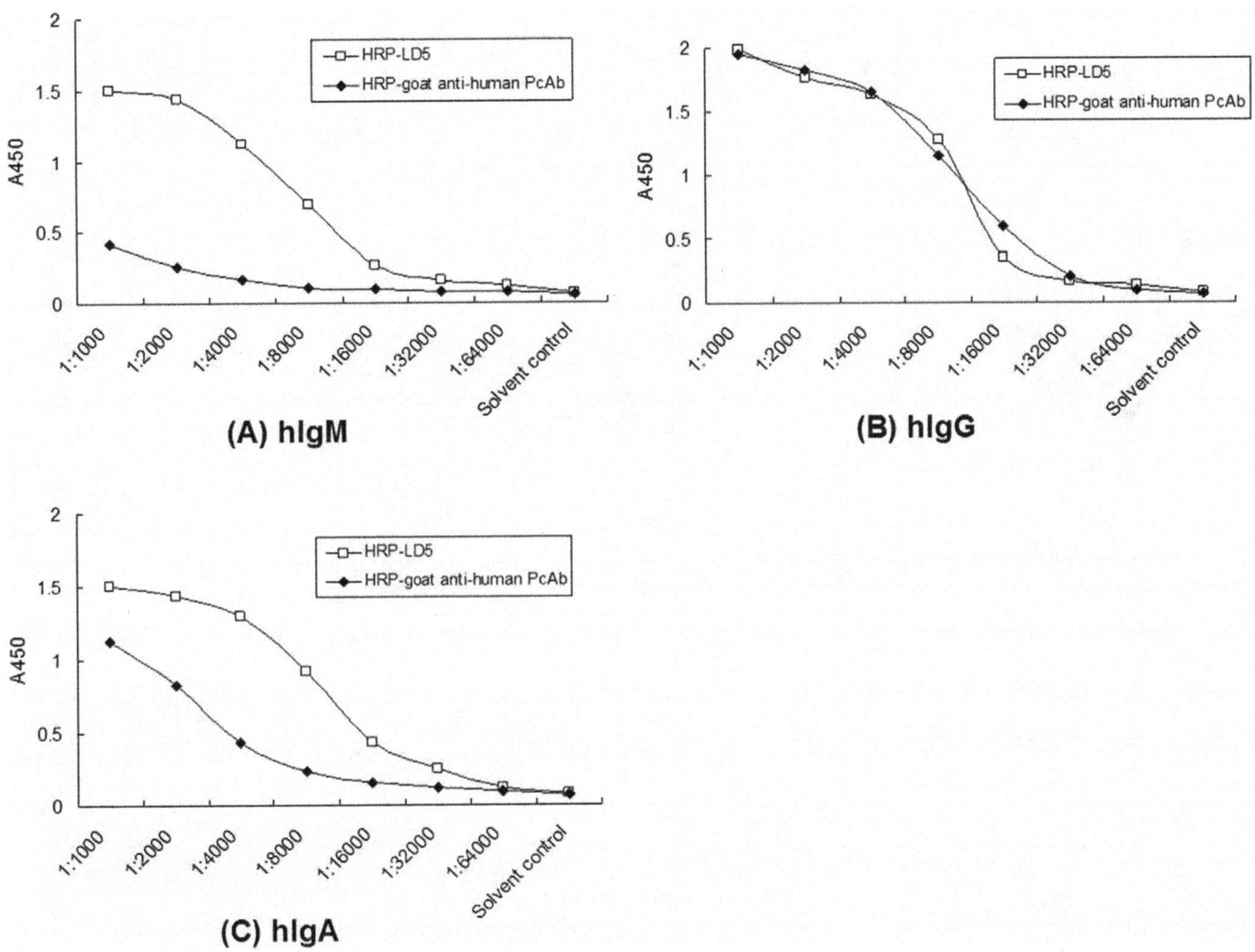

Figure 1. The enzyme-labeled LD5 exhibits enhanced binding activities for IgM and IgA. The binding activities of horseradish peroxidase (HRP)-labeled LD5 (HRP-LD5) or HRP-conjugated goat anti-human polyclonal antibodies (HRP-goat anti-human PcAb) to coated hIgM (A), hIgG (B) or hIgA (C) were examined by ELISA. The coating buffer was used as solvent control.

Discussion

The serologic window between HCV infection and the detection of specific antibodies varies from patient to patient. With current assays, seroconversion occurs on average between 7 and 8 weeks after onset of an infection [13–15]. About 30% to 50% of patients have undetectable anti-HCV antibodies at the onset of clinical symptoms [16]. It is widely accepted that IgM provides a first line of defense during microbial infections and IgM detection has proven valuable for early diagnosis of many viral infections [17]. Therefore, it is predicted that improved IgM detection by an anti-HCV EIA assay may narrow this serologic window.

The IgM detection efficacy of current anti-HCV assays using monoclonal or polyclonal HRP-labeled anti-human Ig antibodies as conjugates has not been evaluated. In this study, we used a NEIBM, LD5 which showed high affinity for IgM in addition to

Table 2. Comparison of anti-HCV detection against the national reference panel of HRP-LD5 assay with three commercial diagnostic kits.

HRP-conjugated molecules	True positive(a)	False negative(b)	True negative(c)	False positive (d)	Sensitivity(%) a/(a+b) (95% CI)[1]	Specificity(%) c/(c+d) (95% CI)[1]	Relative accuracy (%) (a+c)/(a+b+c+d)
Abbott 3.0 kit	30	0	29	1	100 (0.88–1.00)	96.66 (0.83–1.00)	98.33
Ke Hua kit	29	1	30	0	96.66 (0.83–1.00)	100 (0.88–1.00)	98.33
Chang Zheng kit	29	1	30	0	96.66 (0.83–1.00)	100 (0.88–1.00)	98.33
HRP-LD5 assay	30	0	29	1	100 (0.88–1.00)	96.66 (0.83–1.00)	98.33

[1]95% CI, 95% confidence interval.

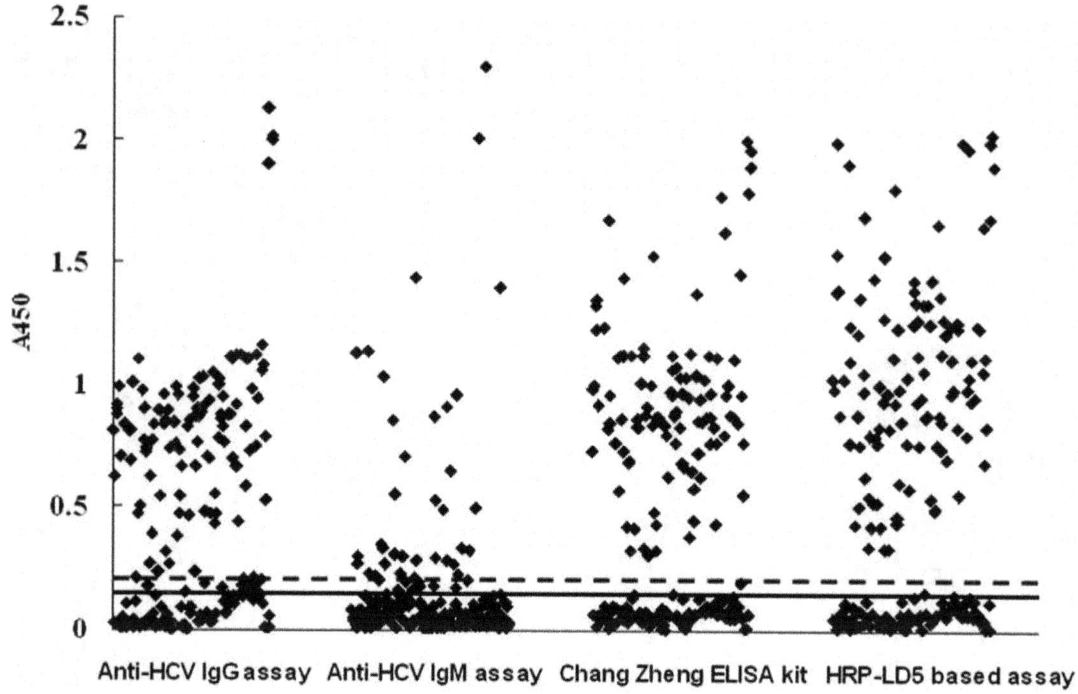

Figure 2. Anti-HCV detection in 195 serum specimens from hemodialysis patients by different ELISA assays. ◆, A_{450} values, with ELISA cut-off values of either 0.150 indicated in solid line (established anti-HCV IgG assay and Chang Zheng anti-HCV diagnostic ELISA kit) or 0.200 indicated in dotted line (established anti-HCV IgM assay and HRP-LD5 based assay).

IgG (Table 1) [8], to make conjugates, HRP-LD5. The HRP-LD5 also expressed a much stronger binding capacity to hIgM than did HRP-goat anti-human PcAb (Fig. 1). Consistently, the established HRP-LD5-based anti-HCV assay showed a higher detection rate than that of the commercial diagnostic kit (Chang Zheng) in hemodialysis patients (Table 3, Fig. 2), and it was attributed to the enhanced IgM detection (Table 3, Table 4).

Hemodialysis patients are a high-risk population for HCV infection. The anti-HCV prevalence seen in these patients varied from 3.3% in New Zealand [18], 39% in South America [19], 44%–60% in Far-Eastern countries [20] to as high as 80.0% in Egypt [21]. HCV is highly transmissible among these patients, and HCV infections at many different stages, including recent infections, are observed in this population. Therefore, a comparison study was conducted among them. Our results showed that the HRP-LD5 based anti-HCV assay had a statistical significant higher detection efficacy (55.9% positive detection rate) than did the domestic diagnostic kit (Chang Zheng) (positive detection rate

Table 3. Comparison of anti-HCV antibody detection in serum samples from 195 hemodialysis patients of HRP-LD5 based assay with Chang Zheng anti-HCV kit.

The established anti-HCV IgG assay or IgM assay		Chang Zheng kit		HRP-LD5 assay	
		+	−	+	−
IgG(+) or gM(+)[1]	108(55.4%)	104(53.3%)	4 (2.1%)	108(55.4%)	0
95% CI[2]	0.484–0.624	463–0.603	0.001–0.041	0.484–0.624	
IgG(+), IgM(+)[1]	33(16.9%)	33(16.9%)	0	33(16.9%)	0
95% CI[2]	0.116–0.222	0.116–0.222		0.116–0.222	
IgG(+), IgM(−)[1]	71(36.4%)	71(36.4%)	0	71(36.4%)	0
95% CI[2]	0.296–0.432	0.296–0.432		0.296–0.432	
IgG(−), IgM(+)[1]	4(2.1%)	0	0	4(2.1%)	0
95% CI[2]	0.001–0.041			0.001–0.041	
IgG(−), IgM(−)[1]	87(44.6%)	0	87(44.6%)	1(0.5%)	86(44.1%)
95% CI[2]	0.376–0.516		0.376–0.516	−0.005–0.015	0.371–0.511
Total samples	195	104	91	109	86

[1]Data shown are the number of cases with each test result. Data shown in parentheses are the percentages of detected cases in the 195 total serum samples.
[2]95% CI, 95% confidence interval.

Table 4. IgM confirmation detection of five cases of HRP-LD5 assay positive alone serum samples*.

No. of individual serum	First collected samples						Second collected samples (after three weeks)					
	Chang Zheng kit		HRP-LD5 based assay		anti-HCV IgM assay		Chang Zheng kit		HRP-LD5 based assay		anti-HCV IgM assay	
	BME		BME		BME		BME		BME		BME	
	−	+	−	+	−	+	−	+	−	+	−	+
1	0.110	0.078	0.433	0.054	0.216	0.048	0.503	0.258	1.354	0.372	1.121	0.053
2	0.178	0.060	0.358	0.047	0.187	0.064	0.280	0.263	0.957	0.675	0.565	0.042
3	0.021	0.045	0.465	0.049	0.312	0.071	0.287	0.117	1.255	0.136	1.010	0.039
4	0.142	0.076	0.876	0.068	0.550	0.055	0.803	0.426	1.876	0.463	1.233	0.064
5	0.090	0.053	0.332	0.032	0.228	0.051	0.652	0.289	1.479	0.244	0.980	0.057

*Serum samples treated without (−) or with (+) β-mercaptoethanol (BME) were used to test anti-HCV IgM antibodies. Data shown are the A_{450} values, and the cut-off values of the ELISA were either 0.200 (HRP-LD5 based assay and established anti-HCV IgM assay) or 0.150 (Chang Zheng kit).

of 53.3%) (Table 3).These positive detection rates are consistent with the 59.7% and 58.8% anti-HCV prevalence reported in other Chinese hemodialysis patient studies [22,23].

The five patients who tested positive using the HRP-LD5 based assay alone were demonstrated to have anti-HCV IgM antibodies and HCV RNA. Follow-up samples taken from these patients three weeks later were positive using both the HRP-LD5-based assay and the Chang Zheng kit (Table 4). These results indicate that these five patients were likely to be newly HCV infected cases, which account for 2.56% of the 195 hemodialysis patients in this study, consistent with the result in a follow-up study of Chinese Shanghai hemodialysis patients that showed the anti-HCV seroconversion rates at 6, 12, 18, 24 and 30 months were 6.4%, 11.9%, 20.7%, 35.4% and 54.5%, respectively [22].

Indirect EIAs have been developed to detect IgM against many microbes. Low sensitivity or specificity is common problem for IgM detection, and the lack of applicable anti-hIgM monoclonal and polyclonal antibodies is a major obstacle for effective IgM detection [24,25]. An indirect anti-HCV IgM EIA assay has also been developed and extensively studied. Many reports have shown it to be useful for early diagnosis of HCV infection [26–29], whereas others do not support this conclusion [30,31]. For unknown reasons, commercially available anti-IgM antibodies have low affinity constants (Ka), varying from 2×10^5 to 5.34×10^8 M^{-1} [32], which is much lower than that of anti-hIgG monoclonal and polyclonal antibodies, which is usually above 1×10^9 M^{-1} [33–35]. Unlike the anti-IgM antibodies used in anti-HCV IgM ELISA assay, LD5 has well defined binding mode, i.e., simultaneously bound to the κ light chain and V_H3 of hIgM. Consequently, it showed a high binding affinity to hIgM with the affinity constant (Ka) of 3.23×10^9 M^{-1} and an equilibrium dissociation constant (K_D) of 0.31 nM, which was as high as that of SpA to hIgG with the Ka of 3.45×10^9 M^{-1} and the K_D of 0.29 nM (Table 1). Consistent with this binding property, the HRP-LD5 based assay displayed a higher IgM detection efficacy than the established IgM assay (Table 3, Table 4).

To our knowledge, this is the first report of the application of an NEIBM, LD5, to establish an anti-HCV detection assay with enhanced detection efficacy due to improved IgM detection. Our results also imply that NEIBMs with a high affinity to IgM could have potential application for detection of antibodies against other viral infections, such as hepatitis E virus or dengue virus, to improve of detection efficacy and early diagnosis.

Author Contributions

Conceived and designed the experiments: WP SS. Performed the experiments: JC QC HZ PQ CL XY JW SJ HY. Analyzed the data: WP JC HZ SS. Contributed reagents/materials/analysis tools: NW BQ JW. Wrote the paper: JC WP.

References

1. Kuo G, Choo QL, Alter HJ, Gitnick GL, Redeker AG, et al. (1989) An assay for circulating antibodies to a major etiologic virus of human non-A, non-B hepatitis. Science 244: 362–364.
2. Abdel-Hamid M, El-Daly M, El-Kafrawy S, Mikhail N, Strickland GT, et al. (2002) Comparison of second- and third-generation enzyme immunoassays for detecting antibodies to hepatitis C virus. J Clin Microbiol 40: 1656–9.
3. Alter HJ (1992) New kit on the block: evaluation of second-generation assays for detection of antibody to the hepatitis C virus. Hepatology 15: 350–353.
4. Kleinman S, Alter H, Busch M, Holland P, Tegtmeier G, et al. (1992) Increased detection of hepatitis C virus (HCV)-infected blood donors by a multiple-antigen HCV enzyme immunoassay. Transfusion 32: 805–813.
5. Glynn SA, Wright DJ, Kleinman SH, Hirschkorn D, Tu Y, et al. (2005) Dynamics of viremia in early hepatitis C virus infection. Transfusion 45: 994–1002.
6. Aach RD, Stevens CE, Hollinger FB, Mosley JW, Peterson DA, et al. (1991) Hepatitis C virus infection in post-transfusion hepatitis. An analysis with first- and second-generation assays. N Engl J Med 325: 1325–1329.
7. Gretch DR (1997) Diagnostic tests for hepatitis C. Hepatology 26 (Suppl. 1): 43S–47S.
8. Jiang SH, Wang JF, Xu R, Liu YJ, Wang XN, et al. (2008) Alternate Arrangement of PpL B3 Domain and SpA D Domain Creates Synergistic Double-Site Binding to V_H3 and V_κ Regions of Fab. DNA and Cell Biology 27: 423–431.
9. Yang H, Cao J, Li LQ, Zhou X, Chen QL, et al. (2008) Evolutional selection of a combinatorial phage library displaying randomly-rearranged various single domains of immunoglobulin (Ig)-binding proteins (IBPs) with four kinds of Ig molecules. BMC Microbiology August 13, 2008,;doi:10.1186/1471-2180-8-137.
10. León P, López JA, Elola C, Domingo CJ, Echevarria JM (1996) Detection of antibody to hepatitis C virus E2 recombinant antigen among samples indeterminate for anti-HCV after wide serological testing and correlation with viremia. The Spanish Study Group for Blood Donors at Risk of Transmission of HCV. Vox Sang 70: 213–216.
11. Garson JA, Tedder RS, Briggs M, Tuke P, Glazebrook JA, et al. (1990) Detection of hepatitis C viral sequences in blood donations by "nested" polymerase chain reaction and prediction of infectivity. Lancet 335: 1419–1422.
12. Okamoto H, Okada S, Sugiyama Y, Tanaka T, Sugai Y, et al. (1990) Detection of hepatitis C virus RNA by a two-stage polymerase chain reaction with two pairs of primers deduced from the 5'-noncoding region. Jpn J Exp Med 60: 215–222.
13. Farci P, Alter HJ, Wong D, Miller RH, Shih JW, et al. (1991) A long-term study of hepatitis C virus replication in non-A, non-B hepatitis. N Engl J Med 325: 98–104.

14. Puoti M, Zonaro A, Ravaggi A, Marin MG, Castelnuovo F, et al. (1992) Hepatitis C virus RNA and antibody response in the clinical course of acute hepatitis C virus infection. Hepatology 16: 877–881.
15. Hino K, Sainokami S, Shimoda K, Niwa H, Iino S (1994) Clinical course of acute hepatitis C and changes in HCV markers. Dig Dis Sci 39: 19–27.
16. National Institutes of Health (1997) National Institutes of Health Consensus Development Conference Panel statement: management of hepatitis C. Hepatology 26: 2S–10S.
17. Racine R, Winslow GM (2009) IgM in microbial infections: taken for granted? Immunol Lett 125: 79–85.
18. Wang NS, Liao LT (1998) Hemodialysis and hepatitis C virus. Guowai Yixue Liuxingbingxue Chuanranbingxue Fence (Chinese) 25: 115–118.
19. Boero R, Martina G, Bosio P, Devos S, Bertolo P, et al. (1995) HCV viremia in hemodialysis patients: detection by a DNA enzyme immunoassay for amplified HCV sequences. Renal Failure 17: 565–573.
20. Souqiyyeh MZ, Shaheen FAM, Huraib SO, Al-Khader AA (1995) The annual incidence of seroconversion of antibodies to the hepatitis C virus in the hemodialysis population in Saudi Arabia. Saudi J Kidney Dis Transplant 6: 167–173.
21. Al-Faleh FZ (1995) Hepatitis C virus infection: an update. Saudi J Kidney Dis Transplant 6: 118–121.
22. Wang NS, Liao LT, Zhu YJ, Pan W, Fang F (2000) Follow-up study of hepatitis C virus infection in uremic patients on maintenance hemodialysis for 30 months. World J Gastroenterol 6: 888–892.
23. Huang CS, Ho MS, Yang CS, Lee CL, Tan CA (1993) Hepatitis C markers in hemodialysis patients. J Clin Microbiol 31: 1764–1769.
24. Liesenfeld O, Press C, Montoya JG, Gill R, Isaac-Renton JL, et al. (1997) False-positive results in immunoglobulin M (IgM) toxoplasma antibody tests and importance of confirmatory testing: the Platelia Toxo IgM test. J Clin Microbiol 35: 174–178.
25. Verhofstede C, Van Renterghem L, Plum J (1989) Comparison of six commercial enzyme linked immunosorbent assays for detecting IgM antibodies against Toxoplasma gondii. J Clin Pathol 42: 1285–1290.
26. Akbar SM, Onji M, Horiike N, Ohta Y (1993) Anti-HCV immunoglobulin M antibody in patients with acute and fulminant hepatitis C. Gastroenterol Jpn 28(Suppl 5): 71–75.
27. Yamaguchi N, Tokushige K, Yamauchi K, Hayashi N (2000) Humoral immune response in Japanese acute hepatitis patients with hepatitis C virus infection. Can J Gastroenterol 14: 593–598.
28. Quinti I, Hassan NF, El Salman D, Shalaby H, El Zimatty D, et al. (1995) Hepatitis C virus-specific B cell activation: IgG and IgM detection in acute and chronic hepatitis C. J Hepatol 23: 640–647.
29. Kikuchi T, Onji M, Michitaka K, Saito I, Miyamura T, et al. (1992) Anti-HCV immunoglobulin M antibody in patients with hepatitis C. J Gastroenterol Hepatol 7: 246–248.
30. Zaaijer HL, Mimms LT, Cuypers HT, Reesink HW, van der Poel CL, et al. (1993) Variability of IgM response in hepatitis C virus infection. J Med Virol 40: 184–187.
31. Quiroga JA, Campillo ML, Catillo I, Bartolomé J, Porres JC, et al. (1991) IgM antibody to hepatitis C virus in acute and chronic hepatitis C. Hepatology 14: 38–43.
32. Rudich SM, Winchester R, Mongini PK (1985) Human B cell activation. Evidence for diverse signals provided by various monoclonal anti-IgM antibodies. J Exp Med 162: 1236–1255.
33. Murphy RM, Slayter H, Schurtenberger P, Chamberlin RA, Colton CK, et al. (1988) Size and structure of antigen-antibody complexes. Electron microscopy and light scattering studies. Biophys J 54: 45–56.
34. Chevrier MC, Châteauneuf I, Guérin M, Lemieux R (2004) Sensitive detection of human IgG in ELISA using a monoclonal anti-IgG-peroxidase conjugate. Hybrid Hybridomics 23: 362–367.
35. Welschof M, Terness P, Kipriyanov SM, Stanescu D, Breitling F, et al. (1997) The antigen-binding domain of a human IgG-anti-F(ab')2 autoantibody. Proc Natl Acad Sci USA 94: 1902–1907.

11

Thrombocytopenia as a Predictor of Severe Acute Kidney Injury in Patients with Hantaan Virus Infections

Meiliang Wang[1*¶], Jiuping Wang[2¶], Tianping Wang[2], Jing Li[2], Ling Hui[1,3], Xiaoqin Ha[1,3]

1 Center for Experimental Medicine, Lanzhou General Hospital, Lanzhou Military Command, Lanzhou, Gansu, China, **2** Department of Infectious Diseases, Tangdu Hospital, the Fourth Military Medical University, Xi'an, Shaanxi, China, **3** Gansu Key Laboratory of Stem Cell and Gene Therapy, Lanzhou, Gansu, China

Abstract

Background: Hematological abnormalities often occur several days before kidney injury in patients with hemorrhagic fever with renal syndrome (HFRS). We aimed to investigate the prevalence and prognostic value of the early hematological markers in patients with HFRS caused by Hantaan virus (HTNV) infection.

Methods: In a retrospective cohort study, we analyzed the case records of 112 patients with acute HTNV infection and evaluated the hematological markers for early prediction and risk stratification of HFRS patients with acute kidney injury (AKI).

Results: Of 112 patients analyzed, 66 (59%) developed severe AKI, defined as either receipt of acute dialysis or increased serum creatinine ≥354 µmol/L. The prognostic accuracy of hematological markers, as quantified by the area under the receiver-operating-characteristic curve (AUC), was highest with the nadir platelet count (AUC, 0.89; 95% CI, 0.83–0.95), as compared with the admission platelet count (AUC, 0.84; 95% CI, 0.77–0.92), and the admission and peak leukocyte counts. The nadir platelet count correlated moderately with the levels of peak blood urea nitrogen ($r = -0.616$) and serum creatinine ($r = -0.589$), the length of hospital stay ($r = -0.599$), and the number of dialysis sessions that each patient received during hospital stay ($r = -0.625$). By multivariate analysis, decreased nadir platelet count remained independently associated with the development of severe AKI (odds ratio, 27.57; 95% CI, 6.96–109.16; $P < 0.0001$).

Conclusions: Thrombocytopenia, rather than leukocytosis, is independently associated with subsequent severe AKI among patients with acute HTNV infection.

Editor: Qianjun Li, University of Alabama at Birmingham, United States of America

Funding: The authors have no support or funding to report.

Competing Interests: The authors have declared that no competing interests exist.

* E-mail: mlwang_2003@yahoo.com

¶ These authors contributed equally to this work.

Introduction

Hemorrhagic fever with renal syndrome (HFRS) is a combination of fever, hemorrhage, thrombocytopenia and acute kidney injury (AKI), among which severe AKI is the leading cause of death in patients with HFRS, particularly in the late stage. The disease is mainly caused by four closely related hantaviruses, Hantaan (HTNV) in Asia, Puumala (PUUV) and Dobrava in Europe, and Seoul virus worldwide. HTNV is the prototypic representative of this genus responsible for most cases of hantavirus infections in Asia. Unlike other hantaviruses, HTNV infections usually result in a severe form of HFRS, but the illness can range from a mild illness without oliguria, to an extremely severe illness requiring hemodialysis.

Currently, there is as yet no vaccine or specific antiviral therapy for HFRS. The treatment for patients with hantavirus infections is supportive care, including intermittent hemodialysis (IHD) and continuous *renal* replacement therapy (CRRT). Expected prognosis whether or when dialysis is started is of great importance to patients with severe HFRS and their clinicians, and for planning of treatment guidelines. Most of the symptoms and signs currently used in classifying HFRS [1,2], such as oliguria, anuria and kidney injury, do not appear until the later stages of illness. Thrombocytopenia is an early, consistent process during hantavirus infection, and is a major diagnostic feature in patients with HFRS [3]. In a cohort of patients infected with PUUV, which causes a mild form of HFRS in Europe, previous study showed that low platelet count ($<60\times10^9$/L) was significantly associated with the subsequent severe AKI [4]. This study used the platelet count obtained at the initial evaluation (1–9 days after symptom onset) to classify thrombocytopenia that may still be normal or have already returned to normal in some patients. Other attempts have provided a list of symptoms, signs, and hematological, biochemical or immunological parameters, that could be associated with severe HFRS [5–9], but how these parameters should be applied for clinical diagnosis is not apparent. To date, no prognostic models are available for patients with HTNV infection in Asia.

Acute hantavirus infection is a highly dynamic process, characterized by a short transient thrombocytopenia followed by mild-to-severe AKI [4]. We therefore assessed the extent to which the early hematological abnormalities, such as thrombocytopenia and leukocytosis, predicted the later biochemical abnormalities, such as the increases in levels of blood urea nitrogen and serum creatinine reflecting the severity of AKI, in patients with HTNV infection.

Methods

Study Population

We retrospectively reviewed the case records of 125 patients with HFRS, diagnosed during the major HTNV epidemic periods, from October through December, in 2008 and 2009, at the Tangdu Hospital of the Fourth Military Medical University in Xi'an. The clinical diagnosis of acute HTNV infection was serologically confirmed by an IgM-capture ELISA (Lanzhou Institute of Biological Products, China) according to the manufacturer's instructions for the detection of virus-specific IgM antibody. The levels of IgM antibodies were scored as follows: 0, negative; 1+, mildly positive; 2+, moderately positive; and 3+, strongly positive. Patients were included if they had a final serological score of 1+ or greater. Exclusion criteria included acute dialysis requirement within 24 h of admission. The study was approved by the ethics committees of the Lanzhou General Hospital and the Fourth Military Medical University. Informed consent was not required as it was a retrospective study and the data were analyzed anonymously. Both ethics committees specifically waived the need for consent.

Clinical Data Collection

Clinical and laboratory data were obtained daily throughout hospitalization and were collected on standardized data collection forms. Data requested from participating patients included demographic information, platelet count, leukocyte count, hematocrit, blood urea nitrogen, serum creatinine, uric acid, albumin, aspartate aminotransferase, alanine aminotransferase, the length of hospital stay, the need for hemodialysis treatment, the number of dialysis sessions, and the presence of shock, proteinuria, hematuria, and severe complications. All subjects were admitted to the hospital and monitored daily until discharged. IHD or CRRT treatment was guided by the ward physician based upon clinical necessity.

Statistical Analysis

Continuous variables were presented as medians with the interquartile range (IQR), and categorical variables as numbers and percentages. Continuous variables were compared with the use of the nonparametric Mann-Whitney U test and categorical variables with the use of the Pearson's χ^2 test or Fisher's exact test when appropriate. Spearman correlations and linear regression analyses were used to evaluate the relations between the early hematological parameters and the later biochemical, hematological, or clinical parameters. Receiver-operating-characteristic (ROC) curves were constructed to assess the sensitivity and specificity of the platelet and leukocyte counts in predicting the development of severe AKI and the need of dialysis. The comparison of areas under the ROC curves (AUC) was performed as recommended by DeLong et al. Multivariate logistic regression model was used to identify hematological factors associated with the development of severe AKI. Covariates entered into the model included age, gender, and the presence of shock, proteinuria and hematuria preceding the development of severe AKI. All P values are two-sided, and P values of <0.05 were considered significant. Analyses were done with PASW statistics, version 18.0 for windows (SPSS), and MedCalc software, version 11.5.0.0 (MedCalc).

Table 1. Characteristics of patients by severe AKI status.

	Severe AKI (n = 66)	No severe AKI (n = 46)	*P* value
Demographic characteristics			
Age (yr)	44 (33–56)	34 (24–45)	0.002
Male sex	57 (86%)	41 (89%)	0.663
Hematological markers			
Admission platelet count ($\times10^9$/L)	24 (11–31)	51 (36–73)	<0.0001
Nadir platelet count ($\times10^9$/L)	14 (9–25)	45 (34–68)	<0.0001
Admission leukocyte count ($\times10^9$/L)	17.9 (11.5–25.1)	11.5 (8.0–15.9)	0.001
Peak leukocyte count ($\times10^9$/L)	21.3 (15.3–31.4)	15.5 (10.4–21.2)	0.0001
Nadir hematocrit (%)	29.5 (24.4–32.8)	36.9 (35.0–38.9)	<0.0001
Renal function			
Peak blood urea nitrogen (mmol/L)	30.2 (25.9–35.4)	11.3 (7.6–16.1)	<0.0001
Peak serum creatinine (μmol/L)	729 (539–956)	181 (132–240)	<0.0001
Peak uric acid (μmol/L)	511 (392–630)	549 (467–659)	0.185
Clinical records			
Shock	16 (24%)	4 (9%)	0.035
Proteinuria	60 (91%)	41 (89%)	0.758
Hematuria	47 (71%)	10 (22%)	<0.0001
Dialysis required	57 (86%)	0 (0%)	<0.0001
Length of hospital stay (days)	21 (14–29)	9 (7–11)	<0.0001

Data are median (IQR) or number (%).

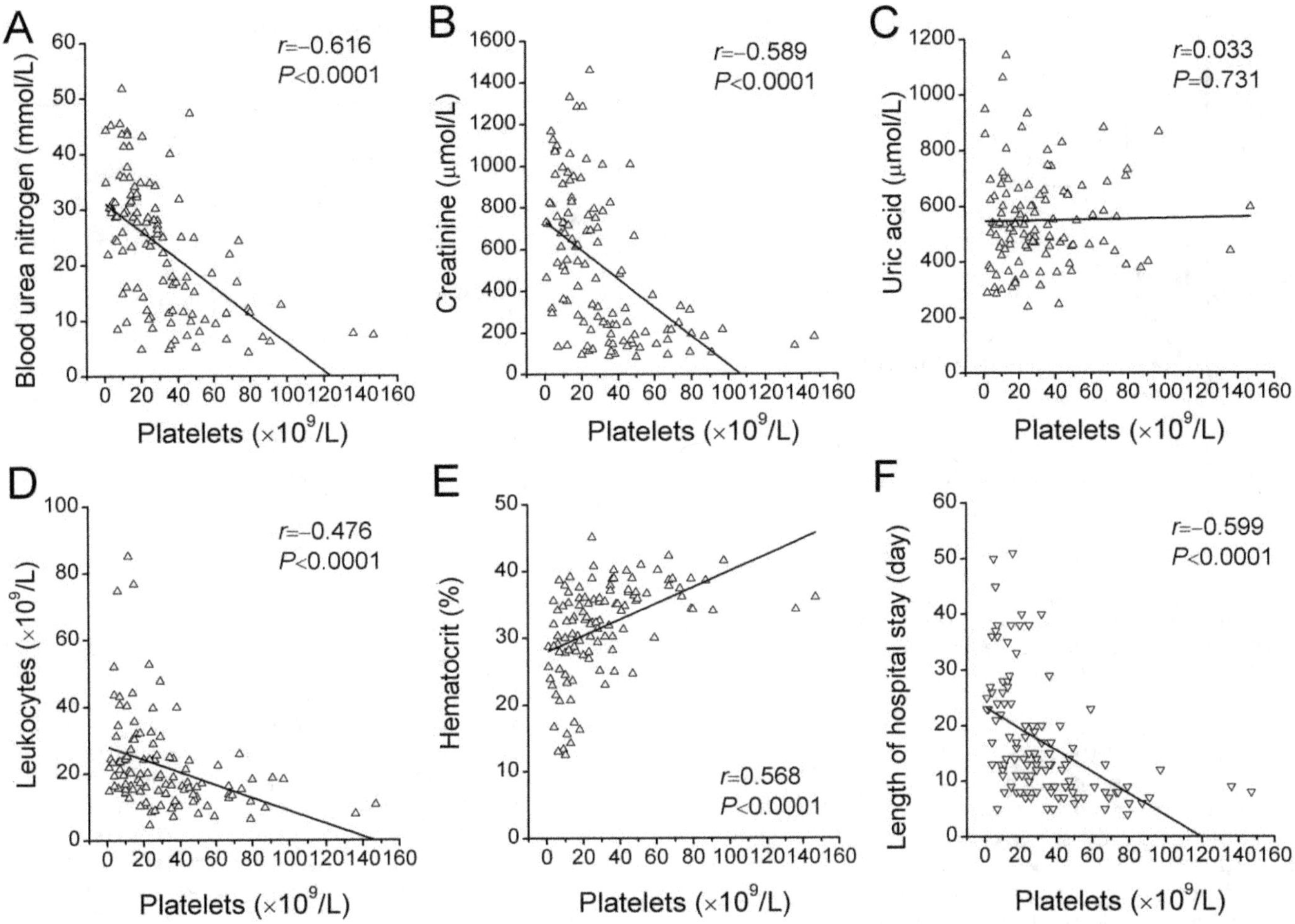

Figure 1. Correlations of nadir platelet count with other laboratory or clinical findings. Shown are the levels of peak blood urea nitrogen (*A*), peak serum creatinine (*B*), peak uric acid (*C*), peak leukocyte count (*D*) and nadir hematocrit (*E*), and lengths of hospital stay (*F*) plotted against the nadir platelet count. The *r* denotes the Spearman correlation coefficient, and the line the linear regression for each comparison.

Results

Characteristics of the Patients

In total, 125 patients were enrolled. Of these patients, 112 (90%) were eligible to be included in the study. The reasons for ineligibility were: patient had an undetermined diagnosis due to the lack of serological HTNV antibodies (n = 2); and patient received acute dialysis on admission due to severe AKI (n = 11).

Patients with acute HTNV infections, 14 females and 98 males, were admitted to the hospital 5 days (IQR 4–6 days) after acute onset of clinical symptoms. The most common laboratory findings were thrombocytopenia, leukocytosis and AKI. Thrombocytopenia (nadir platelet count $<100\times10^9$/L) occurred in 110 (98%) patients, and severe thrombocytopenia ($\leq33\times10^9$/L) in 71 (63%) patients. Leukocytosis (peak leukocyte count $>10\times10^9$/L) was recorded in 102 (91%) patients, and severe leukocytosis in 54 (48%) patients with a leukocyte count of 18.7×10^9/L or more. Moreover, the increases in levels of serum creatinine (>133 μmol/L) were noted in 101 (90%) patients, 66 (65%) of which subsequently developed severe AKI, defined as receipt of acute dialysis or increased serum creatinine ≥354 μmol/L by Acute Kidney Injury Network (AKIN) criteria for stage 3. Fifty-seven patients (51%) received acute dialysis and 2 (2%) died. Patients developing severe AKI were older, and more likely to have shock, hematuria, thrombocytopenia and leukocytosis, need acute dialysis, and therefore stay longer in hospital than patients who did not develop severe AKI (Table 1).

Association of Hematological Markers with Renal Function

Thrombocytopenia is an early, common and consistent laboratory finding in patients with acute HTNV infection. The early decreasing platelet counts reached their nadirs 6 days (IQR, 5–7 days) after the acute onset of fever, followed by consistent rises in levels of blood urea nitrogen and serum creatinine in patients developing severe AKI reaching the maximums 8 days (IQR, 7–11 days), and 11 days (IQR, 8–16 days), respectively. In these patients, platelet count nadirs preceded the peaks of blood urea nitrogen and serum creatinine by 2 days (1–5 days) and 5 days (3–9 days), respectively. Ten days (IQR, 9–11 days) after the onset of symptoms, platelet counts returned to normal in all patients, with values $>100\times10^9$/L. Leukocytosis, reflecting the inflammatory process during hantavirus infection, peaked almost at the same time as thrombocytopenia (median, 7 days; IQR, 5–8 days), but may occur or reoccur at the later stages of the disease.

The nadir platelet count correlated inversely with the peak blood urea nitrogen (r = −0.616, P<0.0001), peak serum creatinine (r = −0.589, P<0.0001), peak leukocyte count (r = −0.476,

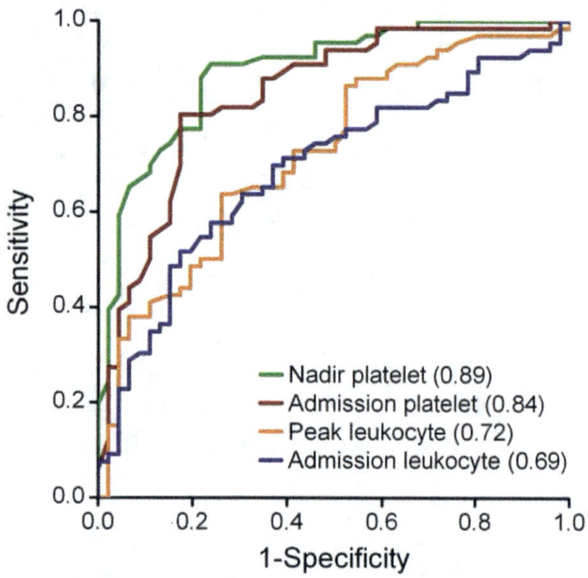

Figure 2. Receiver-operating-characteristic (ROC) curves for hematological markers to predict the development of severe AKI. Severe AKI is defined as the receipt of acute dialysis or increased serum creatinine ≥354 µmol/L.

P<0.0001) and the length of hospital stay ($r=-0.599$, *P*<0.0001), and correlated positively with the nadir hematocrit ($r=0.568$, *P*<0.0001), but not with the peak uric acid ($r=0.033$, $P=0.731$), though hyperuricemia is very common in patients with HFRS (Figure 1).

Significant but weaker correlations were found, moreover, between the peak leukocyte count and the peak blood urea nitrogen ($r=0.344$, $P=0.0002$), peak serum creatinine ($r=0.432$, *P*<0.0001), nadir hematocrit ($r=-0.287$, $P=0.002$) and the length of hospital stay ($r=0.348$, $P=0.0002$).

Association of Hematological Markers with AKI Development

The admission and nadir platelet counts were significantly lower in patients in whom severe AKI subsequently developed than in those without severe AKI (Table 1). In contrast, the admission and peak leukocyte counts were significantly higher in patients who had subsequent severe AKI than in those without. The accuracy for the prediction of severe AKI, as quantified by the AUC, was significantly higher with the nadir platelet count than that with the admission platelet count (AUC for nadir platelet, 0.89; 95% CI, 0.83–0.95; vs. AUC for admission platelet, 0.84; 95% CI, 0.77–0.92; $P=0.028$) and was also significantly higher than that with the admission and peak leukocyte counts (AUC for admission leukocyte, 0.69; 95% CI, 0.59–0.79; and for peak leukocyte, 0.72; 95% CI, 0.63–0.82; *P*<0.0001 and $P=0.0003$, respectively) (Figure 2). At a cut-off value of 33×10^9/L, the sensitivity and specificity to predict severe AKI were 91% and 76% for nadir platelet count, respectively (Table 2). After adjustment for age, gender, peak leukocyte count and for other variables preceding the development of AKI, decreased nadir platelet count (odds ratio, 27.57; 95% CI, 6.96–109.16; *P*<0.0001), and the presence of hematuria (odds ratio, 8.99; 95% CI, 2.32–34.81; $P=0.001$) remained independent predictors of severe AKI (Table 3).

Table 2. Sensitivity, specificity, and predictive values for the development of severe AKI using hematological cut-off values.

	Cut-off value	Sensitivity	Specificity	PPV	NPV
Admission platelet ($\times10^9$/L)	17	0.39	0.96	0.93	0.52
	34	0.80	0.83	0.87	0.75
	62	0.98	0.41	0.71	0.95
Nadir platelet ($\times10^9$/L)	17	0.59	0.96	0.95	0.62
	33	0.91	0.76	0.85	0.85
	49	0.98	0.39	0.70	0.95
Admission leukocyte ($\times10^9$/L)	17.3	0.52	0.83	0.81	0.54
Peak leukocyte ($\times10^9$/L)	18.7	0.64	0.74	0.78	0.59

PPV, positive predictive value; NPV, negative predictive value.

Association of Thrombocytopenia with Dialysis Treatment

Of 112 patients, 57 (51%) received one or more sessions of IHD and/or CRRT treatment. We observed a moderate correlation between the nadir platelet count and the number of dialysis sessions that each patient received during hospital stay ($r=-0.625$, *P*<0.0001) (Figure 3A). The nadir platelet counts were significantly lower in patients receiving acute dialysis compared with those not receiving dialysis (median, 14×10^9/L vs. 39×10^9/L; *P*<0.0001), but there were no differences between nadir platelet counts in patients who received one *versus* more than one dialysis session. The AUC for nadir platelet count in the prediction of dialysis was 0.86 (95% CI, 0.79–0.92) (Figure 3B). At a cut-off level of 33×10^9/L, the sensitivity and specificity of nadir platelet count in predicting dialysis were 93% and 67%, respectively.

Association of Thrombocytopenia with Adverse Outcomes

Patients who had thrombocytopenia during the early stage of infection had more frequently experienced adverse outcomes. Of 71 patients with nadir platelet count $\leq33\times10^9$/L, 7 (10%) developed pulmonary complications including pulmonary *infection*, edema, *hemorrhage, and* respiratory distress or failure, 4 (6%)

Table 3. Multivariable logistic regression for the prediction of severe AKI combining nadir platelet count with other variables.

	Adjusted odds ratio	95% CI	*P* value
Age (per year)	1.04	1.00–1.08	0.071
Gender	0.92	0.16–5.32	0.925
Presence of shock	1.88	0.28–12.64	0.516
Presence of proteinuria	1.09	0.17–7.11	0.932
Presence of hematuria	8.99	2.32–34.81	0.001
Nadir platelet $\leq33\times10^9$/L	27.57	6.96–109.16	<0.0001
Peak leukocyte $\geq18.7\times10^9$/L	1.16	0.33–4.05	0.821

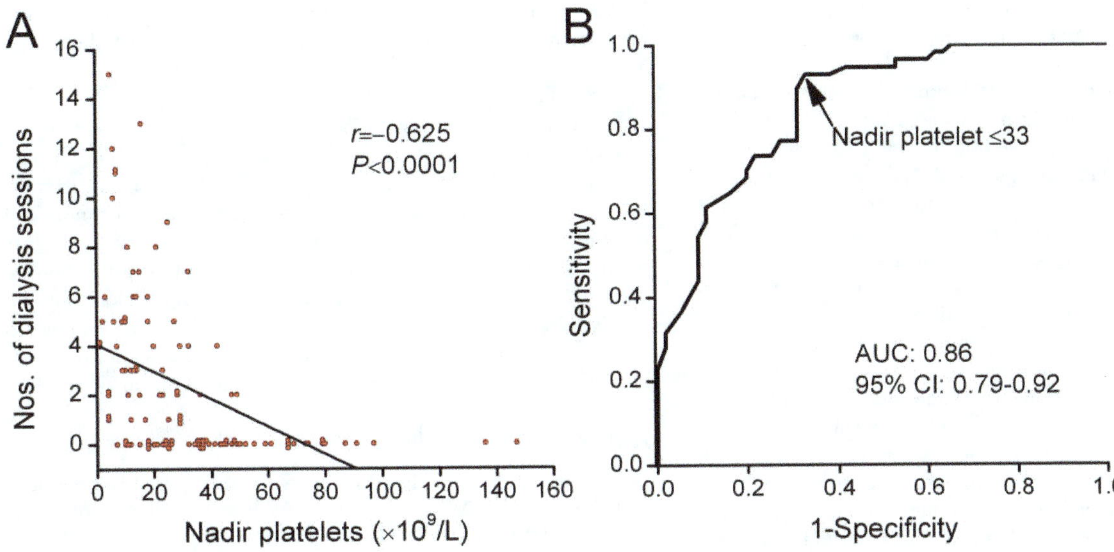

Figure 3. Nadir platelet count associated with dialysis. (A) Nadir platelet count correlated with the number of dialysis sessions each patient received during hospitalization. (B) Shown are receiver-operating-characteristic (ROC) curves for nadir platelet count in predicting the need of dialysis.

experienced severe brain complications including *cerebral* edema, hemorrhage, and uremic encephalopathy, 6 (8%) developed acute pancreatitis, 1 (1%) had multiorgan failure, 10 (14%) received one or more times of urgent rescue medications, and 2 (3%) died. *In contrast, none of 41 patients who had* a nadir platelet count of more than 33×10^9/L developed these complications.

Discussion

In this study, the clinical processes of patients with acute HTNV infection were retrospectively followed throughout hospitalization. During the course of acute HTNV infection, the patients sequentially developed mild-to-severe thrombocytopenia, leukocytosis, and AKI. In these patients, the nadir platelet count negatively correlated with the levels of blood urea nitrogen and serum creatinine, the number of dialysis sessions, and the length of hospital stay reflecting the severity of renal dysfunction. Severe thrombocytopenia in patients with acute HTNV infection, independent of leukocytosis, was strongly associated with a substantially increased risk for development of severe AKI.

Little is known about the prognostic importance of thrombocytopenia in patients with acute hantavirus infections. Approximately half of the patients (7 of 15 or 47% of patients) in the study of PUUV infection had severe thrombocytopenia [4]. These patients also had a higher level of serum creatinine and a higher prevalence of severe AKI. In these patients, thrombocytopenia was defined as an initial platelet count $<60\times10^9$/L, a much higher threshold than that used in our cohort of patients who had a much more severe form of HFRS caused by HTNV infection.

By contrast with this study [4], the platelet count was also measured in one other study of acute HTNV infection in which 24 (39%) of 61 patients had thrombocytopenia, defined as admission platelet count $\leq38\times10^9$/L [6]. The admission leukocyte count, rather than the admission platelet count, was found to be significantly associated with the development of oliguric AKI, which was defined as a urine output <400 mL/24 h (the significant difference of the minimum platelet count between patients with and without AKI was not described further). Similarly, a recent study in a cohort of 36 PUUV-infected patients showed that the maximum leukocyte count, but not the minimum platelet count, was a weak risk factor for severe AKI [10]. The details about the clinical courses of the patients, however, were not available for measuring the discrepancy.

Although most of these studies used a threshold of initial platelet count to define thrombocytopenia, nadir platelet count does reflect the degree of thrombocytopenia more sensitively. Our study shows that in HTNV cohort, up to 71 of 112 (63%) had a nadir platelet count of 33×10^9/L or less. The incidence of thrombocytopenia was higher than previously reported both in the PUUV and HTNV cohorts [4,6].

In our study, the severities of thrombocytopenia and leukocytosis were comparable to those in the previous HTNV study by Kim et al [6], but were more severe than those in the PUUV studies [4,10]. The nadir platelet count, as well as the peak leukocyte count, was found to be correlated with the laboratory and clinical parameters reflecting the severity of the disease (Figure 1). The diagnostic accuracy for severe AKI was highest with the nadir platelet count, as compared with the admission platelet count, and the admission and peak leukocyte counts (Figure 2). Similar to the previous HTNV study [6], the presence of hematuria preceding the development of severe AKI was also an independent predictor (Table 3). We further observed that the nadir platelet count was moderately correlated with the number of dialysis sessions each patient received during hospital stay and ROC curve yielded an AUC of 0.86 for predicting dialysis (Figure 3).

Thrombocytopenia is a consistent finding among viral hemorrhagic fever [11]. Several mechanisms *may be postulated to* explain the cause of thrombocytopenia associated with these diseases, including impaired proplatelet formation and platelet release [12], *coagulation abnormalities* [13,14] and disseminated intravascular coagulation that correlated with a more severe disease [15]. Similar to HFRS, thrombocytopenia has also been shown to be associated with the development of complications in dengue fever [16,17], and a platelet count of 50 $\times10^9$/L or less on days 5 to 7 of illness has been used as a marker of severe disease [18]. Similarly, a significantly lower platelet count was observed in fatal cases than in non-fatal cases with Crimean-Congo hemorrhagic fever [19,20], and a platelet count of $\leq20\times10^9$/L was independently associated with high mortality [14,20]. However, the mechanism underlying thrombocytopenia in patients with severe diseases is not known.

Among the patients with severe AKI, timely initiation of dialysis may reduce subsequent complications and death risk [21]. The platelet count may make it possible both to rule in and to rule out the prognosis of severe AKI and need of dialysis on the basis of the daily measurement. Despite the good performance of the platelet category in the early diagnosis of severe AKI caused by HTNV infection, it should be used only in combination with the initial clinical manifestations of HFRS, such as fever and hemorrhage.

One limitation of this study is its small cohort, therefore, these markers require validation in independent cohorts. Another limitation is that this study can not differentiate the peak levels of blood urea nitrogen and serum creatinine between patients with and without IHD or CRRT treatment. The values were distinctly underestimated in patients who had undergone dialysis; the coefficient was thereby underascertained. Other early abnormalities, such as elevated hematocrit, hypoalbuminemia, and elevated aspartate aminotransferase and alanine aminotransferase indicating the presence of hemoconcentration and liver impairment, were also noted in acute HTNV infection, but were not included in the analysis because they are not measured routinely in patients with HFRS.

In summary, early thrombocytopenia was associated with the development of severe AKI, need of dialysis, and length of hospital stay. Because platelet count is a simple, readily available clinical test that is widely used in medical care, and pronounced thrombocytopenia is an early and consistent laboratory abnormality in HFRS, it might be of value in risk stratification of patients at high risk of developing severe complications for the timely initiation of hemodialysis treatment. Of potential interest to physicians is whether therapeutic increase in platelet count might be useful in the prediction of improvement in clinical severities.

Author Contributions

Conceived and designed the experiments: MW JW. Analyzed the data: MW JW TW JL. Wrote the paper: MW. Participated in revising the manuscript critically: MW JW LH XH.

References

1. Klein SL, Marks MA, Li W, Glass GE, Fang LQ, et al. (2011) Sex differences in the incidence and case fatality rates from hemorrhagic fever with renal syndrome in China, 2004–2008. Clin Infect Dis 52: 1414–1421.
2. Wang M, Wang J, Zhu Y, Xu Z, Yang K, et al. (2009) Cellular immune response to Hantaan virus nucleocapsid protein in the acute phase of hemorrhagic fever with renal syndrome: correlation with disease severity. J Infect Dis 199: 188–195.
3. Denecke B, Bigalke B, Haap M, Overkamp D, Lehnert H, et al. (2010) Hantavirus infection: a neglected diagnosis in thrombocytopenia and fever? Mayo Clin Proc 85: 1016–1020.
4. Rasche FM, Uhel B, Kruger DH, Karges W, Czock D, et al. (2004) Thrombocytopenia and acute renal failure in Puumala hantavirus infections. Emerg Infect Dis 10: 1420–1425.
5. Kim YO, Yoon SA, Ku YM, Yang CW, Kim YS, et al. (2003) Serum albumin level correlates with disease severity in patients with Hemorrhagic Fever with Renal Syndrome. J Korean Med Sci 18: 696–700.
6. Kim YK, Lee SC, Kim C, Heo ST, Choi C, et al. (2007) Clinical and laboratory predictors of oliguric renal failure in haemorrhagic fever with renal syndrome caused by Hantaan virus. J Infect 54: 381–386.
7. Takala A, Lahdevirta J, Jansson SE, Vapalahti O, Orpana A, et al. (2000) Systemic inflammation in hemorrhagic fever with renal syndrome correlates with hypotension and thrombocytopenia but not with renal injury. J Infect Dis 181: 1964–1970.
8. Outinen TK, Makela SM, Ala-Houhala IO, Huhtala HS, Hurme M, et al. (2010) The severity of Puumala hantavirus induced nephropathia epidemica can be better evaluated using plasma interleukin-6 than C-reactive protein determinations. BMC Infect Dis 10: 132.
9. Sane J, Laine O, Makela S, Paakkala A, Jarva H, et al. (2012) Complement activation in Puumala hantavirus infection correlates with disease severity. Ann Med 44: 468–475.
10. Libraty DH, Makela S, Vlk J, Hurme M, Vaheri A, et al. (2012) The Degree of Leukocytosis and Urine GATA-3 mRNA Levels Are Risk Factors for Severe Acute Kidney Injury in Puumala Virus Nephropathia Epidemica. PLoS One 7: e35402.
11. Geisbert TW, Jahrling PB (2004) Exotic emerging viral diseases: progress and challenges. Nat Med 10: S110–121.
12. Pozner RG, Ure AE, Jaquenod de Giusti C, D'Atri LP, Italiano JE, et al. (2010) Junin virus infection of human hematopoietic progenitors impairs in vitro proplatelet formation and platelet release via a bystander effect involving type I IFN signaling. PLoS Pathog 6: e1000847.
13. Laine O, Makela S, Mustonen J, Huhtala H, Szanto T, et al. (2010) Enhanced thrombin formation and fibrinolysis during acute Puumala hantavirus infection. Thromb Res 126: 154–158.
14. Onguru P, Dagdas S, Bodur H, Yilmaz M, Akinci E, et al. (2010) Coagulopathy parameters in patients with Crimean-Congo hemorrhagic fever and its relation with mortality. J Clin Lab Anal 24: 163–166.
15. Sundberg E, Hultdin J, Nilsson S, Ahlm C (2011) Evidence of disseminated intravascular coagulation in a hemorrhagic fever with renal syndrome-scoring models and severe illness. PLoS One 6: e21134.
16. Balmaseda A, Hammond SN, Perez MA, Cuadra R, Solano S, et al. (2005) Assessment of the World Health Organization scheme for classification of dengue severity in Nicaragua. Am J Trop Med Hyg 73: 1059–1062.
17. Hammond SN, Balmaseda A, Perez L, Tellez Y, Saborio SI, et al. (2005) Differences in dengue severity in infants, children, and adults in a 3-year hospital-based study in Nicaragua. Am J Trop Med Hyg 73: 1063–1070.
18. Tanner L, Schreiber M, Low JG, Ong A, Tolfvenstam T, et al. (2008) Decision tree algorithms predict the diagnosis and outcome of dengue fever in the early phase of illness. PLoS Negl Trop Dis 2: e196.
19. Tasdelen Fisgin N, Tanyel E, Doganci L, Tulek N (2009) Risk factors for fatality in patients with Crimean-Congo haemorrhagic fever. Trop Doct 39: 158–160.
20. Cevik MA, Erbay A, Bodur H, Gulderen E, Bastug A, et al. (2008) Clinical and laboratory features of Crimean-Congo hemorrhagic fever: predictors of fatality. Int J Infect Dis 12: 374–379.
21. Liu KD, Himmelfarb J, Paganini E, Ikizler TA, Soroko SH, et al. (2006) Timing of initiation of dialysis in critically ill patients with acute kidney injury. Clin J Am Soc Nephrol 1: 915–919.

12

Serum Fetuin A and Chemerin Levels Correlate with Hepatic Steatosis and Regional Adiposity in Maintenance Hemodialysis Patients

Hung-Yuan Chen[1,2], Chien-Chu Lin[3], Yen-Lin Chiu[1,2], Shih-Ping Hsu[1,2], Mei-Fen Pai[1,2], Ju-Yeh Yang[1,2], Yu-Sen Peng[1,2]*

1 Division of Nephrology, Department of Internal Medicine, Far Eastern Memorial Hospital, New Taipei City, Taiwan, **2** Division of Nephrology, Department of Internal Medicine, National Taiwan University Hospital and National Taiwan University College of Medicine, Taipei, Taiwan, **3** Division of Gastroenterology and Hepatology, Department of Internal Medicine, Far Eastern Memorial Hospital, New Taipei City, Taiwan

Abstract

Background: A deficiency of fetuin A is linked to cardiovascular calcification and mortality in dialysis patients. But, high levels of fetuin A and chemerin correlate with hepatic steatosis and regional adiposity in general population. The association between hepatic steatosis and fetuin A/chemerin levels in hemodialysis (HD) remains unclear.

Methods: We performed a cross-sectional, observational study; 216 prevalent HD patients from a single center were enrolled. Baseline serum fetuin A, chemerin levels, conicity index and anthropometric parameters were checked. Presence of hepatic steatosis was qualified by liver ultrasound and quantified by the hepato-renal index (HRI); central obesity defined by waist circumference (WC). ROC analyses and multivariate logistic regression analyses for prediction of hepatic steatosis and central obesity on the basis of fetuin A/chemerin levels, anthropometric parameters, and other relevant covariates were performed.

Results: Data from 103 women and 113 men (mean age 60±12 years) were analyzed. Eighty subjects had hepatic steatosis and their HRIs were significantly higher than those without hepatic steatosis ($P<0.001$). Serum fetuin A levels were positively associated with HRIs ($P<0.001$) and chemerin levels ($P<0.001$). Fetuin A, chemerin and WC were predictors for hepatic steatosis and central obesity by ROC curve. In multivariate logistic regression analysis, fetuin A and WC independently predicted hepatic steatosis defined by HRIs. And chemerin predicted central obesity and regional adiposity after covariate adjustments (all $P<0.05$).

Conclusions: Serum fetuin A levels were higher in prevalent HD patients with hepatic steatosis, and positively correlated with chemerin levels. Chemerin levels predicted central obesity as well as regional adiposity in the HD patients.

Editor: Haiyan Xu, Warren Alpert Medical School of Brown University, United States of America

Funding: This study was supported by grant from the Far Eastern Memorial Hospital (FEMH) (FEMH- 2011-C-006), Taiwan. The authors would like to express their thanks to the Ta-Tung Kidney Foundation and to Mrs. Hsin-Chin Lee Kidney Research Fund for supporting this investigation. The funders had no role in study design, data collection and analysis, decision to publish, or preparation of the manuscript.

Competing Interests: The authors have declared that no competing interests exist.

* E-mail: taan70@yahoo.com.tw

Introduction

Fetuin A is a protein exclusively secreted by hepatocytes in humans and a potent inhibitor of vascular calcification [1]. While increased fetuin A levels positively correlated with vascular calcification in diabetic patients and general population [2–3], an inverse relationship was observed in dialysis patients [1,4]. Both chronic inflammation and uremia may contribute to exhausting fetuin A release and a consequent catabolic micro-environment of fetuin A lead dialysis patients to be fetuin A deficiency [5]. Fetuin A deficiency is associated with cardiovascular (CV) calcification and, thereby, a high mortality rate in dialysis patients [1,4]. A link between fetuin A deficiency, progression of vascular calcification and atherosclerosis is thought to be the possible mechanism. A high fetuin A level is now considered to be a strong indicator of better CV outcomes in dialysis patients [4,6–7], however, there are currently no practical management to resolve this critical issue.

Beyond its inhibitory potency on calcium phosphate precipitation, fetuin A also inhibits insulin receptor tyrosine kinase of adipose and muscle cells. In animal models, mice with fatty liver presented with up-regulated fetuin A mRNA expression [8–10]. Moreover, a high fetuin A concentration is associated with liver fat accumulation, visceral adiposity and insulin resistance (IR) in the general population, and possibly in chronic kidney disease (CKD) patients [10–12]. Interestingly, children with non-alcoholic fatty liver disease (NAFLD) have higher fetuin A levels, and in adults, treatment with pioglitazone or ezetimibe seems to decrease fetuin A levels and liver fat simultaneously [13–15]. These studies suggest that this liver-secreted protein responds to hepatic steatosis. However, this relationship has not been investigated in dialysis

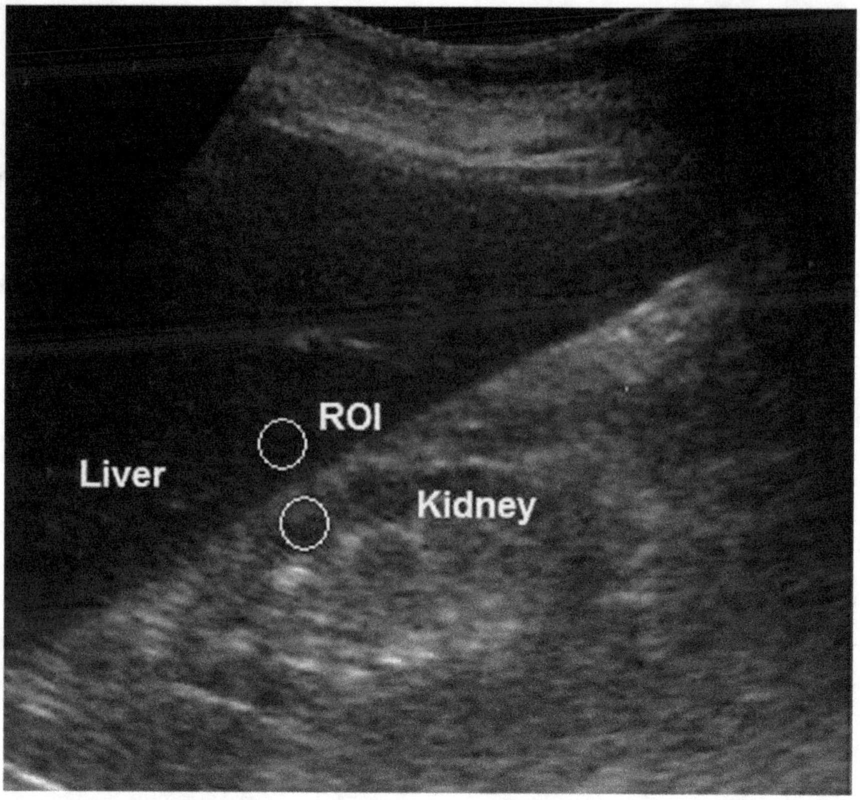

Figure 1. Ultrasound image shows selected regions of interest (ROI) (*circles*).

patients, those with unique catabolism of fetuin A compared with the general population.

Chemerin, a novel adipokine, correlates with NAFLD in obese subjects, and visceral adiposity in the general population [16–17]. In addition, in recent investigations, high chemerin levels have also been shown to correlate with survival benefits in incident hemodialysis (HD) patients [18–19]. Interestingly, serum fetuin A level is negatively associated with another adipokine, adiponectin, in both CKD and non-CKD patients [20–21]. High levels of both fetuin A and chemerin correlate with potential survival benefits in dialysis patients; however, their association has not previously been investigated. Furthermore, whether chemerin levels in dialysis patients also reflect the regional adiposity, that is, central fat, hepatic steatosis or abdominal fat, remains unknown.

The aim of this cross-sectional investigation was to test the hypothesis that patients undergoing maintenance HD and who have hepatic steatosis, have higher serum fetuin A levels. This phenomenon has been shown in the general population, but they have different metabolic process of fetuin A compared with patients under HD. We also intended to explore the relationships between fetuin A and chemerin, chemerin and hepatic steatosis; and to realize the possible connection between fetuin A, chemerin and regional adiposity in prevalent HD patients.

Methods

Subjects and Patients

Two hundred and sixteen patients aged more than 20 years (mean age: 60±12 years; 103 females) who received HD for more than six months at the Far Eastern Memorial Hospital, Taiwan were enrolled. The exclusion criteria were patients: 1) with active infection; 2) who had been recently hospitalized for any major physical or psychiatric illness; 3) with any active malignancy or any status of hepatocellular carcinoma; and 4) who refused to participate.

The enrolled patients received 3.5 to 5 hours of HD three times a week using bicarbonate dialysate. The mean vintage of HD before recruitment was 6.1 years (range: 0.6–25.5 years). The Institutional Review Board of Far Eastern Memorial Hospital approved this study, and all of the participants provided written informed consent.

Central Obesity and Regional Adiposity

Central obesity was defined according to the modified Asian criteria of the National Cholesterol Education Program Adult Treatment Panel III (NCEP ATP III), i.e., WC >90 cm in males and >80 cm in females [22].

Regional adiposity or abdominal fat deposition was assessed by a conicity index (Ci). The Ci was calculated according to the equation defined by Valdez [23], which included waist circumference (WC), weight and height: $WC/[0.109\times$ square root of (weight/height)$]$.

Qualification and Quantification of Hepatic Steatosis

We chose abdominal ultrasound as the method to qualify and quantify the hepatic steatosis in HD patients instead of the invasive procedure, liver biopsy and image studies of liver fat estimation with remarkable complications, magnetic resonance imaging (MRI) or computed tomography (CT). The rationale for this choice was due to the limitations in using MRI due to the potential complications of nephrogenic systemic fibrosis, increased cancer risk through CT, and detrimental impacts of contrast media on the

Table 1. Basic characteristics of all participants.

	All patients (N = 216)	Patients with hepatic steatosis (N = 80)	Patients without hepatic steatosis (N = 136)	P value
Gender (female, male)	103, 113	39,41	64,72	0.8
Age (years)	60±12	62±11	59±12	0.2
HD vintage (years)	6.1±5.0	5.7±4.9	6.3±5.1	0.3
Hepatitis (%)	77 (35.6)	25 (31.3)	52 (38.2)	0.3
DM (%)	87 (40.3)	37 (46)	50 (37)	0.2
Kt/V_{urea}	1.5±0.2	1.5±0.2	1.6±0.2	0.04
nPCR (g/kg/day)	1.05±0.26	1.06±0.24	1.04±0.27	0.5
BMI	22.8±4.0	25.1±4.2	21.4±3.2	<0.001
WC (cm)	85±11	93±11	81±8.1	<0.001
WHR	0.91±0.07	0.95±0.08	0.89±0.06	<0.001
WHtR	0.5±0.1	0.57±0.09	0.51±0.05	<0.001
Central obesity (%)	107 (49.5)	64 (80)	43 (31.6)	<0.001
Conicity index (Ci)	1.29±0.1	1.32±0.1	1.26±0.08	<0.001
Laboratory				
Hemoglobin (g/dl)	11.2±1.4	11.3±1.3	11.1±1.5	0.5
Albumin (g/l)	4.1±0.3	4.1±0.3	4.0±0.3	0.5
Ca (mg/dl)	9.4±0.6	9.4±0.6	9.4±0.6	0.5
P (mg/dl)	5.0±1.4	5.5±1.8	4.8±1.2	<0.001
CaXP	47±13	51±14	45±12	<0.001
iPTH (pg/ml)	241 (116,595)	243 (121,568)	230 (115,609)	0.9
T-CHO (mg/dl)	175±40	185±36	169±41	0.005
TG (mg/dl)	162±121	214±153	131±83	<0.001
LDL-C (mg/dl)	103±33	106±33	101±33	0.3
HDL-C (mg/dl)	40±14	37±11	42±15	0.006
Fetuin A (g/l)	0.63 (0.47,0.79)	0.72 (0.51,0.83)	0.62 (0.44,0.77)	0.03
Adiponectin (ug/ml)	11.5 (7.5, 17.2)	9.8 (6.4,15.3)	13.0 (8.4,17.6)	0.02
Chemerin (ng/ml)	674.7 (494,984)	749 (511,1493)	613.4(479.7,690.9)	0.03
HOMA-IR	2.56 (1.01, 7.7)	3.5 (1.4,12.0)	2.1 (0.8,5.6)	0.01
hs-CRP (mg/dl)	0.28 (0.13, 0.66)	0.34 (0.18,0.78)	0.21 (0.1,0.54)	0.004
Liver fat content				
HRI-S	−11.8 (−26.9, −16)	0.80, (−4.75~8.87)	−22.06, (−34.75~−11.62)	<0.001
HRI-R	0.85 (0.68, 0.97)	1.01, (0.93~1.15)	0.73, (0.63~0.85)	<0.001

Abbreviations: DM, diabetic mellitus; HD, hemodialysis; nPCR, normalized protein catabolic rate; BMI, body mass index; WC: waist circumference; WHR: waist-to-hip ratio; WHtR: waist-to-height ratio; Ca, calcium; P, phosphorus; CaxP, calcium phosphate product; iPTH, intact parathyroid hormone; T-CHO, total cholesterol; TG, triglyceride; LDL-C, low-density lipoprotein; HDL-C, high-density lipoprotein; HOMA-IR, homeostasis model assessment of insulin resistance hs-CRP, highly sensitive C-reactive protein.

Note: Conversion factors for units: hemoglobin in g/dL to g/L, ×10; serum calcium in mg/dL to mmol/L, ×0.2495; serum phosphate in mg/dL to mmol/L, ×0.3229; serum LDL-C in mg/dL to mmol/L, ×0.02586; serum TG in mg/dL to mmol/L, ×0.01129; serum albumin in g/dL to g/L, ×10. No conversion necessary for platelet counts in $\times 10^3$/uL and $\times 10^9$/L; serum iPTH in pg/mL and ng/L; serum potassium in mEq/L and mmol/L.

residual renal function doing CT examinations in the dialysis patients. By the way, owing to the bleeding diathesis of HD patients, the invasive procedure of liver biopsy for measurements of hepatic steatosis was compromised.

Hepatic steatosis was qualified using established criteria, including (1) a definite increase in echogenicity and/or (2) definite impaired visualization of the intra-hepatic vessels and diaphragm, and (3) evidence of focal fatty sparing [24].

Hepatic steatosis was quantified with hepatorenal index (HRI) which was examined by real-time gray-scale ultrasound examinations using a 3.5–5 MHz convex transducer.

All ultrasound examinations were performed by the same hepatologist. Image gain parameters were adjusted identically for all participants so that the right side of the liver, right liver lobe, right kidney, and hepato-renal interface were adequately visualized. Each ultrasound image was composed of segment VI of the liver and adjacent liver parenchyma obtained at the level of the hepato-renal space. After digitization of the ultrasound image as a JPG file, public domain software (ImageJ; National Institutes of Health; http//: rsb.info.nih.gov/ij/index.html) was used for computer-assisted analysis. Values were graded in gray scale using arbitrary units that ranged from 0 to 255 from black to white. For computer-assisted analysis, two circular regions of interest (ROI)

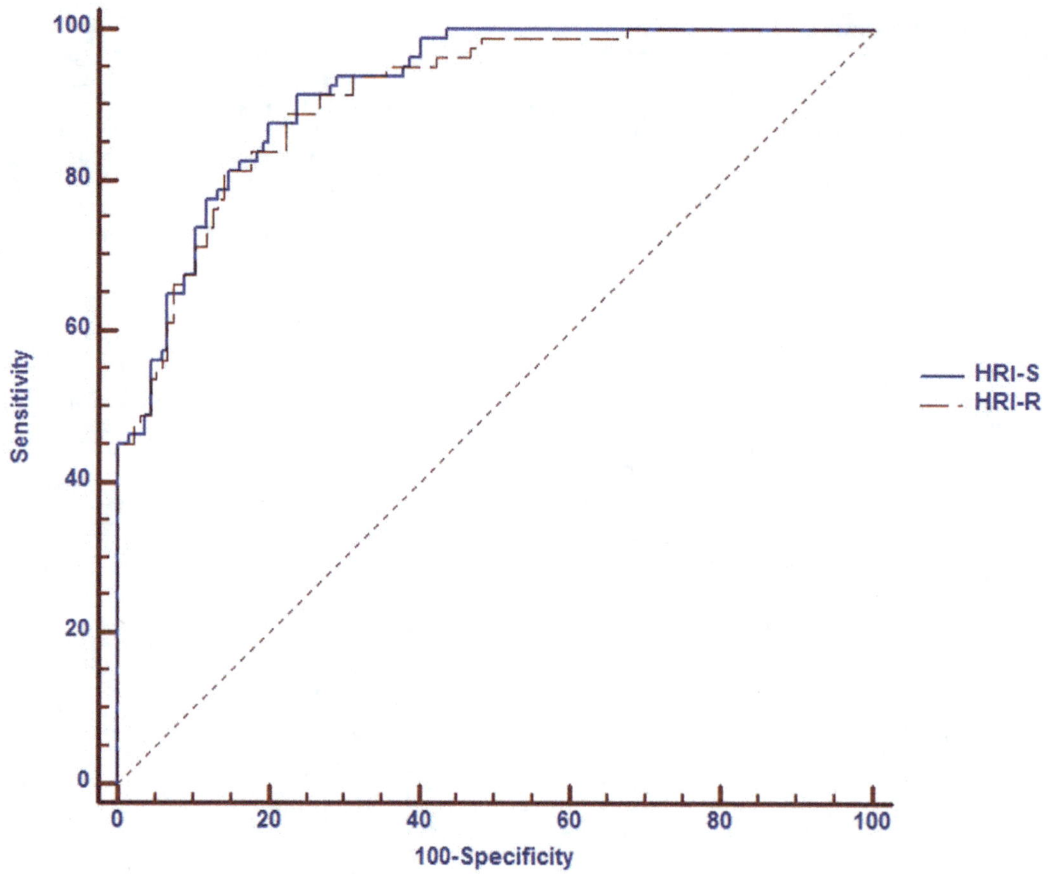

Figure 2. ROC curves for HRI-S and HRI-R versus hepatic steatosis defined by abdominal ultrasound.

were selected as follows (Figure 1): (1) the liver parenchyma, close to the lower border, next to the kidney (area, 400–500 pixels); (2) the corticomedullary junction of the right kidney, (area, 300–450 pixels). The two ROI were selected because they were juxtaposed to each other and on the same axis of the acoustic beam to minimize artifacts in the echogenicity of the acoustic window.

To avoid confounding factors that could modify the liver and kidney echogenicity, after the measurement of echogenicity in the two ROIs, HRIs were calculated using two methods: (1) the value of the kidney echogenicity was subtracted from the value of the liver echogenicity (HRI-S); (2) The ratio of the values of liver and the right kidney echogenicity (HRI-R). This method for estimation of liver fat content has been validated in previous investigations [25–26]. In each case, the calculation of the HRI was repeated at least twice, and the average values were taken as the final results. HRI reproducibility was evaluated on a sample of 40 randomly selected participants who underwent two repeat measures within 14 days. The results of the first and the second HRI (HRI-S and HRI-R) were highly correlated ($r=0.84$, $P<0.001$). The mean differences in HRI between the two examinations were not significant in a paired *t*-test ($P=0.43$).

Measurements of Serum Fetuin A Concentration

Serum fetuin A was measured by a highly sensitive, two-site enzyme linked immuno-assay (Adipo Bioscience, Inc., Santa Clara, CA, USA). Nephelometry for fetuin-A employed the same high specificity antibody as the enzyme-linked immuno-sorbent assay (ELISA) and established reproducible standard curves after testing for appropriate dilution. This was evaluated in a side-by-side comparison with immuno-blot analysis to exclude cross-reactivity of the antibodies with other serum proteins and proteolytic fragments of fetuin-A. The intra-assay coefficient of variation was 4%, and the inter-assay coefficient of variation was 8%. The assay linear measurement range of human fetuin A was 0.003–2.0 g/L.

Measurements of Serum Chemerin Concentration, Adiponectin and Insulin Resistance

Serum concentrations of chemerin (Adipo Bioscience, Inc., Santa Clara, CA, USA) and adiponectin (AssayPro, St. Charles, MO, USA) were analyzed with a commercial enzyme-linked immunosorbent assay kit. Homeostatic model assessment (HOMA-IR) was defined as glucose (mg/dL) × insulin (μU/mL)/405. Serum concentrations of insulin were analyzed with a commercial enzyme-linked immunosorbent assay kit (Mercodia, Inc, Winston Salem, NC, USA).

Baseline Demographic and Clinical Data and Laboratory Parameters

Baseline data, including gender, age, body weight and height, body mass index (BMI), WC, waist-to-hip ratio (WHR), waist-to-height ratio (WHtR), presence of hypertension, diabetes mellitus (DM), underlying renal disease, HD regimen, vintage of HD therapy, and concurrent medications of each patient were recorded.

Venous blood was sampled in the morning after an overnight fast of more than 8 hours before dialysis. Whole blood was used to

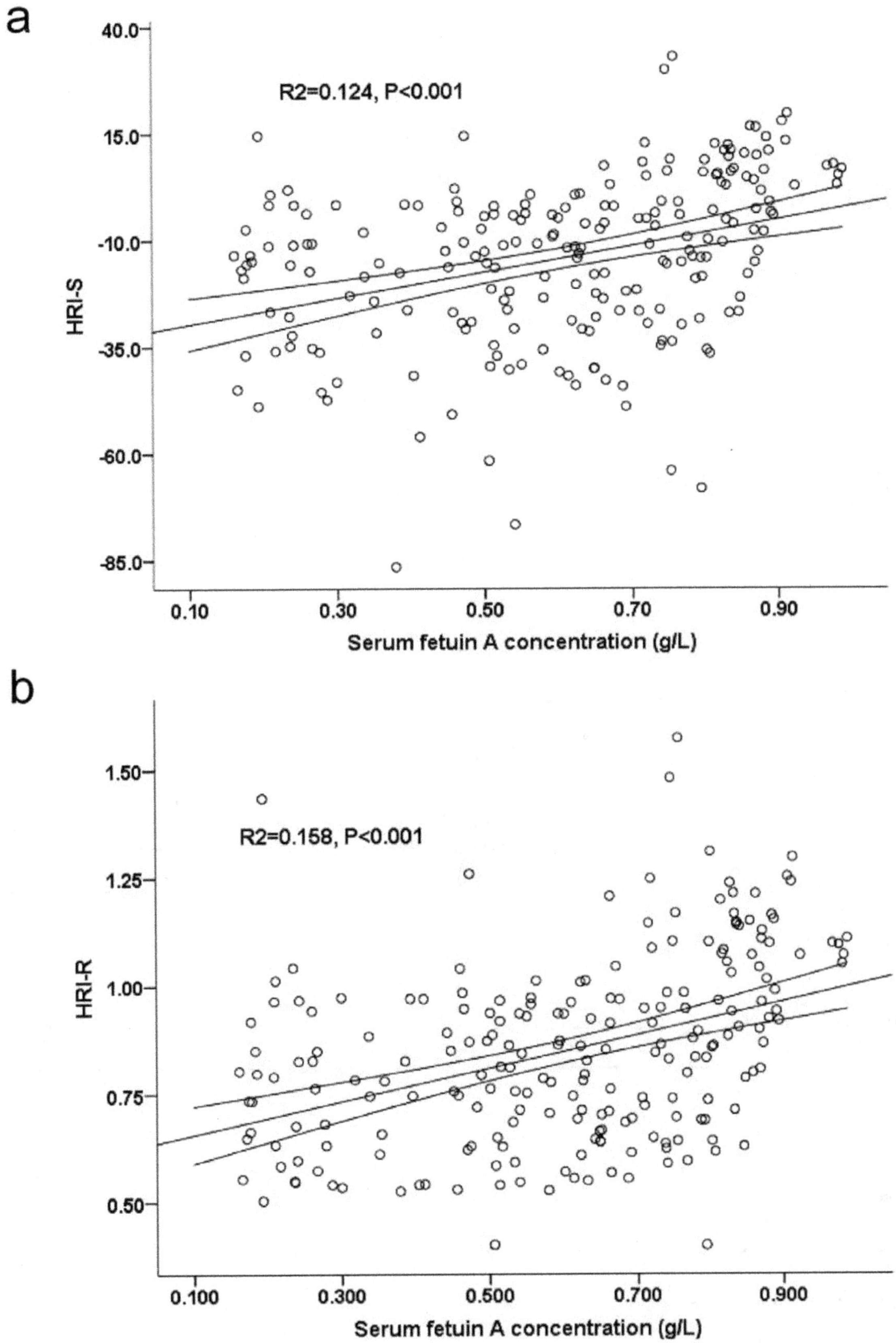

Figure 3. Relationships of serum fetuin A levels with hepato-renal index (HRI-S). (a) and with HRI-R (b) in univariate model (regression line and 95% CI).

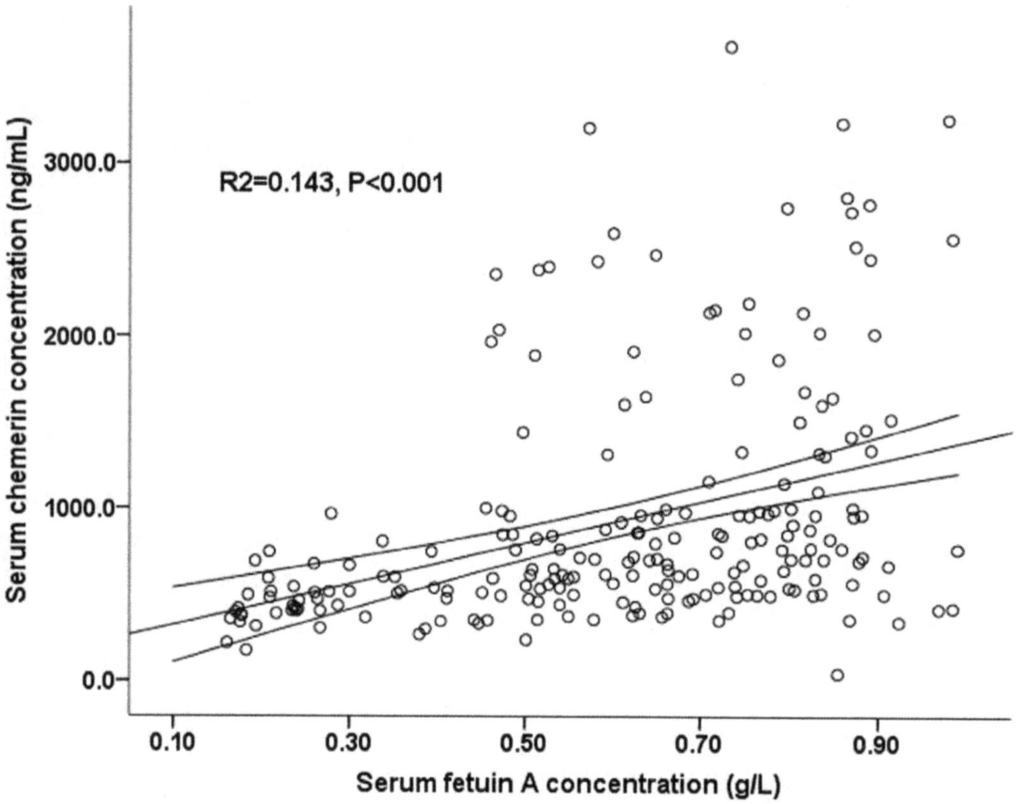

Figure 4. Relationships of serum fetuin A levels with serum chemerin levels in univariate model (regression line and 95% CI).

measure hemoglobin, serum for serum creatinine, calcium, phosphorus, potassium, uric acid, albumin, triglyceride (TG), total cholesterol (T-CHO), low-density lipoprotein cholesterol (LDL-C) and high-density lipoprotein cholesterol (HDL-C).

Intact parathyroid hormone (iPTH) was determined by immunoassay, while the immuno-nephelometric method with a Tina-quant CRP (Latex) ultra-sensitive assay (D & P modular analyzer, Roche Diagnostics GmbH, Mannheim, Germany) was used to determined highly sensitive C-reactive protein (hs-CRP).

Statistical Analysis

Continuous data were presented as mean ± SD or median (interquartile range), and categorical data were reported as percentages. Differences in the baseline characteristics of the patients with and without hepatic steatosis were compared using the Student's *t* test and Mann-Whitney U test accordingly. The chi-square test was used for categorical variables. Sensitivity, specificity, and cutoff levels for HRIs as predictors of the presence of hepatic steatosis and for fetuin A, chemerin levels and

Table 2. AUCs and cutoff values of ROC curves for prediction of hepatic steatosis and prediction of central obesity by fetuin A, chemerin levels, WC, WHR and WHtR.

		Fetuin A	Chemerin	WC	WHR	WHtR
Hepatic steatosis						
HRI-S > −10.8	AUC	0.69±0.04 (0.63~0.77)	0.63±0.04 (0.56~0.71)	0.69±0.04 (0.62~0.76)	0.65±0.04 (0.58~0.72)	0.67±0.04 (0.59~0.74)
	Cutofflevel	0.63 g/L 63.7/61(%)	690 ng/ml 58.8/58.2(%)	83 cm 70/59.3(%)	0.9 61.8/54.6(%)	0.52 65.7/58.3(%)
HRI-R >0.86	AUC	0.72±0.04 (0.66~0.79)	0.67±0.04 (0.59~0.74)	0.7±0.04 (0.63~0.77)	0.64±0.04 (0.57~0.71)	0.68±0.04 (0.61~0.76)
	Cutofflevel	0.63 g/L 65/62 (%)	705 ng/ml 60/64.5(%)	84 cm 62/65.4 (%)	0.91 56.3/57.9(%)	0.53 59.2/66.4(%)
Central obesity						
WC >90 cm in males and >80 cm in females	AUC	0.52±0.04 (0.45~0.57)*	0.65±0.04 (0.58~0.69)*	–	–	–
	Cutofflevel	0.63 g/L 53.3/50.5%	670 ng/ml 58.1/56.3%	–	–	–

Note: Values expressed as AUC ± SE (95% confidence interval) and cutoff level, sensitivity/specificity.
Abbreviations: AUC, area under curve; ROC, receiver operating characteristic; WC: waist circumference; WHR: waist-to-hip ratio; WHtR: waist-to-height ratio.
*AUC of chemerin was greater than that of fetuin A (P = 0.02), which was estimated by means of nonparametric statistical analysis (DeLong test).

Table 3. ORs for fetuin A, chemerin levels and WC to hepatic steatosis and central obesity by logistic regression analysis.

	Hepatic steatosis by HRI-S				Hepatic steatosis by HRI-R				Central obesity			
	Univariate	**P**	**Multivariate***	**P**	**Univariate**	**P**	**Multivariate***	**P**	**Univariate**	**P**	**Multivariate#**	**P**
Fetuin A (every 0.01 g/L increase)	1.03 (1.01~1.05)	<0.001	1.03 (1.01~1.05)	<0.001	1.04 (1.03~1.06)	<0.001	1.04 (1.02~1.06)	<0.001	1.003 (0.99~1.02)	0.6	0.99 (0.98~1.01)	0.6
Chemerin (every 1 ng/ml increase)	1.001 (1.0~1.01)	0.001	1.0 (1.0~1.003)	0.5	1.001 (1.001~1.01)	<0.001	1.0 (1.0~1.001)	0.3	1.002 (1.001~1.01)	0.04	1.01 (1.001~1.02)	0.02
WC (every 1 cm increase)	1.08 (1.04~1.1)	<0.001	1.1 (1.06~1.15)	<0.001	1.09 (1.05~1.13)	<0.001	1.1 (1.07~1.2)	<0.001	-	-	-	-

*Multivariate analysis included fetuin A, chemerin levels, WC, age, hemodialysis vintage, gender, diabetes mellitus, hs-CRP, albumin, Kt/V_{urea} and CaXP levels as covariates.
#Multivariate analysis included fetuin A, chemerin levels, age, gender, diabetes mellitus, albumin and Kt/V_{urea} as covariates.
Abbreviations: ORs: odds ratio; WC: waist circumference.

anthropometric parameters (WC, WHR and WHtR) as the predictors of hepatic steatosis and central obesity were analyzed by means of receiver operating characteristic (ROC) curve. Cutoff levels were estimated by the maximum combination of sensitivity and specificity, and comparisons among areas under the curve (AUCs) were estimated by using the statistical software PASS 2011 (Number Cruncher Statistical Systems, Keysville, UT).

The association of hepatic steatosis/central obesity with fetuin A and chemerin were further evaluated using logistic regression models, with hepatic steatosis (HRI-S and HRI-R) and central obesity as separate outcome variables and fetuin A, chemerin levels and WC as the predictor variables. These models were adjusted for the covariates, including age, HD vintage, gender, presence of DM, hs-CRP, albumin, Kt/V_{urea} and calcium phosphate product (CaXP) levels. Similarly, the association of conicity index with fetuin A and chemerin were checked using linear regression models, with conicity index (Ci) as an outcome variable and fetuin A and chemerin levels as the predictor variables. These models were adjusted for the covariates, including age, HD vintage, gender, presence of DM, albumin and Kt/V_{urea}.

The statistical analyses were performed using SPSS software, version 18.0 (SPSS, Inc., Chicago, IL). A p value of less than 0.05 was considered statistically significant.

Results

Basic Characteristics, Hepatic Steatosis, Fetuin A and Chemerin Levels in all Participants

The basic characteristics of all participants are summarized in Table 1. Eighty subjects had hepatic steatosis by ultrasound diagnosis. HRI-S and HRI-R (both P<0.001) were significantly higher in those with hepatic steatosis than those without. The validity of the HRIs for the estimation of the severity of hepatic steatosis was compared with hepatic steatosis which had been confirmed by liver ultrasound. The area under the ROC curve for HRI-S was 91.9% (95% CI, 88.4–95.3%) and 91.0% (95% CI, 87.3–94.8%) for HRI-R. The cutoff level for the diagnosis of hepatic steatosis was more than −10.8 (sensitivity/specificity: 87.5%/87.3%) by HRI-S and more than 0.86 (sensitivity/specificity: 88.8%/87.8%) by HRI-R (Figure 2). Overall, patients who had hepatic steatosis had significant higher BMI, Ci, WC, WHR and WHtR; besides, they also had significant higher fetuin A, chemerin, HOMAR-IR, hs-CRP, T-CHO, TG and lower adiponectin levels.

HRIs and Fetuin A and Chemerin Concentration

The severity of hepatic steatosis was further quantified by HRIs (HRI-S and HRI-R). The associations between serum fetuin A and HRI-S and HRI-R are shown in Figure 3a and 3b. Participants with higher HRIs had a higher serum fetuin A concentration (HRI-S, $R^2=0.124$, P<0.001; HRI-R, $R^2=0.158$, P<0.001). Also, participants with higher HRIs had a higher chemerin concentration (HRI-S, $R^2=0.071$, P<0.001; HRI-R, $R^2=0.065$, P<0.001).

Association between Fetuin A and Chemerin

The associations between serum fetuin A and chemerin are shown in Figure 4. Participants with higher fetuin A had a higher chemerin concentration ($R^2=0.143$, P<0.001).

ROC Analysis of Fetuin A, Chemerin, WC, WHR and WHtR as Predictors of Hepatic Steatosis

AUC and ROC cut-off levels for fetuin A, chemerin, WC, WHR and WHtR versus hepatic steatosis was shown in Table 2. Hepatic steatosis was defined with HRI-S> −10.8 and HRI-R>0.86 as described above. Fetuin A, chemerin levels, WC, WHR and WHtR were all predictors of the presence of hepatic steatosis (P<0.001). AUC for fetuin A versus hepatic steatosis was greater than that of chemerin; however, AUCs for fetuin A, chemerin, WC, WHR and WHtR were not significantly different (Table 2, all P>0.05).

ROC Analysis of Fetuin A and Chemerin as Predictors of Central Obesity

AUC and ROC cut-off levels for fetuin A and chemerin versus central obesity was shown in Table 2 also. Fetuin A and chemerin levels were both predictors of the presence of central obesity (P<0.001). AUC for chemerin versus central obesity was significantly greater than that of fetuin A (P=0.02).

Conicity Index (Ci) and Fetuin A and Chemerin Concentration

The Ci was positively associated with chemerin concentration ($R^2=0.211$, P=0.002) but was not significantly associated with fetuin A concentration ($R^2 = 0.103$, $P = 0.13$). Using linear regression model, taking Ci as continuous dependent variable, chemerin concentration was independently correlated to Ci (standardized $\beta = 0.26$, $P < 0.001$) after adjusted for fetuin A levels, age, gender, diabetes mellitus status, HD vintage, albumin and Kt/V_{urea}. However, fetuin A concentration was not (standardized $\beta = 0.053$, $P = 0.4$).

Logistic Regression Analysis of the Fetuin A and Chemerin Levels for Prediction of Hepatic Steatosis and Central Obesity

In univariate analysis, fetuin A, chemerin and WC were all predictors of having hepatic steatosis, whether HRI-S or HRI-R evaluated. In multivariate analysis, after adjusting for diabetes status, age, gender, HD vintage, Kt/V_{urea}, WC, fetuin A, chemerin, hs-CRP, albumin and CaXP levels, higher fetuin A levels significantly predicted the diagnosis of hepatic steatosis by HRIs (Table 3, $P < 0.001$).

In univariate analysis, chemerin was the predictor of central obesity, but fetuin A was not (Table 3). In multivariate analysis, after adjusting for diabetes status, age, gender, HD vintage, Kt/V_{urea}, fetuin A, chemerin and albumin levels, only higher chemerin level had significant power to predict the diagnosis of central obesity (Table 3, $P = 0.02$).

Discussion

The main finding of this study is that prevalent HD patients with hepatic steatosis, as quantified by HRIs, have higher fetuin A concentrations. To the best of our knowledge, this is the first investigation to identify this relationship. A high level of fetuin A could be meaningfully found in HD patients with hepatic steatosis. Moreover, fetuin A level positively correlates with chemerin in dialysis patients. We also demonstrate the interesting finding that chemerin independently correlates with central obesity and regional adiposity in this population.

Fetuin A deficiency is a critical issue in dialysis patients, owing to its close relationship with CV calcification and mortality. Beyond the known factors leading to fetuin A deficiency in dialysis patients such as inflammation, aging and malnutrition [27], investigators have been trying to clarify the factors linked to enhanced fetuin A synthesis in dialysis populations. In a non-CKD human longitudinal study, fetuin A levels increased with the accumulation of liver fat [10]. In our previous study, we identified a link between higher fetuin A levels and central obesity and different degrees of lipid derangement in non-diabetic HD patients [28]. Assuming that the consumption of fetuin A is similar, fetuin A concentrations should be higher in HD patients with greater fetuin A synthesis. In the present study, we adjusted the parameters related to fetuin A consumption in multivariate analysis in order to satisfy the presumption of equal fetuin A consumption in the participated HD patients. In case of similar inflammatory and dialysis conditions, our data implied the fetuin A synthesis was in concordance with the hepatic steatosis, and suggested that fetuin A levels would be higher in HD patients with hepatic steatosis.

The current study also demonstrated a novel association between fetuin A and chemerin in HD patients. Both fetuin A and chemerin are associated with visceral fat in non-CKD patients with NAFLD [15,17,21]. In addition, they both correlate with lipoproteins and inflammation in CKD and non-CKD patients [12–13,15,28]. Our results showed a positive correlation between fetuin A and chemerin and the association between chemerin levels and regional adiposity in HD patients. The proposed mechanism by which increased adiposity and the concomitant increase of chemerin level in patients with hepatic steatosis might be the output of infiltration of macrophages in adipose tissue [29]. Nevertheless, fetuin A synthesis responds directly to liver fat accumulation and it indirectly enhances liver fat accumulation by inhibiting adiponectin synthesis in the adipocytes [10,21]. The underlying mechanism by which fetuin A and chemerin respond to hepatic steatosis seems to be different, and the pathophysiologic link between them needs further investigation. But interestingly, in a recent study, a high chemerin level potentially predicted better all-cause mortality in incident dialysis patients [19]. This survival benefit is parallel to dialysis patients with a high fetuin A level, and this further strengthens the linkage between fetuin A and chemerin. However, longitudinal data are needed to support the potential association between the regional adiposity, manifested as hepatic steatosis or central obesity, and survival benefits in prevalent HD patients.

In the general population, liver or visceral fat content is usually evaluated with MRI or CT [12,30]. To the best, liver biopsy is the gold standard of estimation of the severity of hepatic steatosis. However, in CKD patients, especially in HD patients, these two imaging modalities have a limited role in the evaluation of visceral and liver fat content due to the potential harms. The diathesis of bleeding also limited the role of liver biopsy for evaluating the severity of hepatic steatosis in dialysis patients. Abdominal ultrasound is a non-invasive, portable and safe tool to evaluate the status of hepatic steatosis, and it can be used to quantify accurately with an assistant image analyzer (ImageJ). This method has been validated in several investigations comparing the results of liver biopsies [25–26]. In our results, both HRI-S and HRI-R had good sensitivity and specificity for the diagnosis of hepatic steatosis in HD patients (Figure 1). Therefore, we suggested that abdominal ultrasound would be a practical, safe and cost-effective tool to both qualify and quantify the severity of hepatic steatosis in patients under HD.

There some limitations to this study. First, we used the HRIs for the quantification of hepatic steatosis but not liver histological measurements due to the consideration of potential harms. Besides, kidney echogenicity in the ROI can be variable in CKD patients, especially in dialysis patients, due to the different ranges of parenchymal fibrosis and atrophy. Therefore, the precision of the HRIs may not be robust. Nevertheless, we showed the good validity of HRI, either HRI-S or HRI-R, in assessing hepatic steatosis in our results. Moreover, the outstanding intra-observer reproducibility of HRIs further strengthens the reliability of our evaluations. Second, the study has a cross-sectional design, and, therefore, causality could not be established. Further longitudinal changes of liver fat content and fetuin A levels should be investigated in future studies. Third, exact visceral adiposity can not be measured by ultrasound precisely. Therefore, we did not evaluate the visceral adiposity directly and used WC and Ci instead in this study, which might attenuate the strength of the conclusion regarding the association between chemerin and visceral obesity.

In summary, our results suggest that prevalent HD patients who have hepatic steatosis have higher fetuin A concentrations. In addition, fetuin A and chemerin levels positively correlate with each other; and chemerin, but not fetuin A, is a better predictor of regional adiposity in our HD patients. The longitudinal changes of hepatic steatosis and its impact on survival in dialysis patients need to be tested in future studies.

Author Contributions

Conceived and designed the experiments: HYC YSP. Performed the experiments: HYC CCL YSP. Analyzed the data: HYC JYY. Contributed reagents/materials/analysis tools: HYC CCL YLC SPH MFP JYY. Wrote the paper: HYC.

References

1. Ketteler M, Bongartz P, Westenfeld R, Wildberger JE, Mahnken AH, et al. (2003) Association of low fetuin-A (AHSG) concentrations in serum with cardiovascular mortality in patients on dialysis: a cross-sectional study. Lancet 361: 827–833.
2. Weikert C, Stefan N, Schulze MB, Pischon T, Berger K, et al. (2008) Plasma fetuin-a levels and the risk of myocardial infarction and ischemic stroke. Circulation 118: 2555–2562.
3. Tuttolomondo A, Di Raimondo D, Di Sciacca R, Casuccio A, Bivona G, et al. (2010) Fetuin-A and CD40 L plasma levels in acute ischemic stroke: differences in relation to TOAST subtype and correlation with clinical and laboratory variables. Atherosclerosis 208: 290–296.
4. Westenfeld R, Schafer C, Kruger T, Haarmann C, Schurgers LJ, et al. (2009) Fetuin-A protects against atherosclerotic calcification in CKD. J Am Soc Nephrol 20: 1264–1274.
5. Ketteler M (2005) Fetuin-A and extraosseous calcification in uremia. Curr Opin Nephrol Hypertens 14: 337–342.
6. Reynolds JL, Joannides AJ, Skepper JN, McNair R, Schurgers LJ, et al. (2004) Human vascular smooth muscle cells undergo vesicle-mediated calcification in response to changes in extracellular calcium and phosphate concentrations: a potential mechanism for accelerated vascular calcification in ESRD. J Am Soc Nephrol 15: 2857–2867.
7. Schlieper G, Aretz A, Verberckmoes SC, Kruger T, Behets GJ, et al. (2010) Ultrastructural analysis of vascular calcifications in uremia. J Am Soc Nephrol 21: 689–696.
8. Kelley DE, McKolanis TM, Hegazi RA, Kuller LH, Kalhan SC (2003) Fatty liver in type 2 diabetes mellitus: relation to regional adiposity, fatty acids, and insulin resistance. Am J Physiol Endocrinol Metab 285: E906–916.
9. Lin X, Braymer HD, Bray GA, York DA (1998) Differential expression of insulin receptor tyrosine kinase inhibitor (fetuin) gene in a model of diet-induced obesity. Life Sci 63: 145–153.
10. Stefan N, Hennige AM, Staiger H, Machann J, Schick F, et al. (2006) Alpha2-Heremans-Schmid glycoprotein/fetuin-A is associated with insulin resistance and fat accumulation in the liver in humans. Diabetes Care 29: 853–857.
11. Axelsson J, Wang X, Ketteler M, Qureshi AR, Heimburger O, et al. (2008) Is fetuin-A/alpha2-Heremans-Schmid glycoprotein associated with the metabolic syndrome in patients with chronic kidney disease? Am J Nephrol 28: 669–676.
12. Ix JH, Wassel CL, Chertow GM, Koster A, Johnson KC, et al. (2009) Fetuin-A and change in body composition in older persons. J Clin Endocrinol Metab 94: 4492–4498.
13. Chan DC, Watts GF, Gan SK, Ooi EM, Barrett PH (2010) Effect of ezetimibe on hepatic fat, inflammatory markers, and apolipoprotein B-100 kinetics in insulin-resistant obese subjects on a weight loss diet. Diabetes Care 33: 1134–1139.
14. Mori K, Emoto M, Araki T, Yokoyama H, Lee E, et al. (2008) Effects of pioglitazone on serum fetuin-A levels in patients with type 2 diabetes mellitus. Metabolism 57: 1248–1252.
15. Reinehr T, Roth CL (2008) Fetuin-A and its relation to metabolic syndrome and fatty liver disease in obese children before and after weight loss. J Clin Endocrinol Metab 93: 4479–4485.
16. Bozaoglu K, Segal D, Shields KA, Cummings N, Curran JE, et al. (2009) Chemerin is associated with metabolic syndrome phenotypes in a Mexican-American population. J Clin Endocrinol Metab 94: 3085–3088.
17. Sell H, Divoux A, Poitou C, Basdevant A, Bouillot JL, et al. (2010) Chemerin correlates with markers for fatty liver in morbidly obese patients and strongly decreases after weight loss induced by bariatric surgery. J Clin Endocrinol Metab 95: 2892–2896.
18. Weigert J, Neumeier M, Wanninger J, Filarsky M, Bauer S, et al. (2010) Systemic chemerin is related to inflammation rather than obesity in type 2 diabetes. Clin Endocrinol (Oxf) 72: 342–348.
19. Yamamoto T, Qureshi AR, Anderstam B, Heimburger O, Barany P, et al. (2010) Clinical importance of an elevated circulating chemerin level in incident dialysis patients. Nephrol Dial Transplant 25: 4017–4023.
20. Hennige AM, Staiger H, Wicke C, Machicao F, Fritsche A, et al. (2008) Fetuin-A induces cytokine expression and suppresses adiponectin production. PLoS One 3: e1765.
21. Ix JH, Sharma K (2010) Mechanisms linking obesity, chronic kidney disease, and fatty liver disease: the roles of fetuin-A, adiponectin, and AMPK. J Am Soc Nephrol 21: 406–412.
22. Heng D, Ma S, Lee JJ, Tai BC, Mak KH, et al. (2006) Modification of the NCEP ATP III definitions of the metabolic syndrome for use in Asians identifies individuals at risk of ischemic heart disease. Atherosclerosis 186: 367–373.
23. Valdez R (1991) A simple model-based index of abdominal adiposity. J Clin Epidemiol 44: 955–956.
24. Saadeh S, Younossi ZM, Remer EM, Gramlich T, Ong JP, et al. (2002) The utility of radiological imaging in nonalcoholic fatty liver disease. Gastroenterology 123: 745–750.
25. Soder RB, Baldisserotto M, Duval da Silva V (2009) Computer-assisted ultrasound analysis of liver echogenicity in obese and normal-weight children. AJR Am J Roentgenol 192: W201–205.
26. Webb M, Yeshua H, Zelber-Sagi S, Santo E, Brazowski E, et al. (2009) Diagnostic value of a computerized hepatorenal index for sonographic quantification of liver steatosis. AJR Am J Roentgenol 192: 909–914.
27. Hermans MM, Brandenburg V, Ketteler M, Kooman JP, van der Sande FM, et al. (2007) Association of serum fetuin-A levels with mortality in dialysis patients. Kidney Int 72: 202–207.
28. Chen HY, Chiu YL, Hsu SP, Pai MF, Lai CF, et al. (2009) Association of serum fetuin A with truncal obesity and dyslipidemia in non-diabetic hemodialysis patients. Eur J Endocrinol 160: 777–783.
29. Cancello R, Tordjman J, Poitou C, Guilhem G, Bouillot JL, et al. (2006) Increased infiltration of macrophages in omental adipose tissue is associated with marked hepatic lesions in morbid human obesity. Diabetes 55: 1554–1561.
30. Nguyen-Duy TB, Nichaman MZ, Church TS, Blair SN, Ross R (2003) Visceral fat and liver fat are independent predictors of metabolic risk factors in men. Am J Physiol Endocrinol Metab 284: E1065–1071.

13

In Vivo Evaluation of the Biocompatibility of Surface Modified Hemodialysis Polysulfone Hollow Fibers in Rat

Ganpat J. Dahe[1]⁹, Sachin S. Kadam[1]⁹, Siddharth S. Sabale[2], Dattatray P. Kadam[2], Laxman B. Sarkate[3], Jayesh R. Bellare[1]*

1 Department of Chemical Engineering, Indian Institute of Technology Bombay, Powai, Mumbai, India, **2** Department of Veterinary Pathology, Bombay Veterinary College, Parel, Mumbai, India, **3** Department of Surgery & Radiology, Bombay Veterinary College, Parel, Mumbai, India

Abstract

Polysulfone (Psf) hollow fiber membranes (HFMs) have been widely used in blood purification but their biocompatibility remains a concern. To enhance their biocompatibility, Psf/TPGS (d-α-tocopheryl polyethylene glycol 1000 succinate) composite HFMs and 2-methacryloyloxyethyl phosphorylcholine (MPC) coated Psf HFMs have been prepared. They have been evaluated for in vivo biocompatibility and graft acceptance and compared with sham and commercial membranes by intra-peritoneal implantation in rats at day 7 and 21. Normal body weights, tissue formation and angiogenesis indicate acceptance of implants by the animals. Hematological observations show presence of post-surgical stress which subsides over time. Serum biochemistry results reveal normal organ function and elevated liver ALP levels at day 21. Histological studies exhibit fibroblast recruitment cells, angiogenesis and collagen deposition at the implant surface indicating new tissue formation. Immuno-histochemistry studies show non-activation of MHC molecules signifying biocompatibilty. Additionally, Psf/TPGS exhibit most favorable tissue response as compared with other HFMs making them the material of choice for HFM preparation for hemodialysis applications.

Editor: Aristidis S. Charonis, Biomedical Research Foundation of the Academy of Athens, Greece

Funding: This research was supported by the Department of Science and Technology, Government of India (www.dst.gov.in). The funders had no role in study design, data collection and analysis, decision to publish, or preparation of the manuscript.

Competing Interests: The authors have declared that no competing interests exist.

* E-mail: jb@iitb.ac.in

⁹ These authors contributed equally to this work.

Introduction

Membrane technology has proven vital in blood purification applications, especially hemodialysis. In hollow fiber membranes (HFMs), purification is achieved by regulating blood flow through the lumen as the dialysate flows counter-currently outside. The porous structure of the membrane facilitates diffusion of uremic toxins like urea, creatinine etc. from blood to dialysate without the loss of important blood proteins such as albumin. Desirable characteristics of such HFMs include high flux, selectivity and biocompatibility [1]. However, commercially available and most-widely used polysulfone (Psf) hemodialysis membranes have repeatedly been shown to be associated with clinical complications like hypersensitivity reactions, neutropenia, oxidative stress, contact and complement activation [2–5]. This translates into decreased quality of life, life expectancy and mortality of hemodialysis patients and has limited the success rates of such membranes [6,7]. Thus, there is a need to enhance the biocompatibility of such membranes without compromising flux and selectivity.

Biocompatibility is the most desirable property of a biomaterial, of being biologically compatible by not producing a toxic, injurious and immunological response in living tissues or blood for the case of extra-corporeal devices [8]. The most commonly accepted mode of improving HFM biocompatibility has been modification of surface chemistry. Ishihara et al. achieved improved hemocompatibility of cellulose membranes under in vitro conditions by grafting with 2–methacryloyloxyethyl phosphorylcholine (MPC) polymers [9]. Polyacrylonitrile dialysis membranes, modified by covalent immobilization of chitosan/heparin polyelectrolyte complexes, exhibited improved antithrombogenicity and reduced platelet adhesion, thrombus formation and protein adsorption [10]. In our earlier studies on NIH3T3 cells, we showed that impregnation of d-α-tocopheryl polyethylene glycol 1000 succinate (TPGS) in Psf matrices enhances the biocompatibility of native HFMs [11]. However, definitive in vivo studies are required to assess the biocompatibility of such surface modified HFMs before their practical application in hemodialysis.

During a typical hemodialysis procedure, blood is circulated at 200 ml/min through HFMs (surface areas ~1–2 m^2) for 3–5 h thrice a week and such procedures lasts throughout the life of a renal failure patient [12]. The continuous, long-term exposure of blood to such membranes initiates various cellular reactions and protein conformational changes, depending on the physico-chemical nature of HFM surface. Hence, as per ISO 10993-1, systemic toxicity evaluation of membrane material for a week is necessary before hemodialysis trials [13]. These evaluations require studies on circulating blood for which number of animal models have been used [14]. Intra-peritoneal implantation in rats is a proven method for systemic evaluations, since it exposes the samples to both fluid and a variety of mesenchymal cell types of abdominal cavity [15].

In the present study, we have evaluated the in vivo biocompatibility of modified Psf/TPGS composite HFMs and inner-surface coated MPC/Psf HFMs on Wistar rat model. The effects of implanted membrane material on vital organ systems such as liver, kidney etc. have been studied by hematology, serum biochemistry and peritoneal fluid cytology. Tissue and immunological responses to HFMs have been evaluated using histopathological observations and immuno-histochemistry. These studies exhibit that Psf/TPGS membranes exhibit improved biocompatibility as compared to the other studied membranes and are suitable for practical hemodialysis applications.

Results and Discussion

Gross Observations

In any in vivo implant study the change in body weight is an essential parameter to judge health of animal model. The basal and final weights of rats at the time of implantation and after exposure are shown in Table 1. After HFM exposure for 7 days, the body weights of rats of normal, sham, Psf/TPGS and Hemoflow F6 groups were increased by 20–30 gm and for Psf and Psf/MPC groups, by 8–9 gm. By the 21st day, the increase in body weight was 40–50 gm across all groups indicating healthy condition of rats. Figure 1a and 2b are the camera images of Psf HFMs implants in peritoneal cavity on day 7 and 21, respectively. Both cases exhibit tissue formation on day 7 which becomes distinct and accompanied by angiogenesis on day 21.

Blood Hematology and Serum Biochemistry Study

Blood hematology studies are carried out to determine surgery-associated infections during implantation while serum biochemistry studies indicate functionalities of vital organs such as liver and kidney. CBCs, differential leukocyte counts and serum protein levels in blood of all groups after days 7 and 21 are listed in data S1. CBCs across all groups were within the normal range [20] after 7 and 21 days indicating that the implantation procedures were devoid of any infections.

Slightly increased neutrophil numbers in Leukocyte differential count on day 7 for Psf, Psf/TPGS, Psf/MPC and Hemoflow F6 groups indicated the presence of a mild inflammatory response as compared to control and normal groups. These numbers subsided and reached the normal level on the 21st day of implantation. This is a usual phenomenon, which occurs in response to foreign implants and is characterized by reduction in the inflammatory response with increase in the implantation period [21].

In serum biochemistry measurements (data S1), liver enzymes and serum proteins of all groups were within the normal range on days 7 and 21. However, as compared to day 7, the ALT, AST, and ALP enzyme concentrations for Psf, Psf/TPGS, Psf/MPC and Hemoflow F6 groups were elevated on day 21 and were even greater than the sham group. ALP has been documented as a possible marker for wound healing [22] and may also indicate tissue repair and angiogenesis. The observed ALP increase in implanted groups only may, thus, be due to these processes. The creatinine and blood urea nitrogen (BUN) values were within normal ranges for all groups indicating healthy and functional condition of kidney. Since all the implants are non-biodegradable and non-leachable, so no malfunction of liver and kidney was observed.

Peritoneal Fluid Cytology

Differential leukocyte counts performed on peritoneal fluid collected on days 7 and 21 are listed in Table 2. As an initial response to HFM implants, increased polymorphonucleocyte (PMN) numbers were observed in the peritoneal fluid at day 7 when compared to the sham and normal groups. However at day 21, these numbers were within the normal range. The elevated numbers may be due to the surgical procedure. Similar trends were observed for neutrophils in differential leukocyte counts, indicating the presence of post-surgical stress which subsides with time. The decrease in this stress occurs because of wound healing and tissue formation as the time progresses.

Tissue-HFM interaction study by Scanning Electron Microscopy

SEM provides high resolution direct information on tissue-biomaterial interactions with minimal sample preparation as compared to histology. Further, histological sample preparation causes implant detachment from tissues and this information is preserved during SEM sample preparation. The SEM micrographs of HFM implanted groups at day 21 are shown in Figure 2. Dense tissue integration with the implant was observed in all the cases (see inset micrographs). No masses were observed in the implant bores or lumens. Degradation and material surface changes due to body fluids were not observed. However, it is difficult to extract detailed information about surrounding tissue/cells type from these micrographs because of surface similarities in different types of cells.

Histological Study of Implants

The optical microscopy based histological evaluation of tissues surrounding the implant provides morphological and pathological analysis. Tissue reactions in the implanted groups are summarized in Table 3 and optical micrographs of respective histological sections at day 7 and day 21 are shown in Figure 3. On day 7 post-implantation, a relatively greater infiltration of polymorphonucle-

Table 1. Basal and final weight of normal, sham surgeries and implanted rats.

	Day 7 (in gm)		Day 21 (in gm)	
Sample Type	**Basal Weight**	**Final Weight**	**Basal Weight**	**Final Weight**
Normal	150.00±14.14	169.50±30.60	170.50±30.40	220.50±3.53
Sham Surgeries	150.50±16.26	180.00±5.66	173.00±2.83	220.00±1.41
Psf	156.33±16.77	165.33±22.37	165.33±2.08	213.00±17.35
Psf/TPGS	165.67±15.95	189.33±8.33	154.33±9.07	191.00±9.90
Psf/MPC	164.00±10.15	172.33±0.58	159.67±13.65	206.33±17.62
Hemoflow F6	134.33±22.55	165.33±14.22	180.00±8.00	227.00±6.56

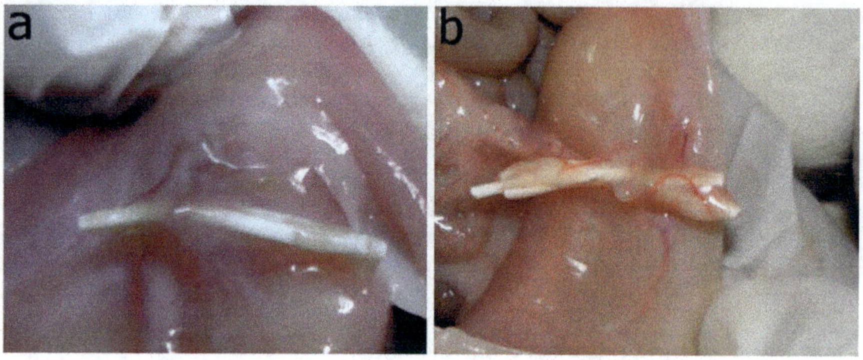

Figure 1. Interaperitoneal implantation of HFM. Images of Psf implants in peritoneum during excision in CO_2 euthanized rat at days 7 (a) and days 27 (b).

ars (PMNs) and macrophages into the surrounding tissues of MPC and Hemoflow F6 implants was observed as compared to the Psf and Psf/TPGS implants. However, infiltration of fibroblasts surrounding the implant and degrees of angiogenesis were more prominent for Psf and Psf/TPGS implants than Psf/MPC and Hemoflow F6 implants. On day 21, fibroblast recruitment was enhanced, while angiogenesis remained the same for all cases as compared to day 7. PMN, macrophage and lymphocyte infiltrations were reduced on day 21 as compared to day 7. Similar trends of reduction in PMNs, macrophages and lymphocytes with time upon implantation of disulfide-crosslinked hyaluronan films have been reported earlier [23].

Collagen deposition is vital for new tissue formation and its distribution and extent can be studied by Masson's trichrome staining. Figure 4 shows the optical micrographs of Masson's trichrome stained sections of different groups at days 7 and 21. On day 7 post-implantation, thin collagen bundles (t) were observed for all implants, while thick collagen bundles (T) were observed on day 21. The increased collagen deposition may be due to increase in fibroblast numbers (Table 3) which secrete collagen and is an indicator of tissue formation. It has also been reported earlier for poly(l-lactide-co-e-caprolactone) scaffolds implanted subcutaneousely [24].

These histological studies exhibit favorable tissue response to all implants indicating biocompatibility. However, the Psf/TPGS group showed minimum lymphocytes and maximum fibroblasts and angiogenesis (Table 3). These observations indicate that Psf/TPGS achieves better tissue response as compared other HFM implants, including commercial HFMs. This may be due to the presence of TPGS, which leaches and cleaves into vitamin E and polyethylene glycol moieties by enzymatic reactions [25]. Vitamin E, a proven anti-oxidant [26], causes a reduction in implant-associated oxidative stress and contributes to the better performance of the Psf/TPGS implant.

Immunohistochemistry by Confocal Microscopy

Studies of immunological response of tissues with HFM implants are vital for assessing host-verses-graft (implant) reactions. HLA-DR is constitutively expressed on antigen-presenting immune system cells like dendritic cells, B cells, and monocytes/macrophages and its expression is further up-regulated upon activation. It is, thus, considered as an essential marker for activation of immune system [27,28]. The confocal micrographs of normal peritoneal tissue and implanted groups stained with DAPI for nuclei and phycoerythrin (PE) conjugated HLA- DR antibody for MHC at day 21 are shown in Figure 5. The micrographs

Table 2. Leukocyte differential counts for peritoneal fluid after HFM implantation.

Sample Type	Incubation Time (days)	PMN*	Mononuclear**	Lymphocytes	Eosinophils	Basophils
Normal (Without Surgery)	7	21±2	61±6	16±3	1±0	1±0
Sham Surgeries	7	30±1	51±2	15±2	1±0	1±0
Psf	7	42±3	40±2	15±3	2±1	1±0
Psf/TPGS	7	39±3	41±1	17±3	2±1	1±0
Psf/MPC	7	42±4	41±4	14±0	2±1	1±0
Hemoflow F6	7	39±3	43±4	15±2	2±1	1±0
Normal (Without Surgery)	21	19±2	61±4	18±3	1±0	1±0
Sham Surgeries	21	20±1	66±2	11±2	2±1	1±0
Psf	21	21±2	61±5	15±2	2±0	1±0
Psf/TPGS	21	25±2	57±4	16±3	2±1	0±0
Psf/MPC	21	24±2	60±2	13±3	2±1	1±0
Hemoflow F6	21	19±2	65±4	15±2	1±0	0±0

(*PMN = polymorph nucleocytes, i.e. granulocytes; **Mononuclear = monocytes, macrophages, and mesothelial).

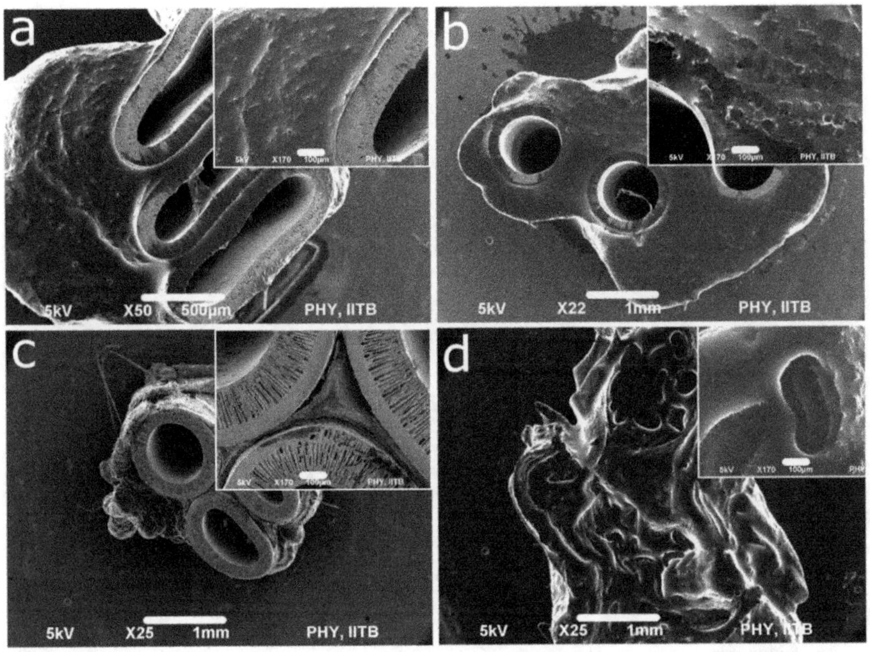

Figure 2. Tissue-HFM interaction study by Scanning Electron Microscopy. SEM micrographs of HFMs implants at day 21 (a) Psf (b) Psf/TPGS (c) MPC coated Psf and (d) Hemoflow F6 showing integration developed tissue with HFMs implants [scale bar: (a) 500 µm and (b), (c), (d) 1 mm (inset: (a), (b), (c) and (d) 100 µm)].

showed distinct nuclei of cells surrounding the implants; however, fluorescence due to PE was not observed indicating non-activation of immune cells in the tissues surrounding the implants. Also, peritoneal fluid cytology showed normal leukocyte differential count in implanted rats. This supports non-activation of immune system at the implant site and indicates acceptance of the implants by the animals.

Psf-based implants with different surface charcateristics were evaluated for their in vivo biocompatibility in rat model. These implants exhibited improved biocompatibility over commercially available membranes. The post-implantation CBC, renal and liver function tests indicated normal health of rat signifying absence of infections due to surgical procedures. Peritoneal fluid cytology exhibited elevated PMNs at day 7 post-implantation due to initial inflammation which returned within the normal range by day 21 indicating absence of chronic inflammation. Histopathology studies revealed abundunt fibroblast and angiogenesis in the tissues surrounding Psf/TPGS implants as compared to Psf, Psf/MPC and Hemoflow F6 implants indicating imporved biocompatiblity of Psf/TPGS implants attributable to the cleaved Vitamin E moiety. Immune responses against all the implants were absent. This study may be useful for generation of hollow fiber based vascular grafts which are able to grow within the peritoneal cavity.

Materials and Methods

Ethics Statement

All the animal experimental protocols were approved by Committee for the Purpose of Control and Supervision of Experiments on Animals (CPCSEA), India and animal ethical committee of Mumbai Veterinary College (MVC), Mumbai.

Preparation of Hollow Fiber membrane

Psf (UDELTM P-3500 LCD MB7-BULK) was procured from M/s. Solvay Advanced Polymers, USA and dried in vacuum oven

Table 3. Inflammatory evaluation of intraperitoneal HFMs implants.

Implantation Period (days)	Implant Type	PMC	Macrophages	Lymphocytes	Fibroblast	Angiogenesis	Collagen Bundles
7	Psf	++	+	+	+	++	Thin
21	Psf	+	+	+	++	++	Thick
7	Psf/TPGS	+	+	+	++	++	Thin
21	Psf/TPGS	+	++	+	+++	++	Thick
7	Psf/MPC	+	+	++	++	++	Thin
21	Psf/MPC	+	++	+	+++	++	Thick
7	Hemoflow F6	++	+	++	+	+	Thin
21	Hemoflow F6	+	++	+	++	++	Thick

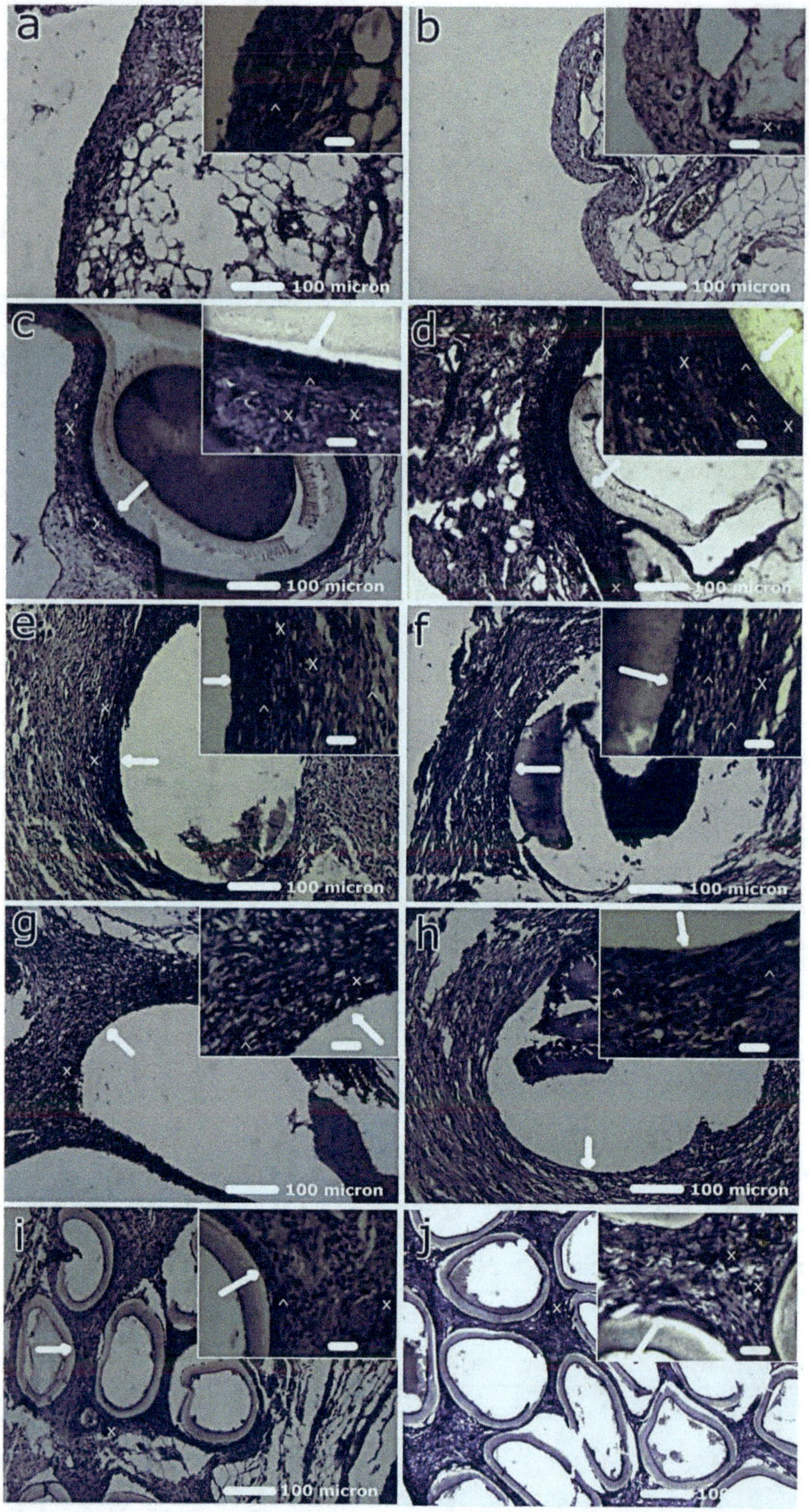

Figure 3. Histopathological analysis of implant by hematoxylin and eosin stain. Optical photomicrograph of hematoxylin and eosin stained tissue section of normal rat peritoneum at day 7 (a) and day 21 (b); Psf HFMs implants at day 7 (c) and day (d); Psf/TPGS HFMs implants at day 7 (e) and day 21 (f); Psf/MPC HFMs implants at day 7 (g) and day 21(h); Hemoflow F6 HFMs implants at day 7 (i) and day 21 (j). Arrow head, cross and big white arrow denotes fibroblast, angiogenesis and interface of implant with tissue respectively. [Scale bar: 100 μm (inset: 20 μm)]. Note: Psf/TPGS (e and f) and Psf/MPC (g and h) implants were detached during tissue processing for histology, but tissue interface with implants are distinctly visible.

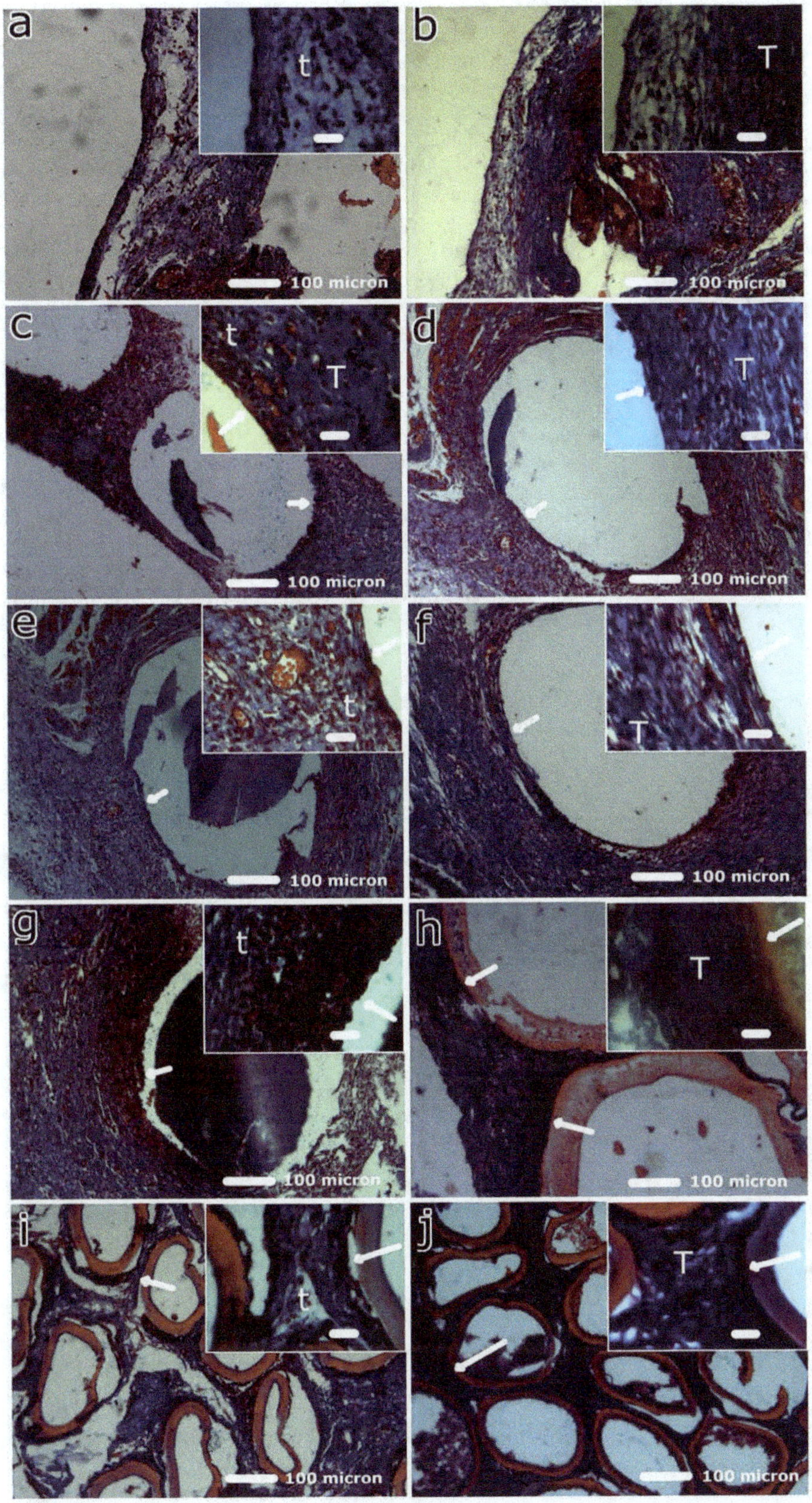

Figure 4. Histopathological analysis of implant by Masson's trichrome stain. Optical photomicrograph of Masson's trichrome stained tissue section of normal normal rat peritoneum at day 7 (a) and day 21 (b); Psf HFMs implants at day 7 (c) and day 21 (d); Psf/TPGS HFMs implants at day 7 (e) and day 21 (f); Psf/MPC HFMs implants at day 7 (g) and day 21 (h); Hemoflow F6 HFMs implants at day 7 (i) and day 21 (j). The symbols t and T denotes thin, thick blue collagen bundles respectively, while arrow shows interface implant with tissue. [Scale bar: 100 μm (inset: 20 μm)]. Note: Some hollow fiber implants are detached (c, d, e, f, and g) during processing for histology.

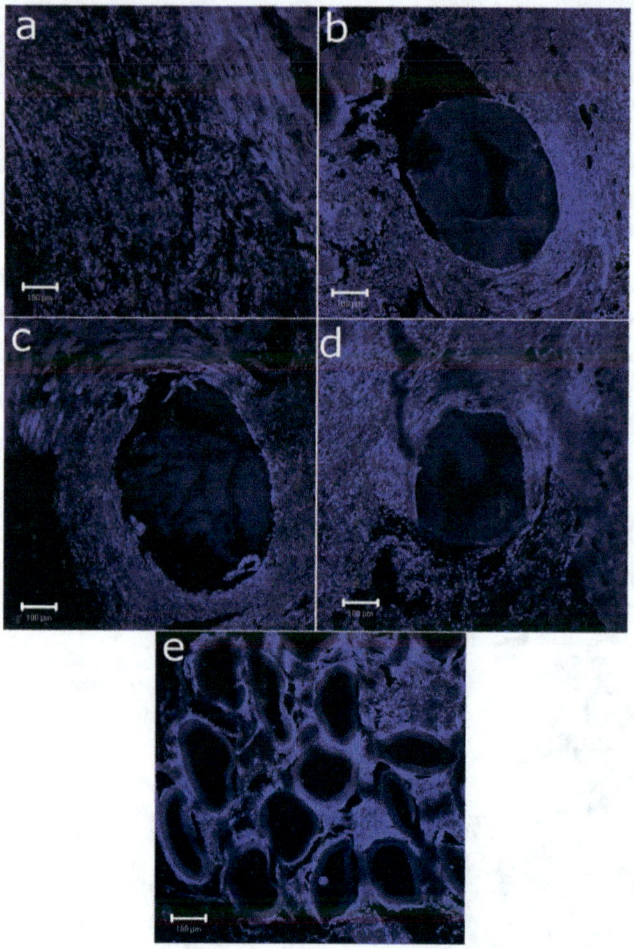

Figure 5. Immunohistochemistry of implants. Confocal laser micrographs of immunohistochemical stained tissue of (a) Psf HFMs, (b) Psf/TPGS HFMs, (c) Psf/MPC HFMs and (d) Hemoflow F6 HFMs implants with DAPI for nuclei (blue) [scale: 100 μm].

for 24 h at 90°C to remove absorbed water. Vitamin E TPGS (NF grade) and MPC polymers PC 2118 [Poly(2-methacryloyloxyethyl)-2′-(trimethylammoniumethyl) phosphate, inner salt)-co-(3-(trimethoxysilyl)propyl methacrylate)-co-(hydroxypropyl methacrylate)] were generously gifted by M/s. Isochem SA (Paris, France) and M/s. Vertellus Specialties Inc., (Basinstoke, UK), respectively. The solvent, N-methyl2-pyrrolidone (NMP), was procured from S.D. Fine-Chem Ltd., India. Psf and Psf/TPGS composite HFMs were prepared as per the conditions and compositions listed in Table 4. The prepared fibers were kept in water for one day to remove the residual solvent and then used for further studies.

Implantation of HFM into Peritoneal Cavity

Wistar female rats (age group of 4–5 weeks) were procured from Bombay Veterinary College animal house and were housed under controlled conditions of light (12 h light and 12 h darkness), temperature (24°C) and humidity (50%) and maintained on normal chow and water.

Recipient rats were anesthetized (ketamine-80 mg/kg and xylazine-8 mg/kg, i.p.), shaved, and cleaned and were subjected to a laparotomy through a 1 cm long incision on the lower right abdominal wall. The exposed area was kept moist with normal saline swab. A bunch of three HFMs (each 1.5 cm long) was slowly delivered inside the peritoneal cavity. Finally, the peritoneum and skin were sutured using absorbable 6–0 catgut sutures (Stericat Gutstrings, Delhi). Approximately 2 mm part of the HFMs was kept above the peritoneum while suturing to avoid implant dislocation.

The study consisted of 6 groups (n = 3) corresponding to Psf, Psf/TPGS, Psf/MPC HFMs and commercial membranes (Hemoflow F6, Fresenius Medical Care), normal (no surgery) and sham (surgery without implant). Samples were assessed on day 7 and day 21. All rats (control and experimental) received an i.p. injection of gentamycin (3 mg/kg body weight), ampicillin and cloxacillin (20 mg/kg body weight) and diclofenac sodium (0.5 mg/kg body weight) for 3 days (starting from the day of operation) in addition to the topical ointments (Soframycin®, Aventis Pharma. Ltd., Pune, India) and placed in a cage on a heating pad.

Table 4. Process parameters used for hollow fiber membrane preparation.

Parameters	**Psf HFMs**	**Psf/TPGS HFMs**	**MPC coated Psf HFMs (Psf/MPC)**
Ambient Temperature (°C)	25	25	25
Relative Humidity (%)	50–60	50–60	50–60
Dope Solution Composition	Psf/NMP (25/75)	Psf/TPGS/NMP (25/20/55)	Psf/NMP (25/75)
Bore Solution Composition	DI Water	DI Water	10 mg/ml PC 2118 in DI water
Dope Solution Temperature (°C)	25	25	25
Bore Solution Temperature (°C)	25	25	25
Dope Flow Rate (ml/min)	2	2	2
Bore Flow Rate (ml/min)	2.5	2.5	2.5
Spinneret ID/OD (mm)	0.8/1.4	0.8/1.4	0.8/1.4
Air Gap (cm)	45	45	45
Coagulation Bath Composition	RO Water	RO Water	RO Water
Rinse Bath Composition	RO Water	RO Water	RO Water
Coagulation Bath Temperature (°C)	25	25	25
Rinse Bath Temperature (°C)	35	35	35
Take-up Drum Velocity (m/min)	3.89	3.01	3.89

Hematology and Serum Biochemistry of transplanted rats

A complete blood count was performed for diagnosis of infections and inflammatory responses. Retro-orbital blood collection was performed in two vials (with and without heparin, 1 ml each) as described by Sorg and Buckner [16] on days 7 and 21. The heparin (2 IU/ml) containing vial was used for hematological studies, while second vial without heparin was used for serum biochemistry study. Complete Blood Count (CBC) was performed using Abacus (Diatron MI PLC, Hungary) hematology analyzer, while serum biochemistry evaluation was done on Erba Chem 7 (Erba Mannheim, Germany) semi-autoanalyzer using commercial reagent kits.

Peritoneal Fluid Cytology

Peritoneal fluid cytology was carried out for evaluating inflammatory responses due to implantation. On days 7 and 21, three rats from each group were scarified by euthanizing in a CO_2 chamber and their abdominal cavities were exposed. The cavities were filled with 5 ml of chilled phosphate buffer saline (PBS) and were massaged gently for 3–5 min. The PBS solution was aspirated; cytospinned and stained using Wright-Giemsa stain (Sigma Aldrich, MO, USA). The slides were then air-dried and a leukocyte differential count was performed by counting the cells in a standard clinical hemocytometer.

Histological Study of Implants

Histopathological evaluation was carried out on days 7 and 21 for sacrificed rats from all the different groups. HFM implants along with the surrounding tissue were excised and fixed with 10% formalin, embedded in paraffin, sectioned (2–3 μm thick) with a microtome at three different distances from the surface, and stained with hematoxylin and eosin (H&E) (Sigma Aldrich, MO, USA) as per standard protocol [17]. Sections were then examined for the presence of fibrin, exudates, induction of vascularization, and formation of fibrous capsule. Sections were also stained with Masson's Trichrome and observed for extent and distribution of collagen fibers in tissue [18].

Scanning electron microscopy (SEM) Study

Fixed HFM implants with tissue were sectioned with a sharp cutter, dehydrated with graded alcohol and dried at room temperature. These samples were coated with gold/palladium using SC7640 Sputter Coater (Quorum Technologies Ltd, UK) and observed under scanning electron microscope (Hitachi, S-3400 N, UK).

Immunohistochemistry Study

Implant sections were prepared as described above. Paraffin was removed using xylene and the sections were hydrated using a series of washes in graded alcohol. The sections were then washed with PBS and heated in 10 mM sodium citrate using microwave oven for antigen retrieval. They were fixed with 4% paraformaldehyde for 20 min, washed with PBS and permeabilized using 0.1% triton-x solution [19]. This was followed by exposure to phycoerythrin (PE) conjugated HLA- DR antibody (Santa Cruz Biotechnology, Inc., CA, USA) (1:200) for 1 h in dark at room temperature to stain major histocompatibility complex (MHC) antigens. Finally, sections on glass slides were mounted using an antifade-containing mounting medium (Vectashield, Vector laboratories, Burlingame, USA) and 4′,6-diamidoino-2-phenylindole (DAPI) (Sigma-Aldrich, USA). Images were captured using a Zeiss-LSM 510 laser scanning confocal microscope (Carl Zeiss Meditec AG, Jena, Germany) using 10× objectives.

Acknowledgments

The authors would like to acknowledge Ms. Ashwini Atre (National Center for Cell Science, Pune) for image acquiring on confocal laser scanning microscopy.

Author Contributions

Conceived and designed the experiments: GD SK. Performed the experiments: GD SK SS. Analyzed the data: GD SK SS DK. Contributed reagents/materials/analysis tools: JB. Wrote the paper: GD SK. Scientifically contributed and reviewed the article: LS JB.

References

1. Clark WR, Gao D, Ronco C (2002) Membranes for Dialysis. In: Hemodialysis Technology. pp 70–77.
2. Cheung AK (1990) Biocompatibility of hemodialysis membranes. Journal of the American Society of Nephrology 1: 150–161.
3. Hakim RM (1993) Clinical implications of hemodialysis membrane biocompatibility. Kidney International 44: 484–494.
4. Janvier G, Baquey C, Roth C, Benillan N, Belisle S, et al. (1996) Extracorporeal Circulation, Hemocompatibility, and Biomaterials. Ann Thorac Surg 62: 1926–1934.
5. Sirolli V, Ballone E, Di Stante S, Amoroso L, Bonomini M (2002) Cell activation and cellular-cellular interactions during hemodialysis: Effect of dialyzer membrane. International Journal of Artificial Organs 25: 529–537.
6. Schiffl H, Lang SM, König A, Strasser T, Haider M, et al. (1994) Biocompatible membranes in acute renal failure: prospective case-controlled study. The Lancet 344: 570–572. doi: DOI: 10.1016/S0140-6736(94)91964-X.
7. Subramanian S, Venkataraman R, Kellum JA (2002) Influence of dialysis membranes on outcomes in acute renal failure: A meta-analysis. Kidney Int 62: 1819–1823.
8. Williams DF (1999) The Williams dictionary of biomaterials. In:Liverpool University Press, Liverpool, UK. 40 p.
9. Ishihara K, Fukumoto K, Miyazaki H, Nakabayashi N (1994) Improvement of hemocompatibility on a cellulose dialysis membrane with a novel biomedical polymer having a phospholipid polar group. Artificial Organs 18: 559–564.
10. Lin WC, Liu TY, Yang MC (2004) Hemocompatibility of polyacrylonitrile dialysis membrane immobilized with chitosan and heparin conjugate. Biomaterials 25: 1947–1957. doi: DOI: 10.1016/j.biomaterials.2003.08.027.
11. Dahe GJ, Teotia RS, Kadam SS, Bellare JR (2011) The biocompatibility and separation performance of antioxidative polysulfone/vitamin E TPGS composite hollow fiber membranes. Biomaterials 32: 352–365. doi: DOI: 10.1016/j.biomaterials.2010.09.005.
12. Pastan S, Bailey J (1998) Medical progress: Dialysis therapy. New England Journal of Medicine 338: 1428–1437.
13. [Anonymous] (2003) ISO 10993-1:2003, Biological evaluation of medical devices Part 1: Evaluation and testing. pp 1–24.
14. [Anonymous] (1999) ISO 10993-5:1999, Biological evaluation of medical devices Part 5: Tests for in vitro cytotoxicity. pp 1–24.
15. Keller JC, Marshall GW, Kaminski EJ (1984) An in vivo method for the biological evaluation of metal implants. J Biomed Mater Res 18: 829–844. 10.1002/jbm.820180713.
16. Sorg D, Buckner D (1964) A simple method of obtaining venous blood from small laboratory animals. Proceedings of the Society for Experimental Biology and Medicine 115: 1131–1132.
17. Luna GL (1968) Manual of histologic staining methods of the Armed Forces Institute of Pathology. In:McGraw-Hill Book Company, New York. pp 82–83.
18. Sheehan D, Hrapchak B (1980) Theory and practice of Histotechnology. In:Battelle Press, Ohio. pp 189–190.
19. Shi SR, Key ME, Karla KL (1991) Antigen retrieval in formalin-fixed, paraffin-embedded tissues: an enhancement method for immunohistochemical staining based on microwave oven heating of tissue sections. J Histochem Cytochem 39: 741–748.
20. Bolliger AP, Everds NE, Zimmerman KL, Moore DM, Smith SA, et al. (2010) Hematology of Laboratory Animals. In: Weiss DJ, Wardrop KJ, eds. Schalm's Veterinary Hematology. pp 852–862.

21. Andorson JM (2004) Inflammation, wound healing and the foreign body response. Biomaterials Science: An Introduction to Materials in Medicine. pp 296–304.
22. Alpaslan G, Nakajima T, Takano Y (1997) Extracellular alkaline phosphatase activity as a possible marker for wound healing: a preliminary report. J Oral Maxillofac Surg 55: 56–62. S0278-2391(97)90447-X [pii].
23. Liu Y, Zheng S, X, Prestwich GD (2005) Biocompatibility and stability of disulfide-crosslinked hyaluronan films. Biomaterials 26: 4737–4746. S0142-9612(05)00004-9 [pii]; 10.1016/j.biomaterials.2005.01.003 [doi].
24. Jeong SI, Kim BS, Kang SW, Kwon JH, Lee YM, et al. (2004) In vivo biocompatibilty and degradation behavior of elastic poly(L-lactide-co-epsilon-caprolactone) scaffolds. Biomaterials 25: 5939–5946. 10.1016/j.biomaterials.2004.01.057 [doi]; S0142961204001127 [pii].
25. Traber MG, Thellman CA, Rindler MJ, Kayden HJ (1988) Uptake of intact TPGS (d-alpha-tocopheryl polyethylene glycol 1000 succinate) a water-miscible form of vitamin E by human cells in vitro. Am J Clin Nutr 48: 605–611.
26. Yan A, Von Dem BA, Kane AB, Hurt RH (2007) Tocopheryl Polyethylene Glycol Succinate as a Safe, Antioxidant Surfactant for Processing Carbon Nanotubes and Fullerenes. Carbon N Y 45: 2463–2470. 10.1016/j.carbon.2007.08.035 [doi].
27. Oczenski W, Krenn H, Jilch R, Watzka H, Waldenberger F, et al. (2003) HLA-DR as a marker for increased risk for systemic inflammation and septic complications after cardiac surgery. Intensive Care Med 29: 1253–1257. 10.1007/s00134-003-1826-8 [doi].
28. Voggenreiter G, Leiting S, Brauer H, Leiting P, Majetschak M, et al. (2003) Immuno-inflammatory tissue reaction to stainless-steel and titanium plates used for internal fixation of long bones. Biomaterials 24: 247–254. S0142961202003125 [pii].

14

Determinants of Compliance Behaviours among Patients Undergoing Hemodialysis in Malaysia

Yoke Mun Chan[1,2]*, Mohd Shariff Zalilah[2], Sing Ziunn Hii[3]

1 Institute of Gerontology, University Putra Malaysia, Serdang, Malaysia, **2** Department of Nutrition and Dietetics, Faculty of Medicine and Health Sciences, University Putra Malaysia, Serdang, Malaysia, **3** Viva Life Science Private Limited, Petaling Jaya, Malaysia

Abstract

Background: Patients with end stage renal disease often fail to follow prescribed dietary and fluid regimen, leading to undesirable outcomes. This study aimed to examine and identify factors influencing dietary, fluid, medication and dialysis compliance behaviours in patients undergoing hemodialysis.

Methods: This was a cross-sectional study which employed purposive sampling design. A total of 188 respondents were recruited from 14 dialysis centres in Malaysia between 2008–2011. Self-reported compliance behaviours and biochemical measurements were used as evaluation tools.

Results: Compliance rates of dietary, fluid, medication and dialysis were 27.7%, 24.5%, 66.5% and 91.0%, respectively. Younger, male, working patients and those with longer duration on hemodialysis were found more likely to be non-compliant. Lacks of adequate knowledge, inadequate self-efficacy skills, forgetfulness and financial constraints were the major perceived barriers towards better compliance to fluid, dietary, medication and dialysis, respectively.

Conclusions: Healthcare professionals should recognise the factors hindering compliance from the patients' perspective while assisting them with appropriate skills in making necessary changes possible.

Editor: Emmanuel A. Burdmann, University of Sao Paulo Medical School, Brazil

Funding: The authors have no funding or support to report.

Competing Interests: One of the authors, SZH is YMC's spouse who has contributed significantly to the study, as clarified in the Author's Contributions of the Cover Letter. The company (Viva Life Science Private Limited) however had no role in the funding, study design, data collection and analysis, decision to publish, or preparation of the manuscript. This does not alter the authors' adherence to all the PLoS ONE policies on sharing data and materials.

* E-mail: yokemun@medic.upm.edu.my

Introduction

In Malaysia, there is consistent increase in the incidence of newly-diagnosed individuals with end-stage renal disease (ESRD) which requires renal replacement therapy each year, fuelled by the expansion of the aged population as well as the rapid emergence of diabetic nephropathy [1]. While peritoneal dialysis is the preferred treatment modality in Hong Kong [2] and Mexico [3], hemodialysis is still the predominant mode of treatment for ESRD patients in most countries [4–5] including Malaysia [1]. Peritoneal dialysis is grossly underutilized in Malaysia despite the conscious effort by the government to promote peritoneal dialysis as the dialysis modality of choice. This is largely attributed to the readily available hemodialysis centres provided by non-government organisations (NGOs) and private sectors besides better survival rate for hemodialysis patients [1]. Successful hemodialysis is highly dependent on the lifetime commitment of patients to four aspects of regimens, namely dietary guidelines, fluid restriction, medication and dialysis [6]. Although compliance to hemodialysis regimens is critical in the management of hemodialysis patients as failure to do so has been associated with increased risk of medical complications including higher risk of cardiac disease [7], poorer quality of life and decreased life expectancy [8–9], nonadherence to one or more aspects of hemodialysis treatment regimen has been widely reported [10–11].

The reported prevalence of non-compliance rates among hemodialysis patients varies widely, ranging from 30–74%, 2–81%, 17–46% and 0–32% for compliance to fluid restrictions [12–14], diet restrictions [11–12,15], medication [14,16–17] and dialysis [17–19], respectively. These variations were partly attributed to the different population being studied and most likely the inconsistency in the measures used to define compliance rates. A number of variables have been identified to influence compliance rate among hemodialysis patients, with varying degrees of agreement between different studies. More consistent reported demographic correlates of non compliant were younger age [15,17,20] and male patients [12,15,21]. Other variables include education [15,22], employment status [22–23], duration on dialysis [24–26], health locus of control and social support [27].

In view of the rapidly increased of ESRD in Malaysia, there is a need to determine the compliance rate to therapeutic regimen among patients undergoing hemodialysis. Previous study identified non-compliance to fluid intake was prevalent among patients undergoing hemodialysis in a single centre in Malaysia [28]. Data on compliance to other treatment regimes (dietary, medication and dialysis attendance) is however not available. Hence this present study aimed to determine the overall compliance behaviour to therapeutic regimens among patients undergoing hemodialysis and to determine the factors contributing to compliance among these subjects.

Materials and Methods

This was a cross-sectional study with respondents recruited from 14 hemodialysis centres in Malaysia. A total of 346 subjects were screened, 217 were found meeting the selection criteria while eventually 188 respondents consented to participate, giving a response rate of 87%. The study employed purposive sampling as the selection of respondents was based on several eligible criteria. The inclusion criteria entailed receiving hemodialysis for four hour thrice weekly; attended routine hemodialysis treatment for a minimum of three months prior to the study; at least 18 years of age, suffers from no major acute diseases or major psychological disorders. The study protocol was approved by the Medical Research Ethics Committee of Faculty of Medicine and Health Sciences, Universiti Putra Malaysia, in accordance with current guidelines on Good Clinical Practice and the Declaration of Helsinki. Following ethics review board approval, the researchers explained the study to potential participants. Anonymity and confidentially were assured before signed individual consents were obtained from all subjects.

A set of structured questionnaire was developed to ascertain information on patients' demographic characteristics. Treatment conditions, medical history and proxy clinical measures include mean serum potassium and phosphorus levels for the last three measurements were retrospectively obtained from medical record. The modified Charlson's Comorbidity Index which has been validated in dialysis patients [29] was used to quantify subject's comorbidity score. Mean interdialytic weight gain (IDWG) which is defined as weight gain between two consecutive dialysis sessions for the past three months was obtained from subject's dialysis record. A 25-item dietary knowledge questionnaire, which was modified from Durose et al. (2004) [11], was used to assess subjects' knowledge on diet and fluid regimen including food sources for nutrients (e.g., chocolate is good food source for phosphorus), recommended dietary preparation/restriction (e.g., dark green leafy vegetables should be cut small before washing and immerse in water), and possible consequences of noncompliance to dietary recommendation (e.g., excessive intake of sodium and fluid is harmful to the heart). The answers were prepared in yes or no format with an additional "don't know" category to avoid bias attributable to guessing. Each correct response was given a score of one while zero score was given to incorrect or "don't know" response. The scores were weighted and converted to standardized normal distribution, giving a maximum score of 100 for the knowledge scale. The internal consistency (Cronbach's alpha) was 0.8, denoting a reasonable internal consistency of this instrument. A combination of objective and subjective measures was used to access the compliance rates in order to increase the reliability and validity of the compliance results [6].

Objective measures

Interdialytic weight gain (IDWG), serum potassium and phosphorus which have been widely used in many studies [12–13,30] were used as indicators of fluid and dietary compliance. In view of the absence of validated international cut-off values, the existing acceptable limits used in the dialysis units were applied to identify non-adherers. Subjects were considered as dietary compliant when both serum potassium and phosphorus were within the acceptable ranges. Fluid compliant of subject was defined when mean IDWG for the past three months were within the acceptable range. Predialysis serum phosphate was selected as compliance indicator for medication [14,22]. Dialysis compliance was determined as the number of appointment or dialysis session skipped compared to the prescribed sessions in a given duration. The data was gathered retrospectively from the subjects' dialysis record books. Attendance to dialysis was classified arbitrarily as non-compliant if subjects skipped at least one dialysis treatment in the month before enrolment into the study.

Subjective Measures

To evaluate patients' compliance behaviour, a modified dialysis diet and fluid non-adherence questionnaire (DDFQ) [31] was used. There were eight subscales: two each (frequency and intensity) to measure the patients' compliance behaviour to dietary guidelines, fluid, prescribed phosphate binding medication and hemodialysis treatment, respectively. The frequency of non-compliance was assessed for the last 14 days while intensity of non-compliance was evaluated on a 5-point rating scale, where responses ranged from 0 as "very severe deviation" to 4 as "no deviation".

Data Analysis

Analyses were performed using the SPSS Windows Version 18 (Chicago, IL). Data were presented as mean standard deviation for continuous variables and percentages for categorical variables. Pearson's product moment correlation coefficients were computed to determine the associations between continuous variables. Stepwise multivariate linear regression analysis was performed to identify variables that predict the compliance indicators. Statistical significance was defined at $p<0.05$.

Results

Subjects' characteristics are presented in Table 1. The mean age of subjects was 58 years old. There were 48.9% male and 51.1% female. A majority were married (80.3%) with more than half (51.1%) had at least completed secondary education. Approximately three-quarters were either retired or unemployed. Diabetes mellitus and glomerulonephritis were the two major known etiology of renal failure. The presence of co-morbidities was common in this sample, with hypertension being the most prevalent (67.0%) and followed by diabetes mellitus (46.3%).

As depicted in Table 2, while a total of 48.4% and 36.2% of the subjects perceived themselves as fluid or dietary compliant, approximately one-quarter of the subjects were actually adhered to dietary (27.7%) and fluid (24.5%) restrictions. Based on self-reported data, 16 subjects missed at least one dialysis session while the dialysis record book indicated 17 subjects actually skipped at least one dialysis session. This gave a high consistency in dialysis compliance rates between self-reported data and data retrieved from patients' dialysis record. On the other hand, self-reported compliance to medication was 50.5%, while clinically determined rate using serum phosphorus was 66.5%. The percentage of self-reported non-compliance (mild to very severe) to prescribed dialysis, medication, fluid and dietary recommendation were 8.5%, 49.5, 51.6% and 63.8%, respectively (Table 3). According to the degree of deviation, majority of the subjects deviated either mildly or moderately from the recommended regimens. There were however a total of 19.7% and 11.7% of the subjects reported severe and very severe degrees of deviation from dietary and medication recommendation, respectively.

Perceived barriers contributing to non-complaint to treatment regimens were identified and are shown in Table 4. A total of 86.2% of the subjects admitted compliant to fluid prescription was

Table 1. Demographics and clinical characteristics of subjects.

Characteristics		Mean (SD)	Range	%
Age (years)		58.2 (10.5)	23 – 75	
Sex	Male			48.9
	Female			51.1
Marital status	Single			12.8
	Married			80.3
	Divorced/Widowed			6.9
Education	No formal education			10.6
	Primary school			38.3
	Secondary school and above			51.1
Employment	Employed			25.5
	Unemployed			66.0
	Retired			8.5
Primary diagnosis of renal failure	Diabetes mellitus			25.5
	Glomerulonephritis			8.5
	Unknown cause			29.8
	Others			37.1
Duration of dialysis (months)		63.2 (39.3)	5 – 162	
Presence of co-morbidity	Hypertension			67.0
	Diabetes mellitus			46.3
	Ischaemic heart disease			14.9
Dry weight (kg)		56.8 (14.0)		
Interdialytic weight gain (kg)		2.8 (0.7)		

the most difficult and challenging aspect, especially during hot weather while 72.9% reported difficulty following their dietary prescription. This was followed by 52.1% who reported had difficulty taking medications as prescribed. The need to change eating habits and inability to resist favourite foods (88.1%) and the highly complexity of dietary recommendation (87.0%) were the major factors cited for dietary non-compliance, superimposed the knowledge factor (74.7%). On the other hand, lacking of knowledge or information pertaining to fluid management was the major factor cited for fluid non-compliance (92.8%) followed by the complexity of fluid management. Forgetfulness, associated side effects/complications and complexity of the prescribed medications treatment were the three major factors perceived by patients contributing to non-compliance to medications. A majority (70.6%) of the subjects reported they had difficulty adhering to phosphate binder *per se* due to its associated side effects such as constipation and the unpleasant experience to take large quantities with meals. Large tablet burden was reported as barrier to compliance for 60.6% of the subjects. There were 12.2% of the subjects admitted having difficulty to comply with dialysis attendance attributed by financial constraint and lacks of transportation facility.

Table 2. Comparison between clinically determined and self-reported compliance rates.

Compliance Indicator	Clinically Determined compliance rates (%)	Self-reported compliance rates (%)
Dietary	27.7[1]	36.2
Fluid	24.5[2]	48.4
Medication	66.5[3]	50.5
Attendance to dialysis	91.0[4]	91.5

[1]Both serum potassium and phosphorus achieved compliance criteria.
[2]IDWG achieved compliance criteria.
[3]Serum phosphorus achieved compliance criteria.
[4]17 subjects skipped at least one dialysis session (data derived from dialysis record).
[5]16 patients self-reported missing at least one dialysis session.

As shown in Table 5, there were positive correlations between age and compliance on dietary ($r = 0.186, p < 0.05$), fluid ($r = 0.385, p < 0.01$) and medication ($r = 0.271, p < 0.01$), respectively, indicating younger subjects were more non-compliant to the therapeutic regimen compared to their older age counterparts. Female subjects were statistically more compliant to dietary ($r = 0.252, p < 0.05$) and fluid restriction ($r = 0.310, p < 0.01$). There was however no significant different between male and female subjects on medication compliance ($r = 0.172, p > 0.05$). Employment status was found to be inversely related to dietary ($r = -0.355, p < 0.01$) and fluid ($r = -0.441, p < 0.01$) compliances. These results suggested that subjects who were employed were more likely to be non-compliant to dietary and fluid restrictions. Longer hemodialysis vintage was associated with poorer compliances on fluid ($r = -0.410, p < 0.01$) and medication ($r = -0.368, p < 0.01$), implying that patients who had longer lengths of time on dialysis were more likely to have hyperphosphatemia and gained more IDWG. Knowledge scores on potassium and phosphorus

Table 3. Self-reported of intensity of treatment compliance.

Deviation of Regimen		Degree of deviation	Mean Compliance Score	Frequency	%
Dietary			2.73		
	No deviation			68	36.2
	With deviation			120	63.8
		Mild		50	26.6
		Moderate		33	17.5
		Severe		25	13.3
		Very Severe		12	6.4
Fluid*			3.06		
	No deviation			90	48.4
	With deviation			96	51.6
		Mild		34	18.3
		Moderate		50	26.9
		Severe		8	4.3
		Very Severe		4	2.1
Medication			3.03		
	No deviation			95	50.5
	With deviation			93	49.5
		Mild		34	18.1
		Moderate		37	19.7
		Severe		14	7.4
		Very Severe		8	4.3
Dialysis			3.91		
	No deviation			172	91.5
	With deviation			16	8.5
		Mild		16	8.5
		Moderate		0	0
		Severe		0	0
		Very Severe		0	0

*Two subjects refused to disclosure information.

were negatively correlated with compliance on dietary ($r=-0.345$, $p<0.01$) and medication ($r=-0.278$, $p<0.05$), respectively. On the other hand, there were no significant correlations between knowledge scores on fluid or sodium with dietary, fluid or medication compliance. These findings suggest that higher knowledge on dietary aspects may not associated with better compliance rates.

Self-reported dietary compliance score was positively correlated with compliance on dietary ($r=0.236$, $p<0.05$) and medication ($r=0.197$, $p<0.05$), while self-reported medication compliance score was correlated with compliance on medication ($r=0.412$, $p<0.01$). There were also significant correlations between fluid compliance with self-reported compliance score on fluid ($r=0.342$, $p<0.05$) and dialysis ($r=0.213$, $p<0.05$). These data may suggest that the self-reported data can be used to determine the compliance behaviors of hemodialysis patients, in the absence of clinical measures. On the other hand, there were no significant associations between compliance indicators and education level or family income.

Stepwise multivariate linear regression analyses were performed to identify variables that predict the compliance behaviours. As displayed in Table 6, higher fluid compliant was predicted by female gender ($\beta=0.207$, $p<0.05$), older age ($\beta=0.195$, $p<0.05$), higher self-reported fluid compliance score ($\beta=0.168$, $p<0.05$), shorterhemodialysis vintage ($\beta=-0.155$, $p<0.01$) and being not employed ($\beta=-0.125$, $p<0.05$). Meanwhile, higher dietary compliance was predicted by higher self-reported dietary compliance score ($\beta=0.250$, $p<0.05$), female gender ($\beta=0.162$, $p<0.05$), older age ($\beta=0.147$, $p<0.05$) and no employment ($\beta=-0.142$, $p<0.05$) while higher medication compliance was significantly predicted by higher self-reported medications compliance score ($\beta=0.353$, $p<0.01$), shorter hemodialysis vintage ($\beta=-0.224$, $p<0.05$) and older age ($\beta=0.181$, $p<0.05$). The variation for these three models ranged from 21.5–39.2%.

Discussion

Diabetes mellitus accounted for the primary renal disease in this cohort of study, which is also a characteristic reported by the national renal registry of Malaysia [1]. A high proportion of hemodialysis patients in Malaysia had difficulty in following diet and fluid restriction. This finding is consistent with the range of compliance behaviours reported in other studies among dialysis patients [12–13,28]. Compared to a recent study conducted in Hong Kong [26], our compliance rates on dietary and dialysis

Table 4. Perceived barriers contributing to non-compliance on treatment regimens.

		Dietary (%)	Fluid (%)	Medication (%)	Dialysis Attendance (%)
Non-compliance Rate[1]		63.8	51.6	49.5	8.5
Difficult to comply [2]		72.9	86.2	52.1	12.2
Perceived barriers	Lacks of knowledge or information[3]	74.7	92.8	55.4	NA
	Affects food preference	88.1	64.2	36.1	NA
	Alters lifestyle[4]	69.2	56.8	54.7	NA
	Complexity[5]	87.0	75.4	75.8	NA
	Side effects/Complications	NA	NA	78.3	NA
	Forgetfulness	NA	NA	80.6	NA
	Large tablet burden	NA	NA	60.6	NA
	Financial constraint and lacks of transportation facility	NA	NA	NA	100

[1]Data derived from Table 2.
[2]Percentage of subjects who admitted having difficulty adhering to the treatment regimens (multiple responses were possible).
[3]Lacks of knowledge (e.g. water allowance for different weather conditions, type of foods to be consumed or restricted).
[4]Alters lifestyle (e.g. the need to consume mega dosage of supplements and medicines).
[5]Complexity (e.g. Nutrient composition of different foods; when and how to consume phosphate binders).

were comparable, but the compliance rates on fluid and medication were 24% and 39% lower. We compared with another study in United States [24] and found that their compliance rates of diet, fluid and medication were 26–47% higher than those reported in our study. A recent publication on the diabetes control also revealed that there was poor compliance on diet, exercise and self-monitoring blood glucose among type 2 diabetics in Malaysia [32]. Although evidence is still lacking to generalise whether Malaysians are less likely to adhere to medical regimes than other populations, the available data suggest that extra efforts and appropriate strategies are needed to assist our hemodialysis patients to achieve the desirable recommendations, especially on fluid and medication.

The findings that our subjects perceived themselves as more compliant to dialysis than medication prescription, dietary or fluid restrictions are similar to earlier studies [24,26,33]. This may be attributed by the need for higher willpower, more appropriate knowledge and skill to achieve dietary and fluid recommendations. The mean self-reported compliance rates for fluid and dietary

Table 5. Correlation between compliance behaviors and variables.

Variables		Dietary Compliance	Fluid Compliance	Medication Compliance
Age		0.186*	0.385**	0.271**
Sex[1]		0.252*	0.310**	0.172
Education level		−0.124	−0.102	−0.108
Employment Status		−0.355**	−0.441**	−0.187
Family income		−0.129	−0.138	−0.115
Vintage on hemodialysis		−0.152	−0.410**	−0.368**
Knowledge scores on	Potassium	−0.345**	0.167	0.109
	Phosphorus	0.162	0.134	−0.278*
	Fluid	0.087	0.123	−0.153
	Sodium	0.113	−0.162	0.144
Self-reported Compliance score	Dietary	0.236*	0.166	0.197*
	Fluid	−0.174	0.342*	−0.156
	Medication	−0.151	−0.152	0.412**
	Dialysis	0.137	0.213*	0.102

[1]Female is a reference group in sex.
*p<0.05.
**p<0.01.

Table 6. Standardized coefficients of the linear regression model predicting compliance.

Compliance Behaviors	Variables	Standardized coefficients (β)	Adjusted R^2
Fluid	Age	0.207	0.392
	Sex[1]	0.195	
	Fluid compliance score	0.168	
	Hemodialysis vintage	−0.155	
	Employment[2]	−0.125	
Dietary	Dietary compliance score	0.250	0.341
	Age	0.162	
	Sex[1]	0.147	
	Employment[2]	−0.142	
Medication	Medications compliance score	0.353	0.215
	Hemodialysis vintage	−0.224	
	Age	0.181	

[1]Female is a reference group in sex.
[2]Job engagement is a reference group in employment.

were 9% and 19% higher than the clinically determined rates. Other studies have also reported that hemodialysis patients consistently overestimated their compliance to fluid and dietary recommendations [13,27,34]. There is no clear explanation for this, but it is likely that the long duration of dependence on dialysis (length of time on dialysis) may cause hemodialysis patients to accustom to the restrictions imposed by the disease and perceived themselves as having better compliance than they actually did. Secondly, the use of clinical data for example serum potassium and phosphorus as the direct measures of dietary compliance could be misleading as these clinical data may also be affected by factors such as dialysis adequacy, medication and other factors yet to be identified. On the other hand, self-reported medication compliance was found to be underestimated by 16% as compared to clinically measured compliance indicator. Tomasello et al. (2004) [35] reported a similar finding where non-compliance to treatment was 58% and 31% when assessed using clinical and self-report measures, respectively. This may provide an impetus that using a single indicator to document the overall medication compliance rate could be insufficient and thus more comprehensive assessment tool is therefore needed.

Older age appeared to be the most important predictor among all predictor variables, explaining variance in all three compliance behaviours. Other studies have also reported that older age was associated with higher compliances to fluid restriction and medication prescription [24,36–37]. Possible explanations are older patients may have more structured lifestyle that accommodates the demands of the treatment regimen while younger patients may perceive themselves as less vulnerable to negative health outcomes [38], confirming the existence of an "intentional noncompliance" [39]. The finding that younger patients were more likely to be non-compliant to treatment recommendation may lead to the future poorer quality of life and higher rates of mortality among these dialysis patients. The dialysis patients in Malaysia are perceived as relatively young [40]. In view of the younger cohort of dialysis patients together with the higher tendency of these patients to be non-compliant to treatment, it is highly recommended that action plans need to be formulated to address the projected higher mortality rates and poorer quality of life among our dialysis population. We shared that women were more compliant to diet and fluid restriction than men and this findings are similar to other studies [12,26,31]. Female hemodialsysis patients had consistently reported to have a lower adjusted hazard ratio for mortality compared to their male counterparts in Malaysia [1]. It is likely that women are more health conscious than men. How gender differences in compliance may benefit patients concerning health outcomes in the long run however deserves for longitudinal research.

The correlations between higher self-reported compliance to medication and dietary compliance with lower phosphorus levels are of particular importance. Cardiovascular events are the leading cause of death in dialysis patients. The increased incidence of cardiovascular event in dialysis patients is associated with hyperphosphatemia [30], making phosphate control an important goal of treatment. While dialysis *per se* cannot remove the significant quantities of phosphate from the body, the appropriate restriction in dietary phosphorus intake and use of phosphate binder are therefore critically important to manage hyperphosphatemia. It is then necessary for hemodialysis patients to comply with *both* the dietary phosphorus intake and phosphate binding medication in reducing the risk of adverse clinical outcomes.

We demonstrated that higher knowledge scores were not associated with better compliance rates, which suggest that knowledge is not the sole factor related to compliance rate. This finding is congruent with other studies [11–12,37]. While Zrinyi et al. (2003) [23] showed that employment may improve the dietary compliance and it is associated with better patient-staff relationships, we found that hemodialysis patients who were employed were more likely to be non-compliant to diet and fluid restriction. This concurs with other study [13]. Working dialysis subjects may consume more outside foods that contain generally higher amount of sodium and potassium, which could lead to a higher challenge in handling thirst stimulus and subsequent increased in serum potassium level.

We found that subjects with longer duration on hemodialysis were more non-compliant. This finding concurs with other studies [13,25,41]. It is postulated that end stage renal disease patients may be more eager to change their dietary habits to meet the requirement of a newly-received life-saving hemodialysis treatment. However as time passes, these patients may feel bored and easily get frustrated with the need to comply with long lists of dietary and fluid restrictions [26]. Patients new to dialysis treatment may also receive more social support and were therefore higher degree of compliant is expected [26]. However, over the long run, it may be difficult for patients to resist the wide variety of food available. In view of this, healthcare providers should identified the individual's perceived barrier, explore patients' willingness and readiness to make changes to their dietary habits to achieve the optimum effect of compliance.

In conclusion, the majority of our subjects were compliant to dialysis prescription. However, compliance to other regimens especially for fluid and diet restriction remains poor. Younger male, working patients and those with long experience with dialysis warrant increased scrutiny and deserve for special attention and support. Besides knowledge, lacking of appropriate self-efficacy skills and regimen complexity were the perceived barriers hindering better compliance from the patients' perspective. Healthcare professionals should recognize that the perceived barriers to compliance vary according to types of treatment. For example, while adequate knowledge and information are needed to improve fluid compliance, appropriate self-efficacy skills and coping strategies are needed to enable hemodialysis patients to achieve the optimum effect of dietary compliance. Messages deliver by the healthcare professional should be "simple and practical", allowing the patients to understand and practice the messages within their capabilities. Reinforcement of messages together with more frequent counseling encounters may promote a better understanding of the prescriptions subsequently a higher compliance rates among the patients.

Our study design was cross-sectional in nature and the sample size was relatively small which could limit the cause-effect interpretation and generalisation of finding. Selection bias is also possible where only patients who were generally healthier or more health conscious were more likely to participate in the study. Despite these limitations, the study highlighted several important findings that require further investigations using stronger research design and larger sample size.

Author Contributions

Conceived and designed the experiments: YMC MSZ SZH. Performed the experiments: YMC SZH. Analyzed the data: YMC. Contributed reagents/materials/analysis tools: YMC MSZ SZH. Wrote the paper: YMC. Critically reviewed the paper for important intellectual content and provided technical support: MSZ SZH.

References

1. Lim YN, Ong LM, Goh BL (2011) 18th Report of the Malaysian Dialysis and Transplant Registry 2010. Retrieved from Clinical Research Centre of Ministry of Health Malaysia: http://www.msn.org.my/nrr/documents/nrr_report2011/contents.pdf. Accessed 2012 April 5.
2. Yu AW, Chau KF, Ho YW, Li PK (2007) Development of the "peritoneal dialysis first" model in Hong Kong. Perit Dial Int 27 (Suppl 2): S53–S55.
3. Cueto-Manzano AM, Rojas-Campos E (2007) Status of renal replacement therapy and peritoneal dialysis in Mexico. Perit Dial Int 27(2): 142–148.
4. Tan CC, Chan CM, Ho CK, Wong KS, Lee EJ, et al. (2005) Health economics of renal replacement therapy: perspectives from Singapore. Kidney Int 67 (Suppl 94): S19–S22.
5. United States Renal Data System (USRDS), 2009. USRDS annual data report. Accessed from http://www.usrds.org/adr.html. Accessed 2012 March 18.
6. Wolcott DL, Maida CA, Diamond R, Nissenson AR (1986) Treatment compliance in end-stage renal disease patients on dialysis. Am J Nephrol 6 (5), 329–338.
7. Karamanidou C, Clatworthy J, Weinman J, Horne R (2008) A systematic review of the prevalence and determinants of nonadherence to phosphate binding medication in patients with end-stage renal disease. BMC Nephrology 9: 2.
8. Baines LS, Jindal RM (2000) Non-compliance in patients receiving haemodialysis: an in-depth review. Nephron 85(1): 1–7.
9. Hoover H (1989) Compliance in patients on hemodialysis: a review of the literature. J Am Diet Assoc 89(7): 957–959.
10. Denhaerynck K, Manhaeve D, Dobbels F, Garzoni D, Nolte C, et al. (2007) Prevalence and consequences of nonadherence to hemodialysis regimens. Am J Crit Care 16(3): 222–236.
11. Durose CL, Holdsworth M, Watson V, Przygrodzka F (2004) Knowledge of dietary restrictions and the medical consequences of noncompliance by patients on hemodialysis are not predictive of dietary compliance. J Am Diet Assoc 104(1): 35–41.
12. Kugler C, Vlaminck H, Haverich A, Maes B (2005) Nonadherence with diet and fluid restrictions among adults having hemodialysis. JNurs Scholarsh 37(1): 25–29.
13. Lee SH, Molassiotis A (2002) Dietary and fluid compliance in Chinese hemodialysis patients. Int J Nurs Stud 39(7): 695–704.
14. Lin CC, Liang CC (1997) The relationship between health locus of control and compliance of hemodialysis patients. Kaohsiung J Med Sci 13(4): 243–254.
15. Bame SL, Petersen N, Wray NP (1993) Variation in hemodialysis patient compliance according to demographic characteristics. Soc Sci Med 37(8): 1035–1043.
16. Betts DK, Crotty GD (1988) Response to illness and compliance of long-term hemodialysis patients. J Am Nephrol Nurses Assoc 15(2): 96–100.
17. Leggat JE, Orzol SM, Hulbert-Shearon TE, Golper TA, Jones CA, et al. (1998) Noncompliance in hemodialysis: predictors and survival analysis. Am J Kidney Dis 32(1): 139–145.
18. Bleyer AJ, Hylander B, Sudo H, Nomoto Y, de la Torre E, et al. (1999) An international study of patient compliance with hemodialysis. JAMA 281(13): 1211–1213.
19. Sherman RA, Cody RP, Matera JJ, Rogers ME, Solanchick JC (1994) Deficiencies in delivered hemodialysis therapy due to missed and shortened treatments. Am J Kidney Dis 24(6): 921–923.
20. Kimmel PL, Peterson RA, Weihs KL, Simmens SJ, Boyle DH, et al. (1995) Behavioral compliance with dialysis prescription in hemodialysis patients. J Am Soc Nephrol 5(10): 1826–1834.
21. Everett KD, Sletten C, Carmach C, Brantley PJ, Jones GN, et al. (1993) Predicting noncompliance to fluid restrictions in hemodialysis patients. Dialysis Transplant 22: 614–620.
22. Curtin RB, Svarstad BL, Keller TH (1999) Hemodialysis patients' noncompliance with oral medications. J Am Nephrol Nurses Assoc 26(3): 307–316.
23. Zrinyi M, Juhasz M, Balla J, Katona E, Ben T, et al. (2003) Dietary self-efficacy: determinant of compliance behaviours and biochemical outcomes in haemodialysis patients. Nephrol Dial Transplant 18(9): 1869–1873.
24. Kim Y, Evangelista LS (2010) Relationship between illness perceptions, treatment adherence, and clinical outcomes in patients on maintenance hemodialysis. Nephrol Nurs J 37(3): 271–280.
25. Kimmel PL, Varela MP, Peterson RA, Weihs KL, Simmens SJ, et al. (2000) Interdialytic weight gain and survival in hemodialysis patients: effects of duration of ESRD and diabetes mellitus. Kidney Int 57(3): 1141–1151.
26. Lam LW, Twinn SF, Chan SW (2010) Self-reported adherence to therapeutic regimen among patients undergoing continuous ambulatory peritoneal dialysis. J Adv Nurs 66(4): 763–773.
27. Brown J, Fitzpatrick R (1988) Factors influencing compliance with dietary restrictions in dialysis patients. J Psychosom Res 32(2): 191–196.
28. Barnett T, Tang LY, Pinikahana J, Tan SY (2008) Fluid compliance among patients having haemodialysis: can an educational programme make a difference? J Adv Nurs 61(3): 300–306.
29. Beddhu S, Bruns FJ, Saul M, Seddon P, Zeidel ML (2000) A simple comorbidity scale predicts clinical outcomes and costs in dialysis patients. Am J Med 108:609–613.
30. Block GA, Hulbert-Shearon TE, Levin NW, Port FK (1998) Association of serum phosphorus and calcium x phosphate product with mortality risk in chronic hemodialysis patients: a national study. Am J Kidney Dis 31(4): 607–617.
31. Vlaminck H, Maes B, Jacobs A, Reyntjens S, Evers G (2001) The dialysis diet and fluid non-adherence questionnaire: validity testing of a self-report instrument for clinical practice. J Clin Nurs 10(5): 707–715.
32. Mafauzy M, Hussein Z, Chan SP (2011) The status of diabetes control in Malaysia: Results of DiabCare 2008. Med J Malaysia 66(3): 175–181.
33. Mok E, Tam B (2001) Stressors and coping methods among chronic haemodialysis patients in Hong Kong. J Clin Nurs 10(4): 503–511.
34. Cummings KM, Becker MH, Kirscht JP, Levin NW (1982) Psychosocial factors affecting adherence to medical regiments in a group of hemodialysis patients. Med Care 20(6): 567–580.
35. Tomasello S, Dhupar S, Sherman RA (2004) Phosphate binders, K/DOQI guidelines, and compliance: the unfortunate reality. Dialysis Transplant 33(5): 236–242.
36. Kara B, Caglar K, Kilic S (2007) Nonadherence with diet and fluid restrictions and perceived social support in patients receiving hemodialysis. J Nurs Scholarsh 39(3): 243–248.
37. Park KA, Choi KS, Sim YM, Kim SB (2008) Comparison of dietary compliance and dietary knowledge between older and younger Korean hemodialysis patients. J Ren Nutr 18(5): 415–423.
38. Kutner NG (2001) Improving compliance in dialysis patients: does anything work? Semin Dial 14(5): 324–327.
39. Hussey LC, Gilliland K (1989) Compliance, low literacy, and locus of control. Nurs Clin N Am 24(3): 605–611.
40. Schober-Halstenberg HJ (2009) End-stage renal disease in aging societies: a global perspective. J Ren Nutr 19(5 Suppl): S3–S4.
41. Oka M, Chaboyer W (1999) Dietary behaviors and sources of support in hemodialysis patients. Clin Nurs Res 8(4): 302–314.

Electrocardiographic Left Ventricular Hypertrophy and Outcome in Hemodialysis Patients

Seung Jun Kim[1], Hyung Jung Oh[1], Dong Eun Yoo[1], Dong Ho Shin[1], Mi Jung Lee[1], Hyoung Rae Kim[1], Jung Tak Park[1], Seung Hyeok Han[1], Tae-Hyun Yoo[1], Kyu Hun Choi[1], Shin-Wook Kang[1,2]*

1 Department of Internal Medicine, College of Medicine, Yonsei University, Seoul, Korea, **2** Severance Biomedical Science Institute, Brain Korea 21, Yonsei University, Seoul, Korea

Abstract

Background and Aims: Electrocardiography (ECG) is the most widely used initial screening test for the assessment of left ventricular hypertrophy (LVH), an independent predictor of cardiovascular mortality in patients with end-stage renal disease (ESRD). However, traditional ECG criteria based only on voltage to detect LVH have limited clinical utility for the detection of LVH because of their poor sensitivity.

Methods: This prospective observational study was undertaken to compare the prognostic significance of commonly used ECG criteria for LVH, namely Sokolow-Lyon voltage (SV) or voltage-duration product (SP) and Cornell voltage (CV) or voltage-duration product (CP) criteria, and to investigate the association between echocardiographic LV mass index (LVMI) and ECG-LVH criteria in ESRD patients, who consecutively started maintenance hemodialysis (HD) between January 2006 and December 2008.

Results: A total of 317 patients, who underwent both ECG and echocardiography, were included. Compared to SV and CV criteria, SP and CP criteria, respectively, correlated more closely with LVMI. In addition, CP criteria provided the highest positive predictive value for echocardiographic LVH. The 5-year cardiovascular survival rates were significantly lower in patients with ECG-LVH by each criterion. In multivariate analyses, echocardiographic LVH [adjusted hazard ratio (HR): 11.71; 95% confidence interval (CI): 1.57–87.18; P = 0.016] and ECG-LVH by SP (HR: 3.43; 95% CI: 1.32–8.92; P = 0.011) and CP (HR: 3.07; 95% CI: 1.16–8.11; P = 0.024) criteria, but not SV and CV criteria, were significantly associated with cardiovascular mortality.

Conclusions: The product of QRS voltage and duration is helpful in identifying the presence of LVH and predicting cardiovascular mortality in incident HD patients.

Editor: Giuseppe Schillaci, University of Perugia, Italy

Funding: This work was supported by the Brain Korea 21 Project for Medical Science, Yonsei University, by the National Research Foundation of Korea (NRF) grant funded by the Korea government (MEST) (No. 2011-0030711), and by a grant of the Korea Healthcare Technology R&D Project, Ministry of Health and Welfare, Republic of Korea (A102065). The funders had no role in study design, data collection and analysis, decision to publish, or preparation of the manuscript.

Competing Interests: The authors have declared that no competing interests exist.

* E-mail: kswkidney@yuhs.ac

Introduction

Cardiovascular disease is prevalent and the most common cause of morbidity and mortality in patients with end-stage renal disease (ESRD) [1]. Even though coronary artery disease and arrhythmia are not uncommon, left ventricular hypertrophy (LVH) is the most frequent cardiovascular manifestation in these patients [2,3]. LVH is known to be present in more than 70% of incident ESRD patients and increases the risk for cardiac ischemia and congestive heart failure in patients on dialysis [4,5]. In addition, LVH is a very strong independent predictor of cardiovascular mortality not only among patients with hypertension but also among ESRD patients [6–9].

LVH in ESRD patients is mainly attributed to hypertension and anemia [10,11]. However, accumulating evidence shows that volume overload, arteriovenous fistula, hyperparathyroidism, and oxidative stress also play a role in the pathogenesis of LVH in dialysis patients [12–15]. Moreover, LVH regression by modifying these risk factors is associated with improved all-cause and cardiovascular survival [7], while progression of LVH has independent prognostic value for cardiovascular events in dialysis patients [8]. Therefore, early identification of LVH and aggressive treatment to regress LVH should become an important part of management for ESRD patients.

To date, several imaging modalities, such as echocardiography, magnetic resonance imaging (MRI), and computerized tomography, have been performed to detect LVH [16–18]. In general, however, electrocardiography (ECG) is more widely used for the assessment of LVH [19]. ECG is a noninvasive, convenient, inexpensive, and easily reproducible test, but the clinical utility of traditional, purely voltage-based ECG criteria for the detection of LVH is limited due to poor sensitivity [20]. Therefore, criteria based on the combination of voltage and QRS duration have been developed and have improved the sensitivity for LVH in the hypertensive population [21,22]. In addition, several studies elucidated the relationship between LVH based on different electrocardiographic criteria and echocardiographic LVH [23]. Moreover, a very recent study demonstrated the impact of LVH determined by different ECG criteria on clinical outcome in chronic kidney disease [24]. However, little is known about the association between electrocardiographic and echocardiographic LVH in patients with CKD and ESRD. Furthermore, no study has explored whether the prognostic power of ECG varies in ESRD patients based on the diagnostic criteria for LVH. In this prospective study, therefore, we compared commonly used ECG criteria for LVH to ascertain their prognostic significance and investigated the association between echocardiographic LV mass and ECG-LVH criteria in incident hemodialysis (HD) patients.

Methods

Ethics statement

The study was carried out in accordance with the Declaration of Helsinki and approved by the Institutional Review Board of Yonsei University Health System Clinical Trial Center. We obtained informed written consent from all participants involved in our study.

Patients

For this prospective observational study, we initially recruited a total of 603 patients who consecutively started maintenance HD at Yonsei University Health System, Seoul, Korea, between January 2006 and December 2008 and were regularly followed-up at the outpatient clinic. Echocardiography was not performed in 35 patients due to noncompliance or other personal reasons, and in 44 patients it was undergone before the initiation of HD. Of these patients, 207 patients were also excluded for the following reasons: age <18 years (n = 4) or >75 years (n = 11), previous history of peritoneal dialysis or kidney transplantation before HD (n = 139), severe systolic dysfunction (ejection fraction $<30\%$, n = 7), severe valvular heart disease (n = 11), underlying malignancy (n = 21), decompensated liver cirrhosis (n = 3), complete bundle branch block (n = 9), and pacemaker insertion (n = 2). Thus, a total of 317 patients were included in the final analysis.

Data collection

Demographic and clinical data at the time of HD initiation, including age, gender, and comorbidities, were recorded. The results of the following laboratory tests performed at the same time were also collected: hemoglobin, serum albumin, total cholesterol, calcium, phosphate, and high-sensitivity C-reactive protein levels. The single-pool Kt/V in HD patients was measured with standard Gotch equations on the mid-dialysis day near at the time of discharge [25].

ECG

Upon admission, a standard 12-lead electrocardiogram was recorded using a MAC 5500 machine (GE Medical system, Milwaukee, WI, USA). All of the patients underwent an additional ECG on a nondialysis day, within 24 hours after the last HD and near the time of discharge, and this follow-up ECG was used for analysis. The output from the MAC 5500 provided QRS duration, PR interval, QT interval, and axes in an automated fashion, but not QRS voltage of every lead. Thus, two independent technicians measured the voltage and discrepancies of >2 mm were resolved by a third reader. The cut-off point for LVH by Sokolow-Lyon voltage (RV5/6+SV1) was ≥35 mm and by Cornell voltage (RaVL+SV3) was ≥28 mm in men and ≥20 mm in women [21]. Products of QRS duration multiplied by the Cornell voltage combination (with 6 mm added in women) ≥2440 mm•msec and by the Sokolow-Lyon voltage combination ≥3674 mm•msec in men and ≥3224 mm•msec in women were used to determine LVH [22]. The QTc interval was calculated based on Bazett's formula: QTc interval = $QT/\sqrt{RR}$, and the following criteria were used to determine QTc interval prolongation: QTc$\geq$460 msec in women; QTc$\geq$450 msec in men [26].

Echocardiography

Echocardiography was performed at the time of follow-up ECG based on the imaging protocol recommended by the American Society of Echocardiography using a SONOS 7500 (Philips Ultrasound, Bothell, WA, USA). LV systolic function was defined by LV ejection fraction (LVEF) using a modified biplane Simpson's method from the apical two- and four-chamber views. LV mass (LVM) was determined using the method described by Devereux and Reichek [27], and LV mass index (LVMI) was calculated by dividing LVM by body surface area (BSA). Echocardiographic LVH was defined as a LVMI$>$131 g/m^2 for men and $>$100 g/m^2 for women [28]. Hypertrophy was considered concentric if LV relative wall thickness was >0.43, and patients with normal LV mass were considered to have normal LV geometry if relative wall thickness was ≤0.43 or to have concentric remodeling if relative wall thickness was increased [23]. Left atrial volume was assessed by the biplane area-length method from the apical two- and four-chamber views and was indexed for BSA. Mitral inflow was assessed with Doppler echocardiography from the apical four-chamber view, and pulse-wave tissue Doppler imaging of the septal mitral annulus was also obtained from the apical four-chamber view. Systolic RV pressure was calculated using the modified Bernoulli equation [4×(tricuspid systolic jet)^2+10 mmHg].

Outcome measures

All the patients included in this study were followed-up every 3 months at the outpatient clinic, and all deaths and hospitalizations were recorded in the serious adverse events database. For this study, the mortality events were retrieved from the database and carefully reviewed. Cardiovascular mortality, the primary study endpoint, was considered to be death from myocardial infarction or ischemia, congestive heart failure, pulmonary edema, and cerebral hemorrhage or vascular disorder.

Statistical analysis

Statistical analysis was performed using SPSS version 18.0 (SPSS Inc, Chicago, IL, USA). Continuous variables were expressed as mean ± SD, and categorical variables as percentages. To determine differences between the two groups, Student's t-test or Mann-Whitney U test was used for continuous variables and the chi-square test was used for categorical variables. Pearson's correlation analysis was performed to estimate the association between LVMI and ECG criteria measurements. Cumulative survival curves were generated by the Kaplan-Meier method, and between-group survival was compared by a log-rank test. The independent prognostic values of electrocardiographic and echocardiographic LVH for cardiovascular mortality were ascertained by Cox proportional hazards regression analysis, which included only the significant variables in univariate analysis. Factors of specific interest were also included in another multivariate analysis. However, each ECG-LVH or echocardiographic criterion was entered separately because there was a significant interaction with each other. The hazard ratios (HRs) and 95% confidence intervals (CIs) were calculated using the

Table 1. Clinical and biochemical characteristics according to the presence or absence of electrocardiographic LVH.

	Sokolow-Lyon voltage LVH			Sokolow-Lyon product LVH			Cornell voltage LVH			Cornell product LVH		
	No (n = 257)	Yes (n = 60)	P	No (n = 274)	Yes (n = 43)	P	No (n = 279)	Yes (n = 38)	P	No (n = 274)	Yes (n = 43)	P
Age (years)	56.4±14.3	58.3±13.8	0.36	56.0±14.2	61.5±13.0	0.018	56.6±14.4	58.0±12.1	0.57	56.5±14.4	58.4±12.6	0.42
Male gender	130 (51%)	40 (67%)	0.024	144 (53%)	26 (61%)	0.33	152 (54%)	22 (58%)	0.40	144 (53%)	26 (61%)	0.33
Diabetes	143 (56%)	31 (52%)	0.58	149 (54%)	25 (58%)	0.65	151 (54%)	23 (61%)	0.46	148 (54%)	26 (61%)	0.43
Hypertension	227 (88%)	54 (90%)	0.71	239 (87%)	42 (98%)	0.045	245 (88%)	36 (95%)	0.21	240 (88%)	41 (95%)	0.14
Coronary artery disease	39 (15%)	15 (25%)	0.07	44 (16%)	10 (23%)	0.24	46 (17%)	8 (21%)	0.48	41 (15%)	13 (30%)	0.01
History of smoking	36 (14%)	12 (20%)	0.24	40 (15%)	8 (19%)	0.50	43 (15%)	5 (13%)	0.72	40 (15%)	8 (19%)	0.50
Primary renal disease			0.54			0.77			0.88			0.52
Diabetes	143 (56%)	30 (50%)		149 (54%)	24 (56%)		150 (54%)	23 (61%)		147 (54%)	26 (61%)	
Glomerulonephritis	24 (9%)	4 (7%)		26 (10%)	2 (5%)		25 (9%)	3 (8%)		24 (9%)	4 (9%)	
ADPKD	7 (3%)	1 (2%)		7 (3%)	1 (2%)		7 (3%)	1 (3%)		6 (2%)	2 (5%)	
Others	83 (32%)	25 (42%)		92 (34%)	16 (37%)		97 (35%)	11 (29%)		97 (35%)	11 (26%)	
Body mass index (kg/m^2)	23.8±3.4	22.5±3.1	0.008	23.7±3.4	22.8±3.2	0.11	23.7±3.5	22.8±2.5	0.12	23.6±3.4	22.9±3.4	0.20
MBP (mmHg)	99.0±14.2	100.5±14.4	0.48	99.1±14.3	100.8±13.9	0.47	98.8±14.0	103.2±15.3	0.08	99.3±14.1	99.4±14.9	0.97
Heart rate (bpm)	73.5±13.5	75.0±13.5	0.44	74.1±13.6	72.4±12.8	0.46	73.7±13.7	75.0±12.6	0.58	74.1±13.4	72.3±14.1	0.42
Blood urea nitrogen (mg/dl)	93.7±32.1	93.4±28.8	0.95	93.3±31.2	95.7±33.3	0.64	94.3±32.2	88.9±25.8	0.32	93.1±31.4	97.2±32.3	0.42
Creatinine (mg/dl)	9.8±4.7	9.9±4.2	0.86	9.8±4.6	9.7±4.3	0.92	9.9±4.7	9.1±3.5	0.32	9.7±4.7	10.2±4.1	0.55
eGFR (ml/min/1.73 m^2)	6.5±3.0	6.3±2.4	0.71	6.5±3.0	6.3±2.5	0.73	6.5±2.9	6.4±2.7	0.82	6.5±3.0	6.1±2.6	0.37
Calcium (mg/dl)	7.8±1.1	8.0±1.1	0.18	7.8±1.1	8.0±1.1	0.18	7.8±1.1	8.1±0.9	0.07	7.8±1.1	7.9±1.2	0.56
Phosphate (mg/dl)	6.2±1.9	6.3±1.7	0.85	6.2±1.9	6.3±1.8	0.78	6.2±1.9	6.1±1.9	0.80	6.2±1.8	6.5±2.1	0.32
Albumin (g/dl)	3.5±0.7	3.6±0.6	0.33	3.5±0.7	3.6±0.5	0.33	3.5±0.7	3.4±0.6	0.26	3.5±0.7	3.5±0.6	0.95
Cholesterol (mg/dl)	161.9±50.0	155.3±41.2	0.34	161.3±49.3	157.0±43.1	0.60	159.0±48.2	173.0±48.8	0.10	160.1±49.0	164.2±45.1	0.61
Hemoglobin (g/dl)	8.4±1.6	8.6±1.3	0.56	8.4±1.6	8.7±1.4	0.34	8.4±1.6	8.8±1.5	0.16	8.4±1.6	8.6±1.6	0.55
C-reactive protein (mg/l)	0.8±0.9	1.1±1.5	0.18	0.8±1.1	0.8±1.0	0.91	0.8±1.1	0.8±0.9	0.88	0.8±1.1	1.0±1.2	0.40
Single-pool Kt/V	1.3±0.3	1.2±0.3	0.76	1.1±0.4	1.2±0.3	0.79	1.2±0.4	1.3±0.3	0.71	1.2±0.3	1.3±0.3	0.81
No of antihypertensive drugs	2.1±1.2	2.2±1.2	0.55	2.1±1.2	2.1±1.1	0.89	2.1±1.2	2.4±1.1	0.13	2.1±1.2	2.2±1.0	0.79
Antihypertensive drugs												
β-blockers	144 (56%)	30 (50%)	0.40	151 (55%)	23 (54%)	0.84	152 (55%)	22 (58%)	0.69	152 (56%)	22 (51%)	0.60
ACE inhibitors or ARBs	148 (58%)	39 (65%)	0.29	160 (58%)	27 (63%)	0.59	158 (57%)	29 (76%)	0.02	159 (58%)	28 (65%)	0.38
Calcium channel blockers	191 (74%)	47 (78%)	0.52	205 (75%)	33 (77%)	0.79	206 (74%)	32 (84%)	0.17	203 (74%)	35 (81%)	0.30
Statin use	74 (29%)	17 (28%)	0.94	74 (27%)	17 (40%)	0.09	77 (28%)	14 (37%)	0.24	72 (26%)	19 (44%)	0.02
Coronary revasculization	31 (12%)	16 (27%)	0.004	31 (11%)	16 (37%)	<0.001	37 (13%)	10 (26%)	0.03	33 (12%)	14 (33%)	<0.001
Stroke	16 (6%)	7 (12%)	0.14	20 (7%)	3 (7%)	0.94	19 (7%)	4 (11%)	0.41	19 (7%)	4 (9%)	0.58

ADPKD, autosomal dominant polycystic kidney disease; MBP, mean arterial blood pressure; BPM, beat per minute; eGFR, estimated glomerular filtration rate; No, number; ACE, angiotensin converting enzyme; ARB, angiotensin II receptor blocker; LVH, left ventricular hypertrophy.
Data are presented as n (%) or mean ± SD.

estimated regression coefficients and standard errors. The positive predictive values for echocardiographic LVH and cardiovascular mortality were also analyzed by receiver operating characteristic (ROC) curve analysis with calculated area under the ROC curve (AUC). The correlation coefficients between LVMI and each ECG criterion measurements and the AUC of each ECG-LVH criterion for echocardiographic LVH and cardiovascular mortality were compared using a two-tailed Z-score. P-values less than 0.05 were considered statistically significant.

Results

Clinical and biochemical characteristics

The baseline patient characteristics according to the presence ECG-LVH are shown in Table 1. The mean age was 56.7±14.2 years (range: 18–75 years), and 53.6% were male. Of the 317 patients, LVH was present in 60 patients (18.9%) by Sokolow-Lyon voltage (SV), 43 (13.6%) by Sokolow-Lyon voltage-duration product (SP), 38 (12.0%) by Cornell voltage (CV), and 43 (13.6%) by Cornell voltage-duration product (CP) criteria. The proportion of male patients was significantly higher in the ECG-LVH group

Table 2. Echocardiographic and electrocardiographic parameters according to the presence or absence of echocardiographic LVH.

	Sokolow-Lyon voltage LVH			Sokolow-Lyon product LVH			Cornell voltage LVH			Cornell product LVH		
	No (n = 257)	Yes (n = 60)	P	No (n = 274)	Yes (n = 43)	P	No (n = 279)	Yes (n = 38)	P	No (n = 274)	Yes (n = 43)	P
Echocardiography												
Ejection fraction (%)	62.2±10.1	57.8±10.5	0.003	62.0±10.0	57.0±11.6	0.003	61.8±10.0	58.4±12.1	0.05	62.3±9.7	55.7±12.1	0.001
LVEDD (mm)	51.5±5.2	53.5±5.5	0.011	51.5±5.0	54.4±6.3	0.001	51.8±5.0	52.9±7.2	0.34	51.5±5.0	54.3±6.7	0.01
IVS thickness (mm)	10.7±1.8	11.6±1.7	<0.001	10.8±1.8	11.7±1.6	0.001	10.8±1.7	11.9±2.2	<0.001	10.7±1.7	12.0±2.1	<0.001
PW thickness (mm)	10.6±1.6	11.5±1.6	0.001	10.7±1.7	11.5±1.5	0.004	10.7±1.6	11.7±1.6	0.001	10.6±1.6	11.8±1.4	<0.001
LV mass index (g/m²)	127.3±27.7	145.0±26.3	<0.001	127.7±27.2	149.7±27.9	<0.001	128.1±27.5	149.5±26.9	<0.001	127.2±27.0	152.6±26.7	<0.001
LA volume index (ml/m²)	34.6± 12.2	40.8±12.7	<0.001	34.6±12.0	43.6±13.0	<0.001	35.2±12.4	39.8±12.5	0.032	34.9±12.2	41.2±13.0	0.002
RV pressure (mmHg)	31.7±10.6	33.4±11.2	0.28	31.7±10.4	34.0±12.2	0.22	31.8±10.8	33.8±10.1	0.31	31.6±10.4	34.5±12.1	0.12
E/E'ratio	16.6±7.1	18.1±8.0	0.17	16.5±6.9	19.6±9.1	0.046	16.3±6.9	21.1±8.1	<0.001	16.4±6.7	19.8±9.6	0.033
Echocardiographic LVH	169 (54%)	49 (60%)	0.017	181 (53%)	37 (65%)	0.009	184 (53%)	34 (69%)	0.003	181 (53%)	37 (70%)	0.009
Relative wall thickness	0.42±0.08	0.43±0.07	0.18	0.42±0.08	0.43±0.07	0.59	0.42±0.07	0.45±0.10	0.12	0.42±0.08	0.44±0.08	0.05
Concentric remodeling/LVH	105 (41%)	31 (52%)	0.13	113 (41%)	23 (53%)	0.13	113 (41%)	23 (61%)	0.019	112 (41%)	24 (56%)	0.07
Electrocardiography												
PR interval (msec)	168.5±30.6	163.8±25.4	0.28	167.4±30.1	169.2±27.3	0.73	168.7±30.1	160.3±25.6	0.11	167.0±28.9	171.9±34.3	0.33
QRS duration (msec)	93.0±14.7	94.0±11.2	0.63	91.4±11.9	104.7±20.4	<0.001	93.0±14.2	94.6±13.2	0.50	91.3±13.4	105.1±12.6	<0.001
QTc interval (msec)	458.0±35.6	467.0±40.8	0.12	457.3±35.7	475.1±39.7	0.003	458.8±35.2	466.6±46.1	0.22	457.1±33.3	476.5±50.9	0.019
ST-T abnormalities	17 (7%)	13 (22%)	<0.001	16 (6%)	14 (33%)	<0.001	15 (5%)	15 (40%)	<0.001	12 (4%)	18 (42%)	<0.001
Sokolow-Lyon voltage (mm)	23.8±6.3	41.3±5.4	<0.001	24.8±7.1	42.0±6.8	<0.001	26.3±8.6	33.3±11.0	0.001	26.0±8.5	34.3±10.6	<0.001
Sokolow-Lyon voltage LVH	-	-	-	24 (9%)	36 (84%)	<0.001	42 (15%)	18 (47%)	<0.001	40 (15%)	20 (47%)	<0.001
Sokolow-Lyon product	2225±743	3888±759	<0.001	2260±694	4322±695	<0.001	2450±914	3194±1264	0.001	2376±862	3583±1121	<0.001
Sokolow-Lyon product LVH	7 (3%)	36 (60%)	<0.001	-	-	-	28 (10%)	15 (40%)	<0.001	23 (8%)	20 (47%)	<0.001
Cornell voltage (mm)	15.0±5.5	21.9±7.1	<0.001	15.4±5.6	21.6±8.5	<0.001	14.8±5.1	26.9±5.2	<0.001	14.6±4.8	26.8±5.3	<0.001
Cornell voltage LVH	20 (8%)	18 (30%)	<0.001	23 (8%)	15 (35%)	<0.001	-	-	-	13 (5%)	25 (58%)	<0.001
Cornell product	1660±553	2270±848	<0.001	1668±531	2458±960	<0.001	1618±480	2931±679	<0.001	1577±423	3036±510	<0.001
Cornell product LVH	23 (9%)	20 (33%)	<0.001	23 (8%)	20 (47%)	<0.001	18 (7%)	25 (66%)	<0.001	-	-	-

LV, left ventricle; IVS, interventricular septum; PW, posterior wall; LA, left atrium; RV, right ventricle; E/E', ratio of early mitral inflow velocity to peak mitral annulus velocity; LVH, left ventricular hypertrophy.
Data are presented as mean ± SD.

by SV criteria, whereas the proportion of patients with hypertension was significantly higher in the ECG-LVH group by SP criteria ($P<0.05$). In addition, there was a significant difference in body mass index (BMI) between patients with and without ECG-LVH only by SV criteria (22.5±3.1 vs. 23.8±3.4 kg/m^2, $P = 0.008$). Moreover, patients with ECG-LVH by CP criteria showed a significantly higher prevalence of coronary artery disease ($P<0.05$). A history of coronary revascularization was significantly more prevalent in patients with ECG-LVH by each criterion than in those without ECG-LVH ($P<0.05$). Blood urea nitrogen, creatinine, albumin, and cholesterol concentrations and Kt/V were also comparable between patients with and without ECG-LVH by each criterion.

Echocardiographic and electrocardiographic findings

As shown in Table 2, LV mass index (LVMI) and left atrial volume index were significantly higher, while LV ejection fraction was significantly lower in patients with LVH by each criterion compared to those without ECG-LVH. In addition, the early mitral inflow velocity to peak mitral annulus velocity (E/E') ratio was significantly higher only in patients with ECG-LVH by QRS voltage-duration product criteria. On the other hand, QT interval was significantly prolonged in patients with ECG-LVH based on SP and CP criteria than in those without ECG-LVH by these criteria.

Pearson's correlation analysis revealed that SP ($r = 0.357$, $P<0.001$) and CP ($r = 0.410$, $P<0.001$) criteria seemed to correlate more closely with LVMI compared to SV ($r = 0.319$, $P<0.001$) and CV ($r = 0.388$, $P<0.001$) criteria, respectively, but the differences did not reach statistical significance (SP vs. SV, Z statistic = 0.542, $P = 0.59$; CP vs. CV, Z statistic = 0.172, $P = 0.86$) (Figure 1). The positive predictive values of SP (86.0%) and CP (89.5%) for echocardiographic LVH were also higher relative to those of SV (81.7%) and CV (86.0%). Among the four ECG criteria, moreover, the CP criteria provided the highest predictive value for echocardiographic LVH in ROC curve analysis (AUC = 0.657, $P<0.001$) (Figure 2). Furthermore, the AUC of the CP criteria was significantly greater than those of the other three ECG-LVH criteria (CP vs. CV, Z statistic = 4.793, $P<0.001$; CP vs. SP, Z statistic = 2.707, $P = 0.007$; CP vs. SV, Z statistic = 2.146, $P = 0.032$).

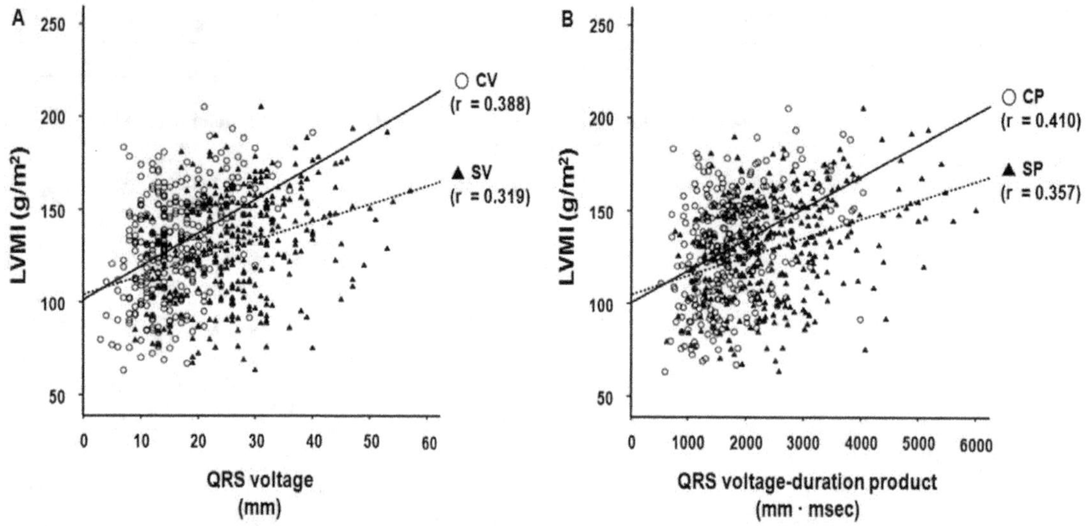

Figure 1. Correlation between electrocardiographic LVH and left ventricular mass index (LVMI). (A) Sokolow-Lyon voltage (SV), Cornell voltage (CV), (B) Sokolow-Lyon voltage-duration product (SP), and Cornell voltage-duration product (CP) correlated significantly with LVMI. Data are correlation coefficients (r).

Clinical outcomes

During the mean follow-up duration of 27.4±17.2 months (3.0–64.0 months), 41 patients (12.9%) died over 725 patient-years of cumulative follow-up, yielding a crude mortality rate of 5.66/100 patient-years. Among them, 25 patients (7.9%) died from cardiovascular causes. Patients with echocardiographic LVH had a significantly lower cardiovascular mortality-free survival than those without echocardiographic LVH (72.2% vs. 98.0%, P=0.003). In addition, the 5-year cardiovascular survival rates were significantly lower in patients with ECG-LVH by SV (60.7% vs. 88.1%, P=0.026), SP (50.6% vs. 87.6%, P=0.001), CV (56.2% vs. 87.0%, P=0.017), and CP criteria (55.7% vs. 87.7%, P=0.001) (Figure 3). Moreover, patients with ST-T wave abnormalities secondary to LVH, including a horizontal or downsloping ST segment and T wave inversion, showed significantly lower cardiovascular survival rates compared to those without these findings (39.5% vs. 87.3%, P=0.005). However, there was no significant difference in cardiovascular mortality between patients with concentric and eccentric LVH and between patients with and without QTc interval prolongation. The overall mortality was also comparable between patients with and without echocardiographic LVH or ECG-LVH.

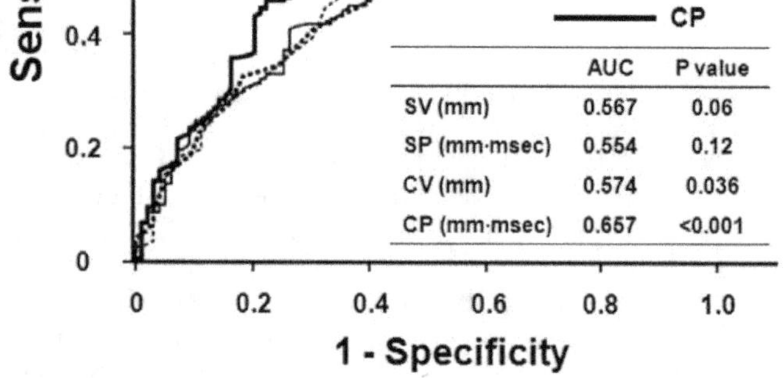

Figure 2. ROC curve analysis for echocardiographic LVH. The ROC curve was constructed by plotting the sensitivity (true positive rate) vs. 1-specificity (false positive rate) for each ECG-LVH criterion. At the highest predicted probability, sensitivities of Sokolow-Lyon voltage (SV), Sokolow-Lyon voltage-duration product (SP), Cornell voltage (CV), and Cornell voltage-duration product (CP) were 27.1%, 40.8%, 32.6%, and 45.9%, respectively.

Table 3 shows the hazard ratios (HRs) for cardiovascular mortality according to the presence of echocardiographic or electrocardiographic LVH. In an unadjusted Cox regression model, there was a significant increased risk for cardiovascular mortality in patients with echocardiographic LVH and ECG-LVH by each criterion. In multivariate analysis adjusted for age, diabetes, and coronary artery disease, which were revealed as significant independent predictors of cardiovascular mortality in univariate analysis, echocardiographic LVH and ECG-LVH based on QRS voltage-duration product were still significantly associated with cardiovascular mortality, but the significant association between ECG-LVH by purely voltage-based criteria and cardiovascular mortality in the unadjusted model disappeared (Model 1). Moreover, even when factors of specific interest, such as ejection fraction, ST-T wave changes, and QTc interval, were included in a multivariate model, echocardiographic LVH (HR: 11.71; 95% CI: 1.57–87.18; P=0.016) and ECG-LVH by SP (HR: 3.43; 95% CI: 1.32–8.92; P=0.011) and CP (HR: 3.07; 95% CI: 1.16–8.11; P=0.024) criteria, but not SV and CV criteria, were significantly associated with cardiovascular mortality (Model 2). In ROC curve analysis, CP criteria provided the highest predictive value for cardiovascular mortality (AUC=0.720, P<0.001), but there were no statistical differences in the AUC among the four ECG-LVH criteria (Figure 4).

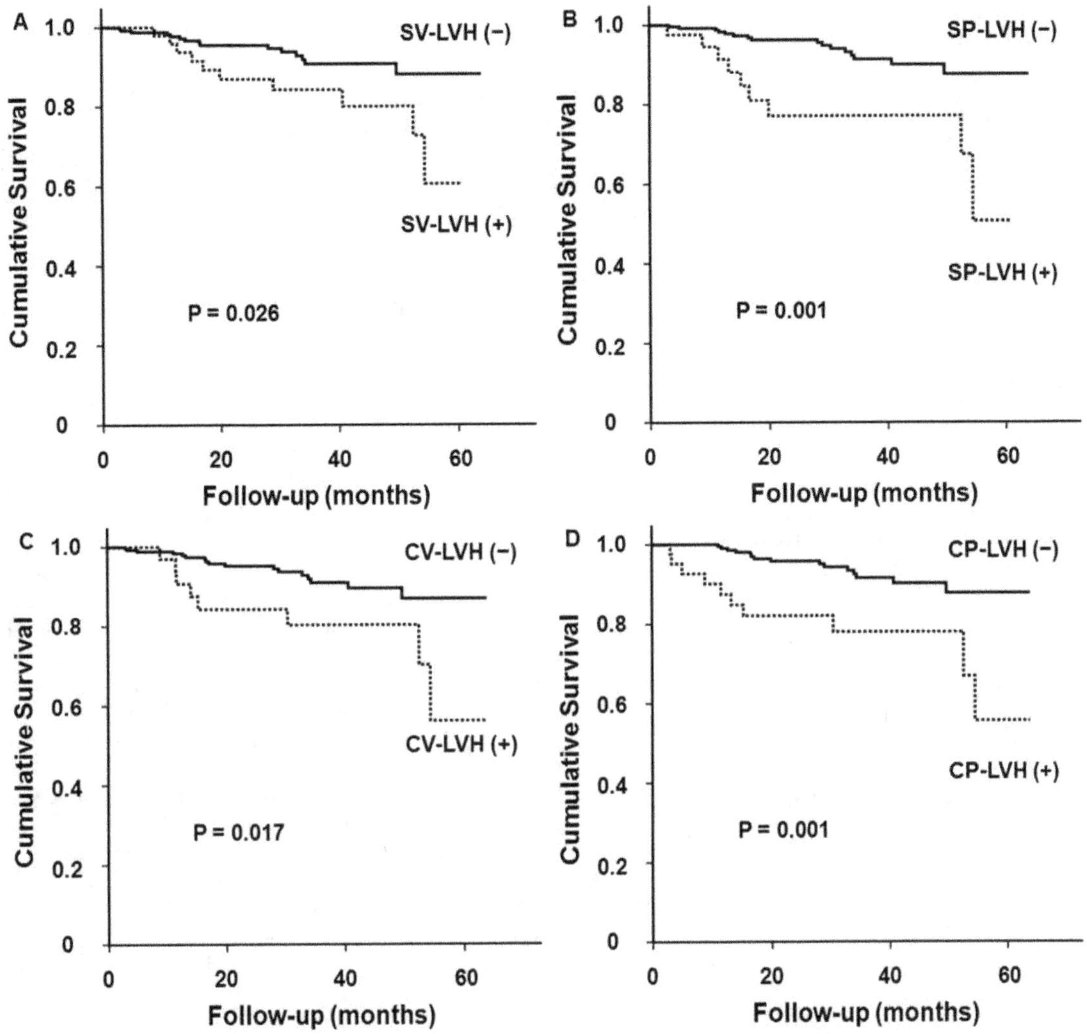

Figure 3. Kaplan-Meier curves for cardiovascular survival. Compared to patients without electrocardiographic LVH, the 5-year cardiovascular survival rates were significantly lower in patients with electrocardiographic LVH based on (A) Sokolow-Lyon voltage (SV), (B) Sokolow-Lyon voltage-duration product (SP), (C) Cornell voltage (CV), and (D) Cornell voltage-duration product criteria (CP).

Discussion

In ESRD patients, LVH detected by ECG or echocardiography is the most common manifestation of cardiovascular disease and strongly predicts cardiovascular morbidity and mortality [2,3,7–9]. In this study, we demonstrate that SP and CP criteria correlated more closely with LVMI determined by echocardiography compared to SV and CV criteria, respectively, and that CP criteria provide the highest predictive value for identification of LVH. In addition, LVH based on QRS voltage-duration product is an independent predictor of cardiovascular mortality in incident HD patients, whereas LVH by QRS voltage-based criteria is not.

Prevalence of LVH

LVH is prevalent in patients with CKD and its prevalence is known to increase as eGFR decreases [4,5,29,30]. However, previous studies show wide variation in the prevalence of LVH in CKD and ESRD patients. A very recent study revealed that the prevalence of ECG-LVH by the Sokolow-Lyon criteria was 10% and by Cornell criteria was 14% in patients with CKD [24]. However, in a Spanish multicenter study on hypertensive patients, more than 20% of the subjects with CKD had ECG-LVH by Cornell criteria [22]. Meanwhile, Foley et al. demonstrated that LVH by echocardiography was present in 74% of ESRD patients at the start of dialysis [4], whereas Levin et al. found the overall prevalence of echocardiographic LVH to be 36% of ESRD patients [5]. In the 4D study, even though all patients were ESRD patients on hemodialysis and had type 2 diabetes, only 12.4% had EKG-LVH by Sokolow-Lyon criteria [31]. The results of the present study also revealed wide variation in the prevalence of LVH: 18.9% by SV, 13.6% by SP, 12.0% by CV, 13.6% by CP criteria, and 68.8% by echocardiography. We surmise that these discrepancies in the prevalence of LVH can be attributed to differences in patient age, gender, ethnicity, BMI, hemoglobin levels, and residual renal function and the proportion of patients with hypertension. Particularly, obesity has been shown to decrease the sensitivity of precordial lead ECG criteria, especially SV criteria, for the identification of LVH because QRS amplitudes are attenuated by interposed tissue, which increases the distance of exploring electrodes from LV [32]. In our study, the prevalence of ECG-LVH by SV criteria might in part be influenced by a relatively low BMI of the subjects, and the

Table 3. Cox regression models for cardiovascular mortality.

	unadjusted		Model 1		Model 2	
	HR (95% CI)	**P-value**	**HR (95% CI)**	**P-value**	**HR (95% CI)**	**P-value**
Echocardiographic LVH	10.88 (1.47–80.43)	0.019	9.11 (1.22–67.82)	0.031	11.71 (1.57–87.18)	0.016
Sokolow-Lyon voltage LVH	2.42 (1.08–5.42)	0.031	1.68 (0.71–3.97)	0.24	2.00 (0.86–4.68)	0.11
Sokolow-Lyon product LVH	3.75 (1.64–8.53)	0.002	2.80 (1.19–6.54)	0.018	3.43 (1.32–8.92)	0.011
Cornell voltage LVH	2.70 (1.16–6.31)	0.022	2.25 (0.95–5.30)	0.06	1.84 (0.68–4.97)	0.23
Cornell product LVH	3.69 (1.65–8.25)	0.001	2.64 (1.14–6.13)	0.024	3.07 (1.16–8.11)	0.024

Data are reported as hazard ratio (HR) and 95% confidence interval (CI).
Model 1: Adjusted for age, diabetes, and coronary artery disease.
Model 2: Adjusted for ejection fraction, ST-T wave abnormalities, and QTc interval.

accuracy of SV criteria might be lessened because they were not gender-based. Whether LVH was assessed by echocardiography or ECG and which ECG criteria were used to define LVH may contribute to this wide variation in the prevalence of LVH.

LVH and cardiovascular outcomes

Mounting evidence indicates that LVH is a powerful independent predictor of cardiovascular mortality in patients with CKD and ESRD [9]. Moreover, the change in LVH has been demonstrated as a strong prognostic factor in these patients. A previous prospective study on prevalent HD patients revealed that the rates of LVMI increase were significantly higher in patients with incident cardiovascular events than in those without such events, and that cardiovascular event-free survival in patients with changes in LVMI below the 25th percentile was significantly higher than in those with changes above the 75th percentile [8]. Similarly, in a cohort study of 153 incident ESRD patients receiving HD, a 10% reduction in LVM during a mean follow-up duration of 54 months resulted in a 22% decrease in all-cause mortality and a 28% decrease in cardiovascular mortality [7]. Furthermore, in that study, LVM regression was independently associated with improved patient survival even after adjustment for age, gender, diabetes, history of cardiovascular disease, and all nonspecific cardiovascular risk factors. While these two studies used echocardiography to assess LVMI or LVM as an indicator of LVH, similar results were observed in hypertensive patients with ECG-LVH [33,34]. With a median interval of 23 days, persistent ECG-LVH at baseline and follow-up identified patients with greater LVM and a higher prevalence of echocardiographic LVH, suggesting that these patients may be at higher risk for subsequent morbidity and mortality [23]. We did not clarify the impact of the changes in LVM or LVMI by echocardiography, newly developed ECG-LVH, and the regression or persistence of ECG-LVH on patients' outcome. Nevertheless, consistent with most previous studies, the baseline echocardiographic LVH at the time of HD initiation was found to be significantly associated with worse cardiovascular survival in incident ESRD patients.

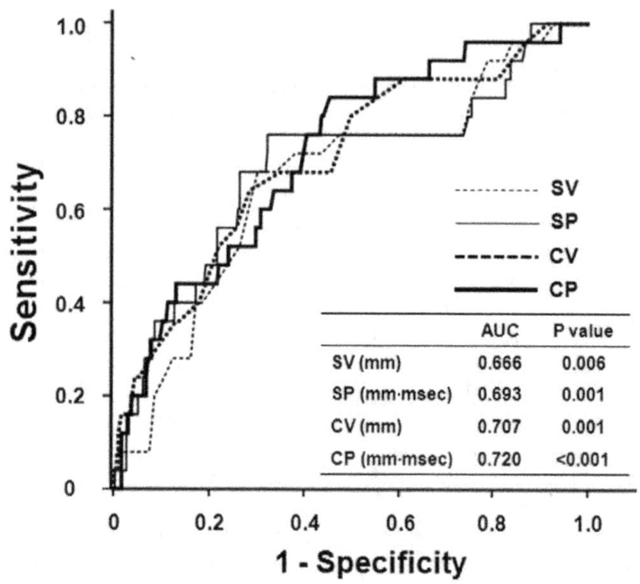

Figure 4. ROC curve analysis for cardiovascular mortality. The ROC curve was constructed by plotting the sensitivity (true positive rate) vs. 1-specificity (false positive rate) for each ECG-LVH criterion. At the highest predicted probability, sensitivities of Sokolow-Lyon voltage (SV), Sokolow-Lyon voltage-duration product (SP), Cornell voltage (CV), and Cornell voltage-duration product (CP) were 68.1%, 72.3%, 64.2%, and 76.0%, respectively.

ECG for the detection of LVH

ECG is a simple tool for the detection of LVH and is widely used in clinical setting [19]. According to the Kidney Disease Outcome Quality Initiative (K/DOQI) practice guidelines, recording of an ECG is recommended in every patient at the initiation of renal replacement therapy and yearly thereafter [35]. Due to the relatively low sensitivity of traditional ECG criteria for the detection of LVH, however, the clinical utility of ECG is limited [20]. On the other hand, prolongation of QRS duration is often observed in patients with LVH [36]. In addition, QRS duration was demonstrated to correlate with LVM [21]. Even though the mechanism for QRS prolongation in LVH has not been clearly determined, it may be related to a longer time required to activate myocardium, decreased conduction velocity in hypertrophic myocardium, and changes in activation sequence or in the relative conductivity of fibrotic intracellular and extracellular spaces [21]. In fact, the VIPE study, which evaluated the effect of candesartan-based treatment on LVH in hypertensive patients, demonstrated that candesartan treatment for 6 months not only reduced LVM, but also shortened the QRS duration [37]. Nevertheless, QRS duration alone has been proven to be poorly sensitive at clinically relevant levels of specificity [36]. For these reasons, there have been many attempts to increase the sensitivity of ECG for the identification of LVH by combining the voltage criteria with QRS duration, and these efforts have modestly improved the performance of ECG for detecting LVH in the general population and hypertensive patients [22]. However, most previous studies on CKD or ESRD patients used voltage criteria to determine ECG-LVH and did not validate ECG-LVH criteria for clinical outcomes [31]. Moreover, few studies have explored the relationship between electrocardiographic and echocardiographic LVH. In this study, we tried to elucidate the correlation between commonly used criteria of ECG-LVH and echocardiographic LVH, and found that SP and CP criteria correlated more closely with LVMI determined by echocardiography than SV and CV criteria, respectively and that CP criteria provided the highest predictive value for echocardiographic LVH. Furthermore, besides echocardiographic LVH, ECG-LVH only by SP and CP criteria was an independent risk factor for cardiovascular mortality in incident HD patients. These findings suggest that the considering QRS duration in addition to voltage may not only improve the identification of LVH but also serve as a more significant predictor of cardiovascular outcome in ESRD patients.

Echocardiography for the detection of LVH

Echocardiography is a noninvasive procedure and provides an accurate assessment of ventricular size, geometry, and function. However, in ESRD patients, echocardiographic measurements, particularly of LVM, are highly dependent on the timing of echocardiography in relationship to dialysis sessions and to intravascular volume [38]. In addition, compared to MRI, echocardiography is known to significantly overestimate LVM in HD patients when LVH and dilation are present [17]. Moreover, the intra-observer and inter-observer variability of echocardiography are significantly higher than those of MRI. Nevertheless, MRI is not routinely performed because it is not widely available, is expensive, and cannot be used in patients with cardiac implantable devices. Consistent with most clinical and research studies, we used LVMI by echocardiography to determine LVH. Furthermore, since the ability to detect LVH in HD patients is improved by performing echocardiography on a nondialysis day, preferably between 12 and 18 hours after the last dialysis session, patients included in the present study underwent echocardiography on a nondialysis day, within 24 hours after the last dialysis, and near the time of discharge to minimize the volume effect on echocardiographic parameters.

Limitations

Our study has several limitations. First, since the study subjects were all Korean ESRD patients on HD, the association between EKG-LVH criteria and clinical outcomes may not be generalizable to other populations. In addition, even though the number of patients was small (18 patients), patients with severe systolic dysfunction and severe valvular heart disease were excluded in this study because we inferred that these cardiac conditions *per se* could not only strongly affect the patient survival but also influence QRS voltage and duration. Nevertheless, we could not completely affirm that there was no selection bias. Second, the 5-year mortality rates in the present study were relatively lower compared to those of previous studies on Western ESRD patients [8,30,31], but they were comparable to those of Japanese patients on HD [29]. Moreover, a small number of events limited the power of the statistical analysis in identifying independent predictors of cardiovascular mortality. Therefore, only 3 factors could be evaluated at a time in the multivariate analysis to maintain the statistical power. Third, we analyzed only the ECG taken at the time of echocardiography. Thus, the possibility of intra-individual variability could not be completely excluded. However, the lower day-to-day variability that has been demonstrated for the measurement of QRS duration could enhance the general use of voltage-duration product criteria to lessen the influence of day-to-day variability [39]. Fourth, LVMI by echocardiography was regarded as the differentiating indicator of LVH in this study. As mentioned earlier, even though MRI is considered to be the "gold standard" technique for the assessment of LVM [17], we were unable to routinely perform MRI in all incident ESRD patients mainly due to its cost. Finally, follow-up ECG and echocardiography were not included for analysis in the present study. It would be worthwhile to investigate the impact of changes in ECG-LVH by different criteria on patient outcomes.

Conclusions

This study shows that ECG-LVH based on QRS voltage-duration product predicts adverse cardiovascular outcomes better than ECG-LVH by QRS voltage-based criteria in incident HD patients. Our findings suggest that standard ECG itself may be of help in risk stratification and in providing therapeutic direction for the management of these patients.

Author Contributions

Analyzed the data: HJO DEY. Wrote the paper: SJK SWK. Carried out data collection: DHS MJL HRK JTP. Participated in the interpretation of data: SHH THY KHC.

References

1. Foley RN, Parfrey PS, Sarnak MJ (1998) Clinical epidemiology of cardiovascular disease in chronic renal disease. Am J Kidney Dis 32: S112–119.
2. Middleton RJ, Parfrey PS, Foley RN (2001) Left ventricular hypertrophy in the renal patient. J Am Soc Nephrol 12: 1079–1084.
3. Levin A, Djurdjev O, Thompson C, Barrett B, Ethier J, et al. (2005) Canadian randomized trial of hemoglobin maintenance to prevent or delay left ventricular mass growth in patients with CKD. Am J Kidney Dis 46: 799–811.
4. Foley RN, Parfrey PS, Harnett JD, Kent GM, Martin CJ, et al. (1995) Clinical and echocardiographic disease in patients starting end-stage renal disease therapy. Kidney Int 47: 186–192.
5. Levin A, Thompson CR, Ethier J, Carlisle EJ, Tobe S, et al. (1999) Left ventricular mass index increase in early renal disease: impact of decline in hemoglobin. Am J Kidney Dis 34: 125–134.
6. Silberberg JS, Barre PE, Prichard SS, Sniderman AD (1989) Impact of left ventricular hypertrophy on survival in end-stage renal disease. Kidney Int 36: 286–290.
7. London GM, Pannier B, Guerin AP, Blacher J, Marchais SJ, et al. (2001) Alterations of left ventricular hypertrophy in and survival of patients receiving hemodialysis: follow-up of an interventional study. J Am Soc Nephrol 12: 2759–2767.
8. Zoccali C, Benedetto FA, Mallamaci F, Tripepi G, Giacone G, et al. (2004) Left ventricular mass monitoring in the follow-up of dialysis patients: prognostic value of left ventricular hypertrophy progression. Kidney Int 65: 1492–1498.
9. Shlipak MG, Fried LF, Cushman M, Manolio TA, Peterson D, et al. (2005) Cardiovascular mortality risk in chronic kidney disease: comparison of traditional and novel risk factors. JAMA 293: 1737–1745.
10. Glassock RJ, Pecoits-Filho R, Barberato SH (2009) Left ventricular mass in chronic kidney disease and ESRD. Clin J Am Soc Nephrol 4 Suppl 1: S79–91.
11. Naito Y, Tsujino T, Matsumoto M, Sakoda T, Ohyanagi M, et al. (2009) Adaptive response of the heart to long-term anemia induced by iron deficiency. Am J Physiol Heart Circ Physiol 296: H585–593.
12. Martin LC, Franco RJ, Gavras I, Matsubara BB, Garcia S, et al. (2004) Association between hypervolemia and ventricular hypertrophy in hemodialysis patients. Am J Hypertens 17: 1163–1169.
13. MacRae JM, Levin A, Belenkie I (2006) The cardiovascular effects of arteriovenous fistulas in chronic kidney disease: a cause for concern? Semin Dial 19: 349–352.
14. Fujii H, Kim JI, Abe T, Umezu M, Fukagawa M (2007) Relationship between parathyroid hormone and cardiac abnormalities in chronic dialysis patients. Intern Med 46: 1507–1512.

15. Gross ML, Ritz E (2008) Hypertrophy and fibrosis in the cardiomyopathy of uremia–beyond coronary heart disease. Semin Dial 21: 308–318.
16. Levy D, Garrison RJ, Savage DD, Kannel WB, Castelli WP (1990) Prognostic implications of echocardiographically determined left ventricular mass in the Framingham Heart Study. N Engl J Med 322: 1561–1566.
17. Stewart GA, Foster J, Cowan M, Rooney E, McDonagh T, et al. (1999) Echocardiography overestimates left ventricular mass in hemodialysis patients relative to magnetic resonance imaging. Kidney Int 56: 2248–2253.
18. Truong QA, Ptaszek LM, Charipar EM, Taylor C, Fontes JD, et al. (2010) Performance of electrocardiographic criteria for left ventricular hypertrophy as compared with cardiac computed tomography: from the Rule Out Myocardial Infarction Using Computer Assisted Tomography trial. J Hypertens 28: 1959–1967.
19. Casale PN, Devereux RB, Kligfield P, Eisenberg RR, Miller DH, et al. (1985) Electrocardiographic detection of left ventricular hypertrophy: development and prospective validation of improved criteria. J Am Coll Cardiol 6: 572–580.
20. Levy D, Labib SB, Anderson KM, Christiansen JC, Kannel WB, et al. (1990) Determinants of sensitivity and specificity of electrocardiographic criteria for left ventricular hypertrophy. Circulation 81: 815–820.
21. Okin PM, Roman MJ, Devereux RB, Kligfield P (1995) Electrocardiographic identification of increased left ventricular mass by simple voltage-duration products. J Am Coll Cardiol 25: 417–423.
22. Calderon A, Barrios V, Escobar C, Ferrer E, Barrios S, et al. (2010) Detection of left ventricular hypertrophy by different electrocardiographic criteria in clinical practice. Findings from the Sara study. Clin Exp Hypertens 32: 145–153.
23. Okin PM, Devereux RB, Jern S, Julius S, Kjeldsen SE, et al. (2001) Relation of echocardiographic left ventricular mass and hypertrophy to persistent electrocardiographic left ventricular hypertrophy in hypertensive patients: the LIFE Study. Am J Hypertens 14: 775–782.
24. Agarwal R, Light RP (2011) Determinants and prognostic significance of electrocardiographic left ventricular hypertrophy criteria in chronic kidney disease. Clin J Am Soc Nephrol 6: 528–536.
25. Gotch FA, Sargent JA (1985) A mechanistic analysis of the National Cooperative Dialysis Study (NCDS). Kidney Int 28: 526–534.
26. Rautaharju PM, Surawicz B, Gettes LS, Bailey JJ, Childers R, et al. (2009) AHA/ACCF/HRS recommendations for the standardization and interpretation of the electrocardiogram: part IV: the ST segment, T and U waves, and the QT interval: a scientific statement from the American Heart Association Electrocardiography and Arrhythmias Committee, Council on Clinical Cardiology; the American College of Cardiology Foundation; and the Heart Rhythm Society. Endorsed by the International Society for Computerized Electrocardiology. J Am Coll Cardiol 53: 982–991.
27. Devereux RB, Alonso DR, Lutas EM, Gottlieb GJ, Campo E, et al. (1986) Echocardiographic assessment of left ventricular hypertrophy: comparison to necropsy findings. Am J Cardiol 57: 450–458.
28. Liao Y, Cooper RS, Durazo-Arvizu R, Mensah GA, Ghali JK (1997) Prediction of mortality risk by different methods of indexation for left ventricular mass. J Am Coll Cardiol 29: 641–647.
29. Goodkin DA, Bragg-Gresham JL, Koenig KG, Wolfe RA, Akiba T, et al. (2003) Association of comorbid conditions and mortality in hemodialysis patients in Europe, Japan, and the United States: the Dialysis Outcomes and Practice Patterns Study (DOPPS). J Am Soc Nephrol 14: 3270–3277.
30. Cheung AK, Sarnak MJ, Yan G, Berkoben M, Heyka R, et al. (2004) Cardiac diseases in maintenance hemodialysis patients: results of the HEMO Study. Kidney Int 65: 2380–2389.
31. Krane V, Heinrich F, Meesmann M, Olschewski M, Lilienthal J, et al. (2009) Electrocardiography and outcome in patients with diabetes mellitus on maintenance hemodialysis. Clin J Am Soc Nephrol 4: 394–400.
32. Okin PM, Jern S, Devereux RB, Kjeldsen SE, Dahlof B (2000) Effect of obesity on electrocardiographic left ventricular hypertrophy in hypertensive patients : the losartan intervention for endpoint (LIFE) reduction in hypertension study. Hypertension 35: 13–18.
33. Mathew J, Sleight P, Lonn E, Johnstone D, Pogue J, et al. (2001) Reduction of cardiovascular risk by regression of electrocardiographic markers of left ventricular hypertrophy by the angiotensin-converting enzyme inhibitor ramipril. Circulation 104: 1615–1621.
34. Okin PM, Devereux RB, Jern S, Kjeldsen SE, Julius S, et al. (2004) Regression of electrocardiographic left ventricular hypertrophy during antihypertensive treatment and the prediction of major cardiovascular events. JAMA 292: 2343–2349.
35. (2005) K/DOQI clinical practice guidelines for cardiovascular disease in dialysis patients. Am J Kidney Dis 45: S1–153.
36. Molloy TJ, Okin PM, Devereux RB, Kligfield P (1992) Electrocardiographic detection of left ventricular hypertrophy by the simple QRS voltage-duration product. J Am Coll Cardiol 20: 1180–1186.
37. Barrios V, Escobar C, Calderon A, Tomas JP, Ruiz S, et al. (2006) Regression of left ventricular hypertrophy by a candesartan-based regimen in clinical practice. The VIPE study. J Renin Angiotensin Aldosterone Syst 7: 236–242.
38. Harnett JD, Murphy B, Collingwood P, Purchase L, Kent G, et al. (1993) The reliability and validity of echocardiographic measurement of left ventricular mass index in hemodialysis patients. Nephron 65: 212–214.
39. Willems JL, Poblete PF, Pipberger HV (1972) Day-to-day variation of the normal orthogonal electrocardiogram and vectorcardiogram. Circulation 45: 1057–1064.

16

Effect of Isovolemic, Isothermic Hemodialysis on Cerebral Perfusion and Vascular Stiffness using Contrast Computed Tomography and Pulse Wave Velocity

Ansgar Reising[1]☯, Saskia Sambale[1]☯, Frank Donnerstag[2], Julius J. Schmidt[1], Carsten Hafer[1], Bernhard M.W. Schmidt[1], Jan T. Kielstein[1]*

1 Department of Nephrology and Hypertension, Medical School Hannover, Hannover, Germany, **2** Institute of Diagnostic and Interventional Neuroradiology, Medical School Hannover, Hannover, Germany

Abstract

Background: Patients undergoing hemodialysis treatment have a six-fold increased risk for stroke relative to the general population. However, the effect of hemodialysis on cerebral blood flow is poorly studied and confounding factors like blood pressure and ultrafiltration as well as temperature changes have rarely been accounted for. The aim of our study was to use state-of-the-art technology to evaluate the effect of a single dialysis session on cerebral perfusion as well as on vascular stiffness.

Methods: Chronic hemodialysis patients (7 male/3 female, mean age 58 years) were recruited. Cerebral blood flow and arterial pulse wave velocity were measured before and immediately after a hemodialysis session. To exclude effects of volume changes we kept ultrafiltration to a minimum, allowing no change in body weight. Isothermic conditions were maintained by using the GENIUS single-pass batch-dialysis system with a high-flux polysulfone dialyser. Cerebral blood flow was measured by contrast-enhanced computed tomography. Pulse wave velocity was measured using the SphygmoCor (AtCor Medical, USA) device by a single operator.

Results: This study shows for the first time that isovolemic, isothermic hemodialysis neither affected blood pressure or heart rate, nor total or regional cerebral perfusion. There was also no change in pulse wave velocity.

Conclusions: Mechanisms other than the dialysis procedure itself might be causative for the high incidence of ischemic strokes in this patient population. Moreover, the sole removal of uremic toxins does not lead to short-term effects on vascular stiffness, underlying the importance of volume control in this patient population.

Editor: Theodore I. Steinman, Harvard Medical School, United States of America

Funding: This study was supported by an unrestricted grant of the Else-Kröner-Fresenius Foundation (P63/06//EKMS 06/03). The funders had no role in study design, data collection and analysis, decision to publish, or preparation of the manuscript.

Competing Interests: JTK recieved unrestricted research support from Fresenius Medical Care Germany. JTK received speaker fees from Fresenius Medical Care Germany. All other authors have declared that no competing interests exist. This does not alter the authors' adherence to all the PLOS ONE policies on sharing data and materials.

* E-mail: Kielstein@yahoo.com

☯ These authors contributed equally to this work.

Introduction

The high prevalence of cardiovascular disease in chronic kidney disease (CKD) stage 5 D, i.e. dialysis patients has been known for decades [1]. Traditional cardiovascular risk markers do not solely explain these events. Functional test like the measurement of pulse wave velocity have been shown to be independent predictor of cardiovascular morbidity and mortality in this patient population [2,3]. Despite an extensive pharmacological treatment the success in preventing or delaying cardiovascular events in CKD 5 D patients is limited [4]. Hence the dialysis procedure itself is thought to play an essential role in the pathophysiology of cardiovascular events, yet their short term impact on vascular function has not been extensively studied. For instance the effect of a single hemodialysis session on the cerebral blood flow is controversially discussed. While one group found an improvement of cerebral blood flow due to dialysis [5] other groups do see either no effect at all [6,7] or even a decrease in cerebral blood flow [8]. Also the effect of a single hemodialysis on arterial stiffness, the result of a complex interaction between structural and functional changes in the vessel wall, has not been the focus of clinical research, making it difficult to dissect the importance of abnormal arterial calcification from volume overload uremic toxins and various endocrine abnormalities [9,10]. Clinical studies on pulse wave velocity measurements are contradicting. Ranging from absent effects [11] to a decrease [12] or even increase [13–14] in pulse wave velocity (PWV) caused by dialysis, a discrepancy that might be due to either temperature effects of dialysis or the hydration status which has been shown to influence PWV [15]. Due to the scarce data about this topic, the unreliable Doppler ultrasound studies of cerebral blood flow, the aim of our study was to analyze the cerebral blood flow and the pulse wave velocity of patients with CKD 5 D before and after a single hemodialysis using the gold standard for the cerebral blood flow measurement, i.e. computer tomography based cerebral perfusion.

Subjects and Methods

The study protocol was approved by the Hannover Medical School Ethics Committee (protocol # 3952). Stable adults undergoing chronic hemodialysis treatment were studied after written informed consent was obtained from the patients.

Participants of the Study

Participants included were undergoing chronic hemodialysis for at least one year with a regimen of at three times per week. None of the patients suffered from instable coronary artery disease or had signs of severe heart failure (>NYHA II). The patients had no signs of infections based on c-reactive protein (CRP) and clinical examination. Exclusion criteria were participation in other studies during the previous three month, allergy against contrast agents or iodine, hyperthyroidism or unclear dysfunction of thyroid gland, premenopausal women, history of radiation of the cranium, residual diuresis (≥500 ml/day), history of stroke within six weeks prior to study participation, taking nutrition supplements containing L-arginine, and any further conditions at the discretion of the treating physician.

Dialysis Procedure

The study participation took place on the patient's midweek dialysis day. After measurement of the predialysis body weight, heart rate, blood pressure and body temperature the dialysis needles (17 Gauge, Bionic Medizintechnik, Friedrichsdorf, Germany) were placed as usual in the dialysis fistula and a blood gas analysis (BGA) including determining sodium and potassium was performed.

Afterwards the patient was taken to the computed tomography (CT) scan in supine and resting position, to rule out influences by altered hemodynamics. The initial CT-scan was performed as described below and the patient was taken back to the dialyis unit. The four hour lasting dialysis session was performed using the Genius® (Fresenius Medical Care, Bad Homburg Germany) single-pass batch-dialysis system with a high-flux polysulfone dialyser FX 60 (Fresenius Medical Care, Bad Homburg Germany). The dialysis solution was composed according to the patient's requirements. The blood flow and the countercurrent dialysate flow ranged between 200 and 250 ml/min, there was no net ultrafiltration. After 4 hours the patients underwent a second pulse wave analysis and subsequently a second CT.

Perfusion CT Imaging Protocol

The method used was described previously and adapted due to modified CT hardware [16]. In brief, all perfusion CT imaging examinations were performed at a Lightspeed 16 row helical CT scanner (GE Medical Systems, Milwaukee, Wis.). The position of the scan region was determined from a previously acquired unenhanced baseline CT. Two adjacent slices at the level of the basal ganglia included the vascular territory of the anterior, middle and posterior cerebral artery. During a scan time of 45s the total number of 90 slices for each position with a thickness of 10-mm sections of continuous (cine) scanning (80 kV, 200 mA) were obtained. CT was initiated 4s after injection (injection rate 2.5 mL/s) of iodinated contrast material with an iodine concentration of 400 mg/dl (Imeron 400, Altana, Konstanz, Germany) with a total volume of 40 mL. The contrast agent was injected via one of the placed dialysis needles followed by a saline flush with the same injection rate with a power injector (Stellant Medrad, Indianola, USA). Parametric maps of brain perfusion parameter were created from the resulting tracer kinetic images using commercially available software (Perfusion 3, AW 4.0, GE Healthcare, Milwaukee, USA). This software algorithm computed the regional cerebral blood flow (CBF) in mL/min/100 g brain tissue with the deconvolution of the parenchymal time-concentration curves by a reference arterial input function (AIF). The region of interest (ROI) that provided the AIF was placed in each anterior cerebral artery (to cover bilateral vessels); the venous outflow function ROI placed in the transverse sinus. Total cerebral perfusion was obtained by averaging blood flow from 4 standardized ROIs in each hemisphere as previously described [17].

Measurement of Pulse Wave Velocity

Carotid-aortic PWV was determined using a validated system (Sphygmocor™; AtCor Medical, Sydney, Australia), which employs high-fidelity applanation tonometry by a pencil-type probe for non-invasive registration of peripheral arterial pressure waves. Pulse waveforms of the common carotid artery and the femoral artery were obtained sequentially and PWV was calculated as the distance between the suprasternal notch and the femoral artery recording site minus the distance between the suprasternal notch and the carotid artery recording site, divided by the time interval between the feet of the flow waves. The device uses the foot-to-foot methods as described previously [18].

Measurement of Body Temperature

Body temperature was measured with an infrared tympanic thermometer (Genius™ 2, Covidien, Mansfield, MA, USA) with an accuracy of +/−0.1°C.

Results

Patient demographics and laboratory data are reported in **Table 1**. Isovolemic conditions could be confirmed by comparing the median [interquartile range] pre dialysis weight (71.15 [65.40–79.88] kg) with the post dialysis weight (71.09 [65.33–79.75] kg), which revealed no difference ($p = 0.9884$). Isothermic hemodialysis could be confirmed by the lack of significant differences comparing pre and post dialysis body temperature (**Figure 1**). Moreover, neither systolic or diastolic blood pressure and heart rate nor pCO_2 or pH changed significantly (**Figure 1**). There was also neither a change in total cerebral blood flow (**Figure 2**), nor in the different territories of the anterior, middle and posterior cerebral artery. Also pulse wave velocity remained unaffected by the dialysis procedure (**Figure 3**). The none-invasively measured blood pressure and heart rate, determined at 30 min intervals, did not show any significant changes over the course of the hemodialysis session (data not shown). The absolute median (range) amount of the removed uremic toxins markers in the collected spent dialysate were 428 (112–630) mmol urea and 15.4 (6.3–22.1) mmol creatinine.

Discussion

The main finding of our study is, that isovolemic, isothermic hemodialysis has neither an effect on cerebral perfusion nor in vascular elasticity in chronic hemodialysis patients.

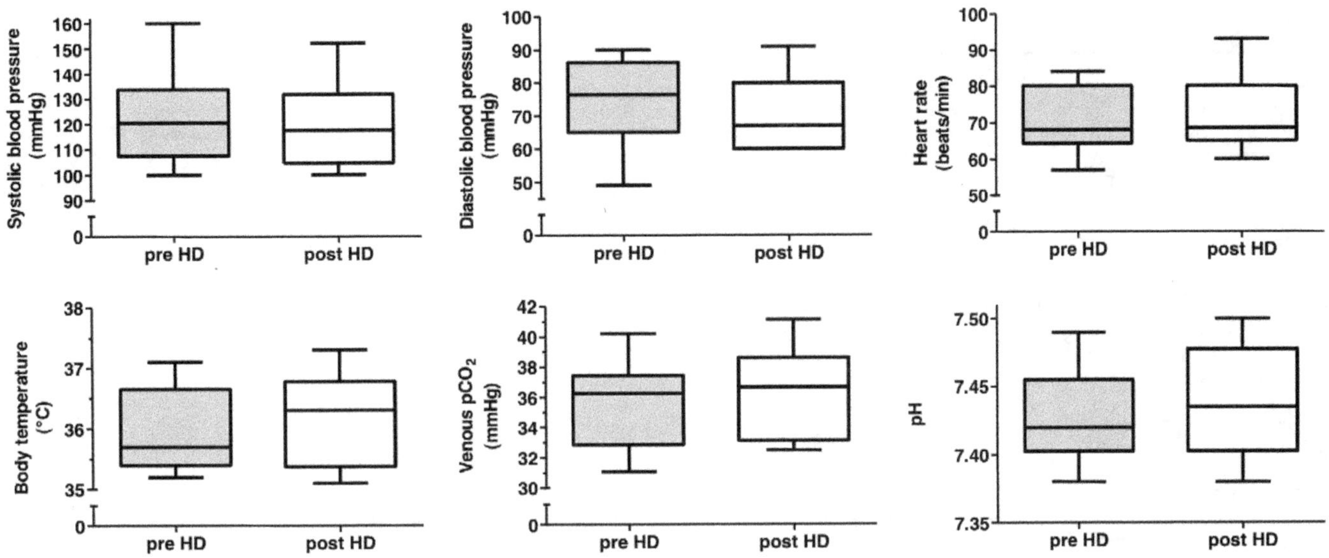

Figure 1. Vital signs and blood gas analysis. Predialysis and postdialysis systolic blood pressure, diastolic blood pressure, heart rate, venous pCO_2 and pH depicted as box and whisker plots. Horizontal bars indicate median values.

Pulse Wave Velocity

Pulse wave velocity is well known as an independent and highly predictive risk marker for cardiovascular events in general population [19] as well as in CKD 5D patients on hemodialysis [2,3]. Thus far the reports on the effect of a single hemodialysis session on PWV are conflicting. Some authors found no effect of hemodialysis on PWV [11,20] while other authors described a significant increase of PWV [13]. The latter group discussed a post-dialytic increase in heart rate and sympathetic nervous activity as causative for these findings [13]. Di Iorio et al found the marked inter- and intradialytic changes of hydration status as the major determinant for a decreasing PWV during dialysis sessions [12]. This finding is supported by our results as we did not perform a net ultrafiltration in our study, specifically to address the potential effect of volume on PWV. Indeed, in all studies investigating the effect of hemodialysis on PWV so far ultrafiltration/weight reduction ranging between ~1500 ml [11] to ~3.2 kg [14]. Nevertheless several of these and other authors discussed effects of the hemodialysis procedure itself, - independent of the hydration or hemodynamic effects due to ultrafiltration - like leukocyte, platelet complement activation and disordered leukocyteendothelial interactions, and increased release of oxidative radicals [11,13,21]. Thermal changes during dialysis strongly influence intradialytic hemodynamics [22] a truth that arose from the pioneering clinical observation of Jonas Bergstroem [23]. Indeed, beside from maintaining peripheral vascular resistance, keeping the body temperature stable also ameliorates the left ventricular dysfunction, which is often associated with hemodialysis [24]. As the sole elimination of uremic toxins in our study did not have any effect on PWV we consider volume changes and body temperature to be of major importance for short term changes in PWV.

Cerebral Blood Flow

In our study we could not detect any effect of isovolemic, isothermic hemodialysis on cerebral blood flow, even by employing an FDA approved method, i.e. computed tomography perfusion technique [16]. Previous published studies on the effect of hemodialysis on cerebral blood flow used transcranial Doppler sonography, which is a poorly reproducible technique. The technique does not directly measure cerebral blood flow but

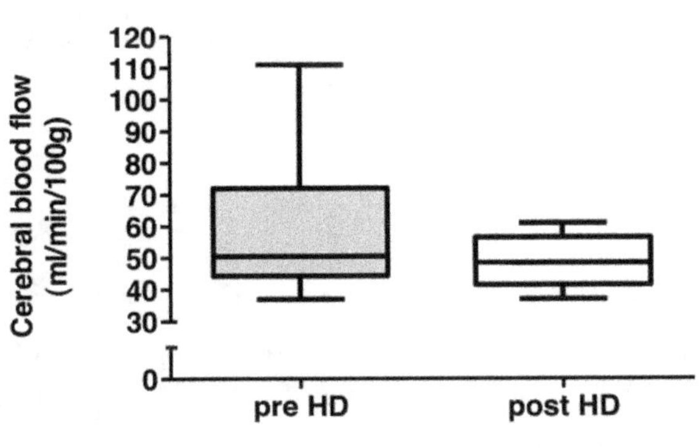

Figure 2. Cerebral blood flow. Predialysis and postdialysis cerebral blood flow depicted as box and whisker plots. Horizontal bars indicate median values. $p = 0.16$ comparing pre- and post-dialysis measurements.

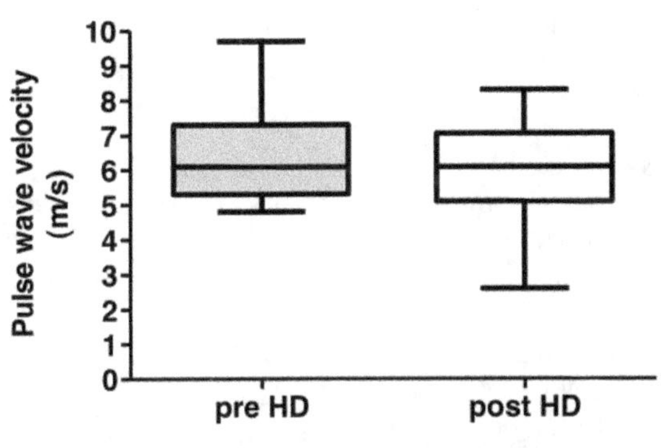

Figure 3. Pulse wave velocity. Predialysis and postdialysis pulse wave velocity depicted as box and whisker plots. Horizontal bars indicate median values. $p = 0.39$ comparing pre- and post-dialysis measurements.

Table 1. Patient characteristics.

Sex	Age (years)	BMI (kg/m^2)	Dialysis (years)	Haemoglobin (g/dl)	Albumin (g/l)	AV fistula	Underlying renal disease
M	71	23.9	10.1	11.8	35	yes	nephrosclerosis
M	39	22.8	4.2	12.2	42	yes	unknown
F	55	28.8	4.5	12.0	29	yes	FSGS
M	49	22.1	4.0	11.0	30	yes	unknown
F	88	29.8	5.5	9.6	25	yes	chronic GN
M	40	23.6	2.3	9.6	41	yes	reflux nephropathy
M	57	22.1	3.5	8.9	28	yes	ADPKD
M	74	26.1	9.5	12.8	46	yes	nephrosclerosis
M	46	27.6	1.3	12.7	46	yes	membranous GN
F	69	18.4	27	12.1	43	yes	IgA nephropathy

Abbreviations: BMI = body mass index; AV-fistula = arteriovenous fistula; FSGS = focal segmental glomerulosclerosis; ADPKD = autosomal dominant polycystic kidney disease; GN = glomerulonephritis.

blood flow velocity. Under conditions of constant vascular resistance cerebral blood flow can be estimated. However we know that the dialysis procedure itself may affect vascular elasticity, either decreasing [12] or increasing it [14]. In contrast to all those studies we could not see a significant change of the cerebral blood flow while eliminating uremic toxins. As we kept blood pressure and the heart rate constant, we could exclude that volume alterations interfered the cerebral blood flow measurements. This could explain the difference to other studies [5,8] in which a marked rate of ultrafiltration of about 2200 ml was performed. Beside ultrafiltration and the loss of body weight the hemoconcentration was associated with change of cerebral flow in this studies. In our study with no net ultrafiltration those parameters were kept stable. Therefore we postulate that the ultrafiltration during dialysis plays a crucial role for the decreased blood flow seen by other authors. Furthermore we conclude that the solute removal itself has no influence on cerebral blood flow. This assumption is supported by data showing that high interdialytic weight gain is associated with a high mortality [25]. Higher rates of ultrafiltration are associated with significant increase in all-cause and cardiovascular mortality, probably induced by repetitive transient cardiac ischemia due to the intravascular hypovolemia [26]. The same effect might happen to the brain that suffers from cyclic states of reduced perfusion following ultrafiltration during hemodialysis. Accelerated aging of the brain due to reduced cerebral blood flow has also been proposed as an important mechanism in the Framingham population [27].

Limitations of the Study

We wish to point out important limitations of our study. Firstly the number of subjects studied is rather small, yet the use of state of the art methodology subjecting patients to an x-ray based procedure. Secondly, we did not perform a net ultrafiltration, as we felt that had been done in several studies performed previously. Thirdly due to methodology it was not possible to measure cerebral blood flow during the dialysis session, therefore we cannot rule out intermediate fluctuations. Fourthly, patients were treated with the GENIUS dialysis system which has some peculiar properties, such as the absence of an in-built heating. Nevertheless, a drop in body temperature had so far not been reported over the course of a four hour treatment [28,29]. Last but not least we specifically excluded patients with diabetic nephropathy.

In summary, during a single hemodialysis session, the removal of uremic toxins alone had neither an effect on vascular stiffness nor on cerebral blood flow. Hence most like the combination of long term changes in the vessel wall anatomy in combination with short term volume shifts might be responsible for the high prevalence of asymptomatic silent cerebral infarction in CKD 5 D patients.

Author Contributions

Conceived and designed the experiments: AR SS JTK. Performed the experiments: AR SS FD CH JS BMWS. Analyzed the data: AR SS JTK. Contributed reagents/materials/analysis tools: FD. Wrote the paper: AR SS JTK.

References

1. Lindner A, Charra B, Sherrard DJ, Scribner BH (1974) Accelerated atherosclerosis in prolonged maintenance hemodialysis. N Engl J Med 290: 697–701.
2. Blacher J, Guerin AP, Pannier B, Marchais SJ, Safar ME, et al. (1999) Impact of aortic stiffness on survival in end-stage renal disease. Circulation 99: 2434–2439.
3. Blacher J, Safar ME, Guerin AP, Pannier B, Marchais SJ, et al. (2003) Aortic pulse wave velocity index and mortality in end-stage renal disease. Kidney Int 63: 1852–1860.
4. Wanner C, Krane V, Marz W, Olschewski M, Mann JF, et al. (2005) Atorvastatin in patients with type 2 diabetes mellitus undergoing hemodialysis. N Engl J Med 353: 238–248.
5. Prohovnik I, Post J, Uribarri J, Lee H, Sandu O, et al. (2007) Cerebrovascular effects of hemodialysis in chronic kidney disease. J Cereb Blood Flow Metab 27: 1861–1869.
6. Metry G, Spittle M, Rahmati S, Giller C, Giller A, et al. (2002) Online monitoring of cerebral hemodynamics during hemodialysis. Am J Kidney Dis

40: 996–1004.

7. Regolisti G, Maggiore U, Cademartiri C, Cabassi A, Caiazza A, et al. (2013) Cerebral blood flow decreases during intermittent hemodialysis in patients with acute kidney injury, but not in patients with end-stage renal disease. Nephrol Dial Transplant 28: 79–85.
8. Stefanidis I, Bach R, Mertens PR, Liakopoulos V, Liapi G, et al. (2005) Influence of hemodialysis on the mean blood flow velocity in the middle cerebral artery. Clin Nephrol 64: 129–137.
9. Chung AW, Yang HH, Kim JM, Sigrist MK, Brin G, et al. (2010) Arterial stiffness and functional properties in chronic kidney disease patients on different dialysis modalities: an exploratory study. Nephrol Dial Transplant 25: 4031–4041.
10. Gusbeth-Tatomir P, Covic A (2007) Causes and consequences of increased arterial stiffness in chronic kidney disease patients. Kidney Blood Press Res 30: 97–107.
11. Kosch M, Levers A, Barenbrock M, Matzkies F, Schaefer RM, et al. (2001) Acute effects of haemodialysis on endothelial function and large artery elasticity. Nephrol Dial Transplant 16: 1663–1668.
12. Di Iorio B, Nazzaro P, Cucciniello E, Bellizzi V (2010) Influence of haemodialysis on variability of pulse wave velocity in chronic haemodialysis patients. Nephrol Dial Transplant 25: 1579–1583.
13. Su HM, Chang JM, Lin FH, Chen SC, Voon WC, et al. (2007) Influence of different measurement time points on brachial-ankle pulse wave velocity and ankle-brachial index in hemodialysis patients. Hypertens Res 30: 965–970.
14. Covic A, Goldsmith DJ, Gusbeth-Tatomir P, Covic M (2004) Haemodialysis acutely improves endothelium-independent vasomotor function without significantly influencing the endothelium-mediated abnormal response to a beta 2-agonist. Nephrol Dial Transplant 19: 637–643.
15. Hogas S, Ardeleanu S, Segall L, Serban DN, Serban IL, et al. (2011) Changes in arterial stiffness following dialysis in relation to overhydration and to endothelial function. Int Urol Nephrol.
16. Bisdas S, Nemitz O, Berding G, Weissenborn K, Ahl B, et al. (2006) Correlative assessment of cerebral blood flow obtained with perfusion CT and positron emission tomography in symptomatic stenotic carotid disease. Eur Radiol 16: 2220–2228.
17. Kielstein JT, Donnerstag F, Gasper S, Menne J, Kielstein A, et al. (2006) ADMA increases arterial stiffness and decreases cerebral blood flow in humans. Stroke 37: 2024–2029.
18. London GM, Pannier B, Agharazii M, Guerin AP, Verbeke FH, et al. (2004) Forearm reactive hyperemia and mortality in end-stage renal disease. Kidney Int 65: 700–704.
19. Mattace-Raso FU, van der Cammen TJ, Hofman A, van Popele NM, Bos ML, et al. (2006) Arterial stiffness and risk of coronary heart disease and stroke: the Rotterdam Study. Circulation 113: 657–663.
20. Georgianos PI, Sarafidis PA, Malindretos P, Nikolaidis P, Lasaridis AN (2011) Hemodialysis reduces augmentation index but not aortic or brachial pulse wave velocity in dialysis-requiring patients. Am J Nephrol 34: 407–414.
21. Himmelfarb J, Stenvinkel P, Ikizler TA, Hakim RM (2002) The elephant in uremia: oxidant stress as a unifying concept of cardiovascular disease in uremia. Kidney Int 62: 1524–1538.
22. Usvyat LA, Kotanko P, van der Sande FM, Kooman JP, Carter M, et al. (2011) Circadian variations in body temperature during dialysis. Nephrol Dial Transplant.
23. Kooman JP, van der Sande F, Leunissen K, Shaldon S (2006) From isolated ultrafiltration to blood-temperature-controlled feedback: an odyssey started by Jonas Bergstrom. Blood Purif 24: 218–221.
24. Selby NM, Burton JO, Chesterton LJ, McIntyre CW (2006) Dialysis-induced regional left ventricular dysfunction is ameliorated by cooling the dialysate. Clin J Am Soc Nephrol 1: 1216–1225.
25. Kalantar-Zadeh K, Regidor DL, Kovesdy CP, Van WD, Bunnapradist S, et al. (2009) Fluid retention is associated with cardiovascular mortality in patients undergoing long-term hemodialysis. Circulation 119: 671–679.
26. Flythe JE, Kimmel SE, Brunelli SM (2011) Rapid fluid removal during dialysis is associated with cardiovascular morbidity and mortality. Kidney Int 79: 250–257.
27. Jefferson AL, Himali JJ, Beiser AS, Au R, Massaro JM, et al. (2010) Cardiac index is associated with brain aging: the Framingham Heart Study. Circulation 122: 690–697.
28. Fliser D, Kielstein JT (2006) Technology Insight: treatment of renal failure in the intensive care unit with extended dialysis. Nat Clin Pract Nephrol 2: 32–39.
29. Lonnemann G, Floege J, Kliem V, Brunkhorst R, Koch KM (2000) Extended daily veno-venous high-flux haemodialysis in patients with acute renal failure and multiple organ dysfunction syndrome using a single path batch dialysis system. Nephrol Dial Transplant 15: 1189–1193.

17

Regional Homogeneity Changes in Hemodialysis Patients with End Stage Renal Disease: *In Vivo* Resting-State Functional MRI Study

Cheng Li[1], Huan-Huan Su[2], Ying-Wei Qiu[2], Xiao-Fei Lv[3], Sheng Shen[1], Wen-Feng Zhan[2], Jun-Zhang Tian[2], Gui-Hua Jiang[2]*

1 Department of Renal Transplantation, Guangdong No.2 Provincial People's Hospital, Guangzhou, People's Republic of China, **2** Department of Medical Imaging, Guangdong No.2 Provincial People's Hospital, Guangzhou, People's Republic of China, **3** State Key Laboratory of Oncology in South China and Department of Medical Imaging and Interventional Radiology, Sun Yat-Sen University Cancer Center, Guangzhou, People's Republic of China

Abstract

Objective: To prospectively investigate and detect early cerebral regional homogeneity (ReHo) changes in neurologically asymptomatic patients with end stage renal disease (ESRD) using in vivo resting-state functional MR imaging (Rs-fMRI).

Methods: We enrolled 20 patients (15 men, 5 women; meanage, 37.1 years; range, 19–49 years) with ESRD and 20 healthy controls (15 men, 5 women; mean age, 38.3 years; range, 28–49 years). The mean duration of hemodialysis for the patient group was 10.7±6.4 monthes. There was no significant sex or age difference between the ESRD and control groups. Rs-fMRI was performed using a gradient-echo echo-planar imaging sequence. ReHo was calculated using software (DPARSF). Voxel-based analysis of the ReHo maps between ESRD and control groups was performed with a two-samples *t* test. Statistical maps were set at *P* value less than 0.05 and were corrected for multiple comparisons. The Mini-Mental State Examination (MMSE) was administered to all participants at imaging.

Results: ReHo values were increased in the bilateral superior temporal gyrus and left medial frontal gyrus in the ERSD group compared with controls, but a significantly decreased ReHo value was found in the right middle temporal gyrus. There was no significant correlation between ReHo values and the duration of hemodialysis in the ESRD group. Both the patients and control subjects had normal MMSE scores (≥28).

Conclusions: Our finding revealed that abnormal brain activity was distributed mainly in the memory and cognition related cotices in patients with ESRD. The abnormal spontaneous neuronal activity in those areas provide information on the neural mechanisms underlying cognitive impairment in patients with ESRD, and demonstrate that Rs-fMRI with ReHo analysis is a useful non-invasive imaging tool for the detection of early cerebral ReHo changes in hemodialysis patients with ESRD.

Editor: Xi-Nian Zuo, Institute of Psychology, Chinese Academy of Sciences, China

Funding: This work was supported by the Guangdong Provincial Science and Technology (Grant number: 2012B031800170). The funders had role in data collection and analysis, decision to publish and preparation of the manuscript.

Competing Interests: The authors have declared that no competing interests exist.

* E-mail: 112662748@qq.com

These authors contributed equally to this work.

Introduction

End stage renal disease (ESRD) is defined as a glomerular filtration rate (GFR) less than 15 mL/min/1.73 m^2, or chronic renal failure that has progressed to the point at which the kidneys are permanently functioning at less than 10% of their capacity. Patients with ESRD usually have central nervous system abnormalities, some related to ESRD itself and others related to problems secondary to hemodialysis [1,2,3,4]. These Patients with ESRD often present with neurological complications such as focal white matter lesions, cerebral atrophy, osmotic demyelination syndrome, dialysis encephalopathy, hypertensive encephalopathy, intracranial hemorrhage, infarction, sinus thrombosis, and infection [1,2,3,4]. Furthermore, among patients with ESRD, depression and cognitive impairment are the most common causes of neuropsychiatric illness [5]. Cognitive deficits may occur in patients with ESRD long before any overt neurological symptoms are observed. Depression and cognitive impairment are considered important factors for the determination of a patient's survival and prognosis. Thus, it is important to elucidate the mechanism of depression and cognitive impairment in Patients with ESRD.

Previous studies of brain changes that accompany or follow ESRD have mainly used brain computed tomography (CT) or conventional magnetic resonance imaging (MRI) [6,7,8,9,10]. Computed tomography can be used to assess neurological complications, such as intracranial hemorrhage and cerebral infarction. MRI is a sensitive imaging tool for the neurological evaluation of patients with ESRD [11]. Because the clinical evaluation and ongoing assessment of ESRD are complicated, so it has been suggested that MRI be used before the onset of therapy, so that these initial findings can serve as a basis for later comparisons [3,4,11]. For example, conventional MRI studies have shown focal white matter lesions to be more common in patients undergoing hemodialysis (56%) than in the normal population (27%) [11]. In the past decade, functional imaging studies about ESRD have consistently demonstrated regional microscopic structure and metabolic abnormalities in the white matter. Hsieh et al, who used diffusion tensor imaging to measure fractional anisotropy (FA) values in patients with ESRD, reported that patients with ESRD have significant lower FA values than healthy control subjects [12]. Chiu et al reported that significant elevations of the choline/phosphatidylcholine (Cho)/total cholesterol (tCr) and myo-inositol (mI)/tCr ratios in the frontal grey matter, frontal white matter, and temporal white matter as well as in the basal ganglia were found in ESRD group compared with controls [13]. However, these brain imaging methods have limitation in that they are not capable of estimation and visualization of neural activity.

Functional brain imaging studies have suggested that the brain is not inactive during rest, but rather shows a default state of activation [14,15,16,17,18]. Low frequency oscillations (ranging from 0.01 to 0.1 Hz) of resting-state functional MRI (Rs-fMRI) time-series are known to show correlated patterns between anatomically separated brain regions [18,19,20]. It has been suggested that these correlations originate from coherency in the underlying neuronal activation patterns of these regions and reflect functional connectivity. Regions that show this kind of coherent functional behavior are said to form a resting-state network (RSN). Regional homogeneity (ReHo) measures the functional coherence of a given voxel with its nearest neighbors and can be used to evaluate resting-state brain activities based on the hypothesis that significant brain activities would more likely occur in clusters than in a single voxel [21]. The Kendall coeffi cient of concordance was used to measure the similarity of the time series of one voxel with that of its nearest neighbors in a voxel-wise analysis [22]. Regional homogeneity does not require the onset time of stimulus and therefore is useful for Rs-fMRI data analysis. Regional homogeneity has been successfully used to study the functional modulations in the resting state in patients with Alzheimer disease [23], Parkinson disease [24], schizophrenia [25], and neuromyelitis optica [26] and in healthy aging subjects [27]. Regional homogeneity could be regarded as a measure for investigating human brain activities in the resting state. It may be helpful to understand the pathophysiology of cognitive deficits in patients with ESRD using the ReHo method, which can reflect the temporal homogeneity of neural activity. In this prospective study, we characterized and compared ReHo differences between hemodialysis patients with ESRD and healthy control subjects

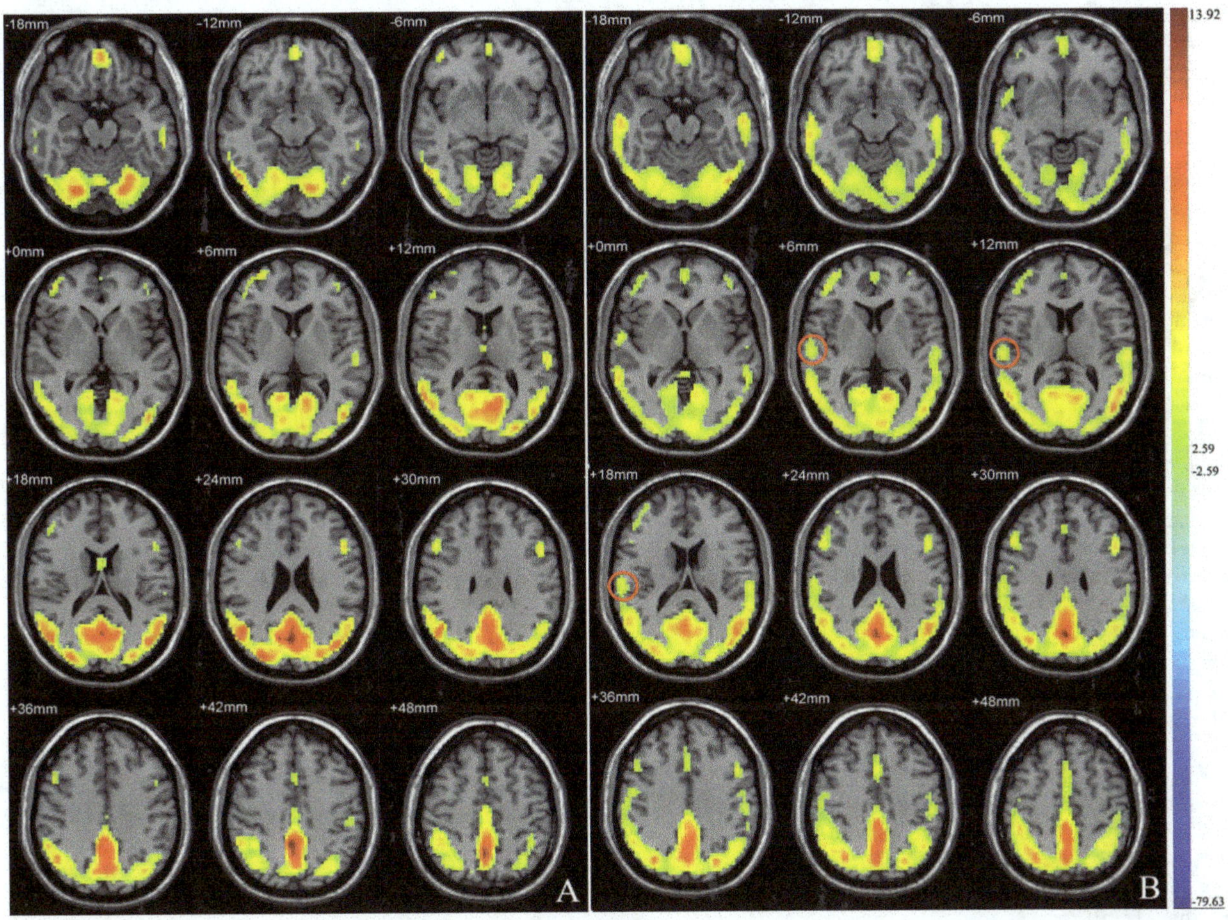

Figure 1. Mean ReHo maps within the ESRD group (A) and healthy controls (B). Left side of the images corresponds to the right side of the subjects. T-score bars are shown on the right. The images illustrate high ReHo in the default network. In the controls group but not the patient group, high ReHo was shown in the right middle temporal gyrus.

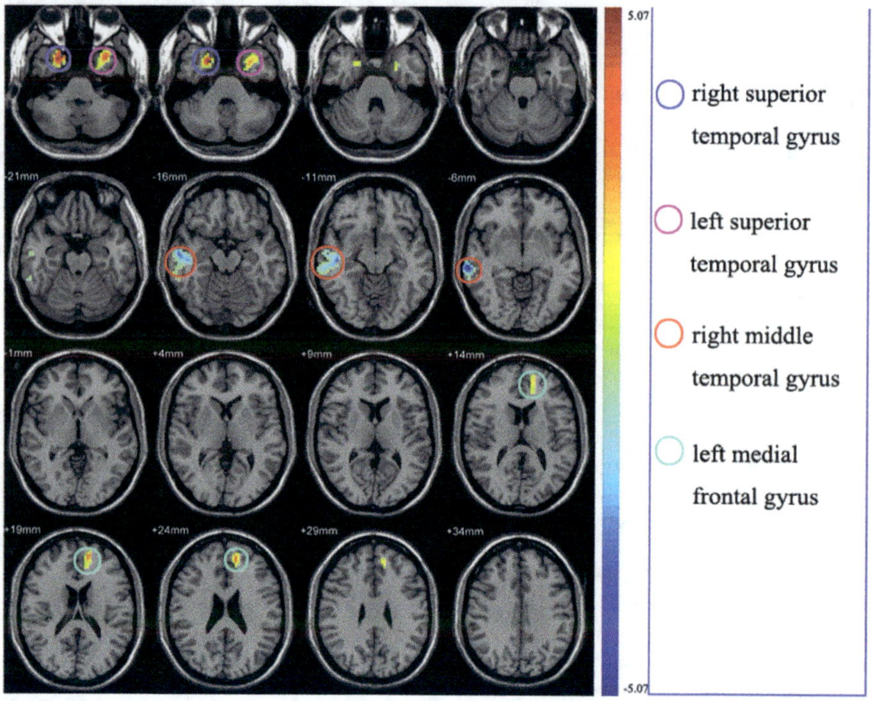

Figure 2. Maps showing statistically significant differences between the ESRD group and the control group. The Patients with ESRD showed a significant ReHo increase in the bilateral superior temporal gyrus and left medial frontal gyrus (warm colors), but a decrease in the right middle temporal gyrus (cold colors) (n = 20, corrected $P<0.05$).

using Rs-fMRI to understand the effect of ESRD on brain function.

Materials and Methods

Subjects

This prospective study was approved by the Research Ethics Review Board of the Institute of Mental Health at the Guangdong No. 2 Provincial People's Hospital. Written informed consent was obtained from all subjects. For this hospitalbased prospective case-control study, we recruited 23 patients with ESRD from the renal transplantation department at our hospital and 20 healthy volunteers with normal renal function between August 2011 and July 2012. To avoid possible confounding effects, all participants were younger than 50 years. They were excluded if they had a history of diabetes, alcoholism, drug abuse, psychiatric disorders, or major neurologic disorders (severe head injury, stroke, epilepsy, or visible lesions). Conventional MR images were interpreted by an experienced radiologist (J.Z.T) with 20 years of experience in neuroradiology who was blinded to whether the images were from the patient group or the control group. Subjects with brain lesions at conventional T1 or T2-fluid-attenuated inversion recovery (FLAIR) MR imaging were excluded. Three patients, whose T2-FLAIR MR images showed abnormal hyperintensities, were excluded because the imaging evidence suggested infarcts, one of the exclusion criteria. The final study population included 20 patients with ESRD (15 men, 5 women) and 20 healthy controls (15 men, 5 women). All patients were diagnosed with renal failure by GFR less than 15 mL/min/1.73 m^2, and underwent regular hemodialysis. Each subject completed a questionnaire before MRI examination, including age, sex, years of education, duration of hemodialysis and Mini-Mental State Examination (MMSE).

Imaging studies

MRI data were obtained using a 1.5T MR scanner (Achieva Nova-Dual; Philips, Best, the Netherlands) in the Department of Medical Imaging, Guangdong No. 2 Provincial People's Hospital. Each subject lay supine with the head comfortably fixed using a belt and foam pads. During Rs-fMRI, subjects were instructed to close their eyes and remain as quiet as possible and to not think of anything systematically or fall asleep. The conventional imaging sequences including T1-weighted images and T2-FLAIR images were obtained for every subject to detect clinically silent lesions. Rs-fMRI data were acquired using a gradient-echo echo-planar sequence sensitive to blood oxygenation level dependent (BOLD) contrast. The Rs-fMRI acquisition parameters were as follows: repetition time (TR) = 3,000 ms, echo time (TE) = 50 ms, flip angle = 90°, field-of-view = 230×230 mm^2, matrix = 64×64, and total volumes = 160. A total of 33 axial slices of 4.5 mm thickness were collected with no intersection gap. In-plane resolution was 3.59×3.59 mm^2. Each Rs-fMRI scan lasted 8 minutes. After the examination, all participants were asked questions to verify the degree of their cooperation.

Data preprocessing and regional homogeneity calculation

The imaging data were preprocessed mainly using a MATLAB toolbox called Data Processing Assistant for Resting-State (DPARSF [28]; http://restfmri.net/forum/DPARSF) for "pipeline" data analysis of Rs-fMRI. DPARSF is based on statistical parametric mapping software functions (SPM8; http://www.fil.ion.ucl.ac.uk/spm) and REST software [29]; http://resting-fmri.sourceforge.net). For each participant, the first 10 time points were discarded to avoid transient signal changes before magnetization reached steady-state and to allow subjects to become accustomed to the fMRI scanning noise. The raw data were corrected for

Table 1. Demographic and clinical characteristics of ESRD and control groups.

Characteristic	ESRD group(n = 20)	Control group(n = 20)	*t* value	*P* value*
Age(y)	37.1±8.6	38.3±6.5	−0.499	0.621
Sex#				1.000
male	15	15		
female	5	5		
Education(y)	12.0±2.9	12.9±3.2	−0.938	0.354
No. of cigarettes/day▲	13.5±9.2	16.7±12.6	−0.325	0.768
Duration of dialysis(mo)$	10.7±6.4	NA		
MMSE score	29.2±0.8	29.5±0.8	−1.189	0.242

Unless otherwise indicated, data are mean±standard deviations.
NA = not applicable. MMSE = Mini-mental status examination.
* *P* values are two sided.
#For sex composition, $\chi^2 = 0.000$ and v = 1.
▲There were two patients in the ESRD group and three persons in the control group with a history of smoking.
$There were 17 inpatients in the ESRD group.

acquisition delay between slices and for the head motion (a least squares approach and a 6 parameter spatial transformation). Subjects with head motion exceeding 1.5 mm in any dimension through the resting-state run were removed. Following the motion correction, all data were spatial normalized to the Montreal Neurological Institute (MNI) template (resampling voxel size $= 3\times3\times3$ mm^3). Subsequent data preprocessing included removal of linear trends and temporal filtering (band pass, 0.01 to 0.08 Hz) to remove the effects of very low-frequency drift and physiological high frequency respiratory and cardiac noise for further ReHo analysis [18].

The ReHo calculation procedure was the same as that reported in a previous study [21]. Briefly, this is accomplished on a voxel-by-voxel basis by calculating Kendall's coefficient of concordance (KCC) [22] for a given voxel time series with those of its nearest 26 neighbors.

$$W = \frac{\sum (R_i)^2 - n(\overline{R})^2}{\frac{1}{12}K^2(n^3 - n)}$$

where W is the KCC among given voxels, ranging from 0 to 1; R_i is the sum rank of the with time point ($R_i = \sum_{j=1}^{k} r_{ij}$ where r_{ij} is the rank of the *i*th time point in the *j*th voxel); $\overline{R} = ((n+1)\,k)/2$ is the mean of the R_i; k is the number of time series within a measured cluster (27, one given voxel plus the number of its neighbors); and n is the number of ranks (n = 150 for this study). The KCC value was calculated to this voxel, and an individual KCC map was obtained for each subject. To reduce the influence of individual variations in the KCC value, ReHo maps normalization was preformed by dividing the KCC among each voxel by the averaged KCC of the whole brain. The resulting data were then spatially smoothed with an 8-mm full-width at half-maximum (FWHM) Gaussian kernel to reduce noise and residual differences in gyral anatomy.

Statistical analysis

Two-sample *t*-tests were performed to assess the differences in age, duration of education and number of cigarettes smoked per day between Patients with ESRD and healthy subjects. Mann-Whitney U tests were used to analyze the differences in sex between the two groups. Pearson correlation coefficient was used to analyze the association between ReHo values and the duration of hemodialysis in the patient group. Analyses were conducted using software (SPSS, version 13.0; Chicago, Ill, USA), and a *P* value less than 0.05 (two-tailed) was considered statistically significant.

Table 2. Brain regions with abnormal ReHo in patients with ESRD compared with control subjects.

			Mean Reho value			MNI coordinate			
Brain area	No. of voxels	Side	Control group	ESRD group	Brodmann area	x	y	z	Peak t value
Superior Temporal gyrus	35	R	−0.440±0.062	−0.329±0.076	38	24	9	−39	5.071
Superior Temporal gyrus	42	L	−0.366±0.074	−0.243±0.101	38	−33	12	−42	4.594
Middle Temporal gyrus	132	R	0.099±0.049	−0.033±0.072	21	66	−30	−6	−5.018
Medial Frontal gyrus	53	L	−0.239±0.058	−0.145±0.082	9	−12	48	21	4.052

L = left, R = right, MNI = Montreal Neurological Institute.

A second-level random-effect one-sample *t*-test ($P<0.01$, with False Discovery Rate (FDR) correction) was performed to show the ReHo results with in each group. To explore the ReHo differences between Patients with ESRD and healthy subjects, a second-level random-effect two-sample *t*-test was performed on the individual normalized ReHo maps in a voxel-by-voxel manner by taking age and years of education as confounding covariates. Significant differences were set at the threshold of a corrected cluster level at *P* less than 0.05. Threshold correction was performed by using a program (AlphaSim; Analysis of Functional NeuroImages, http://afni.nimh.nih.gov/afni/) that applies Monte Carlo simulation to calculate the probability of false positive detection by taking into consideration both the individual voxel probability threshold and cluster size [30]. Using this program, a corrected significance level of *P* less than 0.05 was obtained by clusters with a minimum volume of 1998 mm^3 at an uncorrected individual voxel height threshold of $P<0.01$. This enabled the identification of significant changes in ReHo in the Patients with ESRD compared with the controls. The parameters were as follow: individual voxel *P* value = 0.01, 1,000 simulations, FWHM = 8 mm, and whole brain mask.

Results

After exclusion of three patients with hyperintensities on T2-FLAIR images, we found no other abnormality in morphology or signal intensity on T1-weighted and T2- FLAIR images. The mean age of the patients and healthy controls was 37.1±8.6 years (range, 19–49 years) and 38.3±6.5 years (range, 28–49 years), respectively. Three subjects in the ESRD group were outpatients, we could not collect the duration of hemodialysis of them. The mean duration of hemodialysis for the patient group (n = 17) was 10.7±6.4 monthes. There were no significant differences in age, sex, years of education and number of cigarettes smoked per day between patients with ESRD and control subjects (Table. 1). The mean ReHo maps with in each group are shown in Figure. 1, illustrating high ReHo in the default network. In the controls group, high ReHo in the right middle temporal gyrus was shown, but this was not found in the patient group. Compared with the control group, the Patients with ESRD showed a significant ReHo increase in the bilateral superior temporal gyrus ($P<0.05$, AlphaSim corrected) and left medial frontal gyrus ($P<0.05$, AlphaSim corrected), but a decrease in the right middle temporal gyrus ($P<0.05$, AlphaSim corrected) (Table. 2, Figure. 2). There was no significant correlations between ReHo values and the duration of hemodialysis in the ESRD group. No significantly different score was found between patient and control groups, all subjects had normal MMSE scores (≥28).

Discussion

The ReHo is a data-driven method, which assumes that a given voxel is temporally similar to its neighbors. It measures the ReHo of the time series of the regional BOLD signal. Therefore, ReHo reflects the temporal homogeneity of the regional BOLD signal rather than its density. As the BOLD signal of fMRI may reflect neural activity [31], abnormal ReHo is possibly relevant to the changes of temporal aspects of neural activity in the regional brain. Therefore ReHo may detect the brain regions with abnormal activity.

We found ReHo values in patients with ESRD to be significantly increased in the bilateral superior temporal gyrus and left medial frontal gyrus, but decreased in the right middle temporal gyrus. Interestingly, all of the brain areas with significant ReHo changes were located in the temporal and frontal lobes, which are closely related to the memory and cognition. Our findings are similar to those of many previous brain imaging studies in pre-dialysis patients. Using Tc-99m ethylcysteinate dimer brain single photon emission tomography, Song et al found that prior to beginning dialysis patients with chronic kidney disease have significant hypoperfusion in the right superior and middle temporal gyrus and inferior frontal gyrus [32]. In their previous study using F-18-fluorodeoxyglucose positron emission tomography, they found that several voxel clusters had significantly decreased cerebral glucose metabolism in patients with chronic kidney disease who had not started dialysis, including the prefrontal cortex, superior temporal gyrus and middle temporal gyrus [33]. Kim et al reported that depressive mood and anxiety factors were negatively correlated with regional cerebral blood flow in bilateral superior temporal gyrus, right middle temporal gyrus and left superior frontal gyrus [34]. Thus, all of them cannot reflect the baseline directly as resting-state studies can.

Recently, Xue Liang et al did a similar research to us. They used Rs-fMRI with ReHo algorithm to investigate the pattern of spontaneous neural activity in patients with ESRD. In their study, they found both MNE (minimal nephro-encephalopathy) and non-NE (non-nephro-encephalopathy) patients show decreased ReHo in the multiple areas of bilateral frontal, parietal and temporal lobes [35]. These results have a few difference to ours. It may be relate to the small sample size. Whatever, the differences in ReHo indicate a poor level of coordination and a disorder of communication among neurons in the brain region [21]. These changes in ReHo suggest an abnormality in the resting-state brain function of patients with ESRD and may be early signs for the development of uremic encephalopathy or dialysis encephalopathy.

The temporal and frontal regions are considered as important components of human default-mode networks [15,17,36], and have been shown to exhibit mild cognitive impairment (MCI)-related structural and functional abnormalities [37,38,39,40,41]. James et al reported that hemodialysis patients have a high prevalence of mild cognitive impairment (MCI) despite normal global cognitive function [42]. MCI is a transitional state between normal cognition and the earliest clinical features of dementia. MCI is likely under-diagnosed but highly prevalent in dindividuals with ESRD [43,44,45], and Murray et al described MCI in nearly 64% of hemodialysis patients [46]. In the present study, we found that patients with ESRD have normal global cognitive function (MMSE score >25), but that does not mean that these patients are free of MCI. The greatest defect in our research was that we did not assess the MCI in patients with ESRD.

In our study, there was no significant correlation between ReHo values and the duration of hemodialysis in the ESRD group. This finding may indicate that the significant change in ReHo values relates to ESRD itself but not hemodialysis.

Some limitations of our study are worth mentioning. First, we did not discriminate between neuronal versus vascular effects on changes in ReHo values in patients with ESRD. Second, the sample size in this study is relatively small, and thus the results of the current study may no be representative of ESRD in general. Third, the lack of MCI examinations in our sample is the most serious drawback of our study. Fourth, we did not collect follow-up Rs-fMRI data after renal replacement. In future studies, examinations should include not only fMRI but also arterial spin labeling perfusion imaging, electroencephalograms and other measures to discriminate between neuronal versus vascular effects on changes in neural activity in patients with ESRD. More attention also needs to be paid to mental test and serial changes in neural activity after renal replacement therapy in Patients with ESRD.

In conclusion, we found significant change in ReHo values in patients with ESRD in brain areas located in temporal and frontal lobes, which are closely related to the memory and cognition. The abnormal spontaneous neuronal activity in those areas may be the neural mechanisms underlying the cognitive impairment in patients with ESRD, and suggested that an abnormal ReHo value in certain brain areas may be a potential biomarker to detect the early cerebral ReHo changes in hemodialysis patients with ESRD.

Author Contributions

Conceived and designed the experiments: GJ HS. Performed the experiments: CL HS WZ. Analyzed the data: YQ XL JT. Contributed reagents/materials/analysis tools: HS SS. Wrote the paper: HS.

References

1. Glaser GH (1974) Brain dysfunction in uremia. Res Publ Assoc Res Nerv Ment Dis 53: 173–199.
2. De Deyn PP, Saxena VK, Abts H, Borggreve F, D'Hooge R, et al. (1992) Clinical and pathophysiological aspects of neurological complications in renal failure. Acta Neurol Belg 92: 191–206.
3. Brouns R, De Deyn PP (2004) Neurological complications in renal failure: a review. Clin Neurol Neurosurg 107: 1–16.
4. Tzamaloukas AH, Agaba EI (2004) Neurological manifestations of uraemia and chronic dialysis. Niger J Med 13: 98–105.
5. Kimmel PL, Thamer M, Richard CM, Ray NF (1998) Psychiatric illness in patients with end-stage renal disease. Am J Med 105: 214–221.
6. Fazekas G, Fazekas F, Schmidt R, Kapeller P, Offenbacher H, et al. (1995) Brain MRI findings and cognitive impairment in patients undergoing chronic hemodialysis treatment. J Neurol Sci 134: 83–88.
7. Savazzi GM, Cusmano F, Musini S (2001) Cerebral imaging changes in patients with chronic renal failure treated conservatively or in hemodialysis. Nephron 89: 31–36.
8. Suzuki M, Wada A, Isaka Y, Maki K, Inoue T, et al. (1997) Cerebral magnetic resonance T2 high intensities in end-stage renal disease. Stroke 28: 2528–2531.
9. Kim CD, Lee HJ, Kim DJ, Kim BS, Shin SK, et al. (2007) High prevalence of leukoaraiosis in cerebral magnetic resonance images of patients on peritoneal dialysis. Am J Kidney Dis 50: 98–107.
10. Kamata T, Hishida A, Takita T, Sawada K, Ikegaya N, et al. (2000) Morphologic abnormalities in the brain of chronically hemodialyzed patients without cerebrovascular disease. Am J Nephrol 20: 27–31.
11. Agildere AM, Kurt A, Yildirim T, Benli S, Altinors N (2001) MRI of neurologic complications in end-stage renal failure patients on hemodialysis: pictorial review. Eur Radiol 11: 1063–1069.
12. Hsieh TJ, Chang JM, Chuang HY, Ko CH, Hsieh ML, et al. (2009) End-stage renal disease: in vivo diffusion-tensor imaging of silent white matter damage. Radiology 252: 518–525.
13. Chiu ML, Li CW, Chang JM, Chiang IC, Ko CH, et al. (2010) Cerebral metabolic changes in neurologically presymptomatic patients undergoing haemodialysis: in vivo proton MR spectroscopic findings. Eur Radiol 20: 1502–1507.
14. De Luca M, Beckmann CF, De Stefano N, Matthews PM, Smith SM (2006) fMRI resting state networks define distinct modes of long-distance interactions in the human brain. Neuroimage 29: 1359–1367.
15. Greicius MD, Krasnow B, Reiss AL, Menon V (2003) Functional connectivity in the resting brain: a network analysis of the default mode hypothesis. Proc Natl Acad Sci U S A 100: 253–258.
16. Gusnard DA, Raichle ME, Raichle ME (2001) Searching for a baseline: functional imaging and the resting human brain. Nat Rev Neurosci 2: 685–694.
17. Raichle ME, MacLeod AM, Snyder AZ, Powers WJ, Gusnard DA, et al. (2001) A default mode of brain function. Proc Natl Acad Sci U S A 98: 676–682.
18. Biswal B, Yetkin FZ, Haughton VM, Hyde JS (1995) Functional connectivity in the motor cortex of resting human brain using echo-planar MRI. Magn Reson Med 34: 537–541.
19. Cordes D, Haughton VM, Arfanakis K, Wendt GJ, Turski PA, et al. (2000) Mapping functionally related regions of brain with functional connectivity MR imaging. AJNR Am J Neuroradiol 21: 1636–1644.
20. Fox MD, Raichle ME (2007) Spontaneous fluctuations in brain activity observed with functional magnetic resonance imaging. Nat Rev Neurosci 8: 700–711.
21. Zang Y, Jiang T, Lu Y, He Y, Tian L (2004) Regional homogeneity approach to fMRI data analysis. Neuroimage 22: 394–400.
22. Kendall M GJ (1990) Rank correlation methods. Oxford, England: Oxford University Press.
23. He Y, Wang L, Zang Y, Tian L, Zhang X, et al. (2007) Regional coherence changes in the early stages of Alzheimer's disease: a combined structural and resting-state functional MRI study. Neuroimage 35: 488–500.
24. Wu T, Long X, Zang Y, Wang L, Hallett M, et al. (2009) Regional homogeneity changes in patients with Parkinson's disease. Hum Brain Mapp 30: 1502–1510.
25. Liu H, Liu Z, Liang M, Hao Y, Tan L, et al. (2006) Decreased regional homogeneity in schizophrenia: a resting state functional magnetic resonance imaging study. Neuroreport 17: 19–22.
26. Liang P, Liu Y, Jia X, Duan Y, Yu C, et al. (2011) Regional homogeneity changes in patients with neuromyelitis optica revealed by resting-state functional MRI. Clin Neurophysiol 122: 121–127.
27. Wu T, Zang Y, Wang L, Long X, Li K, et al. (2007) Normal aging decreases regional homogeneity of the motor areas in the resting state. Neurosci Lett 423: 189–193.
28. Chao-Gan Y, Yu-Feng Z (2010) DPARSF: A MATLAB Toolbox for "Pipeline" Data Analysis of Resting-State fMRI. Front Syst Neurosci 4: 13.
29. Song XW, Dong ZY, Long XY, Li SF, Zuo XN, et al. (2011) REST: a toolkit for resting-state functional magnetic resonance imaging data processing. PLoS One 6: e25031.
30. Forman SD, Cohen JD, Fitzgerald M, Eddy WF, Mintun MA, et al. (1995) Improved assessment of significant activation in functional magnetic resonance imaging (fMRI): use of a cluster-size threshold. Magn Reson Med 33: 636–647.
31. Logothetis NK, Pauls J, Augath M, Trinath T, Oeltermann A (2001) Neurophysiological investigation of the basis of the fMRI signal. Nature 412: 150–157.
32. Song SH, Kwak IS, Kim SJ, Kim YK, Kim IJ (2009) Depressive mood in pre-dialytic chronic kidney disease: Statistical parametric mapping analysis of Tc-99m ECD brain SPECT. Psychiatry Res 173: 243–247.
33. Song SH, Kim IJ, Kim SJ, Kwak IS, Kim YK (2008) Cerebral glucose metabolism abnormalities in patients with major depressive symptoms in pre-dialytic chronic kidney disease: statistical parametric mapping analysis of F-18-FDG PET, a preliminary study. Psychiatry Clin Neurosci 62: 554–561.
34. Kim SJ, Song SH, Kim JH, Kwak IS (2008) Statistical parametric mapping analysis of the relationship between regional cerebral blood flow and symptom clusters of the depressive mood in patients with pre-dialytic chronic kidney disease. Ann Nucl Med 22: 201–206.
35. Liang X, Wen J, Ni L, Zhong J, Qi R, et al. (2013) Altered pattern of spontaneous brain activity in the patients with end-stage renal disease: a resting-state functional MRI study with regional homogeneity analysis. PLoS One 8: e71507.
36. Buckner RL, Andrews-Hanna JR, Schacter DL (2008) The brain's default network: anatomy, function, and relevance to disease. Ann N Y Acad Sci 1124: 1–38.
37. Bookheimer SY, Strojwas MH, Cohen MS, Saunders AM, Pericak-Vance MA, et al. (2000) Patterns of brain activation in people at risk for Alzheimer's disease. N Engl J Med 343: 450–456.
38. Dickerson BC, Salat DH, Bates JF, Atiya M, Killiany RJ, et al. (2004) Medial temporal lobe function and structure in mild cognitive impairment. Ann Neurol 56: 27–35.
39. Dickerson BC, Sperling RA (2008) Functional abnormalities of the medial temporal lobe memory system in mild cognitive impairment and Alzheimer's disease: insights from functional MRI studies. Neuropsychologia 46: 1624–1635.
40. Hamalainen A, Pihlajamaki M, Tanila H, Hanninen T, Niskanen E, et al. (2007) Increased fMRI responses during encoding in mild cognitive impairment. Neurobiol Aging 28: 1889–1903.
41. Wang Z, Nie B, Li D, Zhao Z, Han Y, et al. (2012) Effect of acupuncture in mild cognitive impairment and Alzheimer disease: a functional MRI study. PLoS One 7: e42730.
42. Post JB, Jegede AB, Morin K, Spungen AM, Langhoff E, et al. (2010) Cognitive profile of chronic kidney disease and hemodialysis patients without dementia. Nephron Clin Pract 116: c247–c255.
43. Sehgal AR, Grey SF, DeOreo PB, Whitehouse PJ (1997) Prevalence, recognition, and implications of mental impairment among hemodialysis patients. Am J Kidney Dis 30: 41–49.
44. Pereira AA, Weiner DE, Scott T, Chandra P, Bluestein R, et al. (2007) Subcortical cognitive impairment in dialysis patients. Hemodial Int 11: 309–314.
45. Kurella M, Chertow GM, Luan J, Yaffe K (2004) Cognitive impairment in chronic kidney disease. J Am Geriatr Soc 52: 1863–1869.
46. Murray AM, Tupper DE, Knopman DS, Gilbertson DT, Pederson SL, et al. (2006) Cognitive impairment in hemodialysis patients is common. Neurology 67: 216–223.

18

Effects of Hemodiafiltration and High Flux Hemodialysis on Nerve Excitability in End-Stage Kidney Disease

Ria Arnold[1], Bruce A. Pussell[2,3], Timothy J. Pianta[2,3], Virginija Grinius[2], Cindy S-Y. Lin[1], Matthew C. Kiernan[3,4], James Howells[5], Meg J. Jardine[6], Arun V. Krishnan[1]*

1 Translational Neuroscience Facility, University of New South Wales, Sydney, New South Wales, Australia, **2** Department of Nephrology Prince of Wales Hospital, Sydney, New South Wales, Australia, **3** Prince of Wales Clinical School, University of New South Wales, Sydney, New South Wales, Australia, **4** Neuroscience Research Australia, Sydney, New South Wales, Australia, **5** The University of Sydney and Institute of Clinical Neurosciences, Royal Prince Alfred Hospital, Sydney, New South Wales, Australia, **6** Department of Nephrology Concord Repatriation General Hospital and The George Institute for Global Health, Sydney, New South Wales, Australia

Abstract

Objectives: Peripheral neuropathy is the most common neurological complication in end-stage kidney disease. While high flux hemodialysis (HFHD) and hemodiafiltration (HDF) have become the preferred options for extracorporeal dialysis therapy, the effects of these treatments on nerve excitability have not yet been examined.

Methods: An observational proof-of-concept study of nerve excitability and neuropathy was undertaken in an incident dialysis population (n = 17) receiving either HFHD or HDF. Nerve excitability techniques were utilised to assess nerve ion channel function and membrane potential, in conjunction with clinical assessment and standard nerve conduction studies. A mathematical model of axonal excitability was used to investigate the underlying basis of the observed changes. Nerve excitability was recorded from the median nerve, before, during and after a single dialysis session and correlated with corresponding biochemical markers. Differences in nerve excitability were compared to normal controls with longitudinal follow-up over an 18 month period.

Results: Nerve excitability was performed in patient cohorts treated with either HFHD (n = 9) or online HDF (n = 8), with similar neuropathy status. Nerve excitability measures in HDF-treated patients were significantly closer to normal values compared to HFHD patients obtained over the course of a dialysis session ($p<0.05$). Longitudinal studies revealed stability of nerve excitability findings, and thus maintenance of improved nerve function in the HDF group.

Conclusions: This study has provided evidence that nerve excitability in HDF-treated patients is significantly closer to normal values prior to dialysis, across a single dialysis session and at longitudinal follow-up. These findings offer promise for the management of neuropathy in ESKD and should be confirmed in randomised trials.

Editor: Robert Chen, University of Toronto, Canada

Funding: RA and TP were each supported by an Australian Postgraduate Award from the University of New South Wales. AK was supported by a Career Development Award from the National Health and Medical Research Council of Australia (grant 568680). MJ was supported by a Jacquot Research Establishment Award. Grant support was provided by the National Health and Medical Research Council of Australia (grant 630425). The funders had no role in study design, data collection and analysis, decision to publish, or preparation of the manuscript.

Competing Interests: The authors have declared that no competing interests exist.

* E-mail: arun.krishnan@unsw.edu.au

Introduction

Neurological complications are a major cause of physical disability in patients with end-stage kidney disease (ESKD). Of the many neurological complications that can occur in ESKD [1], peripheral neuropathy remains the most common long-term disorder [2–4]. Clinical features of neuropathy include sensory loss, paraesthesia, impaired vibration sense, reduced deep tendon reflexes, muscle wasting and weakness [4,5]. Despite the considerable advances that have occurred in the use of renal replacement therapies (RRT), neuropathy rates remain high affecting 70 to 100% of dialysis patients [2–4,6]. Moreover, neuropathy remains essentially untreatable in the majority of ESKD patients. As such, further investigation into the most beneficial treatment for ESKD patients with neuropathy is a matter of high priority.

The two preferred options for extracorporeal dialysis therapy among renal physicians are high flux hemodialysis (HFHD) and hemodiafiltration (HDF) [7]. While recent ongoing randomized trials have thus far failed to show survival benefit with HDF treatment, there remains widespread interest in the potential clinical advantages of HDF [8,9]. HDF has been reported to achieve better clearance of "clinically relevant" middle molecules [10] and studies have suggested that on-line HDF may have a positive effect on inflammatory status [11,12], oxidative stress [13] and small solute clearance [14–16]. Previous studies have not however addressed neurological function in patients treated with online HDF and HFHD forms of RRT.

While traditional nerve conduction studies demonstrate minimal change over a dialysis session [3], nerve excitability studies have demonstrated prominent abnormalities prior to dialysis that are rapidly reversed by dialysis [17–19]. These techniques are sophisticated neurophysiological measures that provide insights into ion channel function and membrane potential in human peripheral nerves. As such, nerve excitability techniques have been widely used in clinical neurophysiological research and have proven highly sensitive to the alterations in nerve function that occur with therapeutic interventions, such as hemodialysis [17], chemotherapy administration [20] and immunological therapy [21]. The present study was undertaken to investigate whether there were differences in peripheral nerve excitability studies in patients treated with HDF and HFHD.

Methods

Ethics Statement

The studies were approved by the South East Sydney Area Health Service Human Research Ethics Committee (Northern Section) and the Human Research Ethics Committee of the University of New South Wales. Participants gave written informed consent to the procedures in accordance with the Declaration of Helsinki.

An observational, proof-of-concept, clinical study of nerve excitability and neuropathy was undertaken in an incident dialysis population at a tertiary referral centre from 2010–2012. Eligibility criteria included ESKD patients aged 18–75 years, able to give informed consent and who were maintained on HFHD or HDF dialysis modality for a continuous period of at least 6 months. Sensory and motor nerve conduction studies, including sensory comparison studies, were undertaken in all patients to exclude the presence of carpal tunnel syndrome. Patients who had alterations in median sensory or motor conduction, suggestive of carpal tunnel syndrome, were excluded from the study. Study sample size was based on calculations of changes in threshold electrotonus parameters (α error level of 5% and a statistical power of 80%) from previous studies of nerve excitability undertaken in dialysis populations [17–19].

Clinical assessment and neurophysiological studies were undertaken in 17 ESKD patients receiving 4–6 hour, thrice-weekly RRT. Nine patients were treated with HFHD and eight with online post dilution HDF with at least 20 litres of fluid replacement. In order to minimise baseline differences, groups were matched for age, gender, disease duration, presence of diabetes and current neuropathy status. Neurophysiological tests were also undertaken in 20 age and gender matched normal subjects. The two study groups were similar in age, gender, neuropathy status, and diabetic status (Table 1). The causes of ESKD included diabetes, glomerulonephritis, lithium toxicity, amyloid, obstructive nephropathy, interstitial nephritis, reflux nephropathy and in four the cause was unknown. Longitudinal assessment of these tests was undertaken 18 months later in 13 of the 17 patients.

Table 1. Patient Characteristics.

	HDF	HFHD	*p*
Demographics			
Age	61 (14)	62 (14)	0.87
Sex	6M : 2F	7M : 2F	
Diabetes	4Y : 4N	4Y : 5N	
Neuropathy Status			
Total Neuropathy Score	9.9 (3.5)	7.3 (2.7)	0.46
Total Neuropathy Grade	1.7 (0.5)	1.1 (0.4)	0.46
Sural Nerve Amplitude (μV)	6.7 (2.0)	7.5 (2.3)	0.61
Tibial Motor Nerve Amplitude (mV)	4.3 (3.5)	5.8 (5.1)	0.66
RRT measures			
Years on RRT	3.9 (2.4)	4.2 (2.8)	0.79
Hours on RRT (per session)	4.9 (0.5)	4.7 (0.4)	0.54
Equilibrated KT/V	1.81 (0.44)	2.28 (0.76)	0.15
Urea Reduction Ratio	0.79 (0.06)	0.81 (0.13)	0.28
Pre-RRT serum biochemistry			
Sodium (mmol/L)	138(3)	139 (2)	0.70
Potassium (mmol/L)	4.5 (0.7)	5.3 (0.8)	0.03*
Chloride (mmol/L)	100 (3.7)	103 (3.8)	0.14
Bicarbonate (mmol/L)	25.6 (2.4)	23.6 (2.1)	0.08
Serum Urea Nitrogen (mg/dL)	61.1 (30.1)	65.8 (14.0)	0.68
Creatinine (μmol/L))	807 (344)	882 (236)	0.60
Calcium (mmol/L)	2.23 (0.17)	2.27 (0.15)	0.65
Magnesium (mmol/L)	1.01 (0.13)	1.09 (0.14)	0.28
Serum Phosphorus (mmol/L)	1.36 (0.61)	1.53 (0.50)	0.52
Parathyroid hormone (ng/L)	351 (380)	261 (305)	0.56

All values given as mean (±SD). *$p<0.05$ Biochemical values all taken pre-RRT after a 56 hour inter-dialytic period.

Enrolled patients had been maintained on their respective form of RRT consistently for the previous six months. The dialyzers used were Polyflux® 201H (surface area 2.1 m^2) with either a Gambro® 200S dialysis machine for HFHD or a Gambro® AK 200Ultra for online HDF (Gambro, Hechingen, Germany). HDF machines dialysed against ultrapure water, while HFHD used pure water and both modalities used Gambro® Select Bag AX250G dialysis concentrate containing sodium (Na^+) 140 mmol/L, bicarbonate 34 mmol/L, potassium (K^+) 2.0 mmol/L, calcium 1.5 mmol/L, magnesium 0.50 mmol/L and glucose 1.0 g/L. All patients were adequately dialysed as verified by eKT/V (>1.05) and URR (>65%) [9,22].

To ensure groups were matched for severity of pre-existing neuropathy, clinical neurological assessment was undertaken in all patients. Neuropathy was graded using a modified version of the Total Neuropathy Score [23]. This scale is a validated measure of neuropathy severity that assigns a neuropathy grade from 0 (no neuropathy) to 4 (disabling neuropathy), based on clinical features and the results of nerve conduction studies [23]. Nerve conduction studies were conducted using a Medelec Synergy system (Oxford Instruments, Abingdon, United Kingdom).

Motor nerve excitability studies were obtained from the non-fistula arm of ESKD patients before, during and after a single RRT session. All excitability recordings were conducted following a 56-hour interdialytic period. Compound muscle action potentials were recorded from the abductor pollicis brevis muscle following median nerve stimulation using previously published protocols [17,19,24]. Multiple excitability parameters were recorded, including threshold electrotonus and current threshold recordings which provide information on nodal and internodal conductances. The protocol also assessed recovery cycle parameters (refractoriness, superexcitability and late subexcitability), which provide information regarding changes in Na^+ and K^+ channel function and membrane potential [25]. Skin temperature was monitored close to the site of stimulation for the duration of the study. Serum electrolytes, urea, creatinine, calcium, magnesium, phosphate and parathyroid hormone were collected at time intervals corresponding to nerve excitability studies.

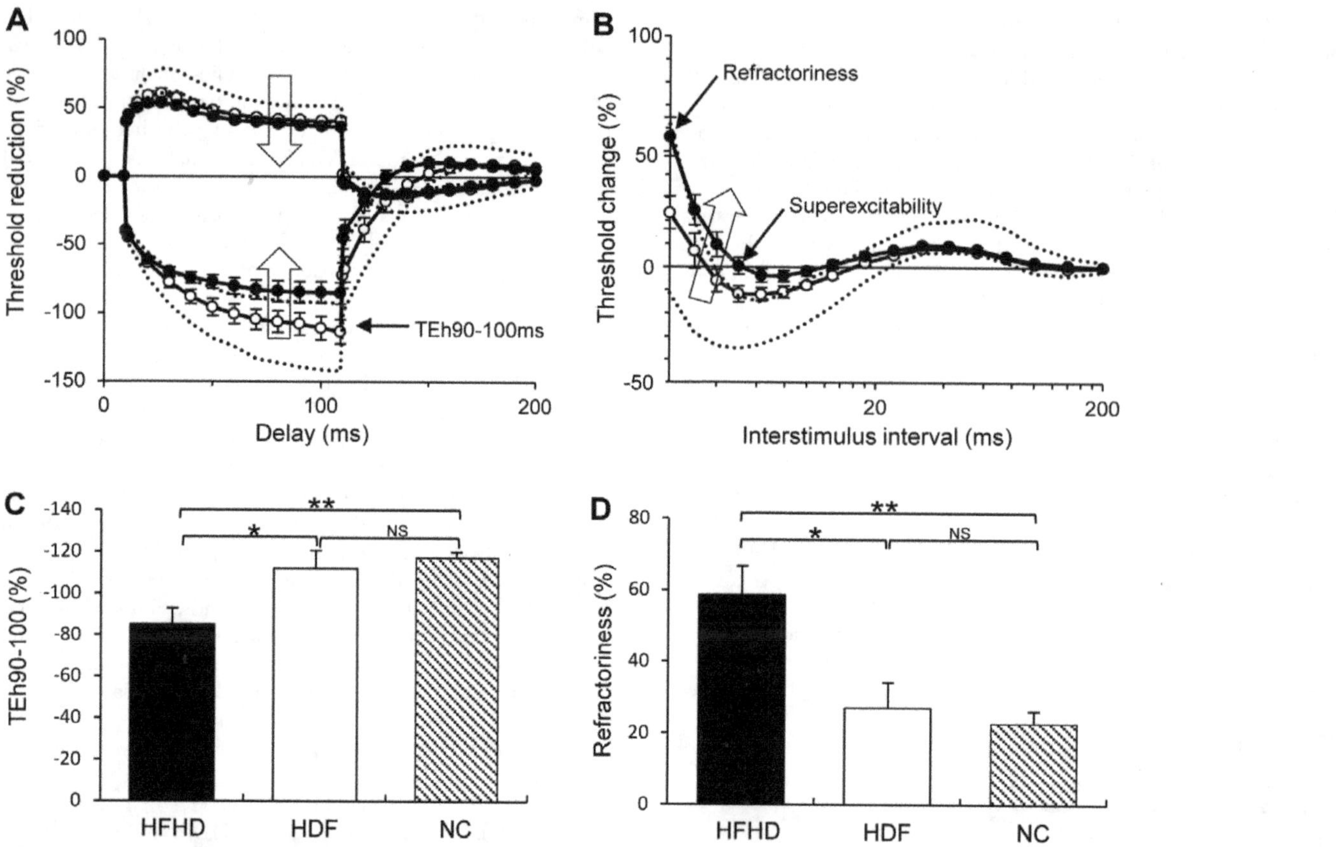

Figure 1. Pre-RRT nerve excitability recordings. Patients receiving hemodiafiltration (HDF) (empty circles) and standard high-flux HD (black filled circles) compared to 95% limits for healthy controls (dashed lines). (A) Depolarising and hyperpolarising threshold electrotonus curves. (B) Recovery cycle curve of excitability, large empty arrows indicate the direction of change with axonal depolarization. In both figures (A) and (B) the HDF group demonstrate results significantly closer to normal values than the HFHD group, specifically at hyperpolarising threshold electrotonus 90–100 ms (TEh90–100 ms), refractoriness and superexcitability. Figures (C) and (D) demonstrate the group differences in TEh90–100 ms and refractoriness in histogram format. **p*<0.05, ***p*<0.001.

Mathematical Modelling

An established model of axonal excitability [26–30] was used to assess whether changes in extracellular K^+ concentration alone could account for the observed differences in excitability between the two groups of patients. This model consists of nodal and internodal compartments linked by a paranodal pathway through and under the myelin sheath [31]. Voltage-gated Na^+ channels (both transient and persistent), K^+ channels (slow and fast) were modelled on the nodal axolemma, while the internode incorporated both slow and fast K^+ channels and the hyperpolarization-activated cation current I_h. Separate leak conductances, Na^+/K^+-ATPase pump currents and axolemmal capacitances were modelled at both the node and internode.

Statistical Analysis

All statistical analyses were performed using IBM SPSS Statistics Package version 20 (SPSS Inc, Chicago, Illinois) with statistical significance defined as $p \leq 0.05$. Clinical variables were expressed as mean±standard deviation (SD) and neurophysiological measures, figures and graphs are expressed as mean±standard error of the mean (SEM). Prior to analysis all nerve excitability data was checked for normality using Shapiro Wilks' test. Direct comparison of pre-RRT recordings with normal controls and analysis of between-group variables was undertaken using ANOVA or Kruskal-Wallis Test. To determine between group differences post-hoc analysis was undertaken. Two-factor mixed model ANOVA analysis was used to investigate differences throughout the dialysis session recordings. Correlation analyses were used to explore relationships between potential uremic toxins and nerve excitability parameters. Longitudinal analyses were undertaken using Wilcoxon Signed Rank test and Mann-Whitney U test was used for intention to treat analyses.

Results

Clinical Findings

Table 1 demonstrates the clinical and biochemical characteristics for HDF and HFHD patient groups. There were no significant differences between the two groups for age, gender, neuropathy status, and diabetic status. Additionally, there were no significant differences between groups for years on dialysis (HDF 3.9±2.4 years; HFHD 4.2±2.8 years), dialysis duration (HDF 4.9±0.5 hours; HFHD 4.7±0.4 hours) or dialysis adequacy as measured by URR (HDF 0.79±0.06; HFHD 0.81±0.13) or eKT/V (HDF 1.81±0.44; HFHD 2.28±0.76). In keeping with previous studies, the prevalence of neuropathy in this ESKD cohort (defined as a total neuropathy score >1) [23] was ~70% [3,4,19]. The groups demonstrated similar severity of pre-existing neuropathy, with no significant baseline differences for total neuropathy score (HDF 9.9±3.5; HFHD 7.3±2.7) or total neuropathy grade (HDF 1.7±0.5; HFHD 1.1±0.4).

Table 2. Pre-RRT nerve excitability results for HDF and HFHD groups compared to controls.

	Normal controls	HDF	HFHD	ANOVA F, *p*
Recovery Cycle				
Refractoriness (%)	19.3 (±2.9)	27.0 (±7.2)	60.4 (±8.4)[a,b]	15.4, <0.001
Superexcitability (%)	−21.7 (±1.5)	−12.2 (±2.3)[a]	−2.0 (±2.5)[a,b]	29.0, <0.001
Threshold Electrotonus				
TEh (90–100 ms) (%)	−117 (±3)	−112 (±9)	−85 (±8)[a,b]	9.7, <0.001
TEd (10–20 ms) (%)	68.4 (±1.0)	59.6 (±3.6)[a]	53.1 (±2.4)[a]	17.7, <0.001
TEd (90–100 ms) (%)	45.4 (±0.7)	40.6 (±2.2)[a]	36.4 (±1.6)[a]	12.2, <0.001
Current Threshold				
Resting I/V slope	0.60 (±0.01)	0.67 (±0.07)	0.84 (±0.07)[a,b]	8.3, 0.001

All values given as mean (±SEM). By convention threshold electrotonus, refractoriness and superexcitability are expressed as percentage change in threshold. TEd, depolarising threshold electrotonus; TEh, hyperpolarising threshold electrotonus; I/V, current threshold.
[a]Significantly different to controls,
[b]significantly different to HDF.

Baseline Nerve Excitability Findings

To assess acute changes in nerve excitability across a dialysis session, recordings were conducted before, during and after a single RRT session. When compared to normal controls (NC), pre-RRT recordings in both groups demonstrated multiple abnormalities with the overall pattern of change consistent with nerve membrane depolarization (Fig. 1) [17,32], a finding that has been previously reported in studies of excitability in ESKD patients dialyzed with conventional semi-permeable membranes [17,19]. Specifically, comparison across the three groups (NC, HDF and HFHD) demonstrated significant differences for multiple nerve parameters; refractoriness, a marker of Na^+ channel inactivation [33], superexcitability, a marker of the function of fast K^+ channels [33], depolarising threshold electrotonus at the 10–20 ms interval (TEd10–20), hyperpolarising threshold electrotonus at the 90–100 ms interval (TEh90–100 ms) and resting current threshold slope (all ANOVA $p = 0.001$), markers of internodal ion channel function and membrane potential [32] (Table 2). Taken together, reductions in these parameters are reflective of nerve membrane depolarization [32].

Critically, further analysis revealed that pre-RRT values in the HDF group were not significantly different to controls for several neurophysiological measures sensitive to alterations in nerve membrane potential (Fig. 1), namely refractoriness, TEh90–100 ms and resting I/V slope (Table 2). In contrast, the HFHD group demonstrated significantly impaired nerve excitability when compared to both normal controls and the HDF group. This was noted for refractoriness (NC; HFHD, $p<0.001$: HFHD; HDF, $p<0.05$), TEh90–100 ms (NC; HFHD, $p<0.001$: HFHD; HDF, $p<0.05$) and resting IV slope (NC;HFHD, $p<0.001$: HFHD; HDF, $p<0.05$) (Fig. 1, Table 2). Superexcitability demonstrated significant differences across all three groups, with a progressive worsening from normal controls to HDF to HFHD (NC −21.7±1.5%; HDF −12.2±2.3%: HD −3.0±2.5%; $p<0.05$).

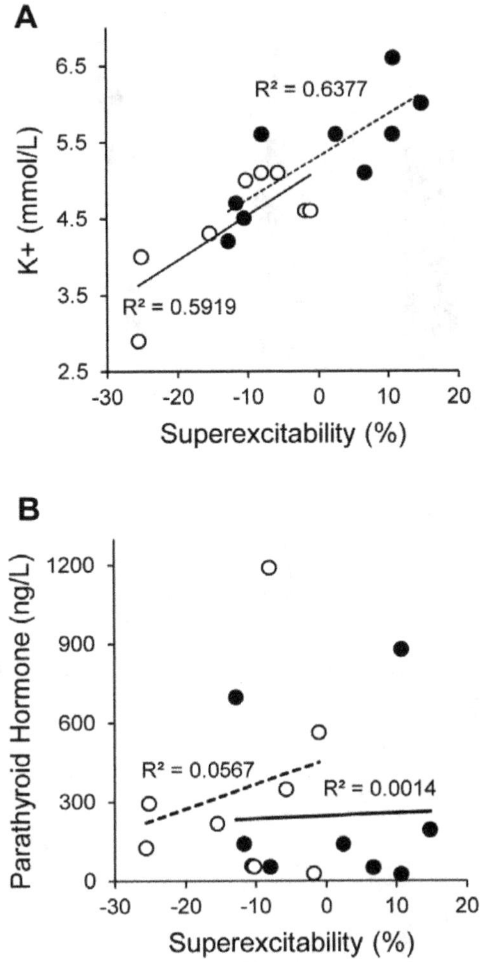

Figure 2. Relationship of pre-RRT bloods and superexcitability; a sensitive measure of membrane potential. (A) Pre-RRT serum K^+ concentrations for both HDF (empty circles) and HFHD (black filled circles) demonstrated multiple significant correlations with nerve excitability parameters including superexcitability. (B) In contrast pre-RRT serum parathyroid hormone concentrations showed no correlation.

While depolarising threshold electrotonus 10–20 and 90–100 ms values also demonstrated a progressive worsening from controls to HDF to HFHD, there was no significant difference between RRT modes (Table 2). Thus, in total, HDF-treated patients demonstrated improved nerve excitability following a 56 hour inter-dialytic period when compared to patients receiving HFHD.

In addition to the pre-RRT findings, the HDF group demonstrated significantly greater normalisation of nerve excitability when assessed across the duration of a dialysis session. While both groups demonstrated significant improvement of nerve excitability abnormalities during and post-RRT, these changes were greater in the HDF group (refractoriness, F = 4.87, $p<0.05$; superexcitability, F = 11.52, $p<0.05$; resting I/V slope, F = 5.39, $p<0.05$), compared to HFHD. This enhanced normalisation in the HDF group was further supported by significantly greater superexcitability in the HDF group when compared to the HFHD group in studies undertaken at the conclusion of RRT (HDF −23.1±2.0: HFHD −18.1±1.4; $p<0.05$).

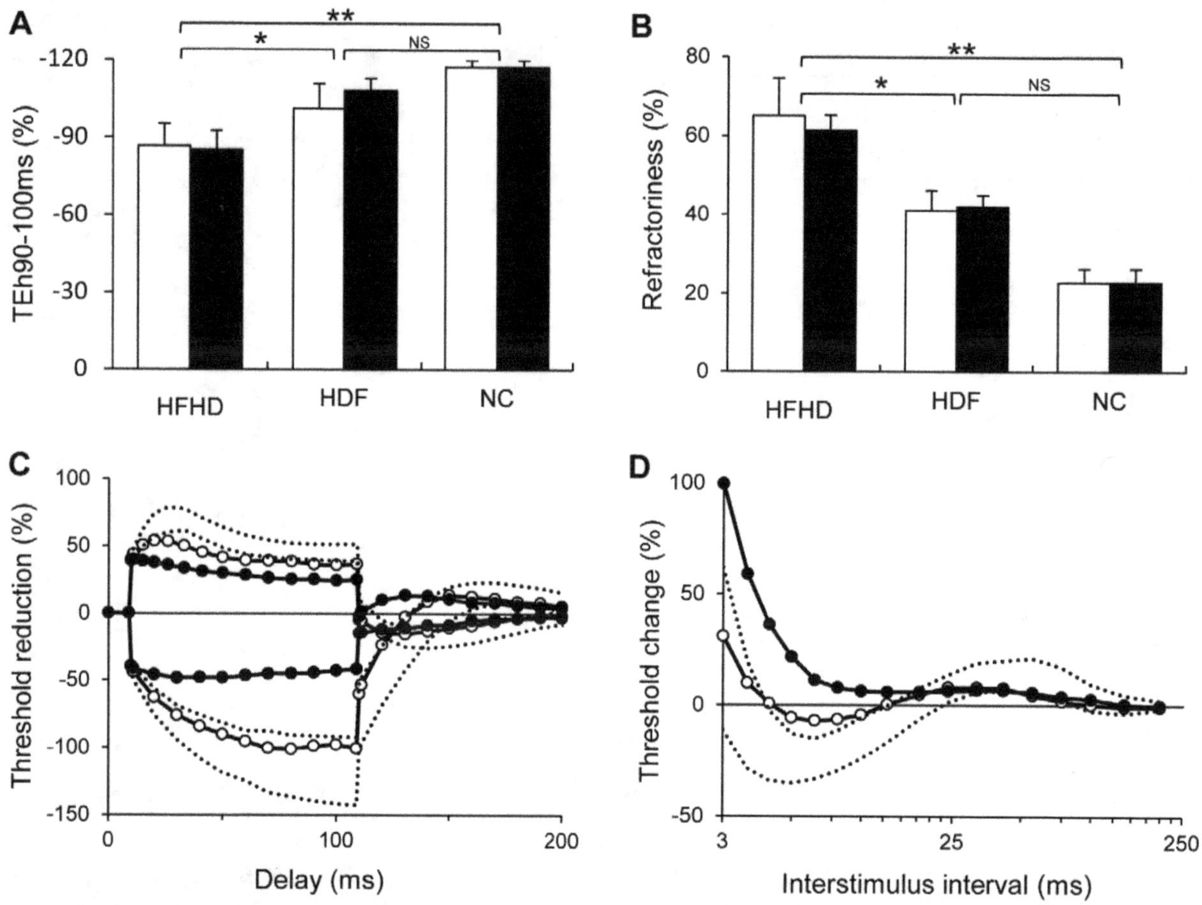

Figure 3. Longitudinal follow-up 18 months of patients who remained on their respective treatment (HDF n = 4 and HFHD n = 7). Panels (A) and (B) demonstrate a relative stability of nerve excitability results in patients who remained on their respective treatments at baseline (white bars) and longitudinal follow-up (black bars). Additionally these graphs depict the sustained significant difference between HDF and HFHD in both hyperpolarising threshold electrotonus 90–100 ms (TEh90–100 ms) and refractoriness. *$p<0.05$, **$p<0.001$. Panels (C) and (D) show the results of a single patient switched from HDF to HFHD. Threshold electrotonus (C) and recovery cycle parameters (D) demonstrate the profound abnormalities at longitudinal follow-up on HFHD.

Correlation between Changes in Nerve Excitability and Levels of Uremic Toxins

Correlations were undertaken to investigate the potential relationship between changes in nerve parameters and potential neurotoxins, including small solutes and middle molecules. There were no significant correlations noted between excitability parameters and concentrations of parathyroid hormone which has previously been suggested as a possible underlying cause of nerve dysfunction in ESKD [34,35]. Pre-dialysis excitability parameters were however strongly correlated with pre-RRT serum K^+ (Fig. 2), a finding that has been demonstrated in more recent studies of nerve excitability in dialysis [17–19]. Specifically, correlations were noted between pre-RRT serum K^+ and refractoriness (HDF $r = 0.76$; $p<0.05$: HFHD $r = 0.69$; $p<0.05$) and superexcitability (HDF $r = 0.77$; $p<0.05$: HFHD $r = 0.80$; $p<0.05$). Serum K^+ also strongly correlated with several threshold electrotonus parameters including TEh90–100 (HDF $r = 0.59$; $p = 0.12$: HFHD $r = 0.74$; $p<0.05$). Importantly, pre-RRT serum K^+ concentration was significantly different between the groups (HDF 4.5±0.7 mmol/L: HFHD 5.3±0.8 mmol/L; $p<0.05$), a finding that was also noted on longitudinal follow-up (HDF 4.7±0.2 mmol/L: HFHD 5.6+0.6 mmol/L; $p<0.05$). Aside from K^+, there were no significant differences between the groups for other biochemical measures (Table 1), including urea (HDF 21.8+3.8 mmol/L; HFHD 23.5+1.7 mmol/L), creatinine (HDF 807.4±121.7 µmol/L; HFHD 882.4±78.7 µmol/L) and parathyroid hormone (HDF 351±380 ng/L; HFHD 261±305 ng/L).

Longitudinal Assessment of Nerve Excitability

Longitudinal assessments were conducted at 18 months on 13 patients. Of the four remaining patients, one received a renal transplant, two died and one declined further testing. There were no significant differences in baseline values between patients lost to follow-up those in whom longitudinal follow-up was undertaken, including serum K^+ (4.9 mmol/L: 5.1 mmol/L), TNS (5.7:9.4) and dialysis hours (4.5 hours: 4.8 hours) respectively. Of the original HDF group, four had remained on HDF while two were switched to HFHD, due to changes in equipment availability. Excitability values in both HDF and HFHD groups demonstrated no significant difference from those obtained at baseline (Fig. 3). Importantly, HDF patients maintained significant improvements in nerve excitability, when compared to the HFHD group, with pre-RRT recordings demonstrating sustained differences in superexcitability ($p<0.05$) and TEh 90–100 ms ($p<0.05$). When these variables were assessed using intention to treat analysis, significant differences remained between the two groups (superexcitability,

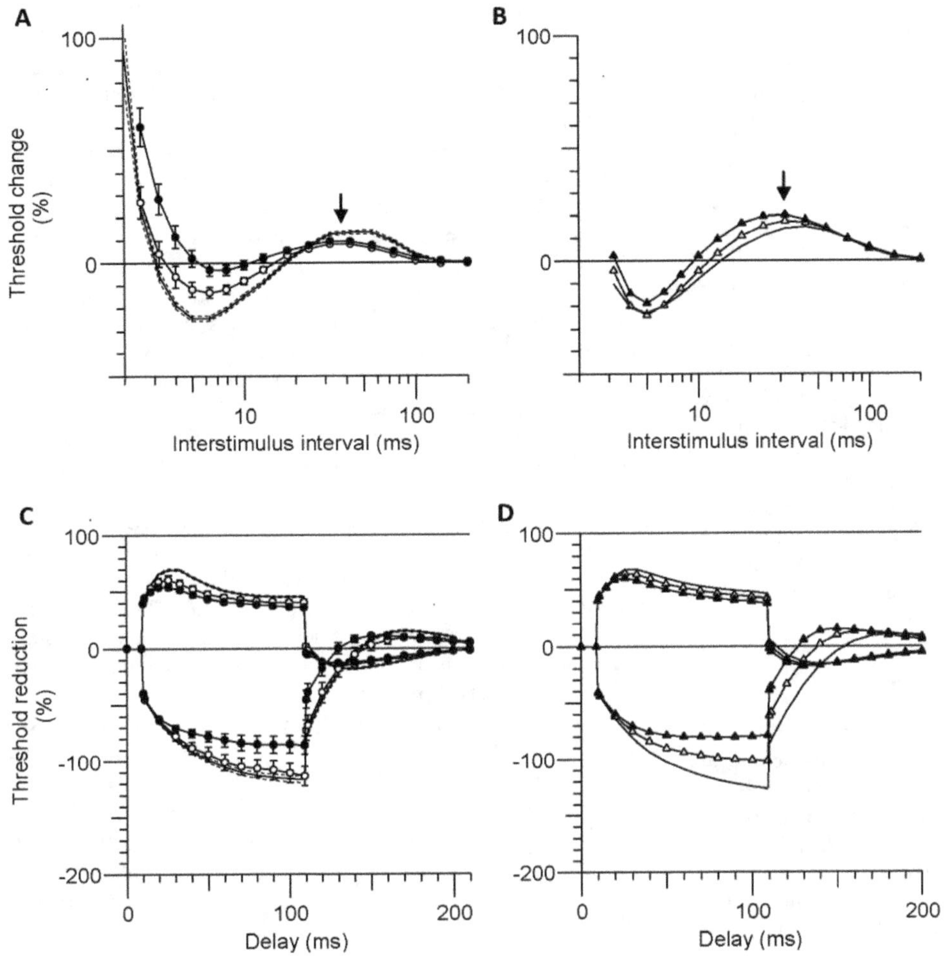

Figure 4. Mathematical model of depolarized axons. The observed excitability (mean ± SEM) is shown in panels (A) and (C) comparing HFHD patients (filled circles) and HDF (empty circles) to the healthy controls (solid and dashed lines). Panels (B) and (D) compare the modelled excitability of a healthy human motor axon (solid line) to the same model with: $[K^+]_o$ increased to 5.3 mmol/L (empty triangles); and with $[K^+]_o$ = 5.3 mmol/L and resting membrane potential further depolarized by 1 mV (filled triangles). The model provides a good fit to the changes in the threshold electrotonus data (C,D) but not the recovery cycle (A,B), particularly the extent of the changes in the refractory period, superexcitability and late subexcitability. Late subexcitability increased in the model (arrow in B) and decreased in the ESKD patients (arrow in A).

$p = 0.05$; TEh90–100, $p = 0.05$). In two patients who were changed from HDF to HFHD, deterioration in nerve excitability was noted at 18-month follow-up, with no change in lower limb motor and sensory nerve conduction amplitudes or latency (Patient #1 Sural 22.4 μV, 57 m/s vs 24.0 μV, 56 m/s and distal tibial motor amplitude 10.8 mV, 4.6 m/s vs 11.6 mV, 4.5 m/s; Patient #2 had no measurable distal tibial motor or sural response at both time points). In patient #1 (a non-diabetic), the deterioration in neurophysiological parameters was accompanied by the onset of diffuse sensory neuropathic symptoms.

Mathematical Modelling

A model of human motor axons was used to explore the underlying mechanisms for the differences between the two patient groups and the healthy controls. In the model, an increase in extracellular K^+ from 4.5 to 5.3 mmol/L alone depolarized resting membrane potential (RMP) by 2.8 mV, with the modelled changes in both threshold electrotonus and the recovery cycle consistent with depolarization (empty triangles in Fig. 4B & D). An additional 1-mV depolarization of RMP modelled threshold electrotonus better for the HFHD data (filled triangles in Fig. 4D). Pure depolarization of RMP however increased late subexcitability, in agreement with the findings of Kiernan and Bostock [2000] [32]. However in the ESKD patients subexcitability was decreased, and there were smaller changes in the other recovery cycle measures (compare arrows in Fig. 4B & A; see discussion).

Discussion

The present study investigated the effects of HDF and HFHD on peripheral nerve excitability in incident ESKD patients. The study has demonstrated that neurophysiological measures of nerve function, specifically those sensitive to changes in nerve membrane potential, were significantly closer to normal in patients receiving HDF compared to the HFHD group. Furthermore, patients who remained on HDF maintained a more normal study profile compared to those on HFHD at long-term follow-up.

Overall, the pattern of change in excitability measures was consistent with nerve membrane depolarisation [32], an abnormality that has been demonstrated in previous studies of ESKD patients, undertaken during the era of conventional semi-permeable membranes [17–19]. Greater normality of nerve excitability results was noted in pre-RRT recordings and following a single RRT session in the HDF group, suggesting that HDF may achieve greater clearance of neurotoxic substances.

The implications of these findings are significant as maintenance of nerve membrane potential is essential for normal biochemical homeostasis and therefore axonal survival. [36,37]. Chronic changes in neural excitability over time may trigger a cascade of events leading to axonal degeneration and development of symptoms of clinical neuropathy, such as numbness and muscle weakness, major causes of disability in ESKD [38]. Moreover, previous studies have demonstrated a direct relationship between neuropathic symptoms and pre-RRT excitability values [18]. The limitations of this study, including the small samples size and the largely cross-sectional nature of the data, suggest that longitudinal studies investigating the effects of nerve excitability changes and dialysis mode on the development of neuropathy are required.

While the HDF group demonstrated greater normality of nerve excitability, the underlying basis for this remains unclear. A potential explanation for the differential effects of HDF and HFHD on nerve excitability relates to the correlation that was noted between parameters of nerve excitability and serum K^+ concentration. This correlation is consistent with the findings of recent studies that have suggested that hyperkalaemia may play an important role in the development of neuropathy in ESKD [17–19,39]. Despite these lines of evidence, a causal relationship between elevated serum K^+ concentration and neurological dysfunction has not yet been established. Moreover, mathematical modelling of data in the present study suggested that while changes in serum K^+ may have played a role in the development of the abnormalities, the changes in excitability in the HFHD group were not explicable solely by increased K^+ concentration. In particular, the significantly reduced super- and late sub- excitability in the ESKD patients may be due to a smaller time-integral of the action current, possibly a consequence of smaller Na^+ currents [27,30].

Given that both HDF and HFHD treatments in this study used the same membrane (Polyflux® 201H), dialysate flow rate (Q_D 500 mL/min) and dialysate concentrations of K^+, Na^+, bicarbonate, calcium, magnesium and glucose, another potential explanation for the differences may relate to the dilutional effects of hemofiltration. The ultrafiltration setting in HDF allows for greater hemofiltration to occur in addition to the hemodialysis component. HDF is achieved with inline fluid replacement and ultrafiltration (UF) of 60 mL/min compared to UF of 0 mL/min for HFHD. Backfiltration of up to 10 litres can be achieved with HFHD whereas the hemofiltration in HDF delivers an average of 20 litres of inline fluid re-infused, which possibly contributes to a dilutional effect on overall clearances.

While previous studies have emphasised the role of middle molecules as a cause of nerve dysfunction in ESKD [40,41], there was no significant correlation between PTH, a middle molecule assayed in this study, and pre-RRT measures of nerve excitability. However, while K^+ was closely related to pre-RRT excitability differences, it cannot explain the during and post-RRT differences between groups. Furthermore, mathematical modelling demonstrated that an additional 1 mV depolarization was required to better model the threshold electrotonus data obtained in HFHD patients, suggesting that a synergistic effect of another neurotoxin may be required to induce nerve dysfunction in ESKD, a view that has been supported by previous neurophysiological studies [19,42]. Given the known superiority of HDF in terms of middle molecule clearance and inflammatory status [12–15], future studies may need to explore a wider range of middle molecules and inflammatory mediators as potential contributors to nerve dysfunction in ESKD patients.

In conclusion, the present study provides evidence that ESKD patients treated with HDF demonstrate more normal nerve excitability both prior to RRT, across a single RRT session and at long-term follow-up compared to HFHD. These results suggest that HDF may help maintain normal nerve excitability in ESKD. The use of HDF for the clinical management of neuropathy in ESKD should be investigated further in large scale randomised trials.

Author Contributions

Contributed to revising the article and approving final version: AK BP VG CL MCK MJJ TJP JH. Conceived and designed the experiments: RA AK BP MK. Performed the experiments: RA VG. Analyzed the data: RA AK CL TJP MCK MJJ JH. Wrote the paper: RA AK BP JH.

References

1. Krishnan AV, Kiernan MC (2009) Neurological complications of chronic kidney disease. Nat Rev Neurol 5: 542–551.
2. Van den Neucker K, Vanderstraeten G, Vanholder R (1998) Peripheral motor and sensory nerve conduction studies in haemodialysis patients. A study of 54 patients. Electromyogr Clin Neurophysiol 38: 467–474.
3. Laaksonen S, Metsarinne K, Voipio-Pulkki LM, Falck B (2002) Neurophysiologic parameters and symptoms in chronic renal failure. Muscle Nerve 25: 884–890.
4. Hojs-Fabjan T, Hojs R (2006) Polyneuropathy in hemodialysis patients: the most sensitive electrophysiological parameters and dialysis adequacy. Wien Klin Wochenschr 118 Suppl 2: 29–34.
5. Krishnan AV, Kiernan MC (2007) Uremic neuropathy: clinical features and new pathophysiological insights. Muscle Nerve 35: 273–290.
6. Tilki HE, Akpolat T, Coskun M, Stalberg E (2009) Clinical and electrophysiologic findings in dialysis patients. J Electromyogr Kinesiol 19: 500–508.
7. Ledebo I, Ronco C (2008) The best dialysis therapy? Results from an international survey among nephrology professionals. NDT Plus 1: 403–408.
8. Canaud B, Bragg-Gresham JL, Marshall MR, Desmeules S, Gillespie BW, et al. (2006) Mortality risk for patients receiving hemodiafiltration versus hemodialysis: European results from the DOPPS. Kidney Int 69: 2087–2093.
9. Eknoyan G, Beck GJ, Cheung AK, Daugirdas JT, Greene T, et al. (2002) Effect of dialysis dose and membrane flux in maintenance hemodialysis. N Engl J Med 347: 2010–2019.
10. Cheung AK, Rocco MV, Yan G, Leypoldt JK, Levin NW, et al. (2006) Serum beta-2 microglobulin levels predict mortality in dialysis patients: results of the HEMO study. J Am Soc Nephrol 17: 546–555.
11. Guth HJ, Gruska S, Kraatz G (2003) On-line production of ultrapure substitution fluid reduces TNF-alpha- and IL-6 release in patients on hemodiafiltration therapy. Int J Artif Organs 26: 181–187.
12. Carracedo J, Merino A, Nogueras S, Carretero D, Berdud I, et al. (2006) On-line hemodiafiltration reduces the proinflammatory CD14+CD16+ monocyte-derived dendritic cells: A prospective, crossover study. J Am Soc Nephrol 17: 2315–2321.
13. Filiopoulos V, Hadjiyiannakos D, Metaxaki P, Sideris V, Takouli L, et al. (2008) Inflammation and oxidative stress in patients on hemodiafiltration. Am J Nephrol 28: 949–957.
14. Ward RA, Schmidt B, Hullin J, Hillebrand GF, Samtleben W (2000) A comparison of on-line hemodiafiltration and high-flux hemodialysis: a prospective clinical study. J Am Soc Nephrol 11: 2344–2350.
15. Schiffl H (2007) Prospective randomized cross-over long-term comparison of online haemodiafiltration and ultrapure high-flux haemodialysis. Eur J Med Res 12: 26–33.
16. Lin CL, Yang CW, Chiang CC, Chang CT, Huang CC (2001) Long-term on-line hemodiafiltration reduces predialysis beta-2-microglobulin levels in chronic hemodialysis patients. Blood Purif 19: 301–307.
17. Kiernan MC, Walters RJL, Andersen KV, Taube D, Murray NMF, et al. (2002) Nerve excitability changes in chronic renal failure indicate membrane depolarization due to hyperkalaemia. Brain 125: 1366–1378.
18. Krishnan AV, Phoon RK, Pussell BA, Charlesworth JA, Kiernan MC (2006) Sensory nerve excitability and neuropathy in end stage kidney disease. J Neurol Neurosurg Psychiatry 77: 548–551.
19. Krishnan AV, Phoon RK, Pussell BA, Charlesworth JA, Bostock H, et al. (2005)

Altered motor nerve excitability in end-stage kidney disease. Brain 128: 2164–2174.

20. Park SB, Goldstein D, Lin CS, Krishnan AV, Friedlander ML, et al. (2009) Acute abnormalities of sensory nerve function associated with oxaliplatin-induced neurotoxicity. J Clin Oncol 27: 1243–1249.
21. Lin CS, Krishnan AV, Park SB, Kiernan MC (2011) Modulatory effects on axonal function after intravenous immunoglobulin therapy in chronic inflammatory demyelinating polyneuropathy. Arch Neurol 68: 862–869.
22. Daugirdas JT, Depner TA, Gotch FA, Greene T, Keshaviah P, et al. (1997) Comparison of methods to predict equilibrated Kt/V in the HEMO Pilot Study. Kidney Int 52: 1395–1405.
23. Cornblath DR, Chaudhry V, Carter K, Lee D, Seysedadr M, et al. (1999) Total neuropathy score: validation and reliability study. Neurology 53: 1660–1664.
24. Kiernan MC, Burke D, Andersen KV, Bostock H (2000) Multiple measures of axonal excitability: a new approach in clinical testing. Muscle Nerve 23: 399–409.
25. Krishnan AV, Lin CS, Park SB, Kiernan MC (2008) Assessment of nerve excitability in toxic and metabolic neuropathies. J Peripher Nerv Syst 13: 7–26.
26. Bostock H, Baker M, Reid G (1991) Changes in excitability of human motor axons underlying post-ischaemic fasciculations: evidence for two stable states. J Physiol 441: 537–557.
27. Kiernan MC, Isbister GK, Lin CS, Burke D, Bostock H (2005) Acute tetrodotoxin-induced neurotoxicity after ingestion of puffer fish. Ann Neurol 57: 339–348.
28. Jankelowitz SK, Howells J, Burke D (2007) Plasticity of inwardly rectifying conductances following a corticospinal lesion in human subjects. J Physiol (Lond) 581: 927–940.
29. Lin CS, Krishnan AV, Lee M-J, Zagami AS, You H-L, et al. (2008) Nerve function and dysfunction in acute intermittent porphyria. Brain 131: 2510–2519.
30. Howells J, Trevillion L, Bostock H, Burke D (2012) The voltage dependence of I(h) in human myelinated axons. J Physiol (Lond) 590: 1625–1640.
31. Barrett EF, Barrett JN (1982) Intracellular recording from vertebrate myelinated axons: mechanism of the depolarizing afterpotential. J Physiol 323: 117–144.
32. Kiernan MC, Bostock H (2000) Effects of membrane polarization and ischaemia on the excitability properties of human motor axons. Brain 123 Pt 12: 2542–2551.
33. Burke D (1993) Microneurography, impulse conduction, and paresthesias. Muscle Nerve 16: 1025–1032.
34. Goldstein DA, Chui LA, Massry SG (1978) Effect of parathyroid hormone and uremia on peripheral nerve calcium and motor nerve conduction velocity. J Clin Invest 62: 88–93.
35. Slatopolsky E, Martin K, Hruska K (1980) Parathyroid hormone metabolism and its potential as a uremic toxin. Am J Physiol 239: F1–12.
36. Vogel W, Schwarz JR (1995) Voltage-clamp studies on axons: macroscopic and single-channel currents. In: Waxman SG, Kocsis JD, Stys PK, editors. The axon: Oxford University Press.
37. Lehning EJ, Doshi R, Isaksson N, Stys PK, LoPachin RM Jr (1996) Mechanisms of injury-induced calcium entry into peripheral nerve myelinated axons: role of reverse sodium-calcium exchange. J Neurochem 66: 493–500.
38. Stys PK (2005) General mechanisms of axonal damage and its prevention. J Neurol Sci 233: 3–13.
39. Bostock H, Walters RJ, Andersen KV, Murray NM, Taube D, et al. (2004) Has potassium been prematurely discarded as a contributing factor to the development of uraemic neuropathy? Nephrol Dial Transplant 19: 1054–1057.
40. Malberti F, Surian M, Farina M, Vitelli E, Mandolfo S, et al. (1991) Effect of hemodialysis and hemodiafiltration on uremic neuropathy. Blood Purif 9: 285–295.
41. Babb AL, Ahmad S, Bergstrom J, Scribner BH (1981) The middle molecule hypothesis in perspective. Am J Kidney Dis 1: 46–50.
42. Krishnan AV, Phoon RK, Pussell BA, Charlesworth JA, Bostock H, et al. (2006) Ischaemia induces paradoxical changes in axonal excitability in end-stage kidney disease. Brain 129: 1585–1592.

19

Two Distinct Functional Patterns of Hepatitis C Virus (HCV)-Specific T Cell Responses in Seronegative, Aviremic Patients

Yoon Seok Choi[1,2], Jung Eun Lee[3], Seung Joo Nam[1], Jung Tak Park[3], Hyon-Suk Kim[4], Kyu Hun Choi[3], Beom Seok Kim[3]*, Eui-Cheol Shin[1]*

1 Laboratory of Immunology and Infectious Diseases, Graduate School of Medical Science and Engineering, KAIST, Daejeon, Republic of Korea, **2** Department of Internal Medicine, Chungnam National University College of Medicine, Daejeon, Republic of Korea, **3** Department of Internal Medicine, Yonsei University College of Medicine, Seoul, Republic of Korea, **4** Department of Laboratory Medicine, Yonsei University College of Medicine, Seoul, Republic of Korea

Abstract

In hepatitis C Virus (HCV) high-risk groups, HCV-specific T cell responses have been detected in seronegative, aviremic persons who have no evidence of HCV infection. Herein, we investigated functional profiles of HCV-specific T-cell responses in seronegative, aviremic patients of a HCV high-risk group. Seventy seven hemodialysis patients with chronic renal disease were analyzed by IFN-γ ELISpot assays, and eight of 71 (11.3%) seronegative, aviremic patients displayed HCV-specific T-cell responses. Their HCV-specific memory T cells were characterized by assessing cytokine polyfunctionality, known to provide antiviral protection. By intracellular staining of IFN-γ, TNF-α, IL-2 and MIP-1β, we identified two distinct populations in the seronegative, aviremic patients: polyfunctional responders and TNF-α-predominant responders. In further analysis, occult HCV infection was excluded as a cause of the HCV-specific T cell response via secondary nested RT-PCR of HCV RNA in peripheral blood mononuclear cell samples. HCV-specific T cells targeted multiple epitopes including non-structural proteins in a single patient, implying that their T cells might have been primed by HCV proteins synthesized within the host. We conclude that HCV-specific memory T cells of seronegative, aviremic patients arise from authentic HCV replication in the host, but not from current occult HCV infection. By functional pattern of HCV-specific T cells, there are two distinct populations in these patients: polyfunctional responders and TNF-α-predominant responders.

Editor: Stacey A. Rizza, Mayo Clinic, United States of America

Funding: This study was supported by a grant of the Korea Healthcare Technology R&D Project, Ministry of Health and Welfare, Republic of Korea (A101923). The funders had no role in study design, data collection and analysis, decision to publish, or preparation of the manuscript.

Competing Interests: Eui-Cheol Shin is a PLOS ONE Editorial Board member, and understand that this does not alter the authors' adherence to all the PLOS ONE policies on sharing data and materials.

* E-mail: ecshin@kaist.ac.kr (ES); docbsk@yuhs.ac (BK)

These authors contributed equally to this work.

Introduction

Hepatitis C virus (HCV) infection is a major cause of chronic viral hepatitis that often progresses to liver cirrhosis and hepatocellular carcinoma [1]. HCV is an enveloped positive-stranded RNA virus of *Flaviviridae* transmitted by parenteral routes [2]. Persons with frequent exposure to blood, blood products, and contaminated needles are at threat of HCV infection [3]. In fact, healthcare workers, hemophiliacs, hemodialysis patients, and injection drug users (IDUs) are all HCV high-risk groups.

HCV infection is determined clinically by the detection of both anti-HCV antibody and HCV RNA. Seropositivity without viremia is considered a sign of past HCV infection. HCV-specific memory T cells have been detected in persons who spontaneously recovered from past HCV infection [4–6]. Intriguingly, HCV-specific T cell responses have been detected not only in persons with past HCV infection but also in seronegative, aviremic persons who have no evidence of current or past HCV infection [7–13]. These studies detected T cells reactive to HCV antigens by secreting cytokines such as IFN-γ ELISpot assay or intracellular cytokine staining. HCV-specific T cell responses in seronegative, aviremic persons have been detected mainly in HCV high-risk groups such as IDUs, residents of HCV-endemic areas, healthy family members of HCV-infected patients, and healthcare workers [7–13]. However, it remains unclear why HCV-specific T cells are primed in seronegative, aviremic persons. In addition, detailed characteristics of HCV-specific T cells have not been previously identified in seronegative, aviremic persons.

HCV-specific T cell responses in seronegative, aviremic persons can be attributed to several possible causes including occult HCV infection with extremely low level viral replication [14,15], heterologous T cell immunity by a cross-reactive epitope [16–18], transient viral replication without seroconversion [19,20] and disappearance of anti-HCV antibody long after prior HCV infection [21].

T cells play a major role in the immune response against HCV. In particular, T cell-mediated protective immunity has been shown in chimpanzees that had recovered from previous HCV infection [22,23]. In these studies, HCV rechallenge resulted in rapid viral clearance with low peak viremia and attenuated liver injury [22–24], and this host protection was mediated by memory T cells as evidenced by T cell-depletion studies [25,26]. Upon HCV rechallenge, depletion of $CD4^+$ T cells resulted in chronic persistent infection [25], while depletion of $CD8^+$ T cells delayed viral clearance [26].

Recently, T cell-mediated host protection has been shown to be associated with polyfunctional T cells, which exert several effector functions simultaneously [27–29]. For example, polyfunctional HIV-specific $CD8^+$ T cells were maintained in human immunodeficiency virus (HIV) long-term nonprogressors [28]. In one vaccination study, Th1 cell polyfunctionality correlated with vaccine efficacy, in terms of protection against Leishmania [27]. Therefore, induction of polyfunctional memory T cells is considered a practical goal in T cell vaccine development.

In the present study, we analyzed HCV-specific T cell responses in seronegative, aviremic hemodialysis patients and tried to reveal possible causes of HCV-specific memory T cell induction. We also characterized HCV-specific memory T cells in detail by assessing T cell polyfunctionality, and demonstrated that HCV-specific T cell responders in seronegative, aviremic hemodialysis patients are classified into two distinct groups, polyfunctional responders and TNF-α-predominant responders.

Materials and Methods

Ethics Statement

All study samples were obtained following acquisition of the study participants' and/or their legal guardians' written informed consent, in accordance with the Declaration of Helsinki. This research protocol was reviewed and approved by the institutional review board of Yonsei University Severance Hospital.

Hemodialysis patients

Seventy-seven patients (48 males and 29 females), who were on maintenance hemodialysis due to chronic kidney disease, were recruited in this study. At the time of enrollment, the mean age (±SD) of patients was 57.0±10.6 years, the mean alanine aminotransferase (ALT) level was 17.3±11.6 U/L, and the median duration of hemodialysis was 39.2 months. All cases were negative for anti-HIV. In sera, anti-HCV antibodies were assayed using Elecsys Anti-HCV Immunoassay (Roche Diagnostics, Basel, Switzerland). HCV RNA was quantitated by COBAS TaqMan HCV assay (Roche Diagnostics). The lower detection limit of HCV RNA assay was 15 IU/mL. Peripheral blood mononuclear cells (PBMCs) were isolated from whole blood by standard Ficoll-Paque (GE Healthcare, Uppsala, Sweden) density gradient centrifugation and cryopreserved. In the case of seronegative, aviremic patients with HCV-specific T cell responses, whole blood was obtained a second time to confirm the T cell responses.

HCV overlapping peptides

Six hundred pentadecamer peptides (Mimotopes, Clayton, Australia), overlapping by 10 amino acids and spanning the complete HCV genotype 1a (H77) sequence, were resuspended at 20 mg/mL in dimethyl sulfoxide (DMSO). Aliquots of each peptide suspension were pooled and diluted with phosphate-buffered saline to obtain 49 mixes designed for a matrix array [30]. Each mix contained 24–25 peptides, and each peptide was present in 2 mixes (Figure S1A). These 49 mixes were used in direct *ex vivo* IFN-γ enzyme-linked immunosorbent spot (ELISpot) assays in each patient.

Direct ex vivo IFN-γ ELISpot assay

Direct *ex vivo* IFN-γ ELISpot assays were performed as previously described [31]. Duplicate cultures of 250,000 PBMCs were set up in RPMI 1640 containing 5% fetal bovine serum (FBS) and 2 mM L-glutamine with 49 peptide mixes (each peptide at a final concentration of 1 μg/ml). DMSO was used as a negative control. After 30 hours in culture, IFN-γ spots were developed. Spots were counted with an ELISpot reader (CTL, Cleveland, OH), and the number of specific spots was calculated by subtracting the mean number of spots in negative control wells of each ELISpot plate from the mean number of spots in each well stimulated with an HCV peptide mix.

Intracellular cytokine staining (ICS) and T cell polyfunctionality assay

Cryopreserved PBMCs were thawed, resuspended in RPMI 1640 containing 5% FBS and 2 mM L-glutamine, and rested overnight at 37°C. PBMCs were stimulated with an epitope peptide or a peptide mix (each peptide at a final concentration of 1 μg/ml) in the presence of anti-CD28 and anti-CD49d (1 μg/ml for each; BD Biosciences, San Jose, CA), and brefeldin A (GolgiPlug, BD Biosciences) and monensin (GolgiStop, BD Biosciences) were added 1 hour later. After another 5 hours of incubation, PBMCs were stained with anti-CD3- V500, anti-CD4-V450 and anti-CD8-APC-H7 (all from BD Biosciences), permeabilized using Cytofix/Cytoperm kit (BD Biosciences) and further stained with either anti-IFN-γ-APC or anti-TNF-α-PE-Cy7 (all from BD Biosciences). In the assay for T cell polyfunctionality, anti-CD107a-PE (BD Biosciences) was included in the initial culture medium and PBMCs were stained with anti-IFN-γ-APC, anti-TNF-α-PE-Cy7, anti-MIP-1β-PerCP-Cy5.5 (all from BD Biosciences) and anti-IL-2-Alexa Fluor 488 (BioLegend, San Diego, CA) after permeabilization. FACS analysis was performed by LSRII flow cytometer (BD Biosciences) and the data were analyzed using FlowJo software (Treestar, San Carlos, CA). T cells positive for the various combinations of cytokines and degranulation were quantified and analyzed using a Boolean gating function in FlowJo software.

Multi-cytokine cytometric bead array (CBA)

PBMCs were stimulated with an epitope peptide or a peptide mix (each peptide at a final concentration of 1 μg/ml) at 300,000 cells/well of a 96-well U-plate. Culture supernatant was harvested after 72 hours of incubation, and the concentration of IFN-γ, TNF-α and IL-2 was simultaneously determined using CBA (BD Biosciences) and LSRII flow cytometer. In selected patients, concentration of granzyme B in culture supernatants was also determined using CBA.

Secondary nested RT-PCR for detection of occult HCV infection

To detect occult HCV infection, secondary nested RT-PCR of the 5′-untranslated region of HCV RNA was performed as described elsewhere [32–34]. Total RNA was extracted from PBMCs using the RNeasy mini kit (Qiagen, Valencia, CA) with on-column deoxyribonuclease digestion. For cDNA synthesis, 200 to 400 ng RNA was reverse transcribed with ReverTraAce-α kit (Toyobo, Osaka, Japan) using an HCV RNA-specific primer. These cDNA samples served as templates in the direct round of PCR amplification (primer pairs used: 5′-CTG TGA GGA ACT ACT GTC TTC and 5′-GCG GTT GGT GTT ACG TTT), and the nested round reaction (primer pairs used: 5′-GCA GAA AGC GTC TAG CCA TGG C and 5′-CTG CAA GCA CCC TAT

CAG GCA GT) was performed with the products of the first round PCR.

For positive cases in secondary nested RT-PCR of HCV RNA, genotypes of HCV were determined as follows. Briefly, the final PCR product of 243 bp was purified and cloned into the TOPO TA cloning vector (Invitrogen, Carlsbad, CA), and genotype was ascertained by automatically sequencing five clones from each patient.

Results

Presence of HCV-specific T cell responses in seronegative, aviremic patients

Among 77 hemodialysis patients with chronic renal disease, one patient was seropositive without viremia, and five patients were seropositive with viremia. The other 71 patients were seronegative and aviremic, meaning they exhibited no clinical evidence of current or past HCV infection. There were no seronegative patients with viremia. HCV-specific T cell responses were evaluated by direct *ex vivo* IFN-γ ELISpot assay of PBMCs in all patients except the seropositive, aviremic patient. For comprehensive analysis, we stimulated PBMCs with 49 matrixed mixes of 600 overlapping peptides covering the complete HCV polyprotein sequence (Figure S1A). All of the viremic patients and a majority of seronegative, aviremic patients exhibited insignificant levels of HCV-specific T cell responses (Figure 1A). In contrast, eight (11.3%) of the seronegative, aviremic patients displayed obvious T cell responses against HCV (Figure 1A). This was an unexpected result as these HCV-specific T cells were detected in patients without evidence of current or past infection. Figure 1B shows results of the IFN-γ ELISpot assay in response to each peptide mix.

Conducting the IFN-γ ELISpot assay with a matrixed mix of overlapping peptides enabled us to identify T cell epitopes within the HCV polyprotein for each patient (Figure S1B and Table 1). T cell responses to the identified epitopes were confirmed by IFN-γ ICS (Figure 1C). We also identified which T cell subset, $CD4^+$ or $CD8^+$, was responsible for the HCV-specific IFN-γ production in each patient (Figure 1C and Table 1).

Cytokine profiles of HCV-specific T cells in seronegative, aviremic patients

We further characterized the HCV-specific T cell responses of the eight seronegative, aviremic patients by examining their cytokine profiles. PBMCs were stimulated with an epitope peptide or a peptide mix, and production of both IFN-γ and TNF-α were investigated in culture supernatants. Intriguingly, five patients (CMI-1 to CMI-5, group I) produced both IFN-γ and TNF-α following HCV-specific stimulation, whereas three patients (CMI-6 to CMI-8, group II) produced only TNF-α (Figure 2A). IL-2 production was also assayed and scarcely detected with exception of one patient (CMI-5, data not shown). In the patients of group II, TNF-α production by HCV-specific T cells was confirmed by ICS (Figure 2B). Thus, HCV-specific cytokine profiles distinguish two unique groups of seronegative, aviremic patients with HCV-specific cellular immune responses.

Two distinct patterns of T cell polyfunctionality in seronegative, aviremic patients

Next, we analyzed T cell polyfunctionality by multi-cytokine ICS to further examine the functional diversity of HCV-specific T cells. In the multi-cytokine ICS of $CD4^+$ T cells, IFN-γ, TNF-α, IL-2, and MIP-1β were simultaneously assessed. In the patients of group I, HCV-specific $CD4^+$ T cells were proven to be polyfunctional, and more than half of HCV-specific $CD4^+$ T cells produced at least three cytokines (group I in Figure 3). In CMI-1, for example, 45.6% of $NS5B_{2966-2980}$-specific $CD4^+$ T cells produced IFN-γ, TNF-α, and MIP-1β simultaneously (Figure 4A and 4B). A similar pattern of polyfunctionality was observed against another epitope, $NS5B_{2921-2935}$, in the same patient (Figure S2A and S2B). In the patient with a $CD8^+$ T cell response (CMI-4), cytotoxic function was also evaluated in a polyfunctionality assay by the addition of CD107a staining. As a result, more than 60% of HCV-specific $CD8^+$ T cells were at least triple-positive, and a major population was quadruple-positive for IFN-γ, TNF-α, MIP-1β, and CD107a (Figure 4C and 4D). In addition, HCV-specific $CD8^+$ T cells secreted granzyme B following epitope peptide stimulation (Figure 4E). In contrast, HCV-specific T cells from group II were not polyfunctional (Figure 3). When HCV-specific $CD4^+$ T cells were analyzed, 80–90% produced only a single cytokine, TNF-α (Figure 5A and 5B). These data demonstrate that there are two distinct groups, polyfunctional responders and TNF-α-predominant responders, in seronegative, aviremic patients who have HCV-specific memory T cells.

Neither occult HCV infection nor heterologous immunity is a cause of the T cell responses seen in seronegative, aviremic patients

Recently, occult HCV infection has been demonstrated in persons negative for HCV RNA by clinical-grade RT-PCR [14]. It was reported not only in patients with cryptogenic liver disease [35] but also in hemodialysis patients [36]. Since a previous study reported HCV-specific T cell responses in occult HCV infection [15], we attempted to detect occult HCV infection in seronegative, aviremic patients with HCV-specific cellular immune responses. We performed secondary nested RT-PCR of PBMC samples in all of the hemodialysis patients and obtained a positive result in three seronegative, aviremic patients as well as in all five of the patients positive for HCV RNA by clinical-grade RT-PCR (COBAS TaqMan HCV assay, Roche Diagnostics) (Table 2). However, the three patients with occult HCV infection were not among the eight patients who displayed HCV-specific T cell responses. All eight of the patients with HCV-specific T cell responses showed no sign of occult HCV infection by nested PCR. Thus, occult HCV infection was not a cause of the HCV-specific T cell responses in seronegative, aviremic patients.

Next, heterologous T cell immunity by a cross-reactive epitope was considered as a possible cause of the T cell responses seen in seronegative, aviremic patients. As shown in Table 1, however, T cells from a single patient were specific for multiple HCV epitopes. At least two epitopes were recognized by T cells from each patient, with exception of one, CMI-4 (Table 1). This finding suggested prior T cell priming by *bona fide* HCV proteins, and not by cross-reactive epitopes from other pathogens. In addition, the identified epitope peptides did not show any significant homology in amino acid sequence with peptides from other known pathogens by NCBI database searches. Of interest, T cell epitopes were found not only in structural proteins but also in non-structural (NS) proteins (Figure 1B and Table 1). T cell responses to HCV NS proteins are evidence of *de novo* synthesis of viral proteins in the host. Therefore, we concluded that the HCV-specific T cell responses observed in seronegative, aviremic patients resulted from prior exposure to HCV, even though there was no serological or clinical-grade RT-PCR evidence of current or past HCV infection.

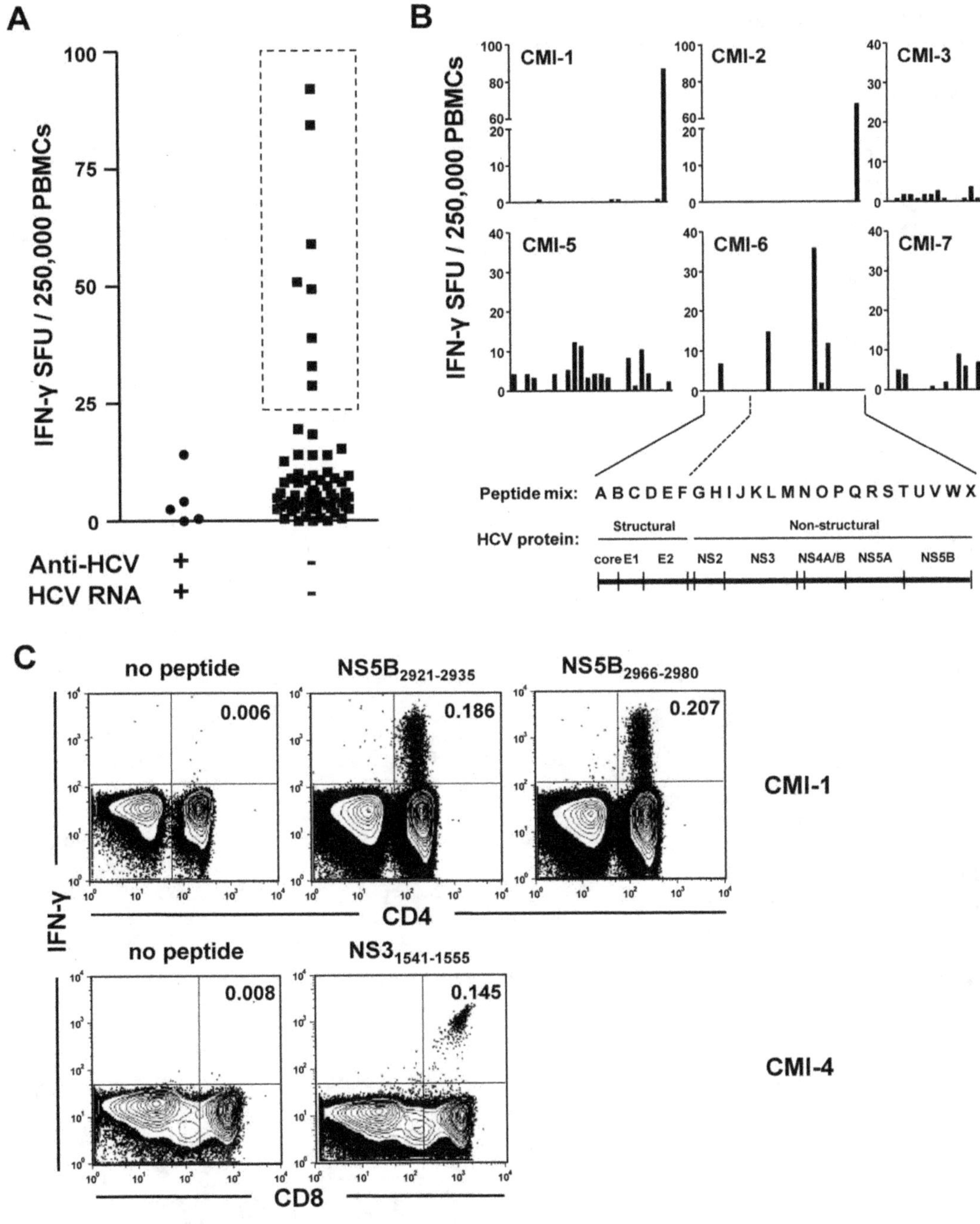

Figure 1. HCV-specific T cell responses in seronegative, aviremic hemodialysis patients. (A) Direct *ex vivo* IFN-γ ELISpot assay was performed to examine HCV-specific T cell responses in PBMCs of 76 hemodialysis patients. Five patients were seropositive with viremia (left side), and 71 patients were seronegative and aviremic (right side). PBMCs were stimulated with the 49 matrix mixes of 600 overlapping peptides covering the complete HCV polyprotein sequence (Materials and Methods and Figure S1A). The sum of A-X mixes and the sum of AA-YY mixes were calculated respectively, and their average value was presented for total HCV-specific T cell responses in each patient. Box with dashed lines denotes seronegative, aviremic patients with obvious T cell responses. **(B)** In the eight seronegative, aviremic patients with obvious T cell responses (CMI-1 to CMI-8), the results of IFN-γ ELISpot assay were presented by each peptide mix (A to X). Relationship between peptide mixes and HCV proteins are also displayed. **(C)** IFN-γ ICS was performed to identify the T cell subset responding to HCV epitopes. PBMCs were stimulated with epitope peptides identified in the IFN-γ ELISpot assay in the each patient. FACS dot plots are representative data from two patients, CMI-1 and CMI-4.

Comparison of different groups of patients in clinical aspects

In the present study, we identified different groups of hemodialysis patients according to HCV infection and immune status. There were chronic HCV-infected group (seropositive and viremic in clinical-grade RT-PCR) and occult HCV-infected group (seronegative and aviremic, but positive in nested RT-PCR). In addition, there were polyfunctional T cell responder group, TNF-α-predominant T cell responder group and non-responder group in seronegative, aviremic patients. We compared the different groups of patients in terms of demographic and clinical information, including duration of hemodialysis and liver enzymes

Table 1. Seronegative, aviremic hemodialysis patients with HCV-specific T cell responses.

Patient	IFN-γ SFU per 250,000 PBMCs	Responding T cells	Epitope peptides
CMI-1	92.0	CD4	$NS5B_{2921-2935}$, $NS5B_{2966-2980}$
		CD8	N.D.*
CMI-2	39.0	CD4	$NS5B_{2921-2935}$, $NS5B_{2966-2980}$
CMI-3	28.8	N.D.	$NS3_{1506-1520}$, $NS3_{1521-1535}$, $NS4B_{1881-1895}$, $NS4B_{1896-1910}$
CMI-4	33.0	CD8	$NS3_{1541-1555}$
CMI-5	84.3	N.D.	$core_{35-43}$, $NS5B_{2426-2440}$
CMI-6	49.3	CD4	$NS3_{1131-1145}$, $NS5A_{2006-2020}$
CMI-7	59.0	CD4	multi-specific
CMI-8	50.9	CD4	multi-specific

*N.D., not determined.

(Table S1). However, there was no significant difference among groups of patients in demographic and clinical aspects.

Discussion

HCV-specific cellular immune responses have been demonstrated in seronegative, aviremic persons with no evidence of current or past HCV infection [7–13]. This phenomenon was reported in HCV high-risk groups such as IDUs, residents of HCV-endemic areas, healthy family members of HCV-infected patients, and healthcare workers [7–13]. Virus-specific T cell responses generated in the absence of apparent infection have also been reported with other viruses. In HIV infection, a portion of seronegative, aviremic persons in the frequent exposure high-risk group displayed strong T cell responses against HIV [37–39]. In the present study, we detected HCV-specific T cell responses in 11.3% of seronegative, aviremic hemodialysis patients by direct *ex vivo* IFN-γ ELISpot assays (Figure 1A). The presence of HCV-specific T cell responses in seronegative, aviremic persons has several possible explanations, including occult HCV infection with extremely low-level viral replication [14,15], and heterologous T cell immunity by a cross-reactive epitope [16–18]. However, we showed that occult HCV infection was not a cause of the T cell responses in seronegative, aviremic patients in this study (Table 2). In addition, memory T cells against multiple HCV epitopes in a single patient (Figure 1B and Table 1) suggest that the T cells were primed by *bona fide* HCV proteins, not by cross-reactive epitopes from other pathogens, which is a key element of heterologous immunity. NCBI database searches also suggest that heterologous immunity is not the cause of the HCV-specific T cell responses seen in our study, because the identified HCV epitope peptides did not exhibit significant homology with peptides derived from other pathogens. Similarity in the three dimensional structure, rather than the primary sequence, also needs to be considered in cross-reactivity of HCV epitopes [40].

Our data indicate that HCV-specific memory T cells in seronegative, aviremic patients arose from previous exposure to

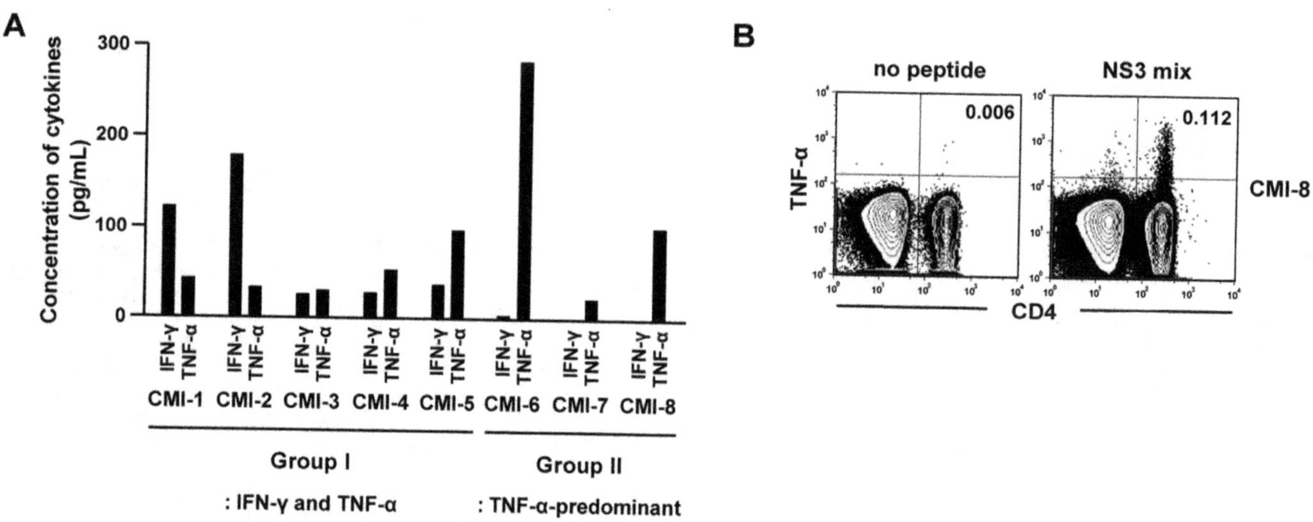

Figure 2. Cytokine profile of HCV-specific T cells in seronegative, aviremic hemodialysis patients. (A) After stimulating PBMCs with an epitope peptide or a peptide mix for 3 days, culture supernatant was harvested, and the concentrations of IFN-γ and TNF-α determined in the culture supernatant by CBA. There are two groups of patients in terms of cytokine profile: group I, patients with IFN-γ and TNF-α responses; group II, patients with TNF-α-predominant responses. **(B)** TNF-α ICS was performed in the patients of group II. FACS dot plots are representative data from two patients, CMI-7 and CMI-8.

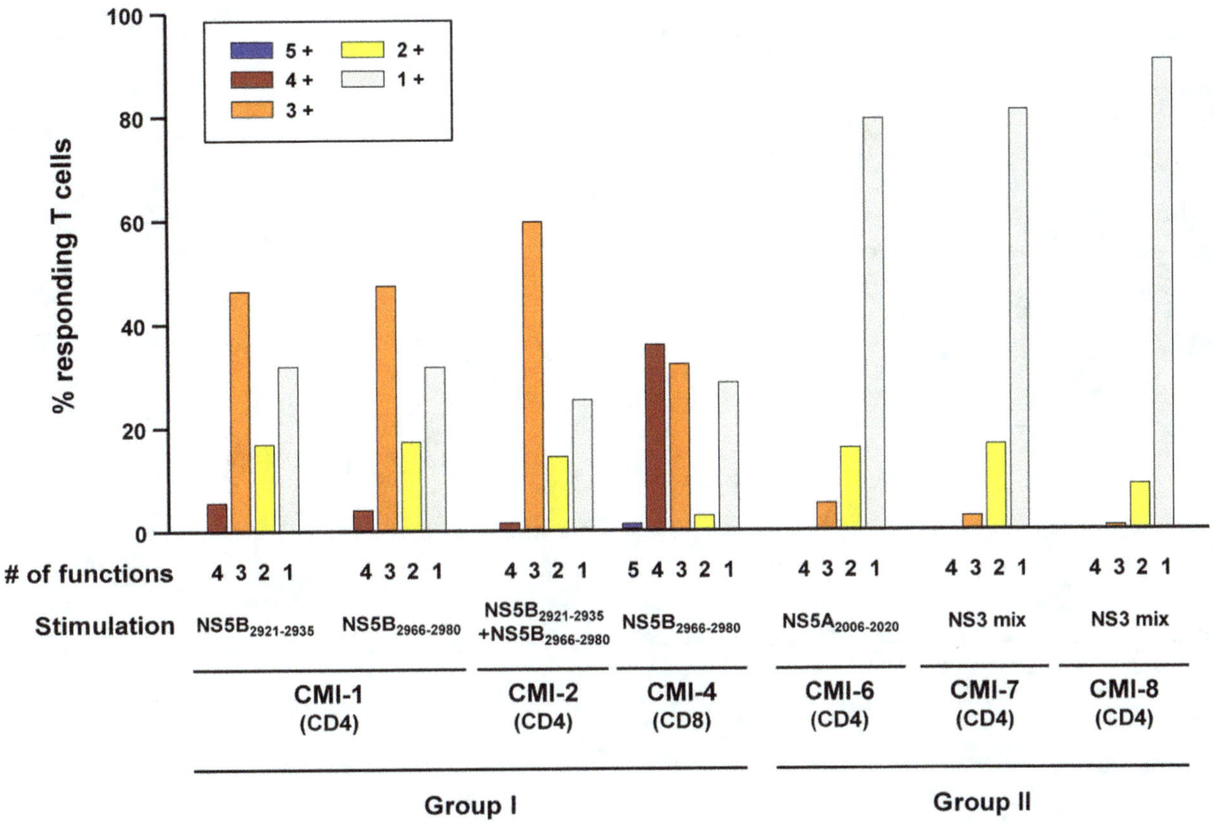

Figure 3. Polyfunctionality of HCV-specific T cells in seronegative, aviremic hemodialysis patients. PBMCs were stimulated with an epitope peptide or a peptide mix, and production of IFN-γ, TNF-α, IL-2, and MIP-1β was simultaneously assessed in multi-cytokine ICS in order to evaluate polyfunctionality of HCV-specific $CD4^+$ T cells. In each patient, the fraction of T cells positive for a given number of functions is presented as bar graphs. In the patient with $CD8^+$ T cell responses (CMI-4), cytotoxic degranulation function was also evaluated by CD107a staining in addition to multi-cytokine ICS for IFN-γ, TNF-α, IL-2, and MIP-1β.

HCV and subclinical transient viral replication without seroconversion. Previous HCV replication in these patients is evidenced by T cell specificity for epitopes derived from HCV NS proteins (Figure 1B and Table 1), which would require *de novo* synthesis of viral proteins in the host. In a previous cohort study, HCV-specific cellular immune responses were detected in self-limited acute HCV infection without seroconversion [19]. In addition, another study directly demonstrated that exposure to low doses of HCV led to HCV-specific T cell responses in chimpanzees, with transient viral replication [20]. The same study found that HCV challenge with 1-10 RNA (+) inoculums resulted in priming of HCV-specific T cells without sustained viremia or seroconversion [20]. It remains possible that in our patients, anti-HCV antibody was generated during an acute infection and has over the course of many years disappeared from circulation. In fact, a previous study demonstrated that anti-HCV disappeared 20 years after recovery from acute HCV infection while cellular immune responses persisted [21]. Clinical implications of HCV-specific T cell response in seronegative, aviremic persons will require further investigation. In addition, phenotypic characteristics of HCV-specific T cells needs to be analyzed in further studies, including memory markers, activation markers and exhaustion markers.

In the present study, we showed two distinct patterns of T cell polyfunctionality in seronegative, aviremic patients (Figures 3, 4, and 5). HCV-specific memory T cells were highly polyfunctional in some patients (group I in Figure 3), whereas they were TNF-α-predominant in the others (group II in Figure 3). Recently, T cell polyfunctionality has been investigated in HIV infection and vaccination studies [27–29] and it was found that polyfunctional HIV-specific $CD8^+$ T cells were maintained in HIV long-term nonprogressors [28]. Furthermore, in a Leishmania vaccination study, the degree of Th1 cell polyfunctionality was shown to correlate with vaccine efficacy [27]. In addition, the profound efficacy of the smallpox vaccine has been attributed to polyfunctionality of virus-specific $CD8^+$ T cells. Taken together, polyfunctional HCV-specific memory T cells in seronegative, aviremic patients would be expected to protect against subsequent exposure to HCV. Intriguingly, a very recent study demonstrated that polyfunctional HCV-specific T cells were associated with vaccine-induced control of HCV [41].

In patients with a TNF-α-predominant response, HCV-specific T cells might not provide antiviral protection upon subsequent HCV exposure. We can infer the absence of a protective role for TNF-α-single-positive T cells from a recent study of tuberculosis. In this study, TNF-α-single-positive *Mycobacterium tuberculosis*-specific $CD4^+$ T cells were preferentially detected in active tuberculosis disease rather than in latent infection [42]. It is possible that TNF-α-single-positive T cell responses might serve solely as evidence of T cell priming by exposure to pathogen.

In the present study, we suggest that HCV-specific memory T cells of seronegative, aviremic patients might result from transient viral replication without seroconversion or, alternately, from disappearance of anti-HCV antibody long after prior HCV infection. If these assumptions prove true, it would suggest that

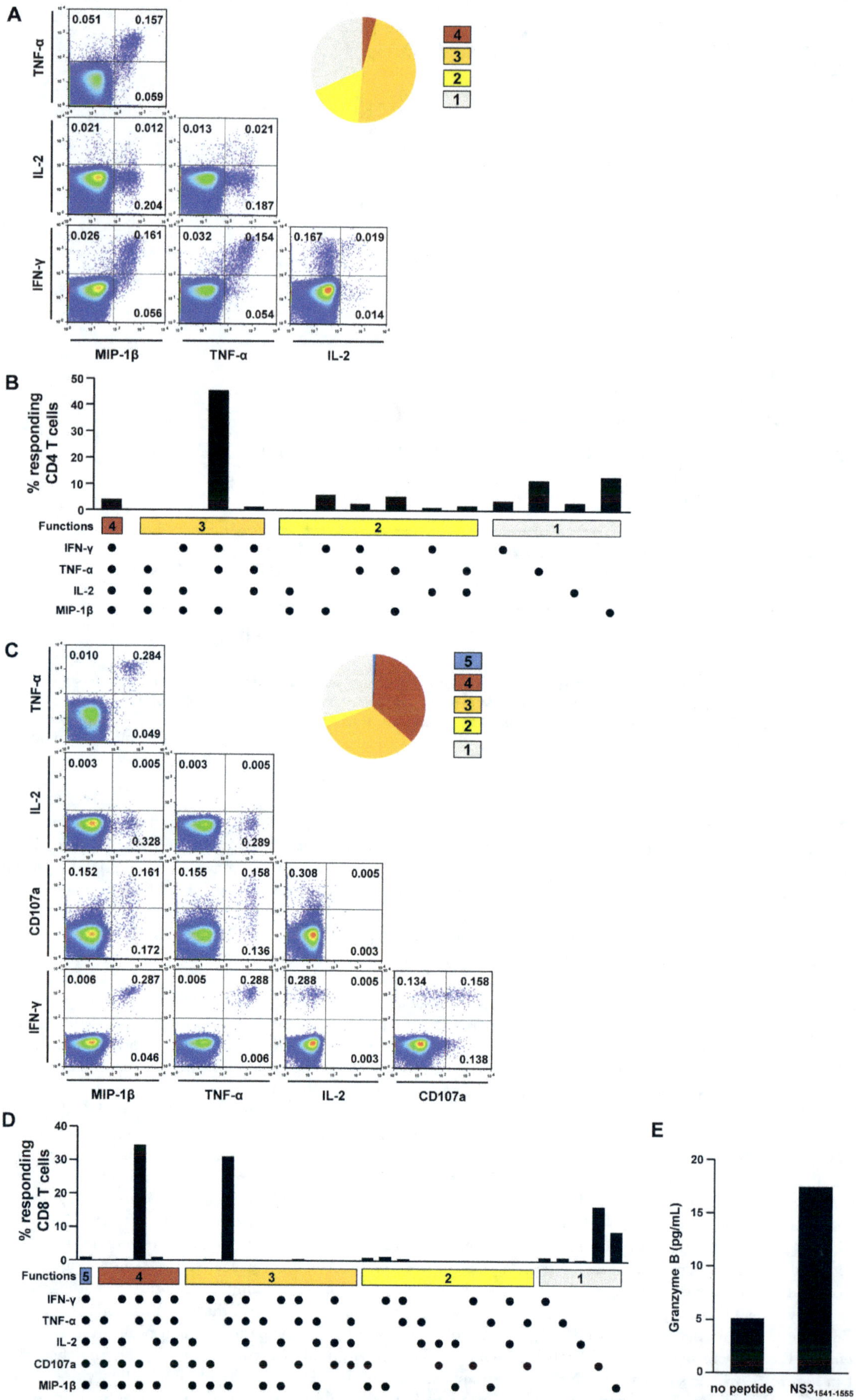
A
TNF-α
IL-2
IFN-γ
MIP-1β
TNF-α
IL-2
0.051 0.157 0.059
0.021 0.012 0.204
0.013 0.021 0.187
0.026 0.161 0.056
0.032 0.154 0.054
0.167 0.019 0.014
4
3
2
1
B
% responding CD4 T cells
Functions
IFN-γ
TNF-α
IL-2
MIP-1β
C
TNF-α
IL-2
CD107a
IFN-γ
MIP-1β
TNF-α
IL-2
CD107a
0.010 0.284 0.049
0.003 0.005 0.328
0.003 0.005 0.289
0.152 0.161 0.172
0.155 0.158 0.136
0.308 0.005 0.003
0.006 0.287 0.046
0.005 0.288 0.006
0.288 0.005 0.003
0.134 0.158 0.138
5
D
% responding CD8 T cells
E
Granzyme B (pg/mL)
no peptide
NS3 1541-1555

Figure 4. Polyfunctionality assay of HCV-specific T cells in the patients of group I. Representative examples of polyfunctionality assays of CD4$^+$ T cells in CMI-1 (A and B) and of CD8$^+$ T cells in CMI-4 (C and D) are presented. In CMI-1, PBMCs were stimulated with NS5B$_{2966-2980}$ epitope peptide, and IFN-γ, TNF-α, IL-2, and MIP-1β production was assessed (A and B). In CMI-4, PBMCs were stimulated with NS3$_{1541-1555}$ epitope peptide, and CD107a, IFN-γ, TNF-α, IL-2, and MIP-1β production was assessed (C and D). In the culture supernatant of NS3$_{1541-1555}$ peptide-stimulated PBMCs, concentration of granzyme B was determined by CBA (E). The data are presented by FACS dot plots and the pie graphs show the fraction of T cells positive for a given number of functions (A and C). Detailed analysis of polyfunctionality is presented with every possible combination of functions (B and D).

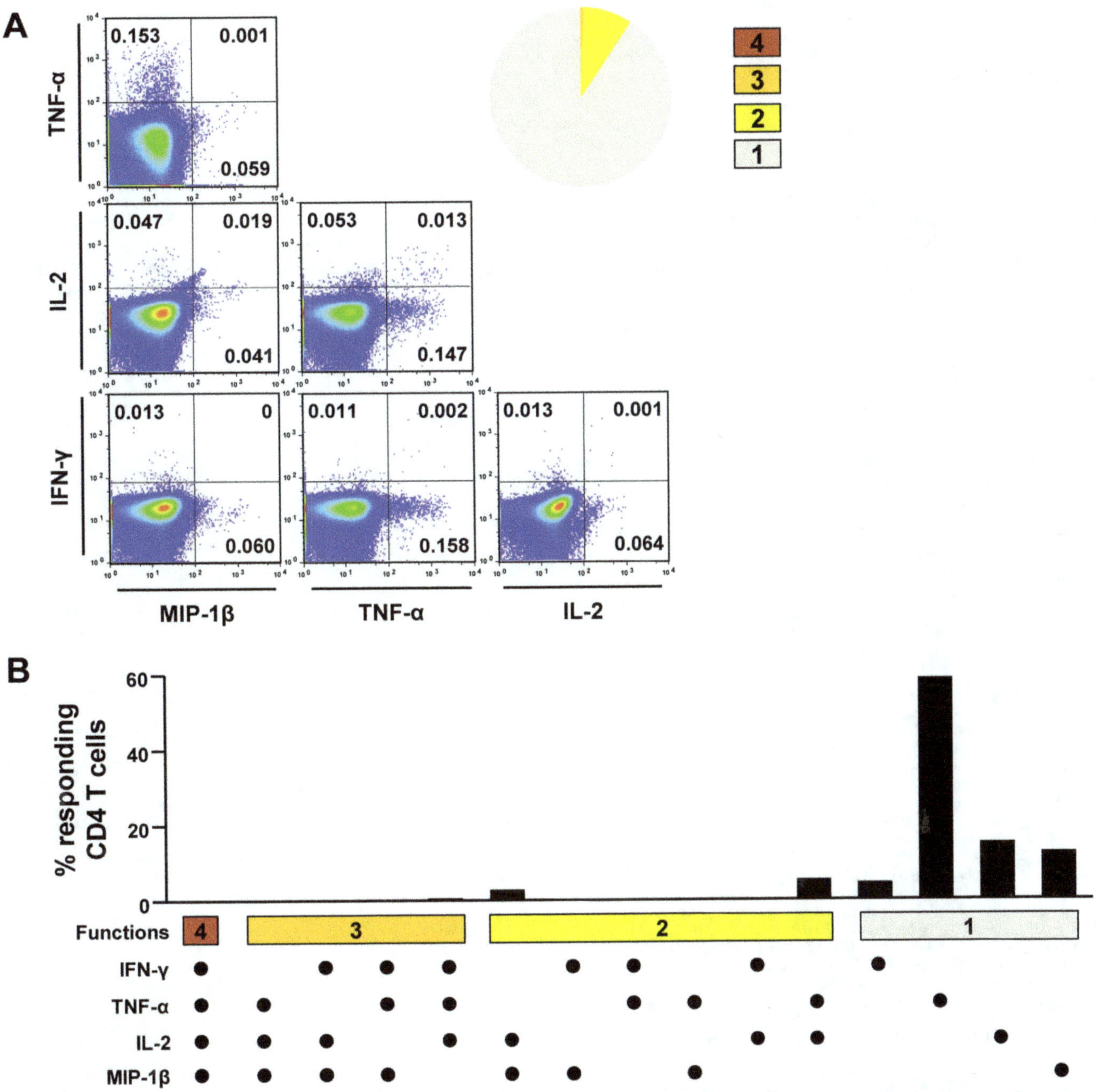

Figure 5. Polyfunctionality assay of HCV-specific T cells in the patients of group II. Representative example of polyfunctionality assays of CD4$^+$ T cells in CMI-8 is presented. PBMCs were stimulated with NS3 peptide mix, and IFN-γ, TNF-α, IL-2, and MIP-1β production were assessed. The data are presented by FACS dot plots and the pie graph shows the fraction of T cells positive for a given number of functions (A). Detailed analysis of polyfunctionality is presented with every possible combination of functions (B).

Table 2. Hemodialysis patients with secondary nested RT-PCR (+).

	Patient	COBAS TaqMan HCV RNA, IU/mL	Nested RT-PCR HCV RNA	Genotype
Seropositive	HepC-1	5.8×10^4	+	1b
	HepC-2	1.0×10^6	+	1b
	HepC-3	4.6×10^5	+	2a
	HepC-4	3.7×10^3	+	1b
	HepC-5	8.1×10^2	+	N.D.*
Seronegative	Occult-1	-	+	2a
	Occult-2	-	+	2a
	Occult-3	-	+	N.D.

*N.D., not determined.

past HCV exposure may be better assessed by HCV-specific T cell responses than by presence of anti-HCV antibody. In fact, HCV-specific T cell assays could confirm HCV exposure in indeterminate blood donors [43–45]. However, T cell assays for IFN-γ responsiveness might underestimate HCV exposure since there are seronegative, aviremic patients who demonstrate a TNF-α-predominant response. Thus, assays specific for a T cell TNF-α response might prove superior to assays examining IFN-γ production.

In summary, we show that HCV-specific T cell responses in seronegative, aviremic hemodialysis patients might result from a prior, transient viral replication without seroconversion or from disappearance of anti-HCV long after acute HCV infection has resolved, but not from current occult HCV infection. We also demonstrate that HCV-specific T cell responders in seronegative, aviremic hemodialysis patients are classified into two distinct groups, polyfunctional responders and TNF-α-predominant responders. Determining the significance of these responses with respect to immunology and vaccinology will require further investigation. In particular, detailed characterization of HCV-specific T cell polyfunctionality might provide a basis for understanding of protective immunity against HCV and a strategy for the development of an HCV vaccine.

Acknowledgments

The Authors thank the patients who participated in the study and Dr. So Rae Choi for clinical help.

Author Contributions

Conceived and designed the experiments: YC HK KC BK ES. Performed the experiments: YC JL SN JP HK. Analyzed the data: YC JL SN HK BK ES. Wrote the paper: YC BK ES.

References

1. Alter HJ, Seeff LB (2000) Recovery, persistence, and sequelae in hepatitis C virus infection: a perspective on long-term outcome. Semin Liver Dis 20: 17–35.
2. Seeff LB (2002) Natural history of chronic hepatitis C. Hepatology 36: S35–46.
3. Shepard CW, Finelli L, Alter MJ (2005) Global epidemiology of hepatitis C virus infection. Lancet Infect Dis 5: 558–567.
4. Lechner F, Wong DK, Dunbar PR, Chapman R, Chung RT, et al. (2000) Analysis of successful immune responses in persons infected with hepatitis C virus. J Exp Med 191: 1499–1512.
5. Rosen HR, Miner C, Sasaki AW, Lewinsohn DM, Conrad AJ, et al. (2002) Frequencies of HCV-specific effector CD4+ T cells by flow cytometry: correlation with clinical disease stages. Hepatology 35: 190–198.
6. Day CL, Lauer GM, Robbins GK, McGovern B, Wurcel AG, et al. (2002) Broad specificity of virus-specific CD4+ T-helper-cell responses in resolved hepatitis C virus infection. J Virol 76: 12584–12595.
7. Mizukoshi E, Eisenbach C, Edlin BR, Newton KP, Raghuraman S, et al. (2008) Hepatitis C virus (HCV)-specific immune responses of long-term injection drug users frequently exposed to HCV. J Infect Dis 198: 203–212.
8. Al-Sherbiny M, Osman A, Mohamed N, Shata MT, Abdel-Aziz F, et al. (2005) Exposure to hepatitis C virus induces cellular immune responses without detectable viremia or seroconversion. Am J Trop Med Hyg 73: 44–49.
9. Bronowicki JP, Vetter D, Uhl G, Hudziak H, Uhrlacher A, et al. (1997) Lymphocyte reactivity to hepatitis C virus (HCV) antigens shows evidence for exposure to HCV in HCV-seronegative spouses of HCV-infected patients. J Infect Dis 176: 518–522.
10. Scognamiglio P, Accapezzato D, Casciaro MA, Cacciani A, Artini M, et al. (1999) Presence of effector CD8+ T cells in hepatitis C virus-exposed healthy seronegative donors. J Immunol 162: 6681–6689.
11. Hashem M, El-Karaksy H, Shata MT, Sobhy M, Helmy H, et al. (2011) Strong hepatitis C virus (HCV)-specific cell-mediated immune responses in the absence of viremia or antibodies among uninfected siblings of HCV chronically infected children. J Infect Dis 203: 854–861.
12. Koziel MJ, Wong DK, Dudley D, Houghton M, Walker BD (1997) Hepatitis C virus-specific cytolytic T lymphocyte and T helper cell responses in seronegative persons. J Infect Dis 176: 859–866.
13. Perrella A, Grattacaso S, d'Antonio A, Atripaldi L, Sbreglia C, et al. (2009) Evidence of hepatitis C virus-specific interferon gamma-positive T cells in health care workers in an infectious disease department. Am J Infect Control 37: 426–429.
14. Welker MW, Zeuzem S (2009) Occult hepatitis C: how convincing are the current data? Hepatology 49: 665–675.
15. Quiroga JA, Llorente S, Castillo I, Rodriguez-Inigo E, Pardo M, et al. (2006) Cellular immune responses associated with occult hepatitis C virus infection of the liver. J Virol 80: 10972–10979.
16. Wedemeyer H, Mizukoshi E, Davis AR, Bennink JR, Rehermann B (2001) Cross-reactivity between hepatitis C virus and Influenza A virus determinant-specific cytotoxic T cells. J Virol 75: 11392–11400.
17. Urbani S, Amadei B, Fisicaro P, Pilli M, Missale G, et al. (2005) Heterologous T cell immunity in severe hepatitis C virus infection. J Exp Med 201: 675–680.
18. Rehermann B, Shin EC (2005) Private aspects of heterologous immunity. J Exp Med 201: 667–670.
19. Post JJ, Pan Y, Freeman AJ, Harvey CE, White PA, et al. (2004) Clearance of hepatitis C viremia associated with cellular immunity in the absence of seroconversion in the hepatitis C incidence and transmission in prisons study cohort. J Infect Dis 189: 1846–1855.

20. Shata MT, Tricoche N, Perkus M, Tom D, Brotman B, et al. (2003) Exposure to low infective doses of HCV induces cellular immune responses without consistently detectable viremia or seroconversion in chimpanzees. Virology 314: 601–616.
21. Takaki A, Wiese M, Maertens G, Depla E, Seifert U, et al. (2000) Cellular immune responses persist and humoral responses decrease two decades after recovery from a single-source outbreak of hepatitis C. Nat Med 6: 578–582.
22. Bassett SE, Guerra B, Brasky K, Miskovsky E, Houghton M, et al. (2001) Protective immune response to hepatitis C virus in chimpanzees rechallenged following clearance of primary infection. Hepatology 33: 1479–1487.
23. Nascimbeni M, Mizukoshi E, Bosmann M, Major ME, Mihalik K, et al. (2003) Kinetics of CD4+ and CD8+ memory T-cell responses during hepatitis C virus rechallenge of previously recovered chimpanzees. J Virol 77: 4781–4793.
24. Lanford RE, Guerra B, Chavez D, Bigger C, Brasky KM, et al. (2004) Cross-genotype immunity to hepatitis C virus. J Virol 78: 1575–1581.
25. Grakoui A, Shoukry NH, Woollard DJ, Han JH, Hanson HL, et al. (2003) HCV persistence and immune evasion in the absence of memory T cell help. Science 302: 659–662.
26. Shoukry NH, Grakoui A, Houghton M, Chien DY, Ghrayeb J, et al. (2003) Memory CD8+ T cells are required for protection from persistent hepatitis C virus infection. J Exp Med 197: 1645–1655.
27. Darrah PA, Patel DT, De Luca PM, Lindsay RW, Davey DF, et al. (2007) Multifunctional TH1 cells define a correlate of vaccine-mediated protection against Leishmania major. Nat Med 13: 843–850.
28. Betts MR, Nason MC, West SM, De Rosa SC, Migueles SA, et al. (2006) HIV nonprogressors preferentially maintain highly functional HIV-specific CD8+ T cells. Blood 107: 4781–4789.
29. Precopio ML, Betts MR, Parrino J, Price DA, Gostick E, et al. (2007) Immunization with vaccinia virus induces polyfunctional and phenotypically distinctive CD8(+) T cell responses. J Exp Med 204: 1405–1416.
30. Shin EC, Park SH, Demino M, Nascimbeni M, Mihalik K, et al. (2011) Delayed induction, not impaired recruitment, of specific CD8 T cells causes the late onset of acute hepatitis C. Gastroenterology 141: 686–695, 695 e681.
31. Shin EC, Protzer U, Untergasser A, Feinstone SM, Rice CM, et al. (2005) Liver-directed gamma interferon gene delivery in chronic hepatitis C. J Virol 79: 13412–13420.
32. Pham TN, MacParland SA, Mulrooney PM, Cooksley H, Naoumov NV, et al. (2004) Hepatitis C virus persistence after spontaneous or treatment-induced resolution of hepatitis C. J Virol 78: 5867–5874.
33. Castillo I, Rodriguez-Inigo E, Bartolome J, de Lucas S, Ortiz-Movilla N, et al. (2005) Hepatitis C virus replicates in peripheral blood mononuclear cells of patients with occult hepatitis C virus infection. Gut 54: 682–685.
34. Castillo I, Bartolome J, Quiroga JA, Barril G, Carreno V (2010) Diagnosis of occult hepatitis C without the need for a liver biopsy. J Med Virol 82: 1554–1559.
35. Castillo I, Pardo M, Bartolome J, Ortiz-Movilla N, Rodriguez-Inigo E, et al. (2004) Occult hepatitis C virus infection in patients in whom the etiology of persistently abnormal results of liver-function tests is unknown. J Infect Dis 189: 7–14.
36. Barril G, Castillo I, Arenas MD, Espinosa M, Garcia-Valdecasas J, et al. (2008) Occult hepatitis C virus infection among hemodialysis patients. J Am Soc Nephrol 19: 2288–2292.
37. De Maria A, Cirillo C, Moretta L (1994) Occurrence of human immunodeficiency virus type 1 (HIV-1)-specific cytolytic T cell activity in apparently uninfected children born to HIV-1-infected mothers. J Infect Dis 170: 1296–1299.
38. Mazzoli S, Trabattoni D, Lo Caputo S, Piconi S, Ble C, et al. (1997) HIV-specific mucosal and cellular immunity in HIV-seronegative partners of HIV-seropositive individuals. Nat Med 3: 1250–1257.
39. Rowland-Jones SL, Dong T, Fowke KR, Kimani J, Krausa P, et al. (1998) Cytotoxic T cell responses to multiple conserved HIV epitopes in HIV-resistant prostitutes in Nairobi. J Clin Invest 102: 1758–1765.
40. Quaratino S, Thorpe CJ, Travers PJ, Londei M (1995) Similar antigenic surfaces, rather than sequence homology, dictate T-cell epitope molecular mimicry. Proc Natl Acad Sci U S A 92: 10398–10402.
41. Park SH, Shin EC, Capone S, Caggiari L, De Re V, et al. (2012) Successful Vaccination Induces Multifunctional Memory T-Cell Precursors Associated with Early Control of Hepatitis C Virus. Gastroenterology.
42. Harari A, Rozot V, Enders FB, Perreau M, Stalder JM, et al. (2011) Dominant TNF-alpha+ Mycobacterium tuberculosis-specific CD4+ T cell responses discriminate between latent infection and active disease. Nat Med 17: 372–376.
43. Semmo N, Barnes E, Taylor C, Kurtz J, Harcourt G, et al. (2005) T-cell responses and previous exposure to hepatitis C virus in indeterminate blood donors. Lancet 365: 327–329.
44. Bes M, Esteban JI, Casamitjana N, Piron M, Quer J, et al. (2009) Hepatitis C virus (HCV)-specific T-cell responses among recombinant immunoblot assay-3-indeterminate blood donors: a confirmatory evidence of HCV exposure. Transfusion 49: 1296–1305.
45. Hitziger T, Schmidt M, Schottstedt V, Hennig H, Schumann A, et al. (2009) Cellular immune response to hepatitis C virus (HCV) in nonviremic blood donors with indeterminate anti-HCV reactivity. Transfusion 49: 1306–1313.

Pre-Dialysis Systolic Blood Pressure-Variability is Independently Associated with All-Cause Mortality in Incident Haemodialysis Patients

Viknesh Selvarajah[1,2]*, Laura Pasea[3], Sanjay Ojha[2], Ian B. Wilkinson[4], Laurie A. Tomlinson[4]

1 Clinical Pharmacology Unit, Department of Medicine, University of Cambridge, Cambridge, United Kingdom, **2** Department of Nephrology, Cambridge University Hospitals NHS Foundation Trust, Cambridge, United Kingdom, **3** Centre for Applied Medical Statistics, Department of Public Health and Primary Care, Institute of Public Health, University of Cambridge, Cambridge, United Kingdom, **4** Cambridge Clinical Trials Unit, University of Cambridge, Cambridge, United Kingdom

Abstract

Systolic blood pressure variability is an independent risk factor for mortality and cardiovascular events. Standard measures of blood pressure predict outcome poorly in haemodialysis patients. We investigated whether systolic blood pressure variability was associated with mortality in incident haemodialysis patients. We performed a longitudinal observational study of patients commencing haemodialysis between 2005 and 2011 in East Anglia, UK, excluding patients with cardiovascular events within 6 months of starting haemodialysis. The main exposure was variability independent of the mean (VIM) of systolic blood pressure from short-gap, pre-dialysis blood pressure readings between 3 and 6 months after commencing haemodialysis, and the outcome was all-cause mortality. Of 203 patients, 37 (18.2%) patients died during a mean follow-up of 2.0 (SD 1.3) years. The age and sex-adjusted hazard ratio (HR) for mortality was 1.09 (95% confidence interval (CI) 1.02–1.17) for a one-unit increase of VIM. This was not altered by adjustment for diabetes, prior cardiovascular disease and mean systolic blood pressure (HR 1.09, 95% CI 1.02–1.16). Patients with VIM of systolic blood pressure above the median were 2.4 (95% CI 1.17–4.74) times more likely to die during follow-up than those below the median. Results were similar for all measures of blood pressure variability and further adjustment for type of dialysis access, use of antihypertensives and absolute or variability of fluid intake did not alter these findings. Diastolic blood pressure variability showed no association with all cause mortality. Our study shows that variability of systolic blood pressure is a strong and independent predictor of all-cause mortality in incident haemodialysis patients. Further research is needed to understand the mechanism as this may form a therapeutic target or focus for management.

Editor: Rudolf Kirchmair, Medical University Innsbruck, Austria

Funding: IBW and VS are supported by the British Heart Foundation and the Cambridge Biomedical Research Centre. The funders had no role in study design, data collection and analysis, decision to publish, or preparation of the manuscript.

Competing Interests: The authors have declared that no competing interests exist.

* E-mail: vs321@cam.ac.uk

Introduction

Mortality is high among patients undergoing haemodialysis treatment for end-stage renal disease (ESRD), and cardiovascular disease is the main cause of death [1]. Hypertension is common in ESRD but, unlike in the general population, is not linearly associated with adverse outcomes [2].

Blood pressure (BP) variability is more closely associated with adverse outcomes in patients with or at risk of vascular disease than 'usual' BP [3] and may play a causal role in the progression of organ damage and in triggering vascular events [4]. BP variability is known to be increased in patients with ESRD [5,6]. Among patients undergoing haemodialysis potential causes of high BP variability such as baroreceptor dysfunction, aortic stiffness and variations in intravascular volume, as well as plausible outcomes such as cerebral small-vessel disease, cerebral haemorrhage and cardiac sudden death are increased compared to the general population [7,8]. Therefore increased BP variability could provide a strong potential explanation for the increased cardiovascular morbidity and mortality among patients undergoing haemodialysis.

BP variability can be quantified over both the short term, using 24-hour ambulatory BP measurements, and long-term using visit-to-visit BP readings [9]. The optimum method for evaluating BP variability for patients with ESRD is unclear. Previous studies have suggested that visit-to-visit pre-dialysis BP variability is associated with mortality among haemodialysis patients [6,10,11]. However, these studies are limited by lack of power and short duration of follow-up, [10,11] inclusion of prevalent haemodialysis patients [6,10] and use of measures of blood pressure variability that are associated with average blood pressure levels [10]. Therefore, we planned to investigate whether visit-to-visit pre-dialysis blood pressure variability was associated with mortality among a cohort of patients commencing incident haemodialysis, independently of confounders including average blood pressure.

Subjects and Methods

Study Design

We performed a longitudinal cohort study of patients who commenced maintenance haemodialysis between January 1st 2005 and December 12th 2010. Patients were from Addenbrookes

Hospital and four satellite units in East Anglia, England. Each underwent haemodialysis three times a week and each dialysis session was at the same time of day and lasted for 3–4 hours.

Inclusion & Exclusion Criteria

We included all patients who were aged over 18 years at the start of dialysis, had no history of prior renal replacement therapy including transplantation, and remained on dialysis for more than 180 days with no recovery of kidney function. To avoid reverse causality (where underlying cardiovascular disease causes variable blood pressure), we excluded patients who died or suffered cardiovascular events (stroke, transient ischaemic attack (TIA), myocardial infarction, angina or heart failure) in the first 180 days after starting haemodialysis.

Exposure: Blood Pressure Measurements

BP was measured was measured at the beginning and end of each dialysis session in a seated position by trained dialysis nurses in accordance with routine unit practice and entered immediately into an electronic database. BP was measured using validated oscillometric BP monitor equipped haemodialysis machines (Fresenius 4008S or Nikisso DBB-05), which were maintained as per dialysis unit protocols. For each patient we analysed pre-dialysis BP readings obtained over a consecutive 3-month period, from the 4th to 6th months after commencing haemodialysis. BP readings from the first 3 months after commencing dialysis were not used because this period is associated with acute illness and frequent adjustments to fluid weight and medications, which may have led to overestimation of BP variability in more unwell patients. We used pre-dialysis BP readings to minimise the effect of change in BP due to fluid removal during haemodialysis. We excluded BP readings taken on the first dialysis session of each week to avoid the possible confounding effects of fluid gains over the extended three-day weekend break. Therefore over the 3-month observation period all patients included in the analysis had almost identical numbers of BP readings included in the measurement of the exposure and these were 2 BP readings per week taken 2 days apart on the same day and same time of day for each individual.

Exposure: Blood Pressure Variability

We measured intra-individual BP variability for both pre-dialysis systolic and diastolic BP using standard deviation, coefficient of variation (standard deviation/mean) and variation independent of the mean (VIM) as previously described [3]. VIM is a transformation of the standard deviation that is uncorrelated with mean BP and is calculated as follows:

$$VIM = \frac{k \times \text{Standard Deviation (SBP)}}{Mean\ (SBP)^x}$$

Where x is calculated from fitting a power model:

$$SD(SBP) = \text{constant} \times \text{Mean(SBP)}^x$$

And $k = \text{Mean(Mean(SBP))}^x$.

(i.e. the mean of all SBP readings across all patients to the power of x).

For this study, $x = 0.789$ and $k = 50.552$.

Outcome: All-cause Mortality

The outcome was all-cause mortality during the study period, i.e. from 6 months after the commencement of haemodialysis (at the end of the 3–6 month measurement of the exposure) until the end of follow-up (May 12th 2011). Follow-up was censored if patients received a kidney transplant, switched to peritoneal dialysis or transferred to a different renal unit.

Demographic data, comorbidities and details and dates of censoring events were obtained from the regional renal electronic database and verified using local medical records. Data on medications, interdialytic weight changes, intradialytic weight changes and type of dialysis access were also available. Previous cardiovascular disease (including clinically evident: stroke, transient ischaemic attack (TIA), myocardial infarction, angina, heart failure or peripheral vascular disease) and diabetes were defined as present if recorded in the medical notes. Data on cause of death was not available so it was not possible to analyse cardiovascular mortality separately.

Statistical Analysis

The definitions of the exposure (including all BP measurements that contributed to the measurement of the exposure and outcome) were defined a priori. The demographic characteristics of groups above and below the median of VIM were compared using Mann-Whitney U tests for continuous variables and chi-squared tests for categorical variables.

We used Cox proportional hazards models to obtain hazard ratios (HR) and 95% confidence intervals (95% CI) for mortality for people with intraindividual visit-to-visit BP variability as a continuous covariate, and also as a categorical covariate, with BP variability dichotomized at the median. We examined whether the proportional hazards assumption was met using partial residual plots for continuous covariates and log (-log) plots for categorical covariates. Kaplan-Meier plots and log-rank tests were also used to compare survival between the two BP variability groups. We carried out univariate analyses of the effect of intraindividual visit-to-visit blood pressure variability on all-cause mortality. We present results adjusted for age and sex as these were considered important a priori confounders. Further covariates examined in multivariate analysis were based on potential evidence of association with mortality among haemodialysis patients; mean systolic BP (SBP), previous cardiovascular events and diabetes. This dataset was complete for all patients. Data on ethnicity was not available but in this region more than 90% of patients are of Caucasian ethnicity. In further separate analyses we adjusted for type of dialysis access (arteriovenous fistula vs indwelling venous catheter), the use of antihypertensive medication (yes vs no) and the number of antihypertensives taken at three months after start of haemodialysis (start of BP variability measurement), the mean intradialytic weight change and the standard deviation of weight change between dialysis sessions as a marker of variability of fluid intake. For this analysis the standard deviation of interdialytic weight change was log transformed due to skewness. We performed the analysis using SPSS version 21.0 (IBM Corp., Armonk, NY).

Ethics Statement

The study received approval from the Hertfordshire Research Ethics Committee (REC 11/H0311/3). Data was anonymised at source so individual patient consent was not required.

Data Availability

We are able to provide anonymized data to researchers upon request.

Results

Patient Demographics

During the study period 219 patients who were eligible for inclusion commenced maintenance haemodialysis in this region with a total follow up time of 409.4 person years. Of these, we did not include in the analysis 7 patients who died or recovered kidney function and 9 who had cardiovascular events within the first 180 days of haemodialysis. Therefore 203 patients were included in the analysis. From a mean of 25 dialysis sessions, the mean number of BP readings used for the analyses was 25 (SD 1.63). Over a mean follow-up period of 2.0 (SD 1.3) years, 37 patients (18.2%) died. Follow-up was censored for 24 (11.8%) patients who underwent kidney transplantation and 5 (2.5%) who switched to peritoneal dialysis. No patients changed renal units during the follow-up period.

Baseline characteristics of the study population and patients above and below the median VIM of intraindividual visit-to-visit BP variability are shown in Table 1. Patients with VIM of BP variability above the median were more likely to have diabetes but otherwise there were no significant difference between the groups.

Intraindividual Visit-to-visit Systolic Blood Pressure Variability

Standard deviation. At an individual level, the mean SD of SBP was 17.4 mmHg (SD 5.1 mmHg). After adjusting for age and sex, the HR for total mortality was 1.07 (95% CI 1.01, 1.13) for every mmHg increase in SD of SBP. This was not attenuated after further adjustment for mean SBP, previous cardiovascular events and diabetes (HR 1.08, 95% CI 1.01, 1.16) (Table 2). After adjusting for age, gender, mean SBP, previous cardiovascular events and diabetes, patients with SD of SBP above the median had a 48% increased risk of death during follow-up but this was not statistically significant (HR 1.48, 95% CI 0.75, 2.91).

Coefficient of variation. For the purpose of regression modelling the coefficient of variation (COV) was multiplied by 100 for each patient to allow sensible interpretation of the hazard ratio. The HR for total mortality, adjusted for age and gender, was 1.13 (95% CI 1.02, 1.24) for every 0.01 increase in COV. After adjusting for age, sex, previous cardiovascular disease, diabetes and mean SBP the HR for total mortality was 1.13 (95% CI 1.02, 1.24) for every 0.01 increase in COV (table 2). After full adjustment, patients with COV of SBP above the median had more than double the risk of death during follow-up (HR 2.08, 95%CI 1.04, 4.16).

Variation independent of the mean. After adjusting for age and sex, the HR for total mortality was 1.09 (95% CI 1.02, 1.16) for a one-unit increase of VIM. Again, this was not attenuated in the fully adjusted model (HR 1.09, 95% CI 1.02, 1.16). Patients with VIM of SBP above the median were 2.4 (95% CI 1.17, 4.74) times more likely to die during follow-up than those below or equal to the median after adjustment for diabetes, prior cardiovascular disease, gender, age and mean SBP (figure 1).

Further Analyses

The relationship between VIM of systolic BP and all-cause mortality was not affected by adjustment for the type of dialysis

Table 1. Demographic characteristics of whole study population and groups above and below the median of blood pressure variability.

	Whole group	VIM below or equal to median	VIM above median	*P*-value*
	n = 203	n = 100	n = 103	
Age (yrs)	66±15	65±17	68±13	0.55
Male	133 (66)	68 (68)	65 (63)	0.46
Diabetes	61 (30)	20 (20)	41 (40)	0.002
Cardiovascular disease	68 (33)	28 (28)	39 (38)	0.14
Number of SBP readings	23.9±2.6	24.0±2.9	23.8±2.3	0.59
Mean SBP (mmHg)	144±16	145±16	144±17	0.78
Mean DBP (mmHg)	75±10	75±11	74±9	0.31
Blood pressure medications at 3 months:				
ACE-I or ARB	69 (34)	31 (31)	38 (37)	0.61
CCB	92 (45)	44 (44)	48(47)	0.90
β-blocker	71 (35)	31 (31)	40 (39)	0.43
Other	109 (54)	46 (46)	63 (61)	0.03
Mean number of agents	2.0±1.3	1.9±1.3	2.2±1.3	0.17
Dialysis access at 3 months:				
Arteriovenous fistula	88 (43)	44 (44)	44 (43)	0.85
Venous catheter	115 (57)	56 (56)	59 (57)	
Interdialytic weight gain (kg)	1.10±0.97	1.04±1.06	1.17±0.87	0.05

Values are expressed as mean ± SD or n (%). ACE-I - Angiotensin Converting Enzyme Inhibitor; ARB - Angiotensin receptor blocker; CCB –Calcium channel blocker, Other – Alpha-blocker, Nitrate, Diuretic, Aldosterone antagonist.

*Mann-Whitney U tests and chi-squared tests were used to compute p-values for continuous and categorical variables respectively.

Table 2. Hazard ratios for one unit increase in measures of systolic BP variability and other covariates from fully adjusted model.

	SD	COV	VIM
	Hazard Ratio (95% CI)	**Hazard Ratio (95% CI)**	**Hazard Ratio (95% CI)**
BP Variability	1.08	1.13	1.09
	(1.01, 1.16)	(1.02, 1.24)	(1.02, 1.16)
Age	1.03	1.03	1.03
	(0.99, 1.06)	(0.99, 1.06)	(0.99, 1.06)
Sex	1.36	1.35	1.35
	(0.65,2.83)	(0.65,2.81)	(0.65,2.82)
Cardiovascular disease	0.91	0.92	0.92
	(0.44,1.90)	(0.44, 1.93)	(0.44, 1.92)
Diabetes	1.33	1.33	1.33
	(0.63,2.81)	(0.63,2.82)	(0.63,2.82)
Mean SBP	0.99	0.99	0.99
	(0.97,1.01)	(0.98, 1.02)	(0.98, 1.02)

SD – standard deviation; COV – coefficient of variation; VIM – Variation independent of the mean; SBP – Systolic blood pressure.

access, the use of antihypertensives, number of antihypertensives used or mean weight change during dialysis sessions (tables S1–S4). In an analysis including the variability of weight change between dialysis sessions (likely to reflect variability of fluid intake) this parameter is also associated with all-cause mortality but does not attenuate the relationship between BP variability and mortality (table S5).

Inclusion of mean diastolic BP in the fully adjusted models made no important difference to the association between any measure of intraindividual visit-to-visit SBP variability and mortality (data not shown).

Intraindividual visit-to-visit diastolic blood pressure variability. Measures of intraindividual visit-to-visit diastolic BP variability were not associated with mortality in univariate or multivariate analyses. The age and sex adjusted HR for a one-unit increase in VIM of DBP is 1.02 [95% CI 0.91, 1.14].

Discussion

Our study shows that intraindividual visit-to-visit variability of systolic BP is associated with all-cause mortality in incident haemodialysis patients, independently of confounders such as age, cardiovascular disease and diabetes. This is seen across measures of BP variability including VIM, which importantly is not correlated with systolic BP. The association between mortality and intraindividual visit-to-visit BP variability is not explained by the type of dialysis access, the use of antihypertensives, absolute fluid intake or variability in fluid intake.

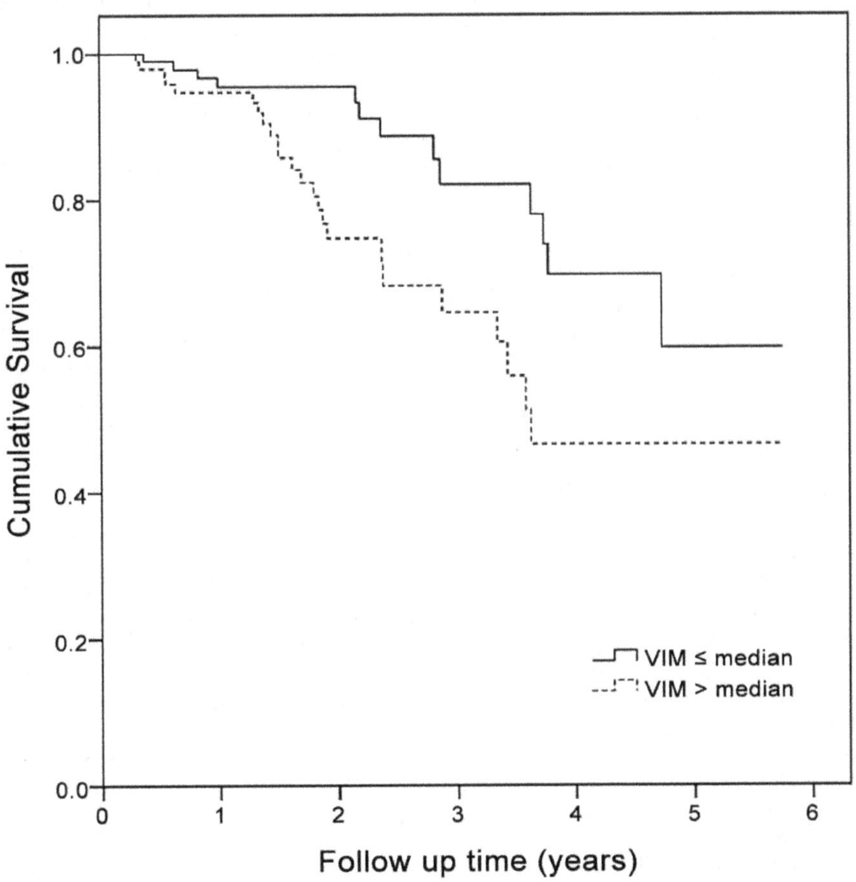

Figure 1. Mortality for patients with high versus low variability of systolic blood pressure.

This study has a number of strengths. Duration of haemodialysis is associated with aortic stiffening and autonomic neuropathy, and thus previous renal replacement therapy may be associated with increased BP variability in prevalent cohorts [12,13]. Therefore, demonstrating these results in a cohort of only incident haemodialysis patients provides greater evidence that this association may be important. We measured intraindividual visit-to-visit BP variability only after 90 days of dialysis, avoiding the early period which may be complicated by acute illness, changes in medications and unstable fluid balance. We only included measurement of pre-dialysis systolic BP taken after the two-day gap to minimize the potential confounding effect of poor compliance with fluid restriction. In addition, we included readings of BP over a prolonged period with very complete data and analyzed the results using three different measures of BP variability. Reverse causality was minimized by excluding patients who had cardiovascular events during measurement of BP variability. This cohort is reasonably large with over two years of follow-up on average and includes all eligible patients in standard clinical care.

However, there are also important limitations. We were not able to adjust for a number of potential cardiovascular risk factors such as smoking, body mass index and cholesterol, as these data were not available. However, among patients with ESRD, the relationship between classic risk factors and risk of adverse events is often weak or reversed and these data may not have affected our findings [14]. We retrospectively analysed routine clinical measurements of blood pressure where technique was as per routine unit practice and not standardized as part of a clinical study protocol. However, it is not clear that use of clinical blood pressure measurements would have led to systematic misclassification of blood pressure variability. Since random measurement error is likely to bias findings to the null, we may have underestimated the strength of the association between BP variability and mortality. Use of routine measurements in an unselected population also means that these results are likely to be generalizable across the United Kingdom and in other countries with similar dialysis schedules and patient populations. In addition, there is potential for selection bias in our findings as follow up was censored when patients received a kidney transplant or transferred to peritoneal dialysis. These people are likely to be healthier, and may have lower BP variability. However, this represents less than 15% of the initial cohort and there was no other loss-to follow-up. Finally, we were not able to examine cause-specific mortality which might have provided greater etiological insight.

Mortality in haemodialysis patients is markedly higher than in the general population and cardiovascular disease is the main cause of death [1]. Conventional measures of BP are linearly associated with cardiovascular risk in the general population [15]. However, among patients undergoing haemodialysis, many studies demonstrate a non-linear relationship between mean BP and mortality [2]. In this group there is increasing evidence that BP variability may be more closely associated with adverse outcomes than conventional measures of BP. Patients with ESRD have greater visit to visit BP variability compared to the general population [5]. Tozawa et al showed that systolic BP variability, quantified by coefficient of variation, predicted all-cause but not cardiovascular mortality in a cohort of 144 Japanese dialysis patients [10]. However, this study was limited by a small number of deaths during the study period (n = 13). A further study by Rossignol and colleagues examined the role of BP variability in a cohort of 397 haemodialysis patients with left ventricular hypertrophy enrolled in an interventional study [16]. They showed that visit-to-visit systolic and diastolic BP variability was associated with a composite end-point of cardiovascular events during follow-up while baseline SBP and DBP were not. A recent study by Chang et al in a cohort of 1844 haemodialysis patients from the HEMO study showed that visit-to-visit SBP variability, quantified by coefficient of variation and average real variability, predicted all-cause and cardiovascular mortality [6]. All three of these studies were limited by inclusion of prevalent haemodialysis patients. Only one study has demonstrated an association between pre-dialysis systolic and diastolic BP variability and all-cause mortality in an incident dialysis cohort [11]. However this study was limited by an extremely short-follow-up (6 months) meaning that reverse causality was a strong potential explanation of their findings. BP variability during haemodialysis has also been associated with all-cause and cardiovascular mortality, as has changing pre-dialysis systolic and diastolic BP over time [17–19]. While examining slightly different hypotheses, it is likely that they reflect similar underlying pathophysiology to studies of pre-dialysis systolic BP variability.

The mechanisms that contribute to increased BP variability in patients with ESRD are complex and poorly understood. They include changes in intravascular volume and vasoactive factors (angiotensin 2, endothelin, nitric oxide), reduced arterial compliance, increased sympathetic innervation and alterations of arterial and cardiopulmonary reflexes [20]. Poor or variable compliance with fluid restriction and antihypertensive therapy could also contribute to BP fluctuations. Whether increased BP variability is causal in cardiovascular events and mortality, or whether it is a marker of vascular disease and autonomic dysfunction, is still subject to debate. Strong arguments have been made for changes in BP as a direct mechanism of event causation in cohorts without CKD [4]. The increased BP variability seen in patients with ESRD as well as the high incidence of outcomes plausibly linked to changes in BP such as dementia due to cerebral small vessel disease, hemorrhagic stroke and sudden cardiac death suggest that changes in BP may directly trigger events among dialysis patients. This is important as the use of antihypertensive drugs associated with reduced BP variability are also associated with reduced incidence of stroke [21]. Evidence for improved outcomes with therapeutic regimes targeted to reduce BP variability and prospective data on the effects of different classes of antihypertensives on BP variability in ESRD are still lacking. However, the growing evidence of a link between BP variability and adverse outcomes among haemodialysis patients raises the hope that future strategies to reduce BP fluctuations may be able to improve outcomes for this vulnerable group of patients.

Conclusions

In summary, this study shows that in standard care, variability of systolic BP from clinical measurements is a strong and independent predictor of all-cause mortality in incident HD patients, even after adjustments for factors such as age, cardiovascular disease and diabetes. This effect is consistent across different measures of BP variability, including VIM, which avoids the confounding effect of average BP. Further research is needed to understand the mechanism as this may form an important therapeutic target or focus for management in this group.

Supporting Information

Table S1 Results of fully adjusted model for analysis examining the effect of type of dialysis access on relationship between VIM and mortality.

Table S2 Results of fully adjusted model for analysis examining the effect of antihypertensive use on relationship between VIM and mortality.

Table S3 Results of fully adjusted model for analysis examining the effect of number of antihypertensives on relationship between VIM and mortality.

Table S4 Results of fully adjusted model for analysis examining the effect of mean intradialytic weight change (kg) on relationship between VIM and mortality.

Table S5 Results of fully adjusted model for analysis examining the effect of interdialytic weight variability on relationship between VIM and mortality.

Acknowledgments

Disclaimer: The results presented in this paper have not been published previously in whole or part, except in abstract format.

Author Contributions

Conceived and designed the experiments: VS LT IBW SO. Analyzed the data: VS LP LT. Wrote the paper: VS LP SO IBW LT.

References

1. Parfrey PS, Foley RN (1999) The Clinical Epidemiology of Cardiac Disease in Chronic Renal Failure. Journal of the American Society of Nephrology 10: 1606–1615.
2. Chang TI (2011) Systolic blood pressure and mortality in patients on hemodialysis. Curr Hypertens Rep 13: 362–369.
3. Rothwell PM, Howard SC, Dolan E, O'Brien E, Dobson JE, et al. (2010) Prognostic significance of visit-to-visit variability, maximum systolic blood pressure, and episodic hypertension. The Lancet 375: 895–905.
4. Rothwell PM (2010) Limitations of the usual blood-pressure hypothesis and importance of variability, instability, and episodic hypertension. The Lancet 375: 938–948.
5. Rohrscheib RM, Myers OB, Servilla KS, Adams CD, DD M, et al. (2008) Age-related Blood Pressure Patterns and Blood Pressure Variability among Hemodialysis Patients. Clinical Journal of the American Society of Nephrology 3: 1407–1414.
6. Chang TI, Flythe JE, Brunelli SM, Muntner P, Greene T, et al. (2013) Visit-to-visit systolic blood pressure variability and outcomes in hemodialysis. J Hum Hypertens: 1–7. doi:10.1038/jhh.2013.49.
7. Lacy P, Carr SJ, O'Brien D, Fentum B, Williams B, et al. (2006) Reduced glomerular filtration rate in pre-dialysis non-diabetic chronic kidney disease patients is associated with impaired baroreceptor sensitivity and reduced vascular compliance. Clinical Science 110: 101–108.
8. Wang AYM, Lam CWK, Chan IHS, Wang M, Lui SF, et al. (2010) Sudden Cardiac Death in End-Stage Renal Disease Patients: A 5-Year Prospective Analysis. Hypertension 56: 210–216.
9. Mallamaci F, Tripepi G (2013) Blood pressure variability in chronic kidney disease patients. Blood Purif 36: 58–62.
10. Tozawa M, Iseki K, Yoshi S, Fukiyama K (1999) Blood pressure variability as an adverse prognostic risk factor in end-stage renal disease. Nephrology Dialysis Transplantation 14: 1976–1981.
11. Brunelli SM, Thadhani RI, Lynch KE, Ankers ED, Joffe MM, et al. (2008) Association between long-term blood pressure variability and mortality among incident hemodialysis patients. Am J Kidney Dis 52: 716–726.
12. Vita G, Bellinghieri G, Trusso A, Costantino G, Santoro D, et al. (1999) Uremic autonomic neuropathy studied by spectral analysis of heart rate. Kidney International 56: 232–237.
13. Blacher J, Guerin AP, Pannier B, Marchais SJ, London GM (2001) Arterial Calcifications, Arterial Stiffness, and Cardiovascular Risk in End-Stage Renal Disease. Hypertension 38: 938–942.
14. Baigent C, Landray MJ, Wheeler DC (2007) Misleading associations between cholesterol and vascular outcomes in dialysis patients: the need for randomized trials. Seminars in Dialysis 20: 498–503.
15. Lewington S, Clarke R, Qizilbash N, Peto R, Collins R, et al. (2002) Age-specific relevance of usual blood pressure to vascular mortality: a meta-analysis of individual data for one million adults in 61 prospective studies. Lancet 360: 1903–1913.
16. Rossignol P, Cridlig J, Lehert P, Kessler M, Zannad F (2012) Visit-to-visit blood pressure variability is a strong predictor of cardiovascular events in hemodialysis: insights from FOSIDIAL. Hypertension 60: 339–346.
17. Flythe JE, Inrig JK, Shafi T, Chang TI, Cape K, et al. (2013) Association of Intradialytic Blood Pressure Variability With Increased All-Cause and Cardiovascular Mortality in Patients Treated With Long-term Hemodialysis. AJKD: 1–9.
18. Di Iorio B, Di Micco L, Torraca S, Sirico ML, Guastaferro P, et al. (2013) Variability of blood pressure in dialysis patients: a new marker of cardiovascular risk. J Nephrol 26: 173–182.
19. Raimann JG, Usvyat LA, Thijssen S, Kotanko P, Rogus J, et al. (2012) Blood pressure stability in hemodialysis patients confers a survival advantage: results from a large retrospective cohort study. Kidney International 81: 548–558.
20. Parati G, Ochoa JE, Bilo G (2012) Blood pressure variability, cardiovascular risk, and risk for renal disease progression. Curr Hypertens Rep 14: 421–431.
21. Webb AJS, Fischer U, Mehta Z, Rothwell PM (2010) Effects of antihypertensive-drug class on interindividual variation in blood pressure and risk of stroke: a systematic review and meta-analysis. Lancet 375: 906–915.

Effectiveness of Influenza Vaccination in Patients with End-Stage Renal Disease Receiving Hemodialysis

I-Kuan Wang[1,2,3], Cheng-Li Lin[4,5], Po-Chang Lin[6], Chih-Chia Liang[2], Yao-Lung Liu[2], Chiz-Tzung Chang[2], Tzung-Hai Yen[7], Donald E. Morisky[8], Chiu-Ching Huang[2]*, Fung-Chang Sung[4,5]*

1 Graduate Institute of Clinical Medical Science, China Medical University College of Medicine, Taichung, Taiwan, **2** Division of Nephrology, China Medical University Hospital, Taichung, Taiwan, **3** Department of Internal Medicine, China Medical University College of Medicine, Taichung, Taiwan, **4** Management Office for Health Data, China Medical University Hospital, Taichung, Taiwan, **5** Department of Public Health, China Medical University, Taichung, Taiwan, **6** Division of Infection, China Medical University Hospital, Taichung, Taiwan, **7** Division of Nephrology, Chang Gung Memorial Hospital, Taipei and Chang Gung Univeristy College of Medicine, Taoyuan, Taiwan, **8** UCLA Fielding School of Public Health, Los Angeles, California, United States of America

Abstract

Background: Little is known on the effectiveness of influenza vaccine in ESRD patients. This study compared the incidence of hospitalization, morbidity, and mortality in end-stage renal disease (ESRD) patients undergoing hemodialysis (HD) between cohorts with and without influenza vaccination.

Methods: We used the insurance claims data from 1998 to 2009 in Taiwan to determine the incidence of these events within one year after influenza vaccination in the vaccine (N = 831) and the non-vaccine (N = 3187) cohorts. The vaccine cohort to the non-vaccine cohort incidence rate ratio and hazard ratio (HR) of morbidities and mortality were measured.

Results: The age-specific analysis showed that the elderly in the vaccine cohort had lower hospitalization rate (100.8 vs. 133.9 per 100 person-years), contributing to an overall HR of 0.81 (95% confidence interval (CI) 0.72–0.90). The vaccine cohort also had an adjusted HR of 0.85 [95% CI 0.75–0.96] for heart disease. The corresponding incidence of pneumonia and influenza was 22.4 versus 17.2 per 100 person-years, but with an adjusted HR of 0.80 (95% CI 0.64–1.02). The vaccine cohort had lowered risks than the non-vaccine cohort for intensive care unit (ICU) admission (adjusted HR 0.20, 95% CI 0.12–0.33) and mortality (adjusted HR 0.50, 95% CI 0.41–0.60). The time-dependent Cox model revealed an overall adjusted HR for mortality of 0.30 (95% CI 0.26–0.35) after counting vaccination for multi-years.

Conclusions: ESRD patients with HD receiving the influenza vaccination could have reduced risks of pneumonia/influenza and other morbidities, ICU stay, hospitalization and death, particularly for the elderly.

Editor: Li-Min Huang, National Taiwan University Hospital, Taiwan

Funding: Executive Yuan National Science Council (grant number NSC 100-2621-M-039 -001), the Department of Health (grant numbers DOH101-TD-B- 111-004 and DOH101-TD-C-111-005) and the China Medical University Hospital (grant number 1MS1). The funders had no role in study design, data collection and analysis, decision to publish, or preparation of the manuscript.

Competing Interests: The authors have declared that no competing interests exist.

* E-mail: fcsung1008@yahoo.com (F-CS); cch@mail.cmuh.org.tw (C-CH)

Introduction

The influenza virus is a common transmissible human respiratory virus that causes significant morbidity and mortality. In the Unites States, influenza can cause hospitalizations of more than 225,000 patients and 36,000 deaths annually [1,2]. The morbidity and mortality of influenza are increased in people of old ages, immunocompromised patients, and those with chronic diseases [3]. Patients with end-stage renal disease (ESRD) are also at increased risk of influenza complications [4]. Infection is the second leading cause of mortality and a major cause of morbidity in ESRD patients [5]. In addition, mortality rate related to pulmonary infection is likely 10-fold higher in ESRD patients than in the general population [6]. Immune dysfunction, older age, and comorbid conditions, such as diabetes mellitus, malnutrition, invasive dialysis procedures, disruption of skin and mucosa barriers, and nosocomial transmission, contribute to the high infection risk for ESRD patients [4,7]. The causes of immune dysfunction in ESRD patients include diminished functions in complement activation, neutrophil, monocyte/macrophage, T-cell, and B-cell [8].

Observation studies have reported that influenza vaccination can reduce the risk of deaths and hospitalizations among elderly and high-risk populations [9,10]. Thus, annual influenza vaccination for ESRD patients is recommended [11]. However, little is known on the effectiveness of influenza vaccine in ESRD patients. Observation studies showed conflicting results.[12,13,14,15,16] The present study aims to investigate the effectiveness of influenza vaccination in reducing morbidity and mortality for ESRD patients receiving hemodialysis (HD) using population-based universal insurance data, derived from the Taiwan National Health Insurance (NHI) program.

Materials and Methods

Data Sources

The Taiwan NHI was integrated from 13 insurance programs in 1995 in Taiwan. This insurance program has covered approximately 99% of the entire 23.74 million people in Taiwan since 1999 [17]. The Taiwan Bureau of National Health Insurance had authorized the National Health Research Institutes (NHRI) to manage reimbursement claims from hospitals and clinics. A committee at the Bureau of National Health Insurance was responsible to randomly select claims and to check the accuracy of claims. NHRI also had been authorized to established data sets for administrative and research uses. We obtained a sub-dataset with one million of population from NHRI for this study. This subset data is similar to the whole population in the distributions in gender and age. The claims data included information on demographic status, date and source of diagnosis, ambulatory care, outpatient and inpatient treatment, dental services, and physicians providing services. Claims data were randomly audited by the insurance system. Data files are linked with scrambled patient identification number to protect the privacy of the patients. The International Classification of Disease, 9th Revision, Clinical Modification (ICD-9-CM) was used to identify individual health status. This study was approved by the Institutional Review Board of China Medical University.

Study Subjects

We identified patients with ESRD newly diagnosed in 1998–2009 yearly from the sub-dataset with one million insured people. The patients who had completed the seasonal influenza vaccination (ICD-9-CM V04.7 and V04.8) were designated in the vaccine cohort, with the date of vaccination defined as the index date for measuring the follow-up period. The patients who received pneumococcal vaccine were excluded (N = 75). Newly diagnosed HD patients without both influenza and pneumococcal vaccinations were also identified annually as the non-vaccine cohort. The corresponding non-vaccine cohort was selected randomly from the same month of the index year.

Outcome Measures

Both cohorts were followed up since the index date for one year or until selected events, death, or withdrawal from the insurance. We were interested in outcome events of total hospitalization, pneumonia or influenza (ICD-9-CM codes 480-487), hospitalization for septicemia, bacteremia, or viremia (ICD-9-CM codes 038.x, 790.7, and 790.8), hospitalization for heart disease (ICD-9-CM codes 401–429), respiratory failure (ICD-9-M codes 518.81, 518.82, 518.83, 518.84, 799.1), or intensive care unit (ICU) admission or death. The history of coronary artery disease (ICD-9-CM codes 410–413, 414.01–414.05, 414.8, and 414.9), congestive heart failure (ICD-9-CM codes 428, 398.91, 402.x1), cancer (ICD-9-CM codes 140–149, 150–159, 160–165, 170–175, 179–189, 190–199, 200, 202, 203, 210–213, 215– 229, 235–239, 654.1, 654.10, 654.11, 654.12, 654.13, 654.14), hyperlipidemia (ICD-9-CM codes 272), hypertension (ICD-9-CM codes 401–405), diabetes (ICD-9-CM codes 250), atrial fibrillation (ICD-9-CM codes 427.31), stroke (ICD-9-CM codes 430–438), chronic hepatitis (ICD-9-CM codes 571, 572.2, 572.3, 572.8, 573.1, 573.2, 573.3, 573.8, 573.9), and chronic obstructive pulmonary disease (ICD-9-CM codes490, 491– 495, 496) were identified as comorbidities before the index date.

Statistical Analysis

Proportion of annual influenza vaccination in HD patients was measured chronologically from 1998–2009. Demographic characteristics of HD patients and prevalence of comorbidities were compared between the vaccine and non-vaccine cohorts, and tested using Chi-square test for categorical variables and t-test for continuous variables. Incidence rates for hospitalization events, infections (pneumonia/influenza, septicemia, bacteremia and viremia), heart disease, respiratory failure, intensive care unit (ICU) admission, and mortality were estimated for each cohort. The vaccine to non-vaccine cohort incidence rate ratio (IRR) and 95% confidence interval (CI) were estimated using Poisson regression. Cox proportional hazards regression model was also used to estimate the hazard ratio (HR) for each of these events and the corresponding 95% CI, within one year after the vaccination. The Cox proportional hazards regression model were also used to estimate pneumonia/influenza-free rates, controlling for age, sex, hyperlipidemia, hypertension, congestive heart failure, chronic hepatitis, chronic obstructive pulmonary disease and calendar year. Similarly, the probability free of respiratory failure, ICU admission, and mortality were plotted using the Cox proportional hazards regression model. The influenza vaccination changed annually, we used the time-dependent Cox model to further evaluate the mortality risk related to the vaccination for multiple years. SAS version 9.1 (SAS Institute, Cary, NC, USA) was used for data analyses; $p < 0.05$ was considered to indicate statistical significance.

Results

From 1998 to 2009, new patients receiving HD increased annually from 264 cases in 1998 to a peak of 368 cases in 2007, and then declined to 347 cases in 2009 (Table 1). The proportion of patients receiving influenza vaccine increased from 1.14% to a peak of 38.0% in 2009. A total of 29 patients received both seasonal influenza and influenza A (H1N1) vaccines in 2009. A total of 103 patients received seasonal influenza vaccination only (data not shown). Overall, 831 patients were in the influenza vaccine cohort, which comprised less portion of women than 3187 patients in the non-vaccine comparison cohort (Table 2). The

Table 1. Proportion of annual influenza vaccination in hemodialysis patients.

	Influenza vaccine			
Year	N	Yes	No	Proportion (%)
1998	264	3	261	1.14
1999	270	16	254	5.93
2000	313	50	263	15.97
2001	315	48	267	15.24
2002	335	80	255	23.88
2003	361	90	271	24.93
2004	363	78	285	21.49
2005	397	89	308	22.42
2006	355	90	265	25.35
2007	368	70	298	19.02
2008	330	85	245	25.76
2009	347	132	215	38.04

Table 2. Demographic status and comorbidity at baseline in hemodialysis patients with and without influenza vaccination.

	Influenza vaccine		p-value
	Yes (n = 831)	No (n = 3187)	
Age, mean ± SD	70.2±9.96	59.4±14.5	<0.0001#
Stratify age			
18–39	8(0.96)	284(8.91)	<0.0001
40–64	127(15.3)	1714(53.8)	
65+	696(83.8)	1189(37.3)	
Gender			
Women	413(49.7)	1635(51.3)	0.41
Men	418(50.3)	1552(48.7)	
Comorbidity			
CAD	401(48.3)	997(31.3)	<0.0001
CHF	253(30.5)	672(21.1)	<0.0001
Cancer	82(9.87)	236(7.41)	0.02
Hyperlipidemia	466(56.1)	1342(42.1)	<0.0001
Hypertension	776(93.4)	2795(87.7)	<0.0001
Diabetes	552(66.4)	1694(53.2)	<0.0001
Atrial fibrillation	26(3.13)	67(2.10)	0.08
Chronic hepatitis	323(38.9)	874(27.4)	<0.0001
COPD	356(42.8)	917(28.8)	<0.0001

Abbreviations: CAD, coronary artery disease; CHF, congestive heart failure; COPD; chronic obstructive pulmonary disease
Chi-square test; #: Two-sample t-test

vaccine cohort mainly included the elderly, with the mean age much higher than that of the non-vaccine cohort (70.2± 9.96 vs. 59.4±14.5 years). The vaccine cohort also tended to be more prevalent with comorbidities. There was no patient who received transplantation or was shifted to peritoneal dialysis during the follow-up period.

The analysis for age-specific hospitalization shows that most of patients hospitalized were the elderly (≥ 65 years) (Table 3). The overall crude hospitalization rate was 11.0% higher in the vaccine cohort than in the non-vaccine cohort (99.4 vs. 89.4 per 100 person-years). However, the vaccine cohort had an adjusted HR of 0.81(95% CI = 0.72–0.90) after controlling for sex, age, coronary artery disease; congestive heart failure; chronic obstructive pulmonary disease, cancer, stroke, and calendar year. The elderly with vaccination had significant lower rate than those without (100.8 vs. 133.9 per 100 person-years), with an adjusted IRR of 0.73 (95% CI 0.64–0.82).

Table 4 shows that the incidence of heart disease, the major cause of hospitalization, was higher in the vaccine cohort than in the non-vaccine cohort (65.3 vs. 51.7 per 100 person-years). However, the adjusted HR of the vaccine cohort was 0.85 (95% CI 0.75–0.96). The incidence rates of pneumonia/influenza, hospitalization for septicemia/bacteremia/viremia, and respiratory failure were also higher in the vaccine cohort than in the non-vaccine cohort. However, adjusted HRs also demonstrated protective association from the vaccination. Compared with the patients in the non-vaccine cohort, those in the vaccine cohort were less likely to be admitted in the ICU [2.6 vs. 6.8 per 100 person-years; adjusted HR 0.2 (95% CI 0.12–0.33)] and to be deceased [18.5 vs. 21.0 per 100 person-years; adjusted HR 0.50 (95% CI 0.41–0.60)].

The evaluation for only the elderly also showed that those with vaccination were at lower risks of pneumonia/influenza, hospitalization for septicemia/bacteremia/viremia, and heart disease, ICU admission, respiratory failure, and death (data not shown). The time-dependent Cox model revealed that the overall adjusted HR for mortality associated with the vaccination reduced to 0.30 (95% CI 0.26–0.35), compared with non-vaccinated persons (Table 5).

Figures 1A trough ID show that, compared with the non-vaccine cohort, the vaccine cohort had significantly lower rates of pneumonia/influenza (*P*-value = 0.02) (Figure 1A), respiratory failure (*P*-value <0.0001) (Figure 1B), ICU stay (Figure 1C) (*P*-value <0.0001), and mortality (Figure 1D) (*P*-value <0.0001).

Discussion

Our study demonstrated that influenza vaccination for ESRD patients receiving HD was associated with lower morbidities, including total hospitalization, ICU admission, pneumonia/influenza, septicemia/bacteremia/viremia, respiratory failure, and heart disease. In addition, influenza vaccination was also associated with lower all-cause mortality risk for 50%. The mortality risk decreased further to have an overall adjusted HR of 0.30 as subjects with vaccinations for multiple years were counted. Consistent with the present study, a previous research in the US reported that the risks of hospitalization and death for HD patients vaccinated against influenza are lower than those of unvaccinated patients, with odds ratios of 0.93 (95% 0.90–0.95) and 0.77 (0.73–

Table 3. Comparison in hospitalization rates between hemodialysis patients with and without influenza vaccination.

	Vaccine			Non-vaccine					
Outcome	Event	PY	Rate#	Event	PY	Rate#	IRR*(95% CI)	Adjusted IRR(95% CI)	Adjusted HR (95% CI)
Total Hospitalization	459	462	99.4	1688	1888	89.4	1.11(0.96, 1.28)	0.80(0.69, 0.94)	0.82(0.73, 0.91)
Age, years									
18–39	1	5	20	113	205	55.1	0.40(0.03, 5.54)	0.36(0.03, 4.76)	0.36(0.05, 2.62)
40–64	59	62	95.2	820	1118	73.3	1.31(0.92, 1.86)	1.22(0.86, 1.74)	1.16(0.89, 1.52)
65+	399	396	100.8	755	564	133.9	0.75(0.64, 0.89)	0.70(0.59, 0.82)	0.73(0.64, 0.82)

Rate#, incidence rate, per 100 person-years; IRR*, incidence rate ratio;
HR, hazard ratio adjusted for sex, age, coronary artery disease; congestive heart failure; chronic obstructive pulmonary disease, cancer, stroke, and calendar year

Table 4. Hospitalization, intensive care unit utilization, and mortality comparison between hemodialysis patients with and without influenza vaccination.

	Vaccine			Non-vaccine					
Outcome	Event	PY	Rate#	Event	PY	Rate#	IRR*(95% CI)	Adjusted IRR (95% CI)	Adjusted HR (95% CI)
Pneumonia/influenza†	139	620	22.4	445	2584	17.2	1.30(1.08, 1.56)	0.77(0.64, 0.93)	0.78(0.64, 0.96)
Septicemia, bacteremia, and viremia†	103	637	16.2	347	2661	13.0	1.24(1.02, 1.50)	0.66(0.47, 0.92)	0.72(0.56, 0.88)
Heart disease†	341	522	65.3	1138	2203	51.7	1.26(1.08, 1.47)	0.83(0.71, 0.97)	0.85(0.75, 0.96)
Respiratory Failure†	66	653	10.1	262	2697	9.7	1.04(0.84, 1.29)	0.52(0.42, 0.64)	0.53(0.41, 0.70)
Intensive care unit admission†	17	660	2.6	184	2696	6.8	0.38(0.27, 0.53)	0.19(0.14, 0.27)	0.20(0.12, 0.33)
Mortality†	123	665	18.5	581	2765	21.0	0.88(0.73, 1.07)	0.49(0.41, 0.59)	0.50(0.41, 0.60)

Rate#, incidence rate, per 100 person-years; IRR*, incidence rate ratio
Hospitalization†: adjusted for age, CAD, CHF, cancer, COPD, stroke, and calendar year
Hospitalization for pneumonia/influenza†: adjusted for age, sex, CAD, CHF, cancer, diabetes, atrial fibrillation, COPD, and calendar year
Hospitalization for septicemia, bacteremia, and viremia†: adjusted for age, cancer, diabetes, atrial fibrillation, and calendar year
Hospitalization for heart disease†: adjusted for age, CAD, CHF, hypertension, diabetes, atrial fibrillation, chronic hepatitis, and calendar year
Respiratory Failure†: adjusted for age, sex, CAD, cancer, CHF, diabetes, hypertension, chronic hepatitis, and calendar year
Intensive care unit†: adjusted for age, cancer, hyperlipidemia, hypertension, diabetes, atrial fibrillation, chronic hepatitis, and calendar year
Mortality†: adjusted for age, sex, CAD, cancer, CHF, diabetes, hyperlipidemia, hypertension, chronic hepatitis, atrial fibrillation, COPD, and calendar year

0.81), respectively [14]. Moreover, they found that vaccination was significantly associated with lower risks of cause-specific mortality, including cardiac and infectious deaths. Recent reports demonstrated that influenza vaccination was associated with a lower mortality risk [12,13]. The mortality hazard was reduced further for patients receiving both pneumococcal and influenza vaccinations. On the contrary, McGrath et al. recently reported little clinical benefits of influenza vaccination on preventing hospitalization and death [16]. However, their study did not consider the confounding effect of pneumococcal vaccination. Therefore, our study observed closely the effectiveness of influenza vaccination, by excluding the effect of pneumococcal vaccine. In addition, these studies analyzed prevalent ESRD patients. Length of time with ESRD may have confounding effect on the outcomes.

Compared with healthy control subjects, ESRD patients possess suboptimal immune response rates but develop satisfying protection rates to influenza vaccination [18,19,20,21,22]. The antibody response rates to influenza vaccination (defined as a four-fold increase in hemagglutination inhibition titers) vary from 7% to 89% [18,19,20,21,22]. The seroprotection rates (defined as hemagglutination inhibition titers≥40) range from 46% to 93%, depending on the specific strain measured [18,19,20,21,22]. Booster vaccination fails to improve the immune response [20,21,23]. Influenza vaccination is safe without causing major adverse effects in HD patients [20,23], and the number of minor adverse reactions is low [20].

Table 5. Time-dependent Cox model estimated hazard ratios and 95% confidence intervals of mortality risk associated with the vaccination.

	Hazard ratio(95% CI)	
	Crude	Adjusted†
Vaccination	0.47(0.41, 0.55)	0.30(0.26, 0.35)

Adjusted HRs†: adjusted for age, sex, CHF, diabetes, hyperlipidemia, hypertension, chronic hepatitis, and atrial fibrillation

Since 1998, the Taiwan NHI program has started to offer influenza vaccinations to high-risk subjects, including ESRD patients and the elderly subjects. Majority of the vaccinated subjects receive this service annually between October 1 and December 31. However, the influenza vaccination rate in this study was low for incident HD patients, especially in the beginning years (1998 and 1999). The higher vaccination rate in 2009 was likely due to the pandemic novel influenza A (H1N1) in April 2009 [24]. The low vaccination rate may be attributed to the lack of awareness on its benefit, fear of adverse reactions, and lack of physician recommendation [25]. The goal of the World Health Organization is to increase the annual influenza vaccination rate to 90% by 2010 for ESRD patients.

Influenza may lead to viral pneumonia and bacterial superinfection. HD patients are susceptible to pulmonary infection. Transient hypoxemia occurs during dialysis because of leukocyte migration in the pulmonary vasculature and loss of carbon dioxide [6]. In addition, HD patients are exposed to other patients and medical staff. Our study demonstrated that influenza vaccination was associated with a lower risk of pneumonia/influenza during the first 3 months after vaccination (data not shown). Seroprotection was maintained at least for 3 months and up to 6 months after influenza vaccination in patients with renal diseases [26].

Consistent with the findings of the present study, Gilbertson reported that influenza vaccination is associated with a lower risk of heart disease in ESRD patients [14]. For patients with chronic kidney disease, an association between influenza vaccination and atherosclerotic heart disease event rates also exists [27]. Systemic inflammation caused by influenza infection may lead to endothelial injury, impaired vasodilatation, and enhanced thrombosis formation [28]. Inflammation is highly associated with increasing cardiovascular mortality [29,30].

The current study has several limitations. First, the NHI database provided limited information on socio-demographic characteristics, with unavailable information on marital status, educational level, smoking habit, body-mass index, and laboratory

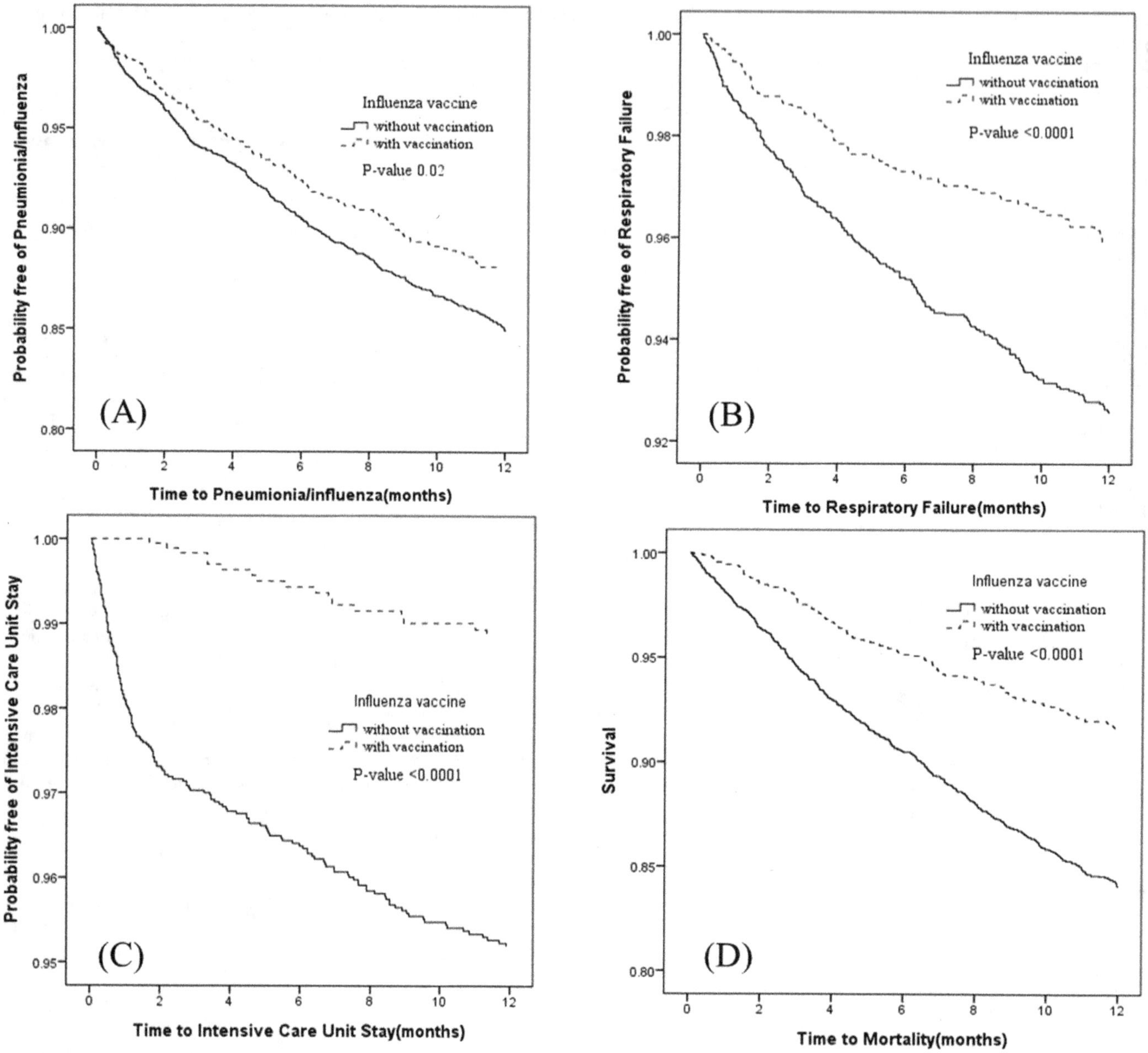

Figure 1. The probability free of pneumonia/influenza, respiratory failure, intensive care unit stay, and mortality for hemodialysis patients with (dashed line) or without (solid line) influenza vaccination.

data, such as hemoglobin, albumin, and residual renal function. These variables cannot be adjusted in the analysis. Furthermore, certain information on chronic conditions, such as hyperlipidemia and hypertension, were not available for some individuals. However, HD patients were visited by health care professionals frequently, the claim data were reliable. Moreover, the decision to receive vaccination may have been affected by socioeconomic status, as well as availability of health care and medical providers. Although multivariate analysis was used, selection bias may occur. Fourth, this study focused only on all-cause mortality because the cause of death cannot be obtained from the database. Finally, the strain and virulence of the predominant virus and the match between the circulating virus strain and the virus strain selected in the vaccine varied from year to year. Therefore, we adjusted the calendar year for temporal effect.

Conclusions

Our study provides evidence that influenza vaccination is associated with the reduction of mortality and morbidity in HD patients. Thus, HD patients should be vaccinated annually. More large-scale prospective studies are necessary to analyze the issue.

Author Contributions

Conceived and designed the experiments: IKW CLL PCL CCL YLL CTC THY. Analyzed the data: CLL. Wrote the paper: IKW CCH FCS DEM.

References

1. Thompson WW, Shay DK, Weintraub E, Brammer L, Cox N, et al. (2003) Mortality associated with influenza and respiratory syncytial virus in the United States. JAMA 289: 179–186.
2. Thompson WW, Shay DK, Weintraub E, Brammer L, Bridges CB, et al. (2004) Influenza-associated hospitalizations in the United States. JAMA 292: 1333–1340.
3. Fiore AE, Uyeki TM, Broder K, Finelli L, Euler GL, et al. (2010) Prevention and control of influenza with vaccines: recommendations of the Advisory Committee on Immunization Practices (ACIP), 2010. MMWR Recomm Rep 59: 1–62.
4. Naqvi SB, Collins AJ (2006) Infectious complications in chronic kidney disease. Adv Chronic Kidney Dis 13: 199–204.
5. Collins AJ, Foley RN, Herzog C, Chavers BM, Gilbertson D, et al. (2010) Excerpts from the US Renal Data System 2009 Annual Data Report. Am J Kidney Dis 55: S1–420, A426–427.
6. Sarnak MJ, Jaber BL (2001) Pulmonary infectious mortality among patients with end-stage renal disease. Chest 120: 1883–1887.
7. Vanholder R, Van Biesen W (2002) Incidence of infectious morbidity and mortality in dialysis patients. Blood Purif 20: 477–480.
8. Descamps-Latscha B (1993) The immune system in end-stage renal disease. Curr Opin Nephrol Hypertens 2: 883–891.
9. Hak E, Nordin J, Wei F, Mullooly J, Poblete S, et al. (2002) Influence of high-risk medical conditions on the effectiveness of influenza vaccination among elderly members of 3 large managed-care organizations. Clin Infect Dis 35: 370–377.
10. Hak E, Buskens E, van Essen GA, de Bakker DH, Grobbee DE, et al. (2005) Clinical effectiveness of influenza vaccination in persons younger than 65 years with high-risk medical conditions: the PRISMA study. Arch Intern Med 165: 274–280.
11. Johnson DW, Fleming SJ (1992) The use of vaccines in renal failure. Clin Pharmacokinet 22: 434–446.
12. Bond TC, Spaulding AC, Krisher J, McClellan W (2012) Mortality of dialysis patients according to influenza and pneumococcal vaccination status. Am J Kidney Dis 60: 959–965.
13. Gilbertson DT, Guo H, Arneson TJ, Collins AJ (2011) The association of pneumococcal vaccination with hospitalization and mortality in hemodialysis patients. Nephrol Dial Transplant 26: 2934–2939.
14. Gilbertson DT, Unruh M, McBean AM, Kausz AT, Snyder JJ, et al. (2003) Influenza vaccine delivery and effectiveness in end-stage renal disease. Kidney Int 63: 738–743.
15. McGrath LJ, Kshirsagar AV (2012) Influenza and pneumococcal vaccination in dialysis patients: merely a shot in the arm? Am J Kidney Dis 60: 890–892.
16. McGrath LJ, Kshirsagar AV, Cole SR, Wang L, Weber DJ, et al. (2012) Influenza vaccine effectiveness in patients on hemodialysis: an analysis of a natural experiment. Arch Intern Med 172: 548–554.
17. Lu JF, Hsiao WC (2003) Does universal health insurance make health care unaffordable? Lessons from Taiwan. Health Aff (Millwood) 22: 77–88.
18. Antonen JA, Hannula PM, Pyhala R, Saha HH, Ala-Houhala IO, et al. (2000) Adequate seroresponse to influenza vaccination in dialysis patients. Nephron 86: 56–61.
19. Cavdar C, Sayan M, Sifil A, Artuk C, Yilmaz N, et al. (2003) The comparison of antibody response to influenza vaccination in continuous ambulatory peritoneal dialysis, hemodialysis and renal transplantation patients. Scand J Urol Nephrol 37: 71–76.
20. Scharpe J, Peetermans WE, Vanwalleghem J, Maes B, Bammens B, et al. (2009) Immunogenicity of a standard trivalent influenza vaccine in patients on long-term hemodialysis: an open-label trial. Am J Kidney Dis 54: 77–85.
21. Song JY, Cheong HJ, Ha SH, Kee SY, Jeong HW, et al. (2006) Active influenza immunization in hemodialysis patients: comparison between single-dose and booster vaccination. Am J Nephrol 26: 206–211.
22. Vogtlander NP, Brown A, Valentijn RM, Rimmelzwaan GF, Osterhaus AD (2004) Impaired response rates, but satisfying protection rates to influenza vaccination in dialysis patients. Vaccine 22: 2199–2201.
23. Tanzi E, Amendola A, Pariani E, Zappa A, Colzani D, et al. (2007) Lack of effect of a booster dose of influenza vaccine in hemodialysis patients. J Med Virol 79: 1176–1179.
24. (2009) 2009 pandemic influenza A (H1N1) virus infections - Chicago, Illinois, April-July 2009. MMWR Morb Mortal Wkly Rep 58: 913–918.
25. Kausz A, Pahari D (2004) The value of vaccination in chronic kidney disease. Semin Dial 17: 9–11.
26. Brydak LB, Roszkowska-Blaim M, Machala M, Leszczynska B, Sieniawska M (2000) Antibody response to influenza immunization in two consecutive epidemic seasons in patients with renal diseases. Vaccine 18: 3280–3286.
27. Snyder JJ, Collins AJ (2009) Association of preventive health care with atherosclerotic heart disease and mortality in CKD. J Am Soc Nephrol 20: 1614–1622.
28. Nichol KL, Nordin J, Mullooly J, Lask R, Fillbrandt K, et al. (2003) Influenza vaccination and reduction in hospitalizations for cardiac disease and stroke among the elderly. N Engl J Med 348: 1322–1332.
29. Engstrom G, Stavenow L, Hedblad B, Lind P, Eriksson KF, et al. (2003) Inflammation-sensitive plasma proteins, diabetes, and mortality and incidence of myocardial infarction and stroke: a population-based study. Diabetes 52: 442–447.
30. Libby P (2002) Inflammation in atherosclerosis. Nature 420: 868–874.

22

Creatinine Index as a Surrogate of Lean Body Mass Derived from Urea Kt/V, Pre-Dialysis Serum Levels and Anthropometric Characteristics of Haemodialysis Patients

Bernard Canaud[1,2], Alexandre Granger Vallée[1], Nicolas Molinari[3], Leila Chenine[1,2], Hélène Leray-Moragues[1,2], Annie Rodriguez[2], Lotfi Chalabi[4], Marion Morena[2,5,6], Jean-Paul Cristol[2,5,6]*

1 Nephrology, Dialysis and Intensive Care Unit, CHRU, Montpellier, France, **2** Dialysis Research and Training Institute, Montpellier, France, **3** UMR 729 MISTEA, DIM, CHRU, Montpellier, France, **4** AIDER, Montpellier, France, **5** Biochemistry Laboratory, CHRU, Montpellier, France, **6** UMR 204, University of Montpellier I, Montpellier, France

Abstract

Background and Objectives: Protein-energy wasting is common in long-term haemodialysis (HD) patients with chronic kidney disease and is associated with increased morbidity and mortality. The creatinine index (CI) is a simple and useful nutritional parameter reflecting the dietary skeletal muscle protein intake and skeletal muscle mass of the patient. Because of the complexity of creatinine kinetic modeling (CKM) to derive CI, we developed a more simplified formula to estimate CI in HD patients.

Design, Setting, Participants & Measurements: A large database of 549 HD patients followed over more than 20 years including monthly CKM-derived CI values was used to develop a simple equation based on patient demographics, predialysis serum creatinine values and dialysis dose ($_{sp}$Kt/V) using mixed regression models.

Results: The equation to estimate CI was developed based on age, gender, pre-dialysis serum creatinine concentrations and $_{sp}$Kt/V urea. The equation-derived CI correlated strongly with the measured CI using CKM (correlation coefficient =0.79, p-value <0.001). The mean error of CI prediction using the equation was 13.47%. Preliminary examples of few typical HD patients have been used to illustrate the clinical relevance and potential usefulness of CI.

Conclusions: The elementary equation used to derive CI using demographic parameters, pre-dialysis serum creatinine concentrations and dialysis dose is a simple and accurate surrogate measure for muscle mass estimation. However, the predictive value of the simplified CI assessment method on mortality deserves further evaluation in large cohorts of HD patients.

Editor: Martin H. de Borst, University Medical Center Groningen and University of Groningen, Netherlands

Funding: The authors have no funding or support to report.

Competing Interests: The authors have declared that no competing interests exist.

* E-mail: jp-cristol@chu-montpellier.fr

Introduction

Protein-energy wasting (PEW) is highly prevalent among the hemodialysis (HD) population [1,2]. Several studies have underlined the prognostic significance of PEW as a strong predictor of morbidity and mortality independently of dialysis adequacy in HD patients [3–5]. Protein nutritional status is determined by markers of visceral and somatic protein stores [6]. Although serum albumin concentration, a visceral protein indicator, is routinely assessed and is inversely associated with mortality in HD patients [3,4,7,8], it is an insensitive confounding factor being an indicator of both inflammation and nutritional status [9,10]. In addition to assessment of visceral proteins, the evaluation of somatic protein status by determination of muscle mass is crucial and commonly used for nutritional assessment of dialysis patients [6]. Reduced muscle mass and lean body mass (LBM) significantly correlate with higher mortality in HD patients [11]. The association of serum creatinine level with LBM and an inverse correlation between serum creatinine concentration and mortality in HD patients [4,8,12] support the use of serum creatinine as a nutritional and muscle mass marker and a predictor of clinical outcomes in these patients [13]. Nevertheless, serum creatinine concentration could be influenced by patient muscle mass, dietary protein intake, hydration status, dialysis clearance and the presence of residual renal function [14,15].

An accurate measure of LBM by using computed tomographic (CT) or magnetic resonance imaging (MRI) of muscle mass, total body potassium counting and deuterium dilution techniques [16,17] is cumbersome, expensive and not readily accessible in clinical practice. The estimation of LBM by creatinine kinetic modeling (CKM) has been validated as a convenient and reliable method of assessment of muscle mass and protein nutritional status in HD patients. CKM is based on the principle that creatinine generation is proportional to LBM in stable dialysis patients who have a constant protein/meat intake. Creatinine index (CI) is defined as normalized creatinine production rate, which is equal to the sum of creatinine excretion rate (dialytic removal and urinary excretion) and metabolic degradation rate in the steady state [18,19]. Furthermore, CI derived from CKM as a marker of muscle mass has been recognized as a powerful prognostic indicator of long-term all-cause and cardiovascular mortalities in HD patients [20,21]. The application of standard CKM requires post-dialysis serum creatinine concentration and dialysate collection to compute creatinine generation rates. Formulas for the prediction of post-dialysis serum creatinine levels and creatinine generation rates have been devised and validated in HD patients [20]. However, the complex mathematical formula requiring computer programs to precisely calculate CI poses a major obstacle to its application in routine clinical practice. Thus, in this study, we aimed to develop and validate a simple formula to substitute the complex equations or formal CKM to calculate CI using patient demographics and classical dialysis dose estimated by $_{sp}Kt/V$ urea in HD patients.

Materials and Methods

Ethics Statement

The manuscript describes an observational non-interventional study, so written informed consent was not required. According to the French Law, the study has been registered at "Ministère de l'Enseignement Supérieur et de la Recherche" after approval by our institution ethical committee (Comité de Protection des Personnes Sud Méditerranée IV, Montpellier, France) with the following number DC-2008-417. The study was conducted according to the principles of the Declaration of Helsinki and in compliance with International Conference on Harmonization/ Good Clinical Practice regulations.

Data sources

We used a large database (available since 1988) of prevalent and incident HD patients treated in two HD units in Montpellier, France (Lapeyronie University Hospital and the AIDER-Montpellier; Association pour l'Installation à Domicile des Épurations Rénales). Dialysis quantification including formal urea kinetic modeling (UKM) and CKM was routinely evaluated on a monthly basis on the mid-week HD sessions. HD charts and laboratory results were collected in an electronic primary care record only available to physicians and nurses from the dialysis centers. These primary data could not be publicly available. The data were collected from 549 patients undergoing HD for more than 3 months including 16,547 monthly assessments of formal UKM and CKM.

Data collection, procedures and laboratory analysis

Medical records were reviewed for age, gender, ethnicity, pre- and post-dialysis weights, treatment modalities and time on dialysis. Formal UKM and CKM were routinely performed during the mid-week dialysis session of the first week of the month in all HD patients in our dialysis units. Pre- and post-dialysis blood samples were collected immediately before, at the end of dialysis sessions (2 minutes after stopping blood pump and before rinsing back of dialyzers) and at the beginning of the following dialysis session. During the first hour of dialysis session, blood samples were drawn from the arterial and venous blood lines and effluent dialysate sample was simultaneously taken. All blood and dialysate samples were measured for urea and creatinine concentrations by an enzymatic method using an automatic analyzer.

Calculations

A single-pool variable-volume model was assumed to calculate creatinine distribution volume (Vc), creatinine appearance rate (Gc) and CI. In this model [18], CI, reflecting creatinine generation rate, is assumed to be equal to the sum of creatinine appearance rate (Gc) and metabolic degradation rate of creatinine (Dc). The dialysis adequacy ($_{sp}Kt/V$ urea) was determined by formal UKM applying a single-pool variable-volume model to pre-dialysis, post-dialysis and pre-dialysis of the next dialysis session serum urea concentrations to calculate urea distribution volume (Vu), urea appearance rate (Gu) using an in vivo hemodialyzer urea clearance (Kdu) and accounting for residual renal function (Kr) [18,22]. Equilibrated Kt/V urea (eKt/V urea) estimated by using simplified equations, as proposed by Daugirdas et al. [23], and urea reduction ratio (URR) were also evaluated to determine dialysis dose. The database, which contained 16,547 values for CKM-derived CI from 549 HD patients, was used to develop and validate the equation. Patients with a significant diuresis (>500 ml urine/24 hours) and/or residual renal function (>2 ml/min) were excluded from the analysis to prevent complicating the final formula.

Mathematical modeling to derive CI formulae from serum creatinine concentrations, $_{sp}Kt/V$ urea and anthropometric parameters

CKM-derived CI was measured at different time points among different HD patients. Mixed regression models were applied to generate formulae for CI prediction from dialysis dose and patient demographics. In this model, measured CI as an outcome variable Y was represented as a function of an intercept, whereas dialysis dose and demographic parameters were represented as predictor variables X. A random error (ε) was assumed in this model. Mixed regression model can be expressed as follows:

$$\boldsymbol{Y}_{ij} = \boldsymbol{\beta}_{0j} + \boldsymbol{\beta}_{1j} \boldsymbol{X}_{ij} + \boldsymbol{\varepsilon}_{ij}$$

where Y_{ij} and X_{ij} are outcome variable and predictor variable at time i for subject j respectively and β_{0j} as well as β_{1j} are regression coefficients. Several predictor variables including patient demographics and dialysis dose were assumed according to an additive model. A regression model and CI estimations were obtained by statistical estimations of regression coefficients. Different formulae were developed and evaluated including those with dry weight and weight loss. We selected the simplest formula that provided the most accurate result. As results, the mixed regression model that best fits in our study is shown as follows:

$$CI_{ij}\ (mg/kg/day) = \beta_{0j} + \beta_{1j}\ age\,(years) + \beta_{2j}\ gender + \beta_{3j}\ pre-dialysis\ creatinine\,(\mu mol/l) + \beta_{4j}\ Kt/V$$

Validation of modeling and error estimate in a large cohort of dialysis patients

We estimated the validity of our equation by examining differences between measured CI and CI predicted using our simplified equation based on 16,547 values for measured CI from

Table 1. Clinical characteristics of hemodialysis patients used for the development of a simplified equation for the calculation of creatinine index.

Parameters	
Number	549
Men, n (%)	330 (60.1)
Age (years)	70.1 [57.0–78.7]
Diabetes, n (%)	143 (26.0)
Chronic obstructive pulmonary disease, n (%)	79 (14.4)
Chronic hepatitis, n (%)	86 (15.7)
History of kidney transplantation, n (%)	89 (16.3)
Ischemic cardiopathy, n (%)	154 (28.1)
Renal replacement modality (%HDF/HD)	59.8/40.2
Post-dialysis weight (kg)	64.7 [55.4–75.2]
Treatment time (min)	219±33
Pre-dialysis serum creatinine concentrations (μmol/l)	733 [616–857]
Residual renal function (ml/min)	0
Urea reduction ratio (%)	78 [75–81]
$_{sp}$Kt/V urea	1.8 [1.6–2.0]
$_{eq}$Kt/V urea	1.6 [1.4–1.7]
Creatinine index (mg/kg/day)	18.9 [15.4–22.9]
C reactive protein (mg/l)	7.1 [3.0–16.7]
Serum albumin (g/l)	36.9±4.6
Total cholesterol (mmol/l)	5.02±1.28
Triglycerides (mmol/l)	1.72 [1.21–2.65]
LDL cholesterol (mmol/l)	2.96±1.00

Note: Qualitative variables expressed as number (percent). Quantitative variables expressed as mean ± SD for normally distributed variables or median [interquartile range] for non normally distributed variables;
Abbreviations: HDF, hemodiafiltration; HD, hemodialysis; min, minutes.

549 HD patients. Regression analysis and Bland-Altman analysis were performed to determine the differences between measured CI and predicted CI and estimate the mean prediction error.

Statistical analyses

Multivariate mixed model analysis was performed using a generalized linear mixed-effect model for repeated measures. Variables were selected if p-value was less than 0.20 in the univariate analysis and a stepwise procedure was used to select potential variables for the final model. Regression and Bland-Altman analyses were performed to validate the equation. The continuous variables were expressed as mean ± standard deviation for normally distributed variables or median [interquartile range] for non normally distributed variables. *P*-values of <0.05 were considered to be statistically significants. Data were analyzed using R version 2.13.0.

Results

General characteristics of the HD population used for equation generation are shown in **Table 1**. The study population included slightly higher proportion of men of Caucasian origin. The median age of the patients was 70.1 years old. Causes of CKD were glomerulonephritis (n = 92, 16.8%), diabetic and hypertensive nephropathy (n = 99; 18.1%), angiosclerosis and hypertensive nephropathy (n = 91; 16.6%), infectious/obstructive interstitial nephropathy (n = 72; 13.1%), renal neoplasia (n = 16; 2.9%), genetic/congenital cause (n = 61; 11.0%), unknown cause (n = 65; 11.8%), systemic disease (n = 49; 8.9%), other cause (n = 4; 0.8%). As previously mentioned, HD patients had no residual renal function at the time of measuring CI. The average creatinine indices (CIs) for men and women were 21.0 and 18.8 mg/kg/day respectively.

The values for CKM-derived CIs in the database (16,547 values) from 549 HD patients were used to develop the equation predicting CI using patient demographic parameters and dialysis dose. Age, gender, pre-dialysis serum creatinine concentrations (Cr_{pre}) and $_{sp}$Kt/V urea were selected as significant variables in the final model by using stepwise procedures. The equation to predict CI was determined as follows:

$$CI\,(mg/kg/day) = 16.21 + 1.12 \times [1 \text{ if male}; 0 \text{ if female}] - 0.06 \times age\,(years) - 0.08 \times {}_{sp}Kt/V\,urea + 0.009 \times Cr_{pre}(\mu mol/l)$$

(Note. To evaluate CI using plasma creatinine concentration in mg/dl, divide the creatinine concentration term by 88.4).

To estimate the validity of the equation, the measured CI using CKM was compared with the equation-derived CI in a large cohort of 549 HD patients. Equation-estimated CIs were closely correlated with CKM-derived CIs as illustrated in **Figure 1** (correlation coefficient = 0.79, P-value <0.001). Bland-Altman analysis confirmed the excellent prediction of CKM-derived CIs

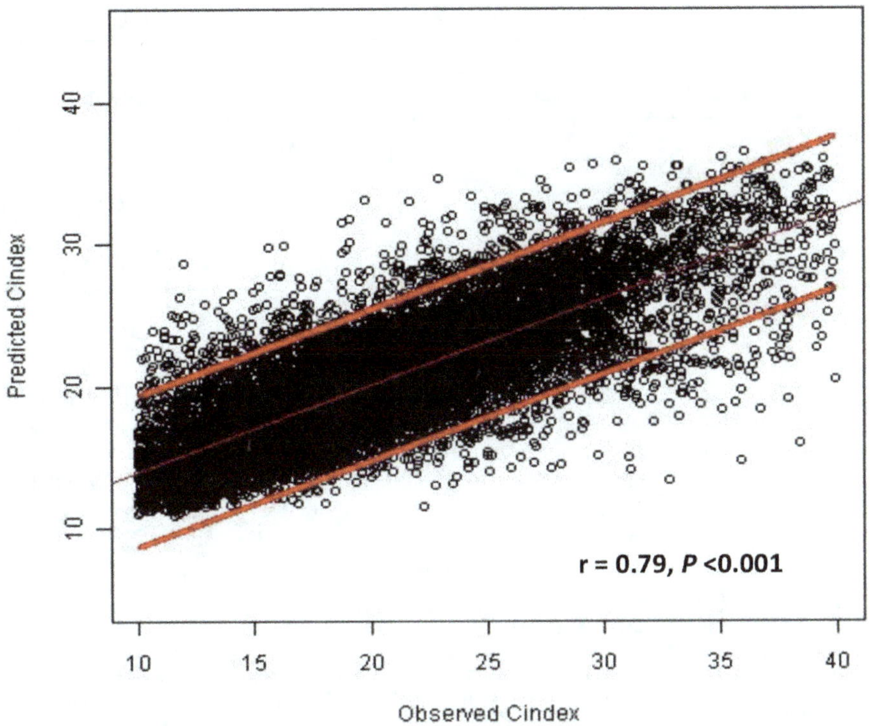

Figure 1. Scatterplot between observed creatinine index and predicted creatinine index. A scatterplot with a regression line and a 95% confidence interval for the line representing the relationship between creatinine kinetic modeling (CKM)-derived creatinine index (Observed Cindex) and creatinine index derived from the equation (Predicted Cindex).

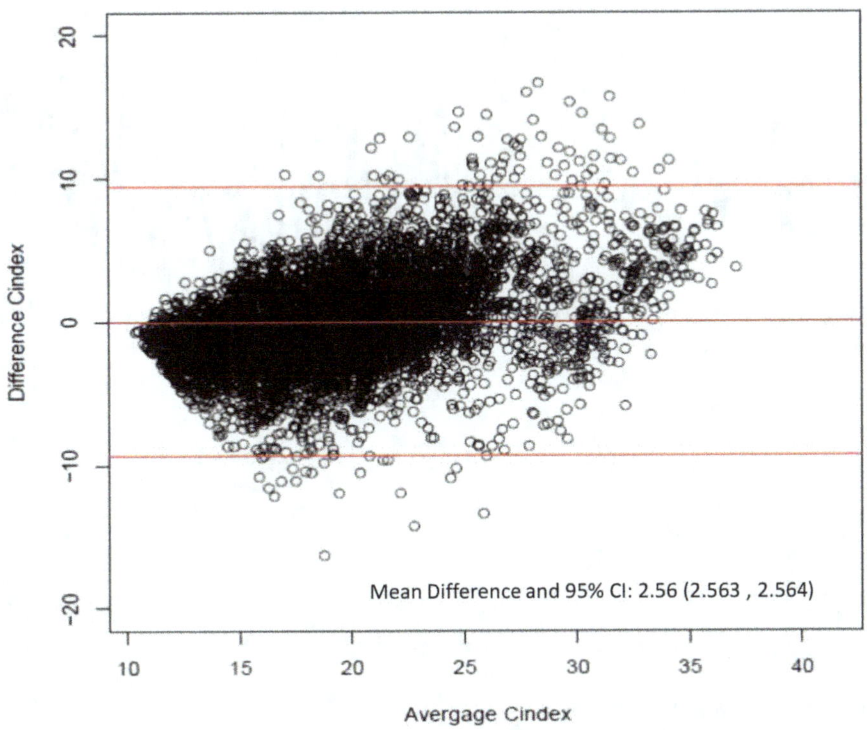

Figure 2. Bland-Altman plot of the difference between equation-derived versus creatinine kinetic modeling-derived creatinine index. The horizontal lines are the mean difference and 95% limits of agreement.

Table 2. Difference plot analysis comparing equation-estimated CI and CKM- derived CI according to gender and age groups.

	Limit of absolute error	Mean difference (95%CI)	Correlation (r)	pP-value
All	0 to 22	2.56 (2.56, 2.56)	0.79	<0.001
Men	0 to 19	2.62 (2.61, 2.62)	0.79	<0.001
Women	0 to 22	2.47 (2.47, 2.47)	0.76	<0.001
Age <65 yrs.	0 to 22	2.56 (2.56, 2.56)	0.79	<0.001
Age ≥65 yrs.	0 to 20	2.25 (2.25, 2.25)	0.75	<0.001

Abbreviations: CI, creatinine index; CKM, creatinine kinetic modeling; 95% CI, 95% confidence interval.

using the equation (**Figure 2**). The mean prediction error was 13.47% (95% confidence interval = 13.46–13.67) which is quite acceptable as a clinical tool. In addition, the developed equation precisely estimated CI in both men and women in all age groups (**Table 2**).

To illustrate the clinical relevance and potential usefulness of this simplified CI formula, a selection of few typical HD patients is presented in **Figures 3, 4, 5, 6, 7.** These cases were selected because they benefit from several years of follow-up and provide appropriate trend analysis. In summary, these cases illustrate different conditions: stable HD patient maintaining CI in normal range according to gender, age and physical activity; improvement in incident HD patient marked by a regular CI increase; deteriorating HD patient with muscle wasting due to intercurrent disease or protein energy wasting condition leading to death. The selection of cases underlines the clinical usefulness and applicability of simplified CI for comforting or alarming physicians on HD patient status. As shown, simplified CI may be easily implemented and used as a nutritional and physical activity assessment tool in the daily life of HD patients helping nephrologist seeking for dialysis adequacy. Time behavior follow-up of simplified CI is a complementary useful and cost effective tool that is easily implemented in the management of HD patient as a combined index with dialysis dose delivery.

Discussion

In a large cohort of 549 hemodialysis patients followed more than 20 years with 16,547 assessments of CKM, we developed a highly simplified formula to predict CI only based on easily-attainable parameters of age, gender, pre-dialysis serum creatinine levels and $_{sp}$Kt/V urea. The formula yielded an accurate estimation of CI with a strong correlation between CKM-derived CI and formula-estimated CI on the basis of both regression and Bland-Altman analyses. Moreover, the CI formula appeared

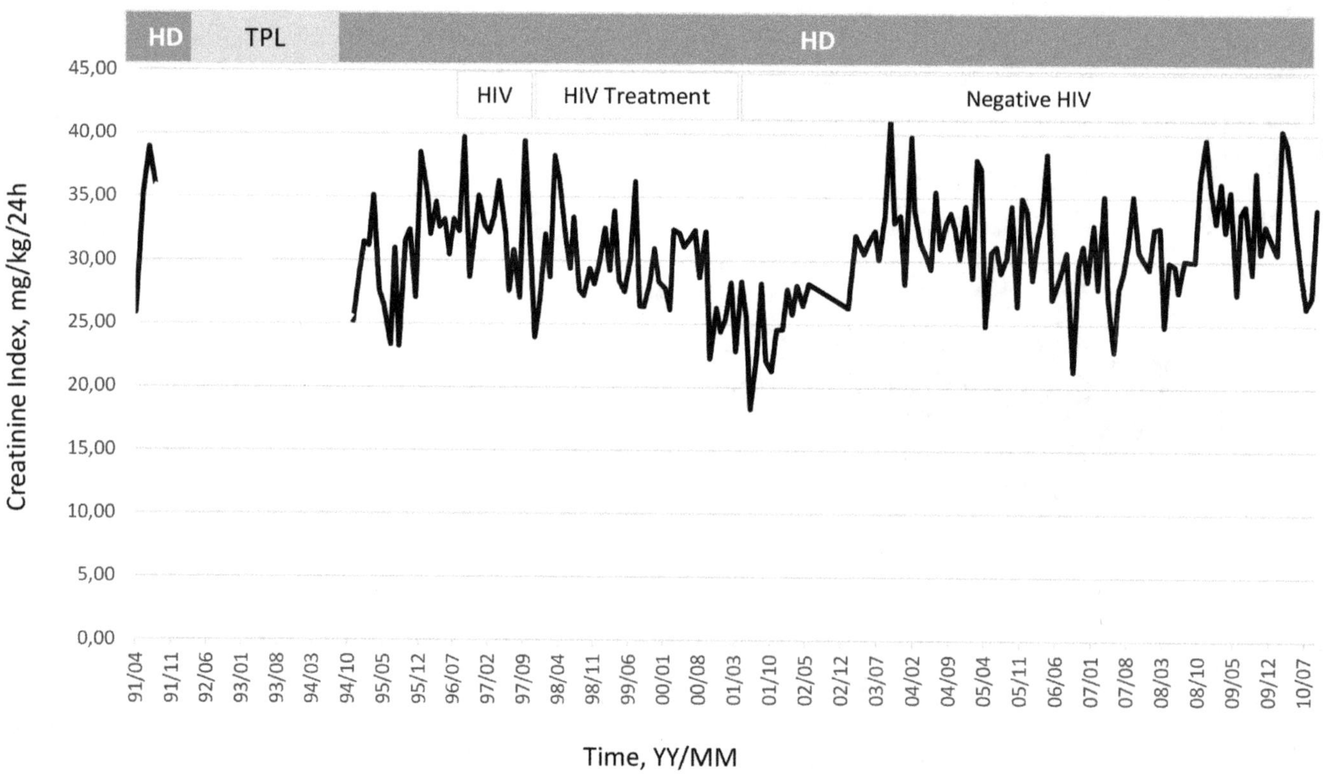

Figure 3. Illustration of clinical relevance and potential usefulness of the simplified CI formula. Case 1: Deteriorating effect of HIV treatment on CI in HD patient with recovery after stopping treatment (Pat. RB, Male, 32 yo, 68.8 Kg, $_{sp}$KT/V 1.61±0.14, CI 30.5±4.7 mg/kg/24 h).

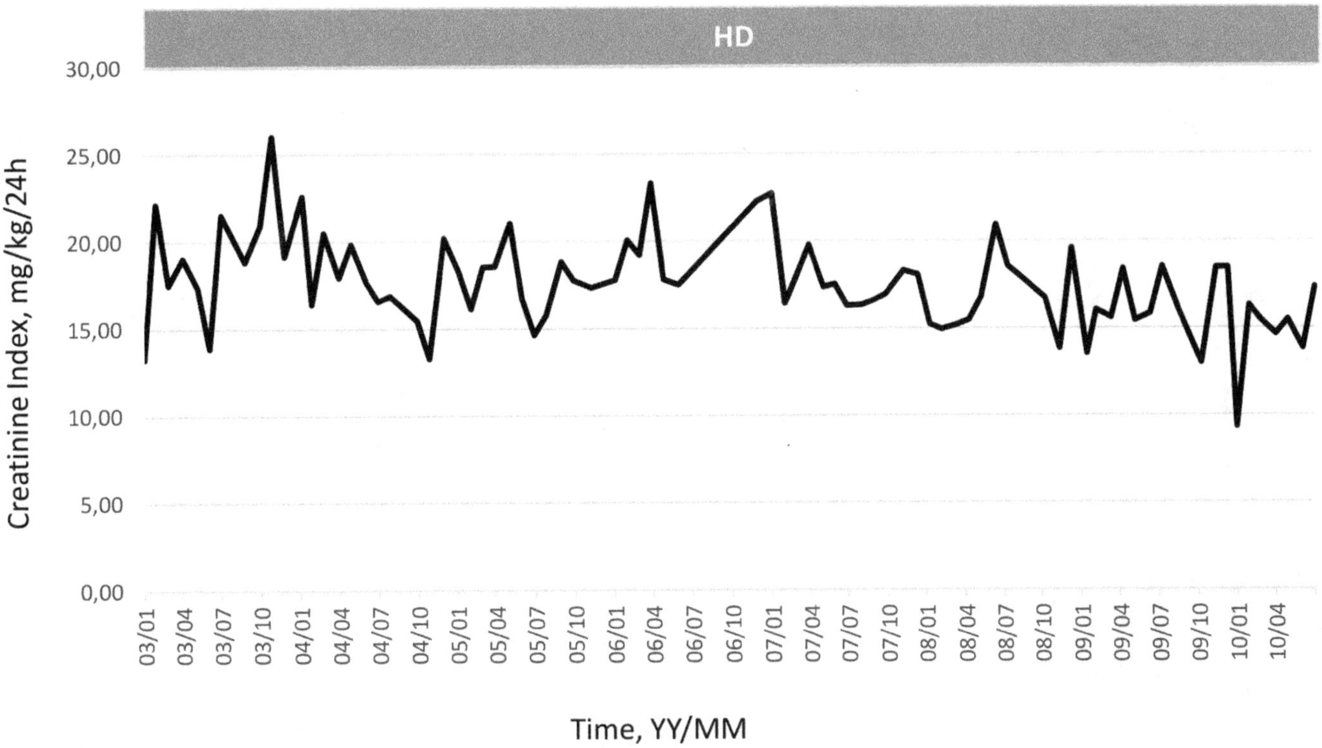

Figure 4. Illustration of clinical relevance and potential usefulness of the simplified CI formula. Case 2: Progressive decline of CI reflecting physiological muscle loss in elderly female HD patient (Pat. BM, Female, 70 yo, 61.7 Kg, $_{sp}$KT/V 1.99±0.16, CI 17.6±2.7 mg/kg/24 h).

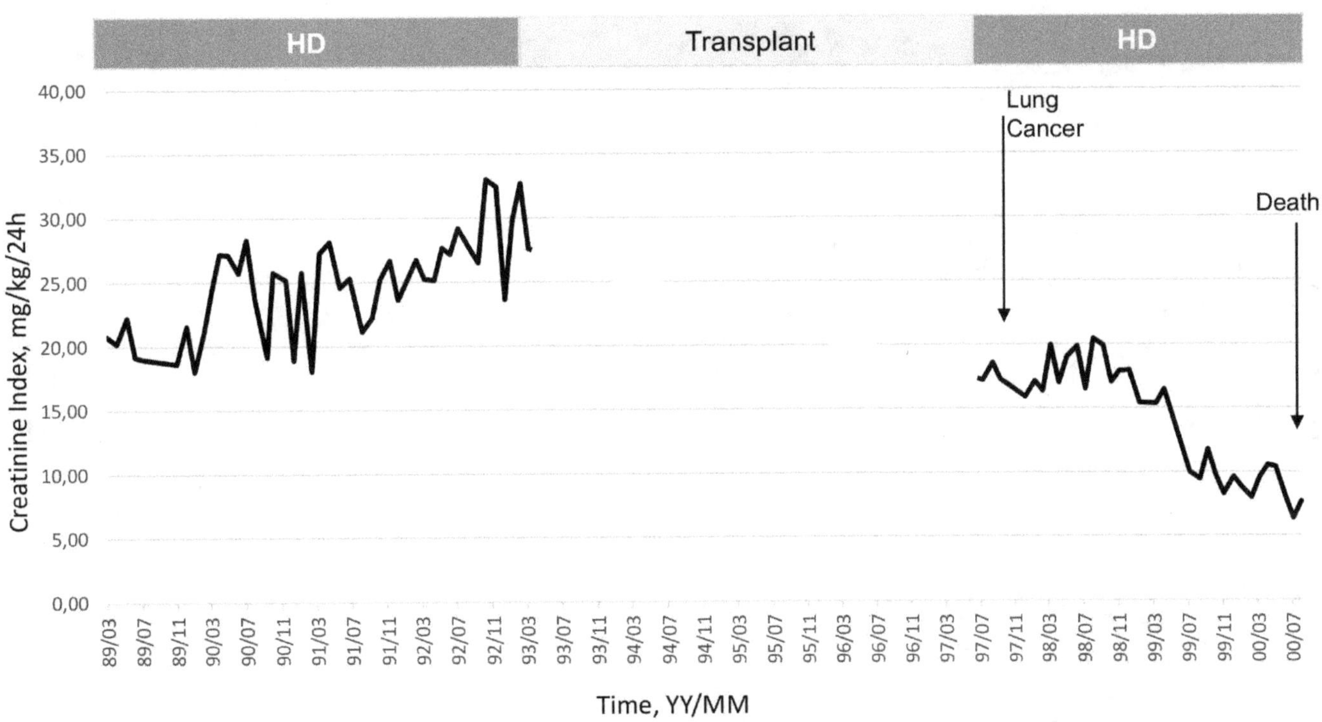

Figure 5. Illustration of clinical relevance and potential usefulness of the simplified CI formula. Case 3: Significant increase of CI and muscle mass after start of hemodialysis (1st phase), loss of muscle mass after renal transplant rejection and rapid deterioration of CI following lung cancer leading to death (Pat. BJ, Male, 58 yo, 76.5 Kg, $_{sp}$KT/V 1.33±0.18, CI 20.2±6.7 mg/kg/24 h).

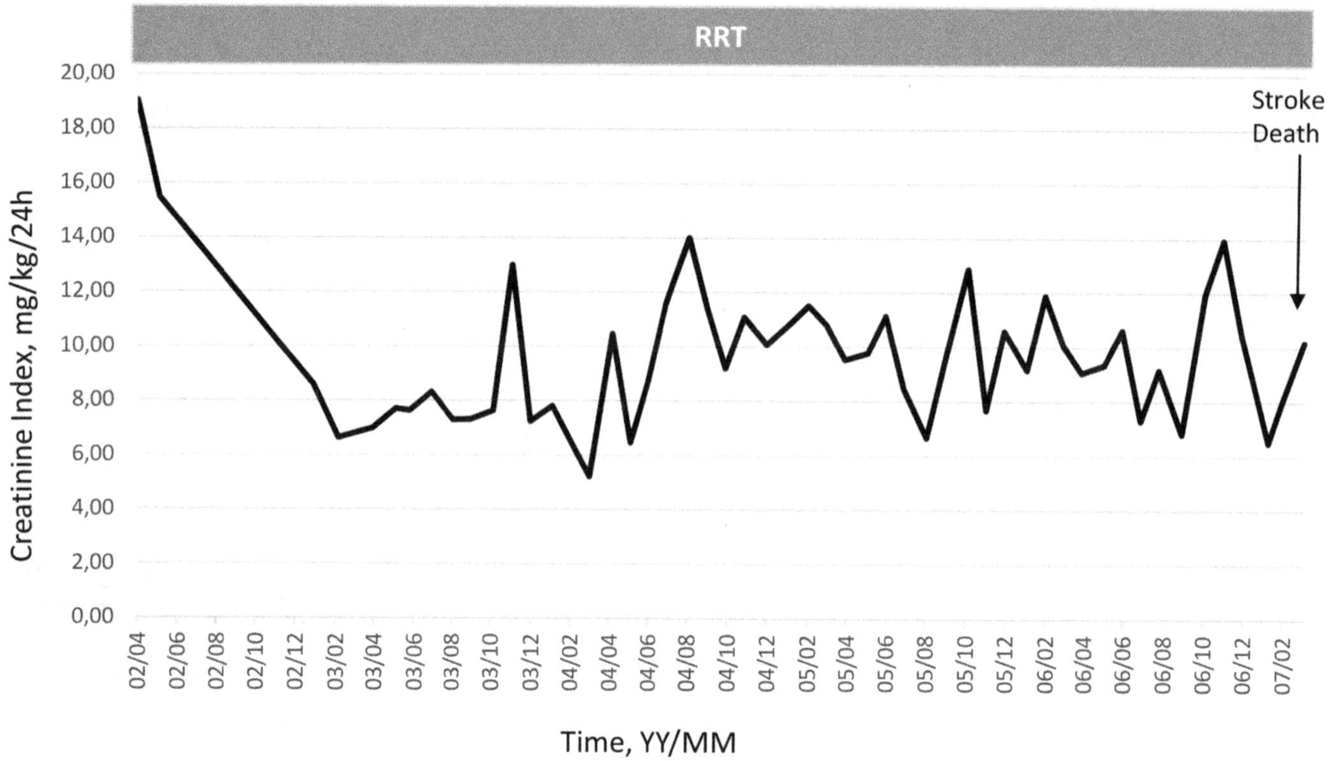

Figure 6. Illustration of clinical relevance and potential usefulness of the simplified CI formula. Case 4: Significant decline of CI and muscle mass in elderly woman after start of dialysis then stability maintenance of CI at low level until stroke and death (Pat. FM, Female, 88 yo, 72.2 Kg, $_{sp}KT/V$ 2.0±0.23, CI 10.2±3.5 mg/kg/24 h).

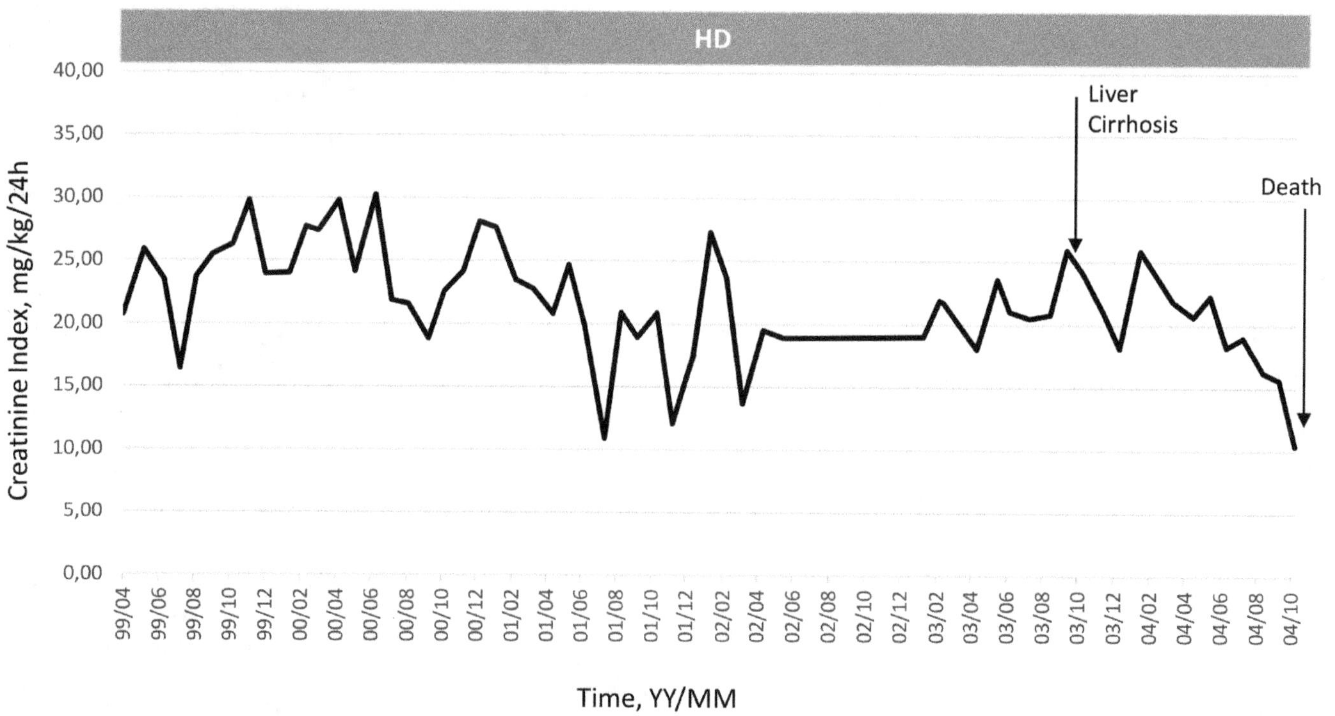

Figure 7. Illustration of clinical relevance and potential usefulness of the simplified CI formula. Case 5: Slow decline of CI reflecting muscle mass loss in young heart transplant man then followed by a rapid CI decline due to development of liver cirrhosis (peliosis hepatitis) leading to death (Pat. KJ, Male, 53 yo, 61.9 Kg, Heart transplant - CV Catheters, $_{sp}KT/V$ 1.62±0.41, CI 22.1±5.9 mg/kg/24 h).

accurate for predicting CI in both men and women in different age groups. Although the study population used for formula development includes mainly Caucasians, the formula is applicable to all HD populations. Ethnicity does not affect the validity of the formula because CI derived from CKM is based on creatinine mass balance determined from the sum of creatinine removal rate and metabolic degradation rate in the steady state that determines creatinine generation rate state [18]. In addition, one must recognize that the range of CIs values found in our population is sufficiently large to cover the wide spectrum of CIs values in different ethnicities.

Evaluation of muscle mass is an important measure for assessing protein nutritional status in HD patients [24–27]. Accurate methods for measuring LBM such as CT or MRI of muscle mass are expensive and their availability is limited in routine clinical practice. In addition, non-invasive techniques such as dual energy X-ray absorptiometry (DEXA) and bioelectrical impedance analysis (BIA) present some limitations in terms of muscle mass measurement. Both DEXA and BIA might not detect malnutrition in overhydrated dialysis patients due to overestimation of LBM [19,28,29]. Conversely, predialysis serum creatinine concentrations or CI obtained by CKM reflecting muscle mass have been recognized as significant predictors of protein nutritional status, all-cause and cardiovascular mortalities in HD patients [18,20,21,30–33]. However, extended use of CI, a more sensitive indicator, based on CKM has been limited by two factors: firstly, the complexity of the mathematical modeling of formal creatinine kinetics for calculating CI is not easily applicable in daily practice; secondly, post-dialysis serum creatinine measurement is not performed in routine clinical dialysis practice for economical reasons. The simplified CI equation using age, gender, pre-dialysis serum creatinine concentrations and $_{sp}$Kt/V urea was therefore developed to overcome these limitations and to provide an additional cost-effective tool for regular LBM nutritional assessment of HD patients. The equation yields serial estimates of CI and trend analysis of CI changes over time provides much more information on patient muscle mass and protein nutritional status than the absolute CI values. Significantly, muscle protein turnover rates are highly variable depending on age, gender and factors affecting protein synthesis and degradation [34]. CI declines with advancing age and is lower for women than men [18]. In addition, several conditions causing loss of muscle mass in chronic kidney disease patients such as catabolic illnesses [35], acidemia [36,37] and resistance to anabolic factors (e.g. insulin, growth hormone and insulin-like growth factor-1) [38–40] could be easily and precisely detected by time reduction of CI values.

Five-year cohort studies of HD patients reported the prognostic significance of CKM-derived CI as an indicator of all-cause and cardiovascular mortalities in HD patients [20,21]. Reduced CI (< 22 mg/kg/day) was significantly associated with poor patient survival [20]. It could be argued from Bland-Altman analysis (**Figure 2**) that the accuracy of this new equation decreases above 30 mg/kg/day. However, the very small number of observations above this value (only 6%) may contribute to decrease estimator accuracy. And, as previously mentioned, only low CI or CI-derived LBM constitutes a high predictive value for mortality in HD population [20,21] or CKD patients [25].

Clinically-relevant and interesting information provided by this simplified CI has been illustrated in selected cases from our cohort. As shown, simplified CI is useful to confirm stability of HD patients maintaining CI in a normal range according to gender and age, while a CI increase may illustrate nutritional improvement in HD patients after start of treatment or, more interestingly, a rapid CI decline would help clinicians to identify and intervene on HD patients undergoing wasting muscle mass.

The main limitation of this study lies in the absence of validation groups for this new equation. The predictive value of this simplified CI equation for long-term mortality in HD patients using routinely collected data (age, gender, pre-dialysis serum creatinine levels and $_{sp}$Kt/V urea) needs to be assessed within large databases. The usefulness of this simplified formula within large databases is needed to ensure the reliability and accuracy of the formula for predicting long-term outcomes of HD patients. Two pilot studies have been conducted in two large cohorts of HD patients with promising results (DOPPS, MONDO) (unpublished data). As a perspective, the development of a website available for physicians may help to easily evaluate CI.

In summary, the simplified CI formula based on age, gender, pre-dialysis serum creatinine concentrations and $_{sp}$Kt/V urea offers a simple, precise and cost-effective tool for CI estimation in HD patients. The predictive value of the equation-estimated CI on patient outcomes needs to be further validated in large epidemiological studies of HD patients but preliminary results appear quite promising.

Author Contributions

Conceived and designed the experiments: BC AGV JPC. Performed the experiments: BC AGV L. Chenine HLM AR L. Chalabi MM JPC. Analyzed the data: BC AGV NM JPC. Wrote the paper: BC AGV NM.

References

1. Aparicio M, Cano N, Chauveau P, Azar R, Canaud B, et al. (1999) Nutritional status of haemodialysis patients: a French national cooperative study. French Study Group for Nutrition in Dialysis. Nephrol Dial Transplant 14(7): 1679–86.
2. Rocco MV, Paranandi L, Burrowes JD, Cockram DB, Dwyer JT, et al. (2002) Nutritional status in the HEMO Study cohort at baseline. Hemodialysis. Am J Kidney Dis 39(2): 245–56.
3. Combe C, Chauveau P, Laville M, Fouque D, Azar R, et al. (2001) Influence of nutritional factors and hemodialysis adequacy on the survival of 1,610 French patients. Am J Kidney Dis 37(1 Suppl 2): S81–8.
4. Dwyer JT, Larive B, Leung J, Rocco MV, Greene T, et al. (2005) Are nutritional status indicators associated with mortality in the Hemodialysis (HEMO) Study? Kidney Int 68(4): 1766–76.
5. Kalantar-Zadeh K, Supasyndh O, Lehn RS, McAllister CJ, Kopple JD (2003) Normalized protein nitrogen appearance is correlated with hospitalization and mortality in hemodialysis patients with Kt/V greater than 1.20. J Ren Nutr 13(1): 15–25.
6. Pupim LB, Ikizler TA (2004) Assessment and monitoring of uremic malnutrition. J Ren Nutr 14(1): 6–19.
7. Mapes DL, Lopes AA, Satayathum S, McCullough KP, Goodkin DA, et al. (2003) Health-related quality of life as a predictor of mortality and hospitalization: the Dialysis Outcomes and Practice Patterns Study (DOPPS). Kidney Int 64(1): 339–49.
8. Pifer TB, McCullough KP, Port FK, Goodkin DA, Maroni BJ, et al. (2002) Mortality risk in hemodialysis patients and changes in nutritional indicators: DOPPS. Kidney Int 62(6): 2238–45.
9. Friedman AN, Fadem SZ (2010) Reassessment of albumin as a nutritional marker in kidney disease. J Am Soc Nephrol 21(2): 223–30.
10. Kaysen GA, Dubin JA, Muller HG, Rosales L, Levin NW, et al. (2004) Inflammation and reduced albumin synthesis associated with stable decline in serum albumin in hemodialysis patients. Kidney Int 65(4): 1408–15.
11. Huang CX, Tighiouart H, Beddhu S, Cheung AK, Dwyer JT, et al. (2010) Both low muscle mass and low fat are associated with higher all-cause mortality in hemodialysis patients. Kidney Int 77(7): 624–9.
12. Lowrie EG, Huang WH, Lew NL (1995) Death risk predictors among peritoneal dialysis and hemodialysis patients: a preliminary comparison. Am J Kidney Dis 26(1): 220–8.
13. Moreau-Gaudry X, Guebre-Egziabher F, Jean G, Genet L, Lataillade D, et al. (2011) Serum creatinine improves body mass index survival prediction in hemodialysis patients: a 1-year prospective cohort analysis from the ARNOS study. J Ren Nutr 21(5): 369–75.

14. (2000) Clinical practice guidelines for nutrition in chronic renal failure. K/DOQI, National Kidney Foundation. Am J Kidney Dis 35(6 Suppl 2): S1–140.
15. Chauveau P, Nguyen H, Combe C, Chene G, Azar R, et al. (2005) Dialyzer membrane permeability and survival in hemodialysis patients. Am J Kidney Dis 45(3): 565–71.
16. Sarkar SR, Kuhlmann MK, Kotanko P, Zhu F, Heymsfield SB, et al. (2006) Metabolic consequences of body size and body composition in hemodialysis patients. Kidney Int 70(10): 1832–9.
17. Ohkawa S, Odamaki M, Yoneyama T, Hibi I, Miyaji K, et al. (2000) Standardized thigh muscle area measured by computed axial tomography as an alternate muscle mass index for nutritional assessment of hemodialysis patients. Am J Clin Nutr 71(2): 485–90.
18. Canaud B, Garred LJ, Argiles A, Flavier JL, Bouloux C, et al. (1995) Creatinine kinetic modelling: a simple and reliable tool for the assessment of protein nutritional status in haemodialysis patients. Nephrol Dial Transplant 10(8): 1405–10.
19. PR, Nolph KD, Moore HL, Prowant B, Emerson PF, et al. (1994) Lean body mass estimation by creatinine kinetics. J Am Soc Nephrol 4(7): 1475–85.
20. Desmeules S, Levesque R, Jaussent I, Leray-Moragues H, Chalabi L, et al. (2004) Creatinine index and lean body mass are excellent predictors of long-term survival in haemodiafiltration patients. Nephrol Dial Transplant 19(5): 1182–9.
21. Terrier N, Jaussent I, Dupuy AM, Morena M, Delcourt C, et al. (2008) Creatinine index and transthyretin as additive predictors of mortality in haemodialysis patients. Nephrol Dial Transplant 23(1): 345–53.
22. P, . Gotch F (1977) Dialysis therapy guided by kinetic modeling: application of a variable-volume single-pool model of urea kinetics. Trans Aust Conf Heat Mass Transfer: 29–37.
23. Daugirdas JT (1995) Simplified equations for monitoring Kt/V, PCRn, eKt/V, and ePCRn. Adv Ren Replace Ther 2(4): 295–304.
24. Kalantar-Zadeh K, Streja E, Molnar MZ, Lukowsky LR, Krishnan M, et al. (2012) Mortality prediction by surrogates of body composition: an examination of the obesity paradox in hemodialysis patients using composite ranking score analysis. Am J Epidemiol 175(8): 793–803.
25. Huang JW, Lien YC, Wu HY, Yen CJ, Pan CC, et al. (2013) Lean body mass predicts long-term survival in Chinese patients on peritoneal dialysis. PLoS One 8(1): e54976.
26. Noori N, Kopple JD, Kovesdy CP, Feroze U, Sim JJ, et al. (2010) Mid-arm muscle circumference and quality of life and survival in maintenance hemodialysis patients. Clin J Am Soc Nephrol 5(12): 2258–68.
27. Park J, Jin DC, Molnar MZ, Dukkipati R, Kim YL, et al. (2013) Mortality predictability of body size and muscle mass surrogates in Asian vs white and African American hemodialysis patients. Mayo Clin Proc 88(5): 479–86.
28. Bhatla B, Moore H, Emerson P, Keshaviah P, Prowant B, et al. (1995) Lean body mass estimation by creatinine kinetics, bioimpedance, and dual energy x-ray absorptiometry in patients on continuous ambulatory peritoneal dialysis. Asaio J 41(3): M442–6.
29. Horber FF, Thomi F, Casez JP, Fonteille J, Jaeger P (1992) Impact of hydration status on body composition as measured by dual energy X-ray absorptiometry in normal volunteers and patients on haemodialysis. Br J Radiol 65(778): 895–900.
30. Rosansky SJ, Clark WF (2011) Low pre-dialysis serum creatinine level and increased incidence of sudden cardiac arrest: a possible explanation of the harm associated with early dialysis initiation. Kidney Int 79(11): 1259.
31. Walther CP, Carter CW, Low CL, Williams P, Rifkin DE, et al. (2012) Interdialytic creatinine change versus predialysis creatinine as indicators of nutritional status in maintenance hemodialysis. Nephrol Dial Transplant 27(2): 771–6.
32. Lertdumrongluk P, Canaud B (2012) Pre-dialysis creatinine and interdialytic change in creatinine as nutritional markers in haemodialysis patients. Nephrol Dial Transplant 27(5): 2130; author reply 2130–1.
33. Park J, Mehrotra R, Rhee CM, Molnar MZ, Lukowsky LR, et al. (2013) Serum creatinine level, a surrogate of muscle mass, predicts mortality in peritoneal dialysis patients. Nephrol Dial Transplant 28(8): 2146–55.
34. Workeneh BT, Mitch WE (2010) Review of muscle wasting associated with chronic kidney disease. Am J Clin Nutr 91(4): 1128S–1132S.
35. Grodstein GP, Blumenkrantz MJ, Kopple JD (1980) Nutritional and metabolic response to catabolic stress in uremia. Am J Clin Nutr 33(7): 1411–6.
36. -Zadeh K, Mehrotra R, Fouque D, Kopple JD (2004) Metabolic acidosis and malnutrition-inflammation complex syndrome in chronic renal failure. Semin Dial 17(6): 455–65.
37. Pickering WP, Price SR, Bircher G, Marinovic AC, Mitch WE, et al. (2002) Nutrition in CAPD: serum bicarbonate and the ubiquitin-proteasome system in muscle. Kidney Int 61(4): 1286–92.
38. Fouque D, Peng SC, Shamir E, Kopple JD (2000) Recombinant human insulin-like growth factor-1 induces an anabolic response in malnourished CAPD patients. Kidney Int 57(2): 646–54.
39. Guebre-Egziabher F, Juillard L, Boirie Y, Laville M, Beaufrere B, et al. (2009) Short-term administration of a combination of recombinant growth hormone and insulin-like growth factor-I induces anabolism in maintenance hemodialysis. J Clin Endocrinol Metab 94(7): 2299–305.
40. Mak RH (1996) Insulin resistance but IGF-I sensitivity in chronic renal failure. Am J Physiol 271(1 Pt 2): F114–9.

Plasma Concentrations of the Vasoactive Peptide Fragments Mid-Regional Pro-Adrenomedullin, C-Terminal Pro-Endothelin 1 and Copeptin in Hemodialysis Patients: Associated Factors and Prediction of Mortality

Ferruh Artunc[1]*, Albina Nowak[2], Christian Mueller[3], Tobias Breidthardt[3], Raphael Twerenbold[3], Robert Wagner[1], Andreas Peter[1], Hans-Ulrich Haering[1], Stefan Ebmeyer[4], Bjoern Friedrich[1,5]

1 Department of Internal Medicine, Division of Endocrinology, Diabetology, Vascular Disease, Nephrology and Clinical Chemistry, University of Tuebingen, Tuebingen, Germany, **2** Division of Internal Medicine, Division of Nephrology, University of Zurich, Zurich, Switzerland, **3** Department of Internal Medicine, Division of Cardiology, University of Basel, Basel, Switzerland, **4** Fisher Scientific, Schwerte, Germany, **5** Dialysis Center, Leonberg, Germany

Abstract

Vasopressin, endothelin and adrenomedullin are vasoactive peptides that regulate vascular tone and might play a role in hypertensive diseases. Recently, laboratory assays have been developed to measure stable fragments of vasopressin, endothelin and adrenomedullin. Little is known about their diagnostic and prognostic value in hemodialysis patients. In this study, we measured the plasma concentration of copeptin, mid-regional-pro-adrenomedullin (MR-pro-ADM) and C-terminal pro-endothelin 1 (CT-pro-ET1) in stable ambulatory hemodialysis patients ($n = 239$) and investigated their associations with clinical factors and mortality. In all patients enrolled, the plasma concentrations of copeptin, MR-pro-ADM and CT-pro-ET1 were largely elevated with a median concentration of 132 pmol/L (interquartile range [IQR] 78–192) for copeptin, 1.26 nmol/L (IQR 1.02–1.80) for MR-pro-ADM and 149 pmol/L (IQR 121–181) for CT-pro-ET1. The plasma concentrations of all vasoactive peptide fragments correlated with time on dialysis and plasma β2-microglobulin concentration and were negatively correlated to residual diuresis. The plasma concentration of MR-pro-ADM was a strong predictor of all-cause (univariate hazard ratio for a 10-fold increase 9.94 [3.14;32], $p<0.0001$) and cardiovascular mortality (hazard ratio 34.87 [5.58;217], $p = 0.0001$) within a 3.8-year follow-up. The associations remained stable in models adjusted for dialysis specific factors and were attenuated in a full model adjusted for all prognostic factors. Plasma copeptin concentration was weakly associated with cardiovascular mortality (only in univariate analysis) and CT-pro-ET1 was not associated with mortality at all. In conclusion, vasoactive peptide fragments are elevated in hemodialysis patients because of accumulation and, most likely, increased release. Increased concentrations of MR-pro-ADM are predictive of mortality.

Editor: Maria A. Deli, Biological Research Centre of the Hungarian Academy of Sciences, Hungary

Funding: The authors have no support or funding to report.

Competing Interests: Stefan Ebmeyer is employed by Fisher Scientific. The company formerly active under the name BRAHMS provided the measurements without charge. This does not alter the authors' adherence to all the PLOS ONE policies on sharing data and materials.

* E-mail: ferruh.artunc@med.uni-tuebingen.de

Introduction

Vasopressin, endothelin and adrenomedullin are vasoactive peptides that regulate vascular tone and perfusion. After being released by vascular endothelial cells (endothelin and adrenomedullin) or pituitary gland (vasopressin), these peptides exert their actions in vascular smooth muscle cells after binding to specific G-protein coupled receptors and generating second messengers. Whereas vasopressin and endothelin lead to vasoconstriction, adrenomedullin exhibits vasodilatory effects [1]. All three have in common a short half-life of a few minutes and ex vivo instability that has precluded valid measurements in humans. To overcome this problem, laboratory assays that detect stable fragments of vasopressin, endothelin and adrenomedullin have been developed, thereby enabling applications in different patient cohorts and diseases [2–4]. Copeptin, the C-terminal portion of pro-vasopressin, C-terminal endothelin 1 (CT-pro-ET1) and mid-regional-pro-adrenomedullin (MR-pro-ADM) are small peptide fragments with 39, 44 and 47 amino acids in length, respectively, that are excised from large precursor peptides during posttranslational processing. They share a low molecular weight (3.4 kDa for copeptin, 5.2 kDa for CT-pro-ET1 and 5.1 kDa for MR-pro-ADM) and because they are stoichiometrically generated they can serve as a good estimate for the plasma concentrations of vasopressin, endothelin and adrenomedullin.

Accurate risk prediction is an important clinical task. In hemodialysis patients, troponins and natriuretic peptides have consistently been shown to be closely associated with patient mortality and improve risk prediction provided by clinical variables alone [5–7]. In this context, the search for new biomarkers reflecting different facts of cardiovascular risk is still ongoing. Among these new biomarkers, the stable fragments MR-pro-ADM, CT-pro-ET1 and copeptin are promising candidates to

Table 1. Patient characteristics of the cohort (N = 239).

median age		70 (61; 77) years (n = 239)
gender distribution		64% male (n = 153)/36% female (n = 86)
renal disease		
	diabetic nephropathy	26% (n = 63)
	hypertension	8% (n = 19)
	glomerulonephritis	30% (n = 71)
	polycystic disease	5% (n = 11)
	other/unknown	31% (n = 75)
cardiac comorbidities		
	coronary heart disease/revascularized	31% (n = 74)/19% (n = 31)
	valvular heart disease	26% (n = 61
	atrial fibrillation	23% (n = 55)
	pulmonary hypertension	7% (n = 16)
	AICD carrier	2% (n = 4)
other comorbidities		
	LV dysfunction	25% (n = 59)
	diabetes mellitus	38% (n = 90)
	peripheral vascular disease	33% (n = 80)
	stroke	16% (n = 38)
	vasculitis	3% (n = 8)
	malignoma	14% (n = 34)
	COPD	8% (n = 19)
length of time on dialysis		46 (19; 85) months (n = 239)
duration of dialysis session		4.0 (4.0; 4.5) hours (n = 239)
dialysis access		
	arteriovenous fistula	71% (n = 169)
	PTFE graft	13% (n = 31)
	tunneled catheter	16% (n = 38)
dialysis membrane		
	high-flux	92% (n = 219)
	low-flux	8% (n = 20)
residual diuresis		250 (0; 1000) mL/day (n = 239)
	anuric patients	39% (n = 93)
interdialytic weight gain		1.85 (1.29; 2.47) kg (n = 239)
blood pump speed		300 (280; 340) mL/min (n = 239)
shunt flow		1080 (733; 1475) mL/min (n = 187)
blood pressure		134 (122; 144)/69 (63; 74) mm Hg (n = 239)
singe pool Kt/V		1.55 (1.40; 1.73) (n = 239)
laboratory data		
	hemoglobin	11.5 (11.1; 12.0) g/dL (n = 239)
	C-reactive protein	8.6 (4.6; 15.0) mg/L (n = 239)
	albumin	37.1 (35.4; 39.3) g/L (n = 239)
	parathormone	204 (130; 348) pg/mL (n = 239)
	β2-microglobulin	23.4 (19.4; 25.4) mg/L (n = 239)
	high sensitive troponin T	49 (31; 73) pg/mL (n = 239)
	NT-pro-BNP	4435 (1687; 16228) pg/mL (n = 223)

Values shown are the median and interquartile range. N indicates number of patients from whom data were available.
Abbreviations:
AICD automatic implantable cardioverter-defibrillator, COPD chronic obstructive pulmonary disease, PTFE polytetrafluorethylene, LV left ventricle.

further improve clinical risk assessment. Interestingly, pilot studies by our group and others [8–12] have shown that in some settings, these novel tools even outperform natriuretic peptides [8;9;12]. However, little is known in hemodialysis patients about the performance and significance of measuring the plasma concentration of MR-pro-ADM, CT-pro-ET1 and copeptin. Two recent studies have shown that increased MR-pro-ADM and copeptin levels were associated with reduced survival [13;14], however, data about the prognostic value of CT-pro-ET1 are not available.

In our study, we analyzed the factors influencing the plasma concentration of copeptin, MR-pro-ADM and CT-pro-ET1 in stable ambulatory hemodialysis patients and analyzed the prognostic value of each vasoactive peptide during a 3.8-year follow-up.

Methods

Patients and cohort

This prospective multicenter study included stable ambulatory hemodialysis patients from four dialysis centers in Southwest Germany between September 2009 and April 2010. Patients were included after they provided written informed consent and when there was no evidence of an acute illness, a cardiac event or a procedure within the previous two months. Patients with cardiac diseases leading to increased cardiac biomarkers concentration (troponin, natriuretic peptides) independent of ESRD, such as amyloidosis were excluded. The study was approved by the local ethics committee of the University of Tuebingen (191/2009BO2).

Laboratory assays

Plasma concentration of copeptin, MR-pro-ADM and CT-pro-ET1 were measured in three independent samples taken within 2 weeks, each one taken to the start of a dialysis session. Blood was collected in lithium-heparinized tubes (Sarstedt, Nuembrecht, Germany), cooled at 4°C and centrifuged within 4 hours; the sera were stored at −80°C for further analysis. The plasma concentrations of copeptin, MR-pro-ADM and CT-pro-ET1 were measured using an automated immunoluminometric assay on a Kryptor system (B.R.A.H.M.S AG, Henningsdorf, Germany) as described in [2–4]. In healthy persons, the normal range defined as the span between the 2.5^{th} and 97.5^{th} percentile was 1.7–11.3 pmol/L for copeptin [3], 0.17–0.49 nmol/L for MR-pro-ADM [2] and 24.8–66.6 pmol/L for CT-pro-ET1 [4].

The plasma concentrations of high sensitive troponin T were measured using an automated Roche assay on an Elecsys 2010 system (Roche, Basel, Switzerland). Plasma concentrations of NT-pro-BNP were measured on a Siemens Immulite 2000 XPi system according to the manufacturers instructions (Siemens Healthcare Diagnostics, Eschborn, Germany). Plasma beta-2-microglobulin concentrations were measured using a turbidimetric assay (Randox Laboratories, Antrim, United Kingdom). All other laboratory values (i.e., parathormone, hemoglobin, albumin and C-reactive protein) were extracted from the patients' medical records and averaged from the available values of the previous year (4–12 values).

Clinical data

From each patient data on residual diuresis (measured by 24 h urine collection), single pool Kt/V (mean of last 4 values), interdialytic weight gain, predialytic systolic and diastolic blood pressure (means from the last 12 values beginning from the first blood draw, resp.), dialysis access and membrane, time on dialysis, blood pump flow and finally shunt flow (measured with a Transonic system, Ithaca, NY, USA) were extracted. The systolic left ventricular (LV) function was classified from available echocardiography examinations.

Statistical analysis

Three plasma samples were available from 87% of the patients and were averaged to calculate the arithmetic mean without excluding possible outliers. Plasma vasoactive peptide concentrations and continuous clinical data were log10 transformed to approximate normal distribution. The association of the plasma

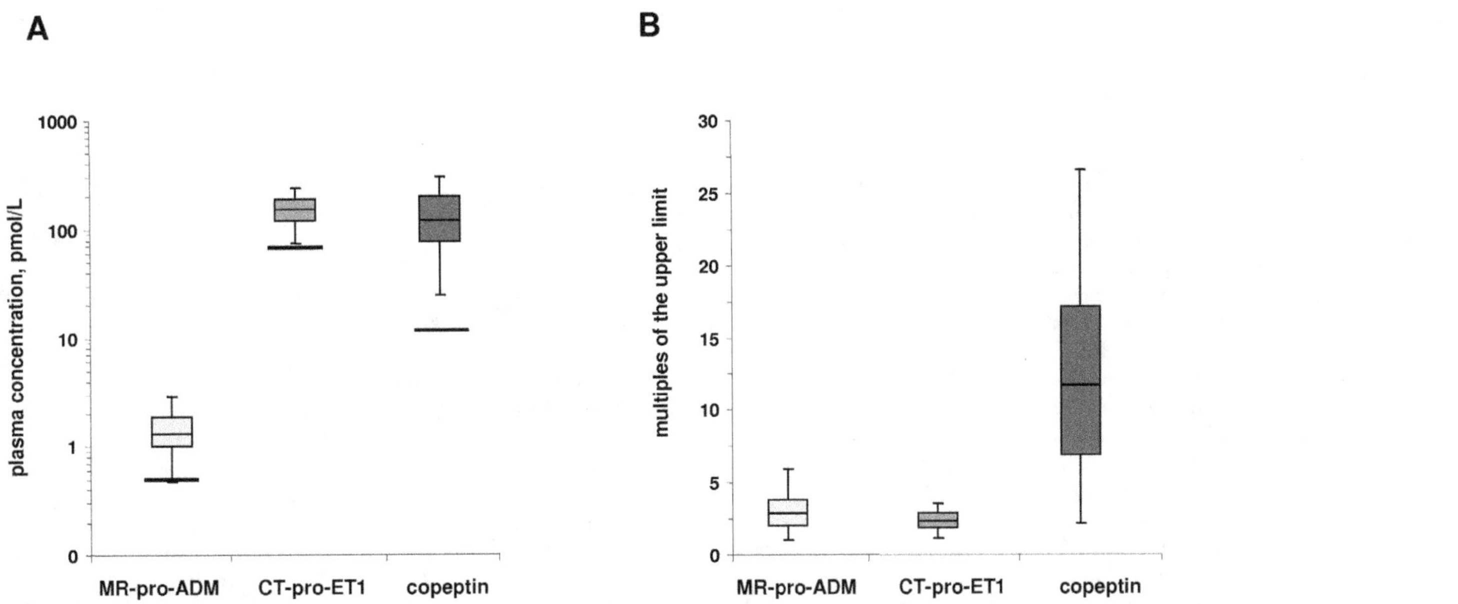

Figure 1. Box-and-Whisker-Plot of the plasma vasoactive peptide concentration indicating median, IQR and the range between the 2.5^{th} and 97.5^{th} percentile (Panel A). Solid lines represent the upper reference limit. Panel B: Box-and-Whisker-Plot of the plasma vasoactive peptide concentration expressed as multiples of the upper reference limit.

Table 2. Univariate correlations (Pearsons r) of the plasma vasoactive peptide concentration with general and dialysis-specific parameters (n = 210–239).

	MR-pro-ADM, pmol/L	CT-pro-ET1, pmol/L	copeptin, pmol/L
dialysis-specific factors			
age, y	n.s.	−0.24 ***	n.s.
time on dialysis, months	0.34 ***	0.33 ***	0.30 ***
residual diuresis, ml/day	−0.25 ***	−0.23 ***	−0.33 ***
interdialytic weight gain, kg	0.13 *	0.12 #	0.16 *
shunt flow, ml/min	n.s.	0.26 ***	0.13 #
systolic blood pressure, mm Hg	−0.18 **	n.s.	n.s.
diastolic blood pressure, mm Hg	n.s.	0.27 ***	n.s.
pulse pressure, mmHg	−0.17 **	−0.25 ***	n.s.
duration of a HD session	n.s.	0.17 *	n.s.
blood pump speed, ml/min	n.s.	n.s.	n.s.
laboratory data			
Kt/V	0.11 #	0.25 ***	0.11 #
hemoglobin, g/dL	n.s.	n.s.	n.s.
plasma albumin, g/L	n.s.	n.s.	n.s.
C-reactive protein, mg/L	0.13 #	−0.11 #	n.s.
parathormone, pg/mL	n.s.	n.s.	n.s.
β2-microglobulin, mg/dL	0.54 ***	0.57 **	0.33 ***
troponin T, pg/mL	0.26 ***	n.s.	0.26 ***
NT-pro-BNP, pg/mL	0.42 ***	0.24 **	0.24 ***
comorbidity (1 = yes)			
systolic LV dysfunction	0.17 *	n.s.	0.13 #
valvular disease	0.28 ***	0.17 **	0.18 **
atrial fibrillation	0.35 ***	n.s.	n.s.
pulmonary hypertension	0.17 **	n.s.	n.s.
peripheral vascular disease	0.21 **	n.s.	n.s.
diabetes mellitus	n.s.	−0.20 ***	n.s.

# $p<0.10$, * $p<0.05$, ** $p<0.01$, *** $p<0.001$, n.s. = not significant ($p>0.10$).

vasoactive peptide concentration with clinical or dialysis-related factors was analyzed by univariate parametric correlation. To identify independent determinants of the plasma vasoactive peptide concentration, multivariate linear regression analyses were performed. Selection of the variables entering the model was derived from forward-stepwise multiple linear regression, and all variables with a p-value<0.20 were subsequently included in the multivariate linear regression models. Finally, the residuals of each model were tested for normality. The follow-up period started on the first day of blood draw and lasted until October 26th, 2013. Causes of death were classified according to the best knowledge of each particular case. Cardiovascular death was considered as sudden death (most probably circulatory or cardiac arrest) and death due to a cardiovascular event or disease (coronary artery disease, hypertensive crisis, stroke, peripheral artery disease). The averaged values of the deceased patients were compared to those from the surviving patients using a t-Test or Wilcoxons test. Kaplan-Meier curves were generated after stratification into tertiles of the variable according to its distribution. Survival curves were compared using the log-rank test. Univariate and multivariate proportional hazards were calculated using the Cox regression analysis. Data analysis was performed using the statistical software package JMP 10.0.1 (SAS Institute, Cary, NC).

Results

Patients

From a total of n = 250 available patients treated in the participating centers, 239 patients (95.6%) were included in the study. 6 patients declined written informed consent, 2 died within the period of blood sampling, 2 had cardiac amyloidosis and one patient was only recently initiated to dialysis. The characteristics of the study cohort are given in table 1.

Plasma concentrations of copeptin, MR-pro-ADM and CT-pro-ET1 in the cohort

In nearly all participating patients, the plasma concentrations of all studied vasoactive peptide fragments were elevated compared to the reference values from healthy persons. The median concentration was 132 pmol/L (IQR 78–192) for copeptin, 1.26 pmol/L (IQR 1.02–1.80) for MR-pro-ADM and 149 pmol/L (IQR 121–181) for CT-pro-ET1 (Figure 1A). Expressed as multiples of the 97.5th percentile taken as the upper end of the reference range obtained from healthy individuals [2–4], the copeptin concentration was elevated 11.7-fold (IQR 6.9–16.9) compared to 2.8-fold for MR-pro-ADM (IQR2.1–3.7) and 2.2-fold for CT-pro-ET1 (IQR 1.8–2.7; Figure 1B).

Table 3. Independent factors determining the plasma vasoactive peptide concentration by multivariate linear modeling (n = 155–201).

	covariate	estimate ± SD	standardized estimate ± SD	p-value
MR-pro-ADM **R^2 = 0.48**	y-intercept	−0.85±0.41	0.13±0.01	
	β2-microglobulin, mg/L	0.97±0.10	0.28±0.03	<0.0001
	duration of a HD session	0.64±0.23	0.13±0.05	0.0069
	atrial fibrillation (1 = yes)	0.13±0.02	0.07±0.01	<0.0001
	systolic blood pressure, mmHg	−0.42±0.17	−0.07±0.03	0.0149
	NT-proBNP, pg/ml	0.03±0.02	0.05±0.03	0.0933
	interdialytic weight gain, kg	−0.03±0.02	−0.04±0.02	0.1196
	peripheral vascular disease (1 = yes)	0.06±0.02	0.03±0.01	0.0061
	valvular disease (1 = yes)	0.03±0.02	0.01±0.01	0.2180
CT-pro-ET1 **R^2 = 0.41**	y-intercept	1.43±0.40	2.17±0.01	
	β2-microglobulin, mg/L	0.56±0.07	0.16±0.02	<0.0001
	NT-proBNP, pg/ml	0.05±0.01	0.07±0.02	0.0009
	age, y	−0.25±0.08	−0.07±0.02	0.0013
	diastolic blood pressure, mmHg	0.43±0.15	0.08±0.02	0.0035
	systolic blood pressure, mmHg	−0.35±0.14	−0.06±0.02	0.0142
	plasma albumin, g/L	0.16±0.12	0.06±0.05	0.1917
	atrial fibrillation (1 = yes)	−0.01±0.02	−0.01±0.01	0.4668
copeptin **R^2 = 0.19**	y-intercept	0.74±0.27	2.08±0.02	
	β2-microglobulin, mg/L	0.68±0.20	0.18±0.05	0.0009
	time on dialysis, months	0.15±0.05	0.14±0.04	0.0014
	systolic LV dysfunction (1 = yes)	0.09±0.04	0.04±0.02	0.0292
	parathormone, pg/mL	0.07±0.05	0.09±0.06	0.1156

Note that all continuous parameter were entered into the model after $\log_{10}$ transformation.

Plasma vasoactive peptide concentrations were moderately correlated to one another, with the highest correlation between MR-pro-ADM and CT-pro-ET1 (0.45, p<0.0001), followed by copeptin and CT-pro-ET1 (0.39, p<0.0001) and MR-pro-ADM and copeptin (0.28, p<0.0001). Within three consecutive samples, the intraindividual variability expressed as the coefficient of variation was the least for CT-pro-ET1 (8±12%), followed by MR-pro-ADM (14±11%) and copeptin (17±14%).

Table 4. Follow-up data after 3.8 (IQR 3.6;3,9) years and causes of death.

continued on HD	138 (57.7%)
transplanted	15 (6.3%)
deceased	86 (36.0%)
sudden death	20 (23% of all deaths)
cardiovascular death[§]	14 (16%)
infection and sepsis	12 (14%)
wasting/cachexia	20 (23%)
malignancy	9 (10%)
others/unknown	11 (13%)

[§]Composite of deaths due to coronary artery disease, hypertension, peripheral artery disease.

Univariate analyses

Table 2 lists the results of the univariate correlation analyses of the plasma vasoactive peptide concentration with the collected parameters. MR-pro-ADM, copeptin and CT-pro-ET1 showed a significant positive correlation to time on dialysis and the β2-microglobulin concentration while they were all negatively correlated to residual diuresis. MR-pro-ADM was negatively correlated to systolic blood pressure, while CT-ET1 was positively correlated to diastolic blood pressure. There was weak correlation of all vasoactive peptides to Kt/V and interdialytic weight gain and almost no correlation to cardiac comorbidity except for MR-pro-ADM (table 2).

Multivariate analyses

To analyze the independent determinants of the plasma vasoactive peptide concentration, a multivariate linear regression model was performed with a stepwise forward approach based on a p-value of <0.20 and all covariates from table 2. Table 3 lists the resulting multivariate models. Plasma β2-microglobulin concentration was the strongest independent determinant of the plasma vasoactive peptide concentration. The modeling was best for

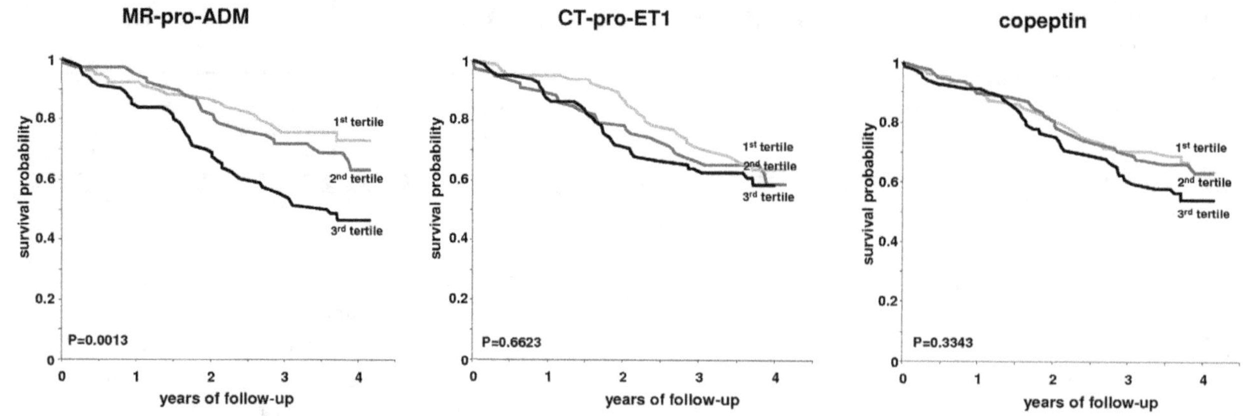

Figure 2. Survival curves of the cohort stratified according to the tertiles (T1, T2 and T3) of MR-pro-ADM (<1.09; 1.09–1.64; >1.64 pmol/L), CT-pro-ET1 (<131; 131–171; >171 pmol/L) and copeptin (<101; 101–171; >171 pmol/L) plasma concentration.

MR-pro-ADM and CT-pro-ET1 with an adjusted r^2 value of 0.48 and 0.41, respectively, and poor for copeptin ($r^2 = 0.18$).

Prognostic value

After 3.8 years of follow-up, data from all 239 patients were available (median follow-up time 1378 days [IQR 1325; 1429]). Of those, 86 had died (36%), 15 (6%) had been transplanted and the rest remained on HD (table 4). The concentration of MR-pro-ADM was significantly ($p<0.0001$) higher in the deceased patients compared to the surviving patients (1.62 pmol/L [IQR 1.19;2.27] vs. 1.26 pmol/L [IQR 0.98;1.66]). The concentrations of CT-pro-ET1 and copeptin were not different in the surviving patients compared to the deceased patients ($p = 0.52$ and $p = 0.07$, respectively).

The survival curves stratified for tertiles of vasoactive peptide concentrations are shown in Figure 2, and the relative risk compared to the first tertile is shown in Figure 3. Using the Cox proportional hazard method, plasma MR-pro-ADM concentration was found to be significantly associated with increased all-cause and cardiovascular mortality in a univariate analysis (hazard ratio for a 10-fold increase 9.94 and 34.87, respectively; table 5). These associations were stable in a model adjusted for dialysis-specific factors and finally attenuated in a model adjusted for all prognostic factors. Plasma copeptin concentration was weakly associated with all-cause ($p = 0.077$) and cardiovascular mortality ($p = 0.033$) in a univariate model, and lost its associations in multivariate analyses. Plasma CT-pro-ET1 concentration was not associated with a significantly increased hazard ratio, both in univariate and multivariate analyses.

Discussion

This study demonstrates that the plasma MR-pro-ADM concentration is a strong predictor of mortality in hemodialysis patients, whereas copeptin was only weakly and CT-pro-ET1 concentrations not at all associated with mortality. Similar results have been published for MR-pro-ADM in hemodialysis patients by Gouya et al. in 2011 [13], who reported a two-threefold increased hazard ratio for mortality of the upper tertile of the patients compared to the lower tertile. The association of the plasma copeptin concentration with mortality has been previously reported in a study with the cohort of the 4D study (German Diabetes Dialysis Study) [14]. In that large study, copeptin was significantly associated with both all-cause and cardiovascular death, however, we could only demonstrate that copeptin was weakly associated with cardiovascular mortality. The reason for this discrepancy could be related to the studied cohort and statistical power since the 4D study comprised 1241 solely diabetic patients reaching the end point by 37–49%. To our knowledge, the results presented on CT-pro-ET1 in this study are reported for the first time and show that the plasma CT-pro-ET1 concentration is not predictive of mortality in hemodialysis patients. Data on

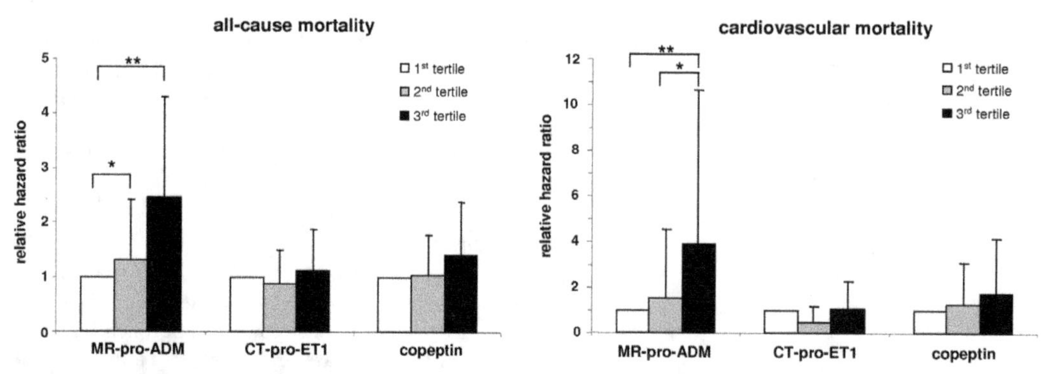

Figure 3. Relative hazard ratios for all-cause mortality and cardiovascular mortality with 95% confidence interval according to the tertiles (T1. T2 and T3) of MR-pro-ADM (<1.09; 1.09–1.64; >1.64 pmol/L), CT-pro-ET1 (<131; 131–171; >171 pmol/L) and copeptin (<101; 101–171; >171 pmol/L) plasma concentration. The risk of the first tertile was set to 1. * $p<0.05$, ** $p<0.01$.

Table 5. Hazard ratios (and 95% CIs) for mortality according to the MR-pro-ADM, CT-pro-ET1 and copeptin levels.

	univariate (crude)		multivariate: model 1		multivariate: model 2	
	HR with 95% CI	**p-value**	**HR with 95% CI**	**p-value**	**HR with 95% CI**	**p-value**
MR-pro-ADM						
all-cause mortality	9.94 [3.14–31.89]	<0.0001	9.54 [1.81–51.17]	0.0079	3.37 [0.82–14.88]	0.0924
cardio-vascular mortality	34.87 [5.58;217]	0.0001	101.26 [5.47;2317]	0.0017	6.14 [0.66; 71.92]	0.1138
CT-pro-ET1						
all-cause mortality	1.21 [0.25–6.18]	0.8185	3.52 [0.29–43.31]	0.3212	3.10 [0.47–21.97]	0.2427
cardio-vascular mortality	2.27 [0.18;32.63]	0.5293	2.75 [0.28;27.29]	0.3813	5.57 [0.26;138.83]	0.2741
copeptin						
all-cause mortality	2.01 [0.92–4.66]	0.0770	2.37 [0.56–11.58]	0.2492	0.97 [0.39–2.60]	0.9550
cardio-vascular mortality	4.24 [1.11;19.57]	0.0334	5.95 [0.81;63.43]	0.0824	2.62 [0.50;17.61]	0.2669

The hazard ratios are displayed for a one-unit increase in the decadic log-transformed (corresponding to a ten-fold increase) of the plasma MR-pro-ADM, CT-pro-ET1 and copeptin concentration. Cardiovascular mortality was considered as sudden death (most probably circulatory or cardiac arrest) and death due to a cardiovascular event or disease (coronary artery disease, hypertensive crisis, stroke, peripheral artery disease).
Model 1: adjusted for demographics, hemodynamic and dialysis-specific risk factors.
- age.
- gender (male).
- time on dialysis.
- residual diuresis.
- shunt flow.
- vascular access on study enrolment (fistula, graft or catheter).
- systolic and diastolic blood pressure.
- interdialytic weight gain.
- pooled Kt/V.

Model 2: adjusted for all factors associated with mortality (significant difference between deceased and surviving patients).
- age.
- body mass index.
- duration of HD session.
- diastolic blood pressure.
- secondary hyperparathyroidism (represented by parathormone concentration).
- inflammatory status (represented by CRP concentration).
- comorbidities: systolic dysfunction (1 = yes), peripheral vascular disease (1 = yes), coronary artery disease (1 = yes), atrial fibrillation (1 = yes).

big endothelin 1, the 38 amino acid precursor molecule of endothelin 1, have shown a modest association with mortality in hemodialysis patients, which was lost during multivariate modeling [15]. The CT-pro-ET1 assay used in this study measures a fragment at the C-terminus comprising amino acid residues 168 through 212 of the initial large precursor molecule pre-pro-ET1 (212 amino acids) [4] from which big endothelin 1 (amino acids residues 53–90) and finally endothelin 1 (amino acid residues 53–73) are derived. The reason why the fragment CT-pro-ET1, although elevated in nearly all studied patients, failed to be associated with mortality in contrast to patients with heart failure [16] or patients after acute myocardial infarction [17] remains unclear.

Both endothelin and vasopressin cause vasoconstriction, while adrenomedullin is a peptide with strong vasodilating effects. The association of MR-pro-ADM with mortality suggests that an increased vasodilatory response in hemodialysis patients is prognostically relevant and that low levels of MR-pro-ADM represent a state of less vasoconstriction and better prognosis. The finding of increased cardiovascular mortality with increased copeptin concentrations supports this notion. In addition, it is also conceivable that there is a resistance to the vasodilatory response of MR-pro-ADM in hemodialysis patients leading to increased secretion. In a study with stable kidney transplant recipients, MR-pro-ADM concentrations correlated with the resistance to antihypertensive treatment which suggests increased vasoconstriction in these patients [18]. Studies from Yoshihara et al. found that MR-pro-ADM plasma concentrations reflected volume overload [19;20]. In this context, increased MR-pro-ADM plasma concentration can be interpreted as a counterregulatory response similar to the increase in the plasma concentration of the natriuretic peptides which are strong predictors of mortality [11] and also exert vasodilating effects [21]. Physiologically, adrenomedullin mRNA is found in the adrenal gland, heart, kidney and blood vessels and up-regulated by inflammation, hypoxia, oxidative and mechanical shear stress, activation of the renin-angiotensin and the sympathetic nervous system [22]. Pharmacological application of adrenomedullin has shown protective effects in models of renal [23] or heart failure [24]. From this perspective, adrenomedullin can be considered as a marker of stress in cardiovascular disease, and particularly in patients with renal failure who have all the above mentioned features.

Our data show that the plasma concentrations of MR-pro-ADM, CT-pro-ET1 and copeptin were greatly increased in hemodialysis patients, most likely reflecting accumulation. This result was particularly true for copeptin, which was increased about tenfold above the upper limit. This finding indicates that the clearance of these peptide fragments is highly impaired during dialysis-dependent chronic kidney disease, which is typical for low molecular weight proteins. A marker of the latter is β2-microglobulin (molecular weight 11.7 kDa), which was a strong independent predictor of the plasma concentration of all vasoactive peptides studied. On the other hand, modern dialysis practices such as high flux dialyzers or hemodiafiltration can remove significant amounts of low-molecular weight proteins as this was known for β2-microglobulin [25] and also was shown for

MR-pro-ADM [19]. In that study the plasma MR-pro-ADM concentration was approximately 25–30% lower after a hemodialysis session. Hence, hemodialysis patients reach a new steady state at a higher level.

The increased plasma concentrations complicate the interpretation of MR-pro-ADM, copeptin and CT-pro-ET1 values, but one has to consider that accumulation can only occur when these peptides are released from their original sites upon biological stimuli, therefore we must assume that there is an increased release of these peptides in hemodialysis patients. The increased plasma concentrations in turn, however, make the interpretation more difficult and only with the aid of studies such as this, clinically meaningful cut-off values can be derived such as the limit of the upper tertile for the prognostic use of MR-pro-ADM (i.e. >1.62 pmol/L). However, more studies are needed to better define cut-off values of the plasma concentration of these peptides for diagnostic and prognostic purposes.

The limitations of the current study might include the incomplete collection of the data relevant to understand the correlation of the studied parameters. In the multivariate regression model, >50% of the variance was not explained by the entered factors, in the case of copeptin even >80%. The study focused on nephrological parameters that are commonly available and accessible during hemodialysis treatment, such as residual diuresis or shunt flow. Furthermore, survival analyses might be limited by the low mortality during the follow-up period.

In conclusion, the fragments of the vasoactive peptides MR-pro-ADM, CT-pro-ET1 and copeptin are largely elevated in hemodialysis patients because of accumulation and, most likely, higher release. Plasma MR-pro-ADM concentration was strongly associated with all-cause and cardiovascular mortality.

Acknowledgments

We thank Andrea Janessa and Claudia Stelzig for their valuable assistance during the study.

Author Contributions

Conceived and designed the experiments: FA BF. Performed the experiments: FA BF. Analyzed the data: AN CM TB RT RW. Contributed reagents/materials/analysis tools: AP SE HUH. Wrote the paper: FA BF.

References

1. Hinson JP, Kapas S, Smith DM (2000) Adrenomedullin, a multifunctional regulatory peptide. Endocr Rev 21: 138–167.
2. Morgenthaler NG, Struck J, Alonso C, Bergmann A (2005) Measurement of midregional proadrenomedullin in plasma with an immunoluminometric assay. Clin Chem 51: 1823–1829.
3. Morgenthaler NG, Struck J, Alonso C, Bergmann A (2006) Assay for the measurement of copeptin, a stable peptide derived from the precursor of vasopressin. Clin Chem 52: 112–119.
4. Papassotiriou J, Morgenthaler NG, Struck J, Alonso C, Bergmann A (2006) Immunoluminometric assay for measurement of the C-terminal endothelin-1 precursor fragment in human plasma. Clin Chem 52: 1144–1151.
5. Apple FS, Murakami MM, Pearce LA, Herzog CA (2002) Predictive value of cardiac troponin I and T for subsequent death in end-stage renal disease. Circulation 106: 2941–2945.
6. Mallamaci F, Zoccali C, Parlongo S, Tripepi G, Benedetto FA, et al. (2002) Troponin is related to left ventricular mass and predicts all-cause and cardiovascular mortality in hemodialysis patients. Am J Kidney Dis 40: 68–75.
7. Khan NA, Hemmelgarn BR, Tonelli M, Thompson CR, Levin A (2005) Prognostic value of troponin T and I among asymptomatic patients with end-stage renal disease: a meta-analysis. Circulation 112: 3088–3096.
8. Potocki M, Breidthardt T, Reichlin T, Morgenthaler NG, Bergmann A, et al. (2009) Midregional pro-adrenomedullin in addition to b-type natriuretic peptides in the risk stratification of patients with acute dyspnea: an observational study. Crit Care 13: R122.
9. Maisel A, Mueller C, Nowak R, Peacock WF, Landsberg JW, et al. (2010): Mid-region pro-hormone markers for diagnosis and prognosis in acute dyspnea: results from the BACH (Biomarkers in Acute Heart Failure) trial. J Am Coll Cardiol 55: 2062–2076.
10. Artunc F, Mueller C, Breidthardt T, Twerenbold R, Peter A, et al. (2012) Sensitive troponins – which suits better for hemodialysis patients? Associated factors and prediction of mortality. PLoS One 7: e47610.
11. Artunc F, Mueller C, Breidthardt T, Twerenbold R, Rettig I, et al. (2012) Comparison of the diagnostic performance of three natriuretic peptides in hemodialysis patients: which is the appropriate biomarker? Kidney Blood Press Res 36: 172–181.
12. Potocki M, Breidthardt T, Mueller A, Reichlin T, Socrates T, et al. (2010) Copeptin and risk stratification in patients with acute dyspnea. Crit Care 14: R213.
13. Gouya G, Sturm G, Lamina C, Zitt E, Freistatter O, et al. (2011) The association of mid-regional pro-adrenomedullin and mid-regional pro-atrial natriuretic peptide with mortality in an incident dialysis cohort. PLoS One 6: e17803.
14. Fenske W, Wanner C, Allolio B, Drechsler C, Blouin K, et al. (2011) Copeptin levels associate with cardiovascular events in patients with ESRD and type 2 diabetes mellitus. J Am Soc Nephrol 22: 782–790.
15. Spinar J, Ludka O, Dusek L, Vitovcova L, Sobotova D, et al. (2007) Neurohumoral activity, heart failure and prognosis in patients with end-stage renal disease treated by hemodialysis. Kidney Blood Press Res 30: 347–357.
16. Jankowska EA, Filippatos GS, von HS, Papassotiriou J, Morgenthaler NG, et al. (2011) Identification of chronic heart failure patients with a high 12-month mortality risk using biomarkers including plasma C-terminal pro-endothelin-1. PLoS One 6: e14506.
17. Khan SQ, Dhillon O, Struck J, Quinn P, Morgenthaler NG, et al. (2007) C-terminal pro-endothelin-1 offers additional prognostic information in patients after acute myocardial infarction: Leicester Acute Myocardial Infarction Peptide (LAMP) Study. Am Heart J 154: 736–742.
18. Suzuki Y, Itoh H, Katagiri F, Sato F, Kawasaki K, et al. (2013) Relationship between plasma mid-regional pro-adrenomedullin level and resistance to antihypertensive therapy in stable kidney transplant recipients. Peptides 48: 45–48.
19. Yoshihara F, Ernst A, Morgenthaler NG, Horio T, Nakamura S, et al. (2007) Midregional proadrenomedullin reflects cardiac dysfunction in haemodialysis patients with cardiovascular disease. Nephrol Dial Transplant 22: 2263–2268.
20. Yoshihara F, Horio T, Nakamura S, Yoshii M, Ogata C, et al. (2005) Adrenomedullin reflects cardiac dysfunction, excessive blood volume, and inflammation in hemodialysis patients. Kidney Int 68: 1355–1363.
21. Federico C (2010) Natriuretic Peptide system and cardiovascular disease. Heart Views 11: 10–15.
22. Ishimitsu T, Ono H, Minami J, Matsuoka H (2006) Pathophysiologic and therapeutic implications of adrenomedullin in cardiovascular disorders. Pharmacol Ther 111: 909–927.
23. Oyar EO, Kiris I, Gulmen S, Ceyhan BM, Cure MC, et al (2012) The protective effect of adrenomedullin on renal injury, in a model of abdominal aorta cross-clamping. Thorac Cardiovasc Surg 60: 5–10.
24. Rademaker MT, Charles CJ, Espiner EA, Nicholls MG, Richards AM (2002) Long-term adrenomedullin administration in experimental heart failure. Hypertension 40: 667–672.
25. Davenport A (2011) Role of dialysis technology in the removal of uremic toxins. Hemodial Int 15 Suppl 1: S49–S53.

Association of Serum Phosphorus Variability with Coronary Artery Calcification among Hemodialysis Patients

Mengjing Wang[1]◔, Haiming Li[1]◔, Li You[1], Xiaoling Yu[1], Min Zhang[1], Ruijiang Zhu[2], Chuanming Hao[1], Zhijie Zhang[3,4], Jing Chen[1]*

1 Division of Nephrology, Huashan Hospital, Shanghai Medical College, Fudan University, Shanghai, China, **2** Division of Radiology, Huashan Hospital, Shanghai Medical College, Fudan University, Shanghai, China, **3** Department of Epidemiology and Biostatistics, School of Public Health, Fudan University, Shanghai, China, **4** Biomedical statistical Center, Fudan University, Shanghai, China

Abstract

Coronary artery calcification (CAC) is associated with increased mortality in patients on maintenance hemodialysis (MHD), but the pathogenesis of this condition is not well understood. We evaluated the relationship of CAC score (CACs) and variability in serum phosphorus in MHD patients. Seventy-seven adults on MHD at Huashan Hospital (Shanghai) were enrolled in July, 2010. CAC of all the patients were measured by computed tomography and CACs was calculated by the Agatston method at the entry of enrollment. Patients were divided into three categories according to their CACs (0~10, 11~400, and >400). Blood chemistry was recorded every 3 months from January 2008 to July 2010. Phosphorus variation was defined by the standard deviation (SD) or coefficient of variation (CV) and it was calculated from the past records. The ordinal multivariate logistic regression analysis was used to analyze the predictors of CAC. The mean patient age (± SD) was 61.7 years (±11.3) and 51% of patients were men. The mean CACs was 609.6 (±1062.9), the median CACs was 168.5, and 78% of patients had CACs more than 0. Multivariate analysis indicated that female gender (OR = 0.20, 95% CI = 0.07–0.55), age (OR = 2.31, 95% CI = 1.32–4.04), serum fibroblast growth factor 23 (OR = 2.25, 95% CI = 1.31–3.85), SD-phosphorus calculated from the most recent 6 measurements (OR = 2.12; 95% CI = 1.23–3.63), and CV-phosphorus calculated from the most recent 6 measurements (OR = 1.90, 95% CI = 1.16–3.11) were significantly and independently associated with CACs. These associations persisted for phosphorus variation calculated from past 7, 8, 9, 10, and 11 follow-up values. Variability of serum phosphorus may contribute significantly to CAC and keeping serum phosphorus stable may decrease coronary calcification and associated morbidity and mortality in MHD patients.

Editor: Elena Aikawa, Brigham and Women's Hospital, Harvard Medical School, United States of America

Funding: This work was supported in part by the Major State Basic Research Development Program of China (973 program, No. 374 2012CB517700), and the China Natural Science Foundation (81170684/30971373) to Jing Chen. The funders had no role in study design, data collection and analysis, decision to publish, or preparation of the manuscript.

Competing Interests: The authors have declared that no competing interests exist.

* E-mail: chenjing1998@fudan.edu.cn

◔ These authors contributed equally to this work.

Introduction

Coronary artery calcification (CAC) is common in patients on maintenance hemodialysis (MHD) therapy [1–3], and such patients have increased risk for cardiovascular disease (CVD) and all-cause mortality [4–9]. Previous research indicated that dialysis patients had a 10- to 20-fold increased risk for death from CVD relative to age- and gender-matched members of the general population [10]. The mechanisms of CAC are not well understood, but advanced age, male sex, hypertension, dyslipidemia, chronic inflammatory state [1–3,11,12], dialysis duration [13], oxidative stress [11], bone-related proteins [14,15], and mineral disturbances [2,16] are associated with increased risk of CAC. However, some studies have refuted these reported associations [17,18].

There is much controversy regarding the mechanism of CAC. Block *et al.* first reported a positive association of hyperphosphatemia and mortality in HD patients [19], and this led to subsequent studies of the association between CAC and phosphorus metabolism in uremic patients, but the results of these studies have been contradictory. In particular, Raggi *et al.* reported that the extent of coronary calcification was greater in MHD patients with higher serum concentrations of phosphorus [2] and Jung *et al.* reported that elevated serum phosphorus was associated with rapid progression of CAC in HD patients [20]. However, other studies reported no association of serum phosphorus and CAC in HD populations [1,11,15,21,22]. Thus, rigorous prospective clinical studies and outcome studies are needed to definitively establish the relationship of elevated serum phosphorus and CAC.

The level of serum phosphorus varies throughout the day under normal physiological conditions [23], but (in the absence of advanced chronic kidney disease [CKD]) is maintained within the range of 2.5 to 4.5 mg/dL (0.8–1.4 mmol/L) by a variety of mechanisms including gastrointestinal absorption, urinary excretion, bone loss and uptake, and transport between the intracellular and extracellular spaces [24]. The level of serum phosphorus has greater daily variation in HD patients due to increased gut absorption from high daily protein intake, high levels of active vitamin D, bone disorders, and decreased urinary excretion [25]. Thus, the serum phosphorus levels of HD patients fluctuate much more than in healthy individuals [26]. However, few studies have examined the relationship between the extent of variation in serum phosphorus and CAC.

The purpose of this study was to investigate the association of serum phosphorus variability with CAC in MHD patients.

Materials and Methods

Patients

This was a retrospective study of 77 consecutive Chinese HD patients in one hemodialysis center (Huashan Hospital, Fudan University, Shanghai, PR China) from January 2008 to July 2010. All patients were over 18 years-old, on HD more than 15 months, and were followed up every 3 months with biochemical and immunological testing on the same day. Patients were excluded if they had severe malnutrition, hepatic insufficiency, active infection, active malignancy, heart failure, prior history of coronary artery revascularization or myocardial infarction, vasculitis, or diabetes mellitus or hypertension that was poorly controlled. The Ethics Committee on Human Research at Huashan Hospital, Fudan University approved this study and all patients provided written informed consent. All patients were undergoing HD (4 h per session, 3 times per week) and were treated with bicarbonate dialysis fluid and low-flux dialysers made of polysulfone (surface area: 1.2 m^2, Diacap α, B. Braun., Melsungen, Germany).

Data collection and evaluation of variability in serum phosphorus, calcium and parathyroid hormone

Data on demographics and dialysis-specific and clinical characteristics were collected at the time of enrollment (July 2010). Two daily urine collections were pooled for the creatinine and urea clearance calculations. The GFR was estimated as the mean of creatinine and urea clearance adjusted for body surface area (ml/min per 1.73 m^2) [25]. Biochemical parameters were also recorded at this time, including: serum hemoglobin, ferritin, transferrin saturation, carbon dioxide combining power (CO_2CP), C-reactive protein (CRP), albumin, serum creatinine, blood urea nitrogen, total, high-density and low-density lipoprotein cholesterol (HDL and LDL), and triglycerides, phosphorus, calcium, parathyroid hormone (PTH), fibroblast growth factor 23 (FGF23), and 1,25$(OH)_2D_3$.

Variability was defined as the standard deviation (SD) or coefficient of variation (SD/mean) [27]. So the past testing results (every 3 months from January 2008 to July 2010, 11 times in total) of serum phosphorus, calcium, and PTH levels were also obtained. For each parameter, we calculated six CVs, six SDs, and six means based on the past 6, 7, 8, 9, 10, and 11 values.

Imaging procedure

All patients were scanned using a 256-detector-row Brilliance iCT scanner (Philips Healthcare, Cleveland, OH) in July 2010. The entire heart was covered in a single breath-hold (20–30 sec). Slices of 3.0-mm thickness were acquired with 150 mA of tube current at 120 kV. Quantification was performed by a single trained reader who was blinded to the clinical data, using software for calcium scoring (Heartbeat-CS, EBW, Philips Medical Systems, Best, The Netherlands). This software can detect calcified lesions with a density of at least 130 Hounsfield units (HU) over a minimal area of 0.5 mm^2. Patients were assigned calcification scores based on the number, area, and peak HU of the calcific lesions, as described by Agatston *et al* [28]. (1: 110–199 HU; 2: 200–299 HU; 3: 300–399 HU; 4: >400 HU). Data obtained during the diastolic phase of the heart cycle were used for image reconstruction. The total score was calculated by summing the calcification scores of the left main, left anterior descending, left circumflex, and right coronary arteries.

Laboratory testing

The patients in the morning shift fasted routinely after 10 pm before the day of laboratory tests. However the patients in the afternoon shift had their lunch after the blood samples were collected. Blood samples were drawn direct from the AV-fistula at 8 am or 1 pm (at the beginning of dialysis) on the day of the mid-week HD session and biochemical parameters were assessed by standard techniques. The formula used to calculate corrected calcium was described in the K/DOQI guidelines [29]: Corr-Ca = Measured serum Ca+[4.0 - measured serum albumin (g/dL)] ×0.8. The single-pool Kt/V_{urea} delivered by HD (sp-dKt/V_{urea}) was estimated by the second-generation Daugirdas formula [30]. The normalized protein nitrogen appearance (nPNA) was calculated as described by Termorshuizen *et al.* and normalized to standard body weight (total body water/0.58) [31]. Total-body water was determined from Watson's formula [32]. The serum levels of intact PTH (Santa Cruz, CA, USA), intact FGF23 (Immutopics, San Clemente, CA, USA), and 1,25$(OH)_2D_3$ (Immunodiagnostic Systems, Boldon, UK) were measured by ELISA according to the manufacturers' protocols. The detection of intact FGF23 guarantees that we measure the biologically active form of human FGF23. FGF23 fragments will not be measured [33].

Statistical analysis

The mean, SD, median, and interquartile range (IQR) or number and percentage were used to characterize variables of the study objects. Ordinal univariate logistic regression was first used to analyze the predictors of CAC, based on CACs. Explanatory variables included two types of data: *(i)* clinical characteristics and biochemical parameters obtained at the time of enrollment (age, sex, smoking, diabetes, dialysis vintage, body mass index [BMI], nPNA, systolic BP, diastolic BP, blood flow, Kt/V, medications, serum hemoglobin, ferritin, transferrin saturation, CO_2CP, CPR, albumin, serum creatinine, blood urea nitrogen, phosphorus, calcium, PTH, FGF23, 1,25$(OH)_2D_3$, total, HDL, LDL, cholesterol, and triglycerides); and *(ii)* variations and means of serum phosphorus, calcium, and PTH calculated from previous records. The explanatory variables were not normally distributed, so the BOX-COX transformation was applied before modeling. Predictors with *p*-values of 0.2 or less were included in the ordinal multivariate logistic regression analysis. Backward selection was used to determine the significant variables in the best fitted model, and a *p*-value less than 0.05 was considered statistically significant. Six models were developed using the same explanatory variables described above except for variations and means of serum phosphorus, calcium, and PTH. The variations and means of six models were calculated from previous 6, 7, 8, 9, 10, and 11 values, respectively. All statistical analysis was performed with SAS version 9.3 (SPSS, Inc., Chicago, IL, USA).

Results

Coronary artery calcification and traditional risk factors

Of the whole patients that met the inclusion criteria, 5 patients were excluded for active infection, prior history of coronary artery

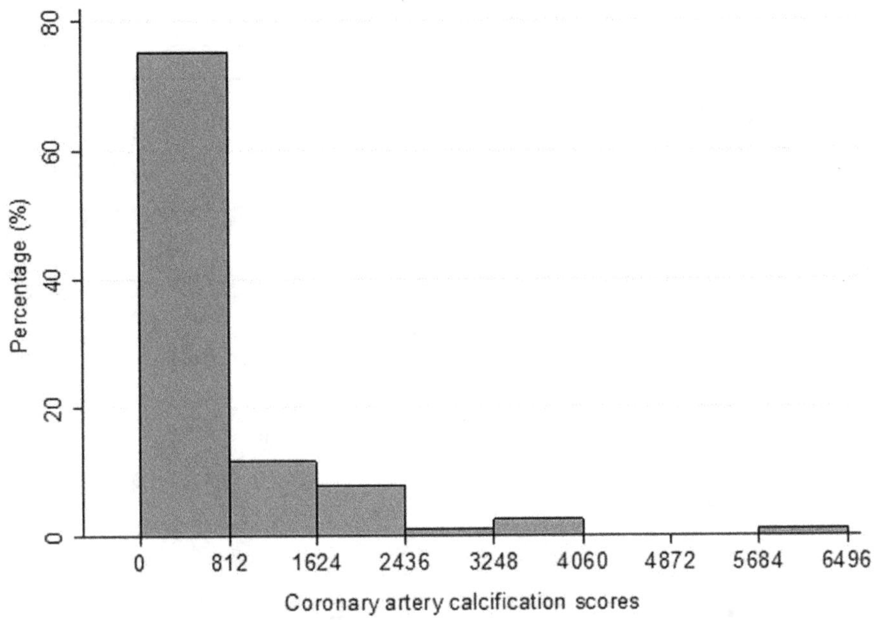

Figure 1. Distribution of coronary artery calcification scores (CACs) in MHD patients. Seventeen patients had no evidence of coronary calcification (CACs = 0) and 60 patients had CACs from 0.5 to 6493.2. Seventy five percent of the CACs were between 0 and 811.6, the mean CACs was 609.6±1062.9, the median CACs was 168.5, and the interquartile range was 2.5 to 788.2.

revascularization and myocardial infarction. Seventy-seven patients were actually enrolled. The mean (±SD) age of the 77 patients was 61.7 (±11.3) years and 51% of patients were men. 82% of female patients were in menopausal or postmenopausal and they did not receive estrogen therapy. The causes of renal failure were diabetes mellitus (n = 11), hypertension (n = 10), glomerulonephritis (n = 45), and other conditions (n = 11). The average time on HD therapy was 5.9 years (±4.4) and the mean Kt/V was 1.47 (±0.21). Figure 1 shows the distribution of CACs for the 77 patients. Seventeen patients had no evidence of CAC and the other 60 patients had CACs from 0.5 to 6493.2. The mean CACs was 609.6 (±1062.9), the median was 168.5, and the IQR was 2.5 to 788.2.

We classified these patients into three coronary calcification groups using the modified categorization proposed by Rumberger *et al.* [34]: mild (CACs = 0 to 10, low risk for CVD), moderate (CACs = 11 to 400, moderate risk for CVD), and severe (CACs> 400, severe risk for CVD). Table 1 shows the baseline

Table 1. Baseline characteristics of MHD patients by CAC score tertile.

	CAC score			
	<10 (n = 23)	**11–400 (n = 26)**	**>400 (n = 28)**	***P***
Male (n %)	6 (26.1)	14 (53.8)	19 (67.8)	<0.001**
Age (years)	56.8±12.5	61.8±11.4	65.5±8.7	0.01**
Dialysis vintage (months)	69.5±63.9	69.5±48.8	74.6±46.7	0.7
Smokers (n)	2	6	9	0.05*
Diabetes (n %)	1 (4.3)	5 (19.2)	5 (17.8)	0.3
GFR (ml/min per 1.73 m^2)	1.04±1.83	0.86±2.76	0.29±0.96	0.2
Systolic BP (mmHg)	117.0±19.1	117.1±28.6	119.3±22.5	0.8
Diastolic BP (mmHg)	71.9±10.8	67.7±12.7	72.4±11.4	0.8
Blood flow rate (mL/min)	226.2±20.9	231.4±30.3	235.9±20.3	0.2
Kt/V urea-dialysis	1.49±0.25	1.46±0.22	1.46±0.17	0.7
Dosage of $CaCO_3$ (g/d)	2.7±2.7	2.9±2.8	2.9±2.9	0.8
Dosage of calcitriol (ug/w)	2.17±4.33	2.42±5.96	2.03±3.69	0.9

Values are expressed as mean ± SD or number (percentage).
MHD, maintenance hemodialysis; CAC, coronary artery calcification; BP, blood pressure.
Data compared by univariate ordinal logistic regressions;
**P*<0.2,
***P*<0.05.

Table 2. Laboratory measures of MHD patients by CAC score tertile at study onset.

	CAC score			
	<10 (n = 23)	11–400 (n = 26)	>400 (n = 28)	P
Hb (g/dL)	10.8±1.2	10.7±1.8	11.2±1.7	0.5
Ferritin (ng/ml)	322.2±188.0	394.4±193.5	408.9±180.4	0.1*
Transferrin saturation (%)	38.7±11.3	40.2±14.6	40.3±15.2	0.7
CO_2CP (mmol/L)	22.6±2.1	21.4±2.1	21.9±3.2	0.4
CRP (mg/L)	3.6±1.6	6.0±5.6	10.1±13.6	0.04**
BMI (kg/m^2)	20.7±3.2	21.1±2.8	20.9±2.3	0.8
nPNA (g/kg per day)	1.06±0.20	1.12±0.15	1.07±0.18	0.9
Scr (umol/L)	864±173	945±236	929±188	0.3
BUN (mmol/L)	23.5±5.0	24.8±3.8	25.1±4.3	0.2
Alb (g/dL)	3.91±0.28	3.73±0.25	3.72±0.29	0.02**
Total cholesterol (mg/dL)	175.6±41.0	160.1±36.0	161.6±36.0	0.2
Triglycerides (mg/dL)	187.8±116.9	154.1±86.8	194.0±118.7	0.7
LDL-cholesterol (mg/dL)	87.8±34.0	81.6±26.3	82.0±24.8	0.5
HDL-cholesterol (mg/dL)	39.8±11.2	36.7±11.6	32.1±8.1	0.03**
Phosphorus (mg/dL)	5.18±1.38	5.23±1.58	5.31±1.32	0.8
Calcium (mg/dL)	9.21±0.91	9.22±0.87	9.52±0.82	0.2
PTH (pg/mL)	160.4±91.7	236.3±244.1	282.7±258.3	0.09*
FGF23 (pg/mL)	250.8±334.5	413.5±352.3	429.5±373.9	0.1*
1,25$(OH)_2VitD_3$ (pg/mL)	3.22±3.93	4.23±4.22	3.23±4.23	0.9

Values expressed as mean ± SD.
MHD, maintenance hemodialysis; CAC, coronary artery calcification; Hb, hemoglobin; CO_2CP, carbon dioxide combining power; CRP, C-reactive protein; BMI, body mass index; nPNA, normalized protein nitrogen appearance; Alb, albumin; Scr, Serum creatinine; BUN, blood urea nitrogen; LDL, low-density lipoprotein; HDL, high-density lipoprotein; PTH, parathyroid hormone; FGF23, fibroblast growth factor 23.
Data compared by univariate ordinal logistic regressions;
*$P<0.2$,
**$P<0.05$.

characteristics of the study subjects based on CAC category. Male gender ($p<0.001$) and advanced age ($p=0.01$) were significantly associated with higher CACs, but the other variables (dialysis vintage, smoking, diabetes, GFR, systolic and diastolic blood pressure, blood flow rate, Kt/V, and medications) had no significant associations with CACs.

Table 2 shows the laboratory measurements of patients in these three groups. The results indicate significant relationships between higher CRP ($p=0.04$), lower serum albumin ($p=0.02$), and lower serum HDL ($p=0.03$) with higher CACs. Other measures of nutritional status (BMI and nPNA), iron parameters (serum ferritin and transferrin saturation), lipid metabolism (total cholesterol, triglycerides, and LDL), mineral metabolism (serum phosphorus, calcium, PTH, FGF23, 1,25$(OH)_2D_3$), serum creatinine, blood urea nitrogen did not differ significantly among the 3 groups at enrollment.

To exclude the possibility that these results may be due to occasional or spurious events, we compared the serum levels of phosphorus, calcium, and PTH of the past 6 follow-ups (including the value at entry) in these three groups (Figure 2). Similarly, there were no significant differences among the three CAC groups in these parameters except for the second follow-up value for calcium.

Variation in serum phosphorus, calcium, and PTH and severity of CAC

Table 3 shows that the mean value of serum phosphorus from the past 6 follow-ups (April 2009 to July 2010) was unrelated to CAC severity. The variability for serum phosphorus, defined by the SD and CV, tended to be greater in high-CACs group, but this was not significant ($p=0.07$ for SD, $p=0.07$ for CV). Similarly, the severity of CAC tended to be greater in patients with higher mean of calcium and PTH, but these differences were not significant ($p=0.2$ for mean of calcium, $p=0.2$ for mean of PTH). There were no significant differences among groups in the variabilities of calcium and PTH. We also performed boxplot analysis of this data (Figure 3).

Independent predictors of CAC

To avoid model overfitting and the possible effects of confounding factors, all variables with p-values less than 0.2 under the univariate analysis (asterisks in Table 1, Table 2, and Table 3) were considered as potential predictors in the multivariate analysis (Table 4). In view of the strong positive correlation between phosphorus SD and CV ($r=0.85$; $p<0.001$), we entered these two variables into separate regression models (Model 1 and 2, respectively). The results of the multivariate analysis indicated that female gend\er (Model 1, $p=0.002$; Model 2, $p=0.003$), age (Model 1, $p=0.003$; Model 2, $p=0.01$), serum FGF23 (Model 1, $p=0.003$; Model 2, $p<0.001$), SD-phosphorus (Model 1, $p=0.007$), and CV-phosphorus (Model 2, $p=0.01$) were significantly and independently associated with CAC. Female gender was associated with a nearly 80% relative risk reduction ($OR_{Model\ 1}=0.20$, $OR_{Model\ 2}=0.21$). In Model 1, an increase of 1 year in age, 1 pg/mL in FGF23, or 1 mg/dL in the SD of serum phosphorus was associated with a 2.31, 2.25, and 2.12 increased risk of being in higher CAC category, respectively.

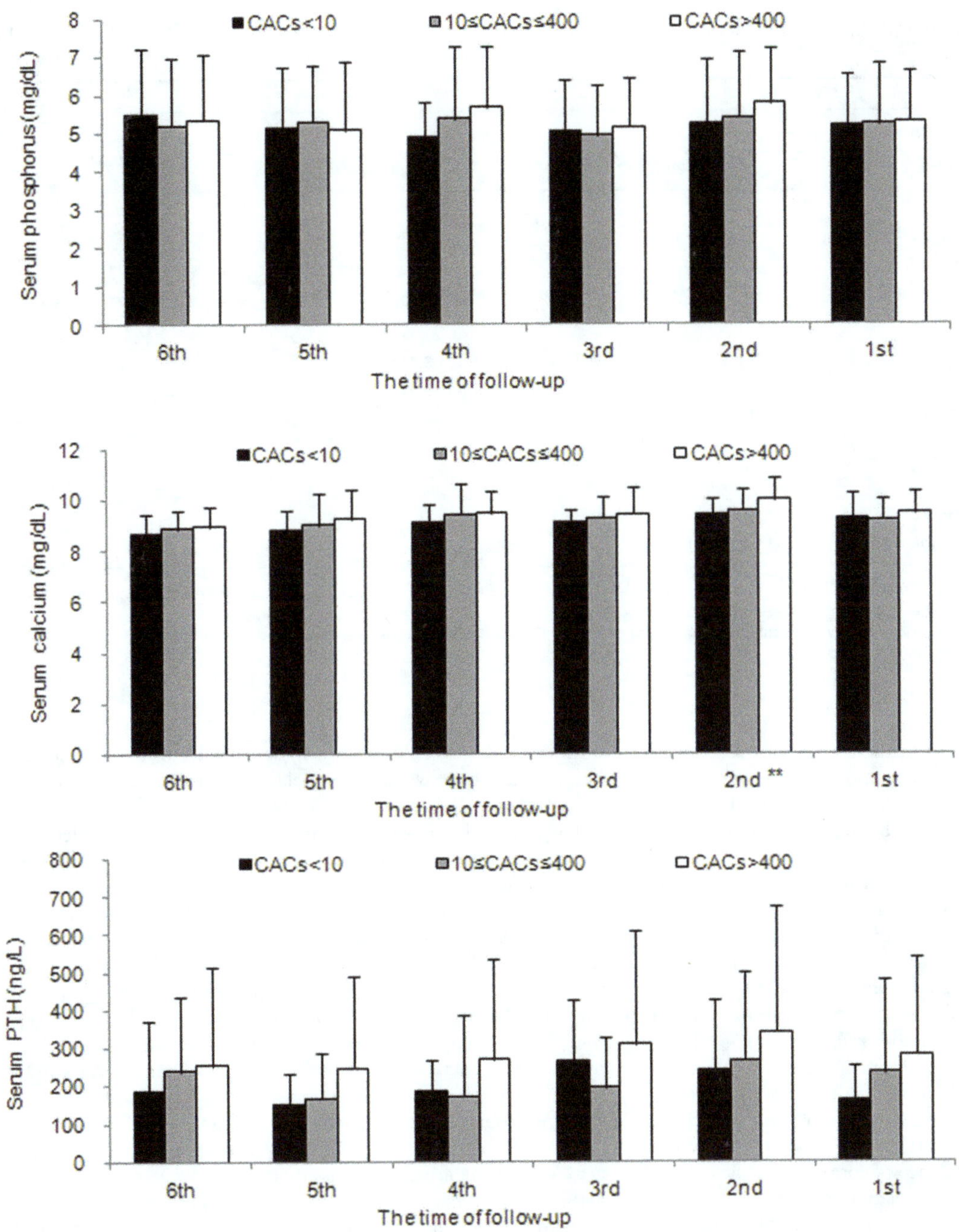

Figure 2. Effect of serum levels of phosphorus (top), calcium (middle), and parathyroid hormone (PTH, bottom) on CAC score during the past 6 follow-ups. The only significant differences were in the 2nd measurement for serum calcium ($^{**}P<0.05$). Each column represents mean±SD. 1st : the value at the entry of study (July, 2010); 2nd: the value of April, 2010; 3rd : the value of January, 2010; 4th : the value of October 2009; 5th : the value of July 2009; 6th : the value of April 2009.

Finally, we analyzed whether mean and variability of serum phosphorus calculated from different follow-up durations affected the results of this multivariate analysis. Thus, we analyzed mean and variability values calculated from past 7 (January 2009 to July 2010), 8 (October 2008 to July 2010), 9 (July 2008 to July 2010), 10 (April 2008 to July 2010), and 11 (January 2008 to July 2010) follow-up values, and developed five other logistic regression models using the same procedures as described in Table 4. The results of multivariate analysis confirmed that age, sex, serum FGF23, and variability of serum phosphorus were independent predictors of CAC in HD patients (Table 5 and Table 6). Interestingly, there were no obvious differences in the ORs of phosphorus variabilities in all six models. This suggests that phosphorus variability calculated from the past 6 records alone might be sufficient.

Discussion

Dialysis patients have a 10- to 20-fold increased mortality in comparison with healthy individuals, cardiomyopathy is one of the most important causes of this increased mortality [35]. The

Table 3. Mean, standard deviation (SD), and coefficient of variation (CV) of serum phosphorus, calcium, and iPTH of MHD patients by CAC score tertile.

	CAC score			
	<10 (n = 23)	11–400 (n = 26)	>400 (n = 28)	*P*
Serum phosphorus				
mean (mg/dL)	5.14±1.17	5.24±1.35	5.37±1.12	0.5
SD (mg/dL)	0.85±0.44	0.88±0.46	1.09±0.43	0.07*
CV	0.16±0.07	0.17±0.08	0.20±0.07	0.07*
Serum calcium				
mean (mg/dL)	9.14±0.51	9.24±0.76	9.44±0.74	0.2*
SD (mg/dL)	0.64±0.25	0.64±0.33	0.63±0.33	0.8
CV	0.07±0.03	0.07±0.04	0.07±0.03	0.7
Serum PTH				
mean (pg/mL)	205.3±99.2	207.1±154.8	281.5±253.5	0.2*
SD (pg/mL)	97.5±73.0	90.8±92.8	103.3±69.8	0.8
CV	0.47±0.26	0.45±0.28	0.44±0.27	0.8

Values expressed as *mean* ± *SD*. SD and CV were calculated from the past 6 follow-up values (April 2009 to July 2010). The *mean* was the average of patients' SD or CV which depended on the variations of patients over time. The *SD* showed how much variation from the average existed in one group.
MHD, maintenance hemodialysis; CAC, coronary artery calcification; SD, standard deviation; CV, coefficient of variation; PTH, parathyroid hormone.
Data compared by univariate ordinal logistic regressions;
$^*P<0.2$.

association between vascular calcification and left ventricular hypertrophy (LVH) had also been reported in many studies, among which the CAC was considered as one of risk factors of promoting the development of LVH [36,37]. CAC occurs more frequently in HD patients than in non-HD subjects of the same age and sex. In CKD patients, CAC can be measured by many ways, among which CT-based CAC score is recommend as a "standard" detection by ISN KDIGO guideline [38]. The Multi-Ethnic Study of Atherosclerosis (MESA) study reported that the prevalence of coronary calcification (Agatston score>0) was 59% in Chinese men and 42% in Chinese women who were 45 to 84 years-old and had no clinical cardiovascular disease [39]. By comparison, other studies reported the prevalence of CAC in HD patients was 72 to 83% [1–3], and that there was a higher prevalence (88%) in young HD patients (20 to 30 years-old) [13]. Our results indicated that 78% of MHD patients had CACs more than 0, supporting the high prevalence of coronary calcification in this population. CAC can be associated with severe clinical consequences, and maybe considered a predictor of CVD [4–7], which could account for approximately half of all deaths among HD patients [8,9]. Previous cross-sectional and prospective clinical studies have investigated the factors that contributed to CAC, such as the classic cardiovascular risk factors and factors related to uremia and the HD treatment itself [1–3,11–17]. The present study is the first to report a significant and independent association between variation of serum phosphorus and CAC. These results may help to identify the presence of modifiable risk factors of HD patients in clinic practice.

In agreement with previous research, we observed that age [3,11,21] and gender [7,39]were the most important risk factors for coronary calcification [40]. Age-linked vascular calcification has been known since the nineteenth century. In particular, CAC appears in the artery wall but not in other soft tissues, as serum calcium and phosphorus levels increase with age [41]. On the other hand, age is also a reflection of the cumulative exposure to all atherogenic risk factors for calcification [42]. Among female hormones, oestrogen has known beneficial effects on lipid and bone metabolism which may delay the process of calcification [43,44].

Patients with diabetes mellitus have a greater prevalence of hyperglycemia, oxidative stress, insulin resistance, and inflammation, and these may play a role in vascular calcification [45–48]. We observed no significant association between diabetes and coronary calcification, although only 11 of our 77 patients had diabetes and the proportion of diabetes patients was higher in the high CACs group. Other studies have also reported no relationship of diabetes and calcification [15,49]. The association between these factors may be clarified by measurement of the serum levels of glucose or metabolism-associated proteins that are responsible for vascular calcification in the presence of diabetes [45–48].

As in some previous studies, we also found no significant associations between dialysis vintage, blood pressure, Kt/V, BMI, acidosis, serum creatinine, blood urea nitrogen, or hemoglobin with coronary calcification [2,13,50,51]. This may be because some of the parameters were strictly controlled in a relatively narrow range among subjects in the current study. Previous research indicated that smoking, medications, iron metabolism, nutritional state, inflammation, and dyslipidemia impact the severity of coronary calcification in HD patients [18,52–55]. However, our multivariate analysis showed that GFR, serum levels of ferritin, transferrin saturation, albumin, CRP, HDL, and medications were not significantly associated with CAC, possibly because of the limited cohort size in this study. Though the smoking showed a marginal trend toward significance ($p = 0.05$) in univariate analysis, it was excluded from the final model possibly because the difference of smoking among the three groups was due to the relationship between smoking and gender, not real smoking and CAC.

At present, mineral disturbances, including hyperphosphatemia and hypercalcaemia, secondary hyperparathyroidism, high FGF23, and adynamic bone disease, are the best known and studied uremic abnormalities associated with development of

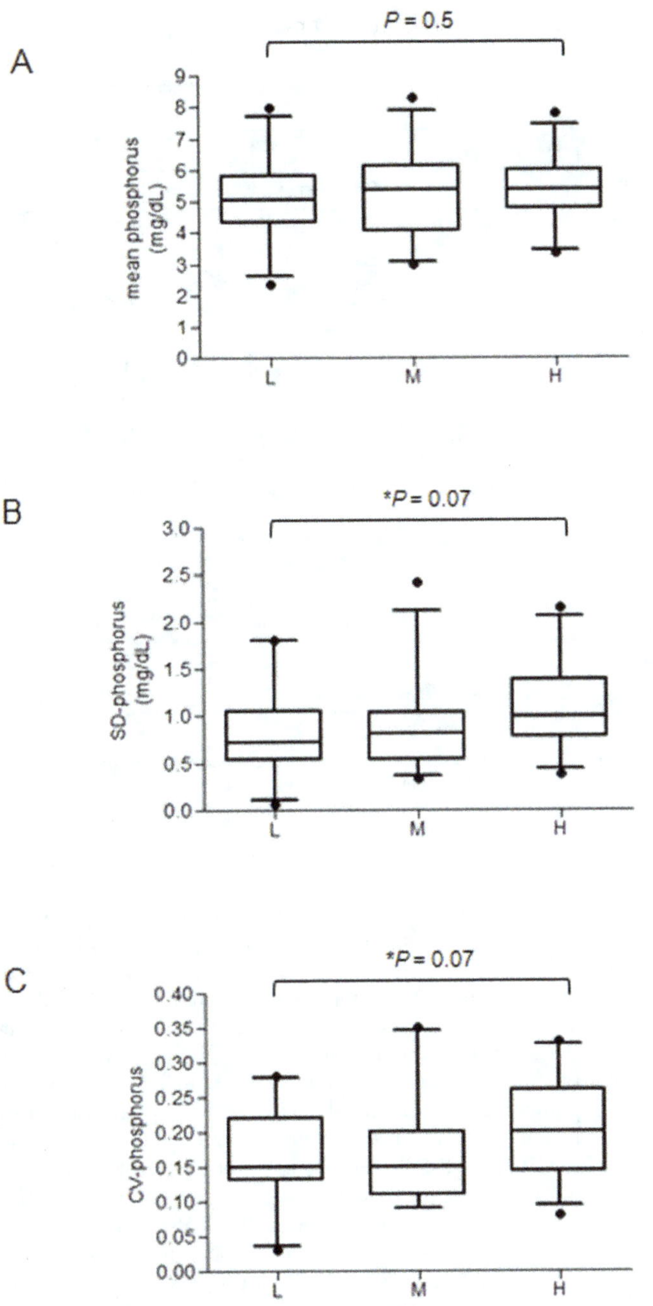

Figure 3. Boxplots of mean serum phosphorus (A), SD of serum phosphorus (B), and CV of serum phosphorus (C) in the three groups. The mean, SD, and CV were calculated from the past 6 follow-up values (April 2009 to July 2010). Data were compared by univariate ordinal logistic regressions. $^*P<0.2$. Box: interquartile range; upper and lower lines: 75th and 25th percentiles; central horizontal line: median; vertical whiskers above and below the boxes: 5th and 95th percentiles; circles beyond the whiskers: outliers.

vascular calcifications. Experimental studies indicated that elevated calcium and phosphorus had direct effects on vascular smooth muscle cells (VSMCs) that promote vascular calcification, including stimulation of osteogenic/chondrogenic differentiation, vesicle release, apoptosis, loss of inhibitors, and extracellular matrix degradation [24]. Indeed, some (but not all) clinical studies of HD patients indicated that serum calcium levels were associated with vascular calcification [1,2,11,15,21,22]. Moreover, a recent meta-analysis showed that serum phosphorus – but not calcium or PTH – was associated with cardiovascular events and mortality in individuals with CKD (N = 327 644) [56]. In agreement with these results, we also found no significant association between serum calcium and CACs. The role of serum calcium in artery calcification of HD patients requires further study.

Some epidemiological evidence suggests a pivotal role for elevated serum phosphorus in driving vascular calcification in ESRD patients [2,13,57,58]. For example, a cross-sectional analysis by Raggi *et al.* [2] indicated that serum phosphorus was significantly and positively correlated with the severity of CAC in adult HD patients. Other studies indicated that this relationship also occurs in pediatric and young HD patients [13,57,58]. However, some other studies reported no significant association between serum phosphorus and CAC in HD patients [1,11,15,21,22]. Our results also indicated no significant association between CAC and hyperphosphatemia.

One possible reason for the disagreement about the role of serum phosphorus in vascular calcification may be that the HD patients of these different studies had different baseline levels of serum phosphorus and calcium. For example, the mean values of serum phosphorus and the calcium–phosphorus product of all patients in the present study were 5.2 mg/dL (±1.4) and 48.9 mg^2/dL^2 (±14.1), respectively; the corresponding values in the Goodman *et al.* [13] study were 6.9 mg/dL (±0.9) and 65.0 mg^2/dL^2 (±10.6) and the values in the Raggi *et al.* [2] study were 5.7 mg/dL (±1.4) and 55.1 mg^2/dL^2 (±13.5). The higher levels of serum phosphorus reported in these two studies may have stimulated phenotypic changes, an osteoblastic transcriptional program, or apoptosis of smooth muscle cells of the vascular system [59–61].

Another possible reason for the disagreement about the role of serum phosphorus in vascular calcification may be that a single measurement or mean value of serum phosphorus does not indicate changes in phosphorus metabolism over time. Our results clearly showed that the variability of serum phosphorus was positively associated with coronary calcification in HD patients, even though the mean serum phosphorus levels were not very high. This suggests that phosphorus variability may better reflect the imbalance of phosphorus metabolism in HD patients. Phosphorus regulates enzymatic activity and serves as an essential component of nucleic acids, adenosine triphosphate, and phospholipid membranes [62], and phosphorus variability may induce cell apoptosis, a key regulator of VSMC calcification [63]. In addition, high variability of serum phosphorus might be associated with low rate of bone turnover, because bone serves as a huge phosphorus reservoir that contributes to serum phosphorus stability *via* bone formation and resorption [24,64]. Under the state of low bone turnover, excess phosphorus cannot be taken up by the adynamic bone, so it might precipitate on vascular tissue, or move into a newly formed exchangeable phosphorus pool that develops as VSMCs transition towards the osteoblastic phenotype during medial calcification in vascular tissues of CKD patients [65]. Preliminary data indicate a negative relationship between low bone turnover and vascular calcification in HD patients [66]. More studies are needed to establish whether phosphorus variability is simply a marker of CAC or whether phosphorus variability is part of the mechanism for vascular calcification in HD patients.

There is disagreement about relationship between serum PTH and vascular calcification. Some previous studies showed that low PTH (median 200 pg/mL) or higher PTH (>300 pg/mL) was associated with increased risk of vascular calcification in HD

Table 4. Multiple logistic regression analysis of factors associated with CAC score tertile in MHD patients.

Variable	Unadjusted		Adjusted			
			Model 1		Model 2	
	OR	*P*	OR_1 (95% CI)	P_1	OR_2 (95% CI)	P_2
Female gender	0.28	<0.001	0.20 (0.07–0.55)	0.002	0.21 (0.07–0.58)	0.003
Age (/1-y)	1.82	0.01	2.31 (1.32–4.04)	0.003	2.04 (1.18–3.53)	0.01
Smoking	2.76	0.05				
Laboratory measurements						
Ferritin (ng/ml)	1.002	0.1				
Alb (/1-g/dL)	0.60	0.02				
CRP (/1-mg/L)	2.40	0.04				
PTH (/1-pg/mL)	1.53	0.09				
FGF23 (/1-pg/mL)	1.45	0.1	2.25 (1.31–3.85)	0.003	2.50 (1.46–4.30)	<0.001
HDL (/1-mg/dL)	0.57	0.03				
Mean and variability measurements						
Mean-PTH (/1-pg/mL)	1.43	0.2				
Mean-Ca (/1-mg/dL)	1.38	0.2				
SD-Pi (/1-mg/dL)	1.54	0.07	2.12 (1.23–3.63)	0.007		
CV-Pi (/1)	1.59	0.07			1.90 (1.16–3.11)	0.01

SD and CV were calculated from the past 6 follow-up values.
MHD, maintenance hemodialysis; CAC, coronary artery calcification; OR, Odds ratio; CI, confidence interval; Alb, albumin; CRP, C-reactive protein; PTH, parathyroid hormone; FGF23, fibroblast growth factor 23; HDL, high-density lipoprotein; SD, standard deviation; CV, coefficient of variation.
P_1 from multiple regression that adjusted for female sex, age, FGF23, and SD-phosphate.
P_2 from multiple regression that adjusted for female sex, age, FGF23, and CV-phosphate.

patients [49,66–69], but whether caused by the related bone disease was difficult to clarify. In addition, some (but not all) studies reported reduction in the rate of progression of vascular calcification after parathyroidectomy [70]. The present study found no association of coronary calcification with serum PTH (mean value in three groups ranged from 150 to 350 pg/mL), possibly because the predictive value of PTH for identifying underlying bone histology had getting weaker [71], and it was difficult to judge whether high or low PTH level was the consequence or cause of calcium salt use, vitamin D analogue use, parathyroidectomy, and hyperphosphataemia, all of which can affect vascular calcification [70].

Our results demonstrated that serum FGF23 was significantly related to the severity of CAC in HD patients, in accordance with previous cross-sectional studies [16,57,68,72–75]. There is no clear evidence indicating a direct pathogenetic effect of FGF23 on vasculature, so previous studies attributed this association to indirect effects. In particular, elevated FGF23 may reflect a higher time-averaged phosphorus burden, vitamin D deficiency, different dose of phosphorus binders [72], lower adiponectin, and dyslipidemia [74]. Recent mechanistic studies indicated that Klotho, a β-glucuronidase that affects calcium homeostasis, was an inhibitor of vascular calcification [76,77]. We observed no differences in phosphorus and vitamin D in our three CACs groups, so we suggest that circulating FGF23 may have a protective effect on arterial wall integrity and that rising FGF23 levels in HD patients are in part a consequence of vascular resistance to FGF23, because of uremia-mediated down-regulation of Klotho expression in vascular cells [77,78]. Future studies are needed to examine the existence of FGF-23/Klotho interactions within the arterial wall in order to more completely characterize the anticalcific effects of FGF23.

We acknowledge several limitations of the present study. First, we cannot infer the causality of the associations identified in current analysis due to the possible presence of unknown confounders. Second, the sample size was rather small and all patients were from a single institution, so there may have been some selection bias. Third, the variability of phosphorus calculated from trimonthly records may not be the most accurate way to assess phosphorus fluctuation. Fourth, we did not measure the level of bone-associated proteins, such as members of the BMP family (BMP-2, BMP-7), which are known to be involved in bone metabolism and vascular calcification [52,79], so we were unable to determine whether phosphorus variability was a marker of bone metabolism or direct affected vasculature. Fifth, the quantification of CAC has only been performed by a single reader, the biased reading may have happened. Finally, we have no data on alcohol consumption which may be a risk factor of vascular calcification [36,80].

In conclusion, variability of serum phosphorus appears to contribute significantly to CAC in MHD patients. Future clinical studies are needed to establish whether maintenance of a stable serum phosphorus level decreases coronary calcification and associated morbidity and mortality in MHD patients.

Acknowledgments

We are grateful to all patients and medical staff who participated in this project.

Author Contributions

Conceived and designed the experiments: JC MJW HML. Performed the experiments: MJW HML LY XLY MZ RJZ CMH. Analyzed the data:

Table 5. Odds ratio (OR) for risk of high CAC score in MHD patients.

Variable	Adjusted									
	SD was calculated from the past									
	7 records		8 records		9 records		10 records		11 records	
	OR	P_1	OR	P_1	OR	P_1	OR	P_1	OR	P_1
Female gender	0.19	0.002	0.18	0.002	0.19	0.002	0.20	0.003	0.20	0.003
Age (/1-y)	2.26	0.005	2.20	0.006	2.22	0.006	2.25	0.006	2.43	0.003
FGF23 (/1-pg/mL)	2.31	0.003	2.29	0.004	2.29	0.004	2.25	0.005	2.25	0.005
SD-Pi (/1-mg/dL)	2.41	0.003	2.34	0.004	2.18	0.006	2.15	0.007	2.09	0.009

Variability in serum phosphorus was defined as the standard deviation.
MHD, maintenance hemodialysis; CAC, coronary artery calcification; OR, Odds ratio; FGF23, fibroblast growth factor 23; SD, standard deviation.
P_1 from multiple regression that adjusted for female sex, age, FGF23, and SD-phosphate.

Table 6. Odds ratio (OR) for risk of high CAC score in MHD patients.

Variable	Adjusted									
	CV was calculated from the past									
	7 records		8 records		9 records		10 records		11 records	
	OR	P_2	OR	P_2	OR	P_2	OR	P_2	OR	P_2
Female gender	0.20	0.003	0.19	0.002	0.20	0.003	0.21	0.003	0.20	0.003
Age (/1-y)	1.97	0.02	1.91	0.02	1.95	0.02	2.03	0.01	2.22	0.007
FGF23 (/1-pg/mL)	2.85	<0.001	2.79	<0.001	2.76	<0.001	2.68	<0.001	2.73	<0.001
CV-Pi (/1)	2.32	0.002	2.25	0.002	2.20	0.003	2.18	0.003	2.12	0.003

Variability in serum phosphorus was defined as the coefficient of variation.
MHD, maintenance hemodialysis; CAC, coronary artery calcification; OR, Odds ratio; FGF23, fibroblast growth factor 23; CV, coefficient of variation.
P_2 from multiple regression that adjusted for female sex, age, FGF23, and CV-phosphate.

ZJZ. Contributed reagents/materials/analysis tools: RJZ ZJZ. Wrote the paper: MJW HML.

References

1. Barreto DV, Barreto FC, Carvalho AB, Cuppari L, Cendoroglo M, et al. (2005) Coronary calcification in hemodialysis patients: the contribution of traditional and uremia-related risk factors. Kidney Int 67:1576–1582.
2. Raggi P, Boulay A, Chasan-Taber S, Amin N, Dillon M, et al. (2002) Cardiac calcification in adult hemodialysis patients. A link between end-stage renal disease and cardiovascular disease? J Am Coll Cardiol 39:695–701.
3. Pencak P, Czerwienska B, Ficek R, Wyskida K, Kujawa-Szewieczek A, et al. (2013) Calcification of coronary arteries and abdominal aorta in relation to traditional and novel risk factors of atherosclerosis in hemodialysis patients. BMC Nephrol 14:10.
4. Kondos GT, Hoff JA, Sevrukov A, Daviglus ML, Garside DB, et al. (2003) Electron-beam tomography coronary artery calcium and cardiac events: a 37-month follow-up of 5635 initially asymptomatic low- to intermediate-risk adults. Circulation 107:2571–2576.
5. Wong ND, Hsu JC, Detrano RC, Diamond G, Eisenberg H, et al. (2000) Coronary artery calcium evaluation by electron beam computed tomography and its relation to new cardiovascular events. Am J Cardiol 86:495–498.
6. Haydar AA, Hujairi NM, Covic AA, Pereira D, Rubens M, et al. (2004) Coronary artery calcification is related to coronary atherosclerosis in chronic renal disease patients: a study comparing EBCT-generated coronary artery calcium scores and coronary angiography. Nephrol Dial Transplant 19:2307–2312.
7. Arad Y, Goodman KJ, Roth M, Newstein D, Guerci AD. (2005) Coronary calcification, coronary disease risk factors, C-reactive protein, and atherosclerotic cardiovascular disease events: the St. Francis Heart Study. J Am Coll Cardiol 46:158–165.
8. Cheung AK, Sarnak MJ, Yan G, Berkoben M, Heyka R, et al. (2004) Cardiac diseases in maintenance hemodialysis patients: results of the HEMO Study. Kidney Int 65:2380–2389.
9. de Jager DJ, Grootendorst DC, Jager KJ, van Dijk PC, Tomas LM, et al. (2009) Cardiovascular and noncardiovascular mortality among patients starting dialysis. JAMA 302:1782–1789.
10. Foley RN, Parfrey PS, Sarnak MJ. (1998) Clinical epidemiology of cardiovascular disease in chronic renal disease. Am J Kidney Dis 32:S112–119.
11. Taki K, Takayama F, Tsuruta Y, Niwa T. (2006) Oxidative stress, advanced glycation end product, and coronary artery calcification in hemodialysis patients. Kidney Int 70:218–224.
12. Ohtake T, Ishioka K, Honda K, Oka M, Maesato K, et al. (2010) Impact of coronary artery calcification in hemodialysis patients: Risk factors and associations with prognosis. Hemodial Int 14:218–225.
13. Goodman WG, Goldin J, Kuizon BD, Yoon C, Gales B, et al. (2000) Coronary-artery calcification in young adults with end-stage renal disease who are undergoing dialysis. N Engl J Med 342:1478–1483.
14. Ozkok A, Caliskan Y, Sakaci T, Erten G, Karahan G, et al. (2012) Osteoprotegerin/RANKL axis and progression of coronary artery calcification in hemodialysis patients. Clin J Am Soc Nephrol 7:965–973.
15. Barreto DV, Barreto Fde C, Carvalho AB, Cuppari L, Draibe SA, et al. (2008) Association of changes in bone remodeling and coronary calcification in hemodialysis patients: a prospective study. Am J Kidney Dis 52:1139–1150.
16. Khan AM, Chirinos JA, Litt H, Yang W, Rosas SE. (2012) FGF-23 and the progression of coronary arterial calcification in patients new to dialysis. Clin J Am Soc Nephrol 7:2017–2022.
17. McCullough PA, Sandberg KR, Dumler F, Yanez JE. (2004) Determinants of coronary vascular calcification in patients with chronic kidney disease and end-stage renal disease: a systematic review. J Nephrol 17:205–215.
18. Hujairi NM, Afzali B, Goldsmith DJ. (2004) Cardiac calcification in renal patients: what we do and don't know. Am J Kidney Dis 43:234–243.
19. Block GA, Hulbert-Shearon TE, Levin NW, Port FK. (1998) Association of serum phosphorus and calcium x phosphate product with mortality risk in chronic hemodialysis patients: a national study. Am J Kidney Dis 31:607–617.
20. Jung HH, Kim SW, Han H. (2006) Inflammation, mineral metabolism and progressive coronary artery calcification in patients on haemodialysis. Nephrol Dial Transplant 21:1915–1920.
21. Braun J, Oldendorf M, Moshage W, Heidler R, Zeitler E, et al. (1996) Electron beam computed tomography in the evaluation of cardiac calcification in chronic dialysis patients. Am J Kidney Dis 27:394–401.
22. Shantouf R, Kovesdy CP, Kim Y, Ahmadi N, Luna A, et al. (2009) Association of serum alkaline phosphatase with coronary artery calcification in maintenance hemodialysis patients. Clin J Am Soc Nephrol 4:1106–1114.
23. Portale AA, Halloran BP, Morris RC, Jr. (1987) Dietary intake of phosphorus modulates the circadian rhythm in serum concentration of phosphorus. Implications for the renal production of 1,25-dihydroxyvitamin D. J Clin Invest 80:1147–1154.
24. Shanahan CM, Crouthamel MH, Kapustin A, Giachelli CM. (2011) Arterial calcification in chronic kidney disease: key roles for calcium and phosphate. Circ Res 109:697–711.
25. Wang M, You L, Li H, Lin Y, Zhang Z, et al. (2013) Association of circulating fibroblast growth factor-23 with renal phosphate excretion among hemodialysis patients with residual renal function. Clin J Am Soc Nephrol 8:116–125.
26. Kestenbaum B, Sampson JN, Rudser KD, Patterson DJ, Seliger SL, et al. (2005) Serum phosphate levels and mortality risk among people with chronic kidney disease. J Am Soc Nephrol 16:520–528.
27. Rothwell PM, Howard SC, Dolan E, O'Brien E, Dobson JE, et al. (2010) Prognostic significance of visit-to-visit variability, maximum systolic blood pressure, and episodic hypertension. Lancet 375:895–905.
28. Agatston AS, Janowitz WR, Hildner FJ, Zusmer NR, Viamonte M, Jr., et al. (1990) Quantification of coronary artery calcium using ultrafast computed tomography. J Am Coll Cardiol 15:827–832.
29. National Kidney Foundation. (2003) K/DOQI clinical practice guidelines for bone metabolism and disease in chronic kidney disease. Am J Kidney Dis 42:S1–201.
30. Daugirdas JT. (1993) Second generation logarithmic estimates of single-pool variable volume Kt/V: an analysis of error. J Am Soc Nephrol 4:1205–1213.
31. Termorshuizen F, Dekker FW, van Manen JG, Korevaar JC, Boeschoten EW, et al. (2004) Relative contribution of residual renal function and different measures of adequacy to survival in hemodialysis patients: an analysis of the Netherlands Cooperative Study on the Adequacy of Dialysis (NECOSAD)-2. J Am Soc Nephrol 15:1061–1070.
32. Watson PE, Watson ID, Batt RD. (1980) Total body water volumes for adult males and females estimated from simple anthropometric measurements. Am J Clin Nutr 33:27–39.
33. Shimada T, Hasegawa H, Yamazaki Y, Muto T, Hino R, et al. (2004) FGF-23 is a potent regulator of vitamin D metabolism and phosphate homeostasis. J Bone Miner Res 19:429–435.
34. Rumberger JA, Brundage BH, Rader DJ, Kondos G. (1999) Electron beam computed tomographic coronary calcium scanning: a review and guidelines for use in asymptomatic persons. Mayo Clin Proc 74:243–252.
35. Foley RN, Parfrey PS, Sarnak MJ. (1998) Epidemiology of cardiovascular disease in chronic renal disease. J Am Soc Nephrol 9:S16–23.
36. Bhan I, Thadhani R. (2009) Vascular calcification and ESRD: a hard target. Clin J Am Soc Nephrol 4 Suppl 1:S102–105.
37. Nitta K, Akiba T, Uchida K, Otsubo S, Otsubo Y, et al. (2004) Left ventricular hypertrophy is associated with arterial stiffness and vascular calcification in hemodialysis patients. Hypertens Res 27:47–52.
38. Kidney Disease: Improving Global Outcomes (KDIGO) CKD-MBD Work Group. (2009) KDIGO clinical practice guideline for the diagnosis, evaluation, prevention, and treatment of Chronic Kidney Disease-Mineral and Bone Disorder (CKD-MBD). Kidney Int Suppl 113:S1–130.
39. Bild DE, Detrano R, Peterson D, Guerci A, Liu K, et al. (2005) Ethnic differences in coronary calcification: the Multi-Ethnic Study of Atherosclerosis (MESA). Circulation 111:1313–1320.
40. Wexler L, Brundage B, Crouse J, Detrano R, Fuster V, et al. (1996) Coronary artery calcification: pathophysiology, epidemiology, imaging methods, and clinical implications. A statement for health professionals from the American Heart Association. Writing Group. Circulation 94:1175–1192.
41. Atkinson J. (2008) Age-related medial elastocalcinosis in arteries: mechanisms, animal models, and physiological consequences. J Appl Physiol 105:1643–1651.
42. Allison MA, Wright CM. (2005) Age and gender are the strongest clinical correlates of prevalent coronary calcification (R1). Int J Cardiol 98:325–330.
43. Kolovou GD, Bilianou HG. (2008) Influence of aging and menopause on lipids and lipoproteins in women. Angiology 59:54S–57S.
44. Terauchi M. (2011) Bone and calcium metabolism in menopause transition. Clin Calcium 21:1353–1359.
45. Chen NX, Duan D, O'Neill KD, Moe SM. (2006) High glucose increases the expression of Cbfa1 and BMP-2 and enhances the calcification of vascular smooth muscle cells. Nephrol Dial Transplant 21:3435–3442.
46. Olesen P, Nguyen K, Wogensen L, Ledet T, Rasmussen LM. (2007) Calcification of human vascular smooth muscle cells: associations with osteoprotegerin expression and acceleration by high-dose insulin. Am J Physiol Heart Circ Physiol 292:H1058–1064.
47. Mody N, Parhami F, Sarafian TA, Demer LL. (2001) Oxidative stress modulates osteoblastic differentiation of vascular and bone cells. Free Radic Biol Med 31:509–519.
48. Wadwa RP, Kinney GL, Ogden L, Snell-Bergeon JK, Maahs DM, et al. (2006) Soluble interleukin-2 receptor as a marker for progression of coronary artery calcification in type 1 diabetes. Int J Biochem Cell Biol 38:996–1003.
49. Noordzij M, Cranenburg EM, Engelsman LF, Hermans MM, Boeschoten EW, et al. (2011) Progression of aortic calcification is associated with disorders of mineral metabolism and mortality in chronic dialysis patients. Nephrol Dial Transplant 26:1662–1669.
50. Dellegrottaglie S, Saran R, Gillespie B, Zhang X, Chung S, et al. (2006) Prevalence and predictors of cardiovascular calcium in chronic kidney disease (from the Prospective Longitudinal RRI-CKD Study). Am J Cardiol 98:571–576.

51. Harris DC, Yuill E, Chesher DW. (1995) Correcting acidosis in hemodialysis: effect on phosphate clearance and calcification risk. J Am Soc Nephrol 6:1607–1612.
52. Nitta K. (2011) Vascular calcification in patients with chronic kidney disease. Ther Apher Dial 15:513–521.
53. Kakuta T, Tanaka R, Hyodo T, Suzuki H, Kanai G, et al. (2011) Effect of sevelamer and calcium-based phosphate binders on coronary artery calcification and accumulation of circulating advanced glycation end products in hemodialysis patients. Am J Kidney Dis 57:422–431.
54. Bas A, Lopez I, Perez J, Rodriguez M, Aguilera-Tejero E. (2006) Reversibility of calcitriol-induced medial artery calcification in rats with intact renal function. J Bone Miner Res 21:484–490.
55. Zarjou A, Jeney V, Arosio P, Poli M, Antal-Szalmás P, et al. (2009) Ferritin prevents calcification and osteoblastic differentiation of vascular smooth muscle cells. J Am Soc Nephrol 20:1254–1263.
56. Palmer SC, Hayen A, Macaskill P, Pellegrini F, Craig JC, et al. (2011) Serum levels of phosphorus, parathyroid hormone, and calcium and risks of death and cardiovascular disease in individuals with chronic kidney disease: a systematic review and meta-analysis. JAMA 305:1119–1127.
57. Srivaths PR, Goldstein SL, Silverstein DM, Krishnamurthy R, BrewerED. (2011) Elevated FGF 23 and phosphorus are associated with coronary calcification in hemodialysis patients. Pediatr Nephrol 26:945–951.
58. Civilibal M, Caliskan S, Kurugoglu S, Candan C, Canpolat N, et al. (2009) Progression of coronary calcification in pediatric chronic kidney disease stage 5. Pediatr Nephrol 24:555–563.
59. Jono S, McKee MD, Murry CE, Shioi A, Nishizawa Y, et al. (2000) Phosphate regulation of vascular smooth muscle cell calcification. Circ Res 87:E10–17.
60. Mathew S, Tustison KS, Sugatani T, Chaudhary LR, Rifas L, et al. (2008) The mechanism of phosphorus as a cardiovascular risk factor in CKD. J Am Soc Nephrol 19:1092–1105.
61. Son BK, Kozaki K, Iijima K, Eto M, Kojima T, et al. (2006) Statins protect human aortic smooth muscle cells from inorganic phosphate-induced calcification by restoring Gas6-Axl survival pathway. Circ Res 98:1024–1031.
62. Kestenbaum B. (2007) Phosphate metabolism in the setting of chronic kidney disease: significance and recommendations for treatment. Semin Dial 20:286–294.
63. Kendrick J, Chonchol M. (2011) The role of phosphorus in the development and progression of vascular calcification. Am J Kidney Dis 58:826–834.
64. Hruska KA, Mathew S, Lund R, Qiu P, Pratt R. (2008) Hyperphosphatemia of chronic kidney disease. Kidney Int 74:148–157.
65. Cannata-Andia JB, Roman-Garcia P, Hruska K. (2011) The connections between vascular calcification and bone health. Nephrol Dial Transplant 26:3429–3436.
66. London GM, Marty C, Marchais SJ, Guerin AP, Metivier F, et al. (2004) Arterial calcifications and bone histomorphometry in end-stage renal disease. J Am Soc Nephrol 15:1943–1951.
67. Coen G, Pierantozzi A, Spizzichino D, Sardella D, Mantella D, et al. (2010) Risk factors of one year increment of coronary calcifications and survival in hemodialysis patients. BMC Nephrol 11:10.
68. Jean G, Bresson E, Lorriaux C, Mayor B, Hurot JM, et al. (2012) Increased levels of serum parathyroid hormone and fibroblast growth factor-23 are the main factors associated with the progression of vascular calcification in long-hour hemodialysis patients. Nephron Clin Pract 120:c132–138.
69. Neves KR, Graciolli FG, dos Reis LM, Graciolli RG, Neves CL, et al. (2007) Vascular calcification: contribution of parathyroid hormone in renal failure. Kidney Int 71:1262–1270.
70. Tomson C. (2003) Vascular calcification in chronic renal failure. Nephron Clin Pract 93:c124–130.
71. Barreto FC, Barreto DV, Moyses RM, Neves KR, Canziani ME, et al. (2008) K/DOQI-recommended intact PTH levels do not prevent low-turnover bone disease in hemodialysis patients. Kidney Int 73:771–777.
72. Nasrallah MM, El-Shehaby AR, Salem MM, Osman NA, El Sheikh E, et al. (2010) Fibroblast growth factor-23 (FGF-23) is independently correlated to aortic calcification in haemodialysis patients. Nephrol Dial Transplant 25:2679–2685.
73. Inaba M, Okuno S, Imanishi Y, Yamada S, Shioi A, et al. (2006) Role of fibroblast growth factor-23 in peripheral vascular calcification in non-diabetic and diabetic hemodialysis patients. Osteoporos Int 17:1506–1513.
74. Masai H, Joki N, Sugi K, Moroi M. (2013) A preliminary study of the potential role of FGF-23 in coronary calcification in patients with suspected coronary artery disease. Atherosclerosis 226:228–233.
75. Desjardins L, Liabeuf S, Renard C, Lenglet A, Lemke HD, et al. (2012) FGF23 is independently associated with vascular calcification but not bone mineral density in patients at various CKD stages. Osteoporos Int 23:2017–2025.
76. Hu MC, Shi M, Zhang J, Quinones H, Griffith C, et al. (2011) Klotho deficiency causes vascular calcification in chronic kidney disease. J Am Soc Nephrol 22:124–136.
77. Lim K, Lu TS, Molostvov G, Lee C, Lam FT, et al. (2012) Vascular Klotho deficiency potentiates the development of human artery calcification and mediates resistance to fibroblast growth factor 23. Circulation 125:2243–2255.
78. Zoppellaro G, Faggin E, Puato M, Pauletto P, Rattazzi M. (2012) Fibroblast growth factor 23 and the bone-vascular axis: lessons learned from animal studies. Am J Kidney Dis 59:135–144.
79. Hruska KA, Mathew S, Saab G. (2005) Bone morphogenetic proteins in vascular calcification. Circ Res 97:105–114.
80. Vliegenthart R, Oei HH, van den Elzen AP, van Rooij FJ, Hofman A, et al. (2004) Alcohol consumption and coronary calcification in a general population. Arch Intern Med 164:2355–2360.

25

The Clinical Significance and Risk Factors of Anti-Platelet Factor 4/heparin Antibody on Maintenance Hemodialysis Patients

Delong Zhao[1☯], Xuefeng Sun[1*☯], Li Yao[2], Hongli Lin[3], Jijun Li[4], Jiuyang Zhao[5], Zhimin Zhang[6], Lide Lun[7], Jianrong Zhang[8], Mingxu Li[9], Qi Huang[1], Yang Yang[1], Shimin Jiang[1], Yong Wang[1], Hanyu Zhu[1], Xiangmei Chen[1*]

1 Department of Nephrology, Chinese PLA General Hospital, State Key Laboratory of Kidney Disease (2011DAV00088), Beijing, China, **2** Department of Nephrology, The First Affiliated Hospital, Chinese Medical University, Shenyang, China, **3** Department of Nephrology, The First Affiliated Hospital, Dalian Medical College, Dalian, China, **4** Department of Nephrology, The First Affiliated Hospital, General Hospital of PLA, Beijing, China, **5** Department of Nephrology, The Second Affiliated Hospital, Dalian Medical College, Dalian, China, **6** Department of Nephrology, General Hospital of the General Headquarters, Beijing, China, **7** Department of Nephrology, General Hospital of the Air Force, Beijing, China, **8** Department of Nephrology, General Hospital of the Force Police Army, Beijing, China, **9** Department of Nephrology, General Hospital of the Navy, Beijing, China

Abstract

Background: Heparin-induced thrombocytopenia is an immune response mediated by anti-PF4/heparin antibody, which is clinically characterized by thrombocytopenia and thromboembolic events. In this study, a prospective and multi-center clinical investigation ① determined the positive rate of anti-PF4/heparin antibody in maintenance hemodialysis patients in China, ② identified the related risk factors, and ③ further explored the effect of the anti-PF4/heparin antibody on bleeding, thromboembolic events, and risk of death in the patients.

Methods: The serum anti-PF4/heparin antibody was measured in 661 patients from nine hemodialysis centers, detected by IgG-specific ELISA and followed by confirmation with excess heparin. Risk factors of these patients were analyzed. Based on a two-year follow-up, the association between the anti-PF4/heparin antibody and bleeding, thromboembolic events, and risk of death in the patients was investigated.

Results: ① The positivity rate of the anti-PF4/heparin antibody in maintenance hemodialysis patients was 5.6%. With diabetes as an independent risk factor, the positivity rate of the anti-PF4/heparin antibody decreased in the patients undergoing weekly dialyses ≥3 times. ② The positivity rate of the anti-PF4/heparin antibody was not related to the occurrence of clinical thromboembolic events and was not a risk factor for death within two years in maintenance hemodialysis patients. ③ Negativity for the anti-PF4/heparin antibody combined with a reduction of the platelet count or combined with the administration of antiplatelet drugs yielded a significant increase in bleeding events. However, the composite determination of the anti-PF4/heparin antibody and thrombocytopenia, as well as the administration of antiplatelet drugs, was not predictive for the risk of thromboembolic events in the maintenance hemodialysis patients.

Conclusions: A single detection of the anti-PF4/heparin antibody did not predict the occurrence of clinical bleeding, thromboembolic events, or risk of death in the maintenance hemodialysis patients.

Editor: Masataka Kuwana, General Hospital of the General Headquarters, China

Funding: This work was supported by the grants from the Major State Basic Research Development Program of China (2013CB530800), http://www.973.gov.cn/AreaMana.aspx; National Natural Science Foundation of China (81270819), http://isis.nsfc.gov.cn; National Key Technology R&D Program (2011BAI10B00), http://kjzc.jhgl.org. The funders had no role in study design, data collection and analysis, decision to publish, or preparation of the manuscript.

Competing Interests: The authors have declared that no competing interests exist.

* E-mail: xfssun@126.com (XS); xmchen301@126.com (XC)

☯ These authors contributed equally to this work.

Introduction

Hemodialysis is currently the major treatment method for end-stage renal disease (ESRD). Hemodialysis is a treatment model of extracorporeal circulation, and the heparin anticoagulants are its main anticoagulant drugs [1]. Heparin-induced thrombocytopenia (HIT) is one of the serious adverse effects of heparin, which often results in severe thrombotic diseases [2,3]. The pathogenesis of HIT mainly involves the binding of heparin to platelet factor 4 (PF4) to form a heparin-PF4 complex that stimulates the body to produce anti-PF4/heparin antibodies and mediates an immune response, which leads to platelet activation and reduction and results in an elevated risk of thromboembolic disease [4–6].

Due to the long-term administration of heparin, hemodialysis patients have a high risk [7]of positivity for the anti-PF4/heparin antibody with a reported positivity rate of 1.2% – 10.3% for the anti-PF4/heparin antibody [8–12]; by contrast, other researchers determined that the positivity rate of the anti-PF4/heparin antibody is as high as 47% [13]. Several studies suggested that the anti-PF4/heparin antibody increases the occurrence of thrombotic events in maintenance hemodialysis (MHD) patients [14,15], but these results were different. The main reason for the variations in the results from most of the investigations was the use of a single center and a small sample size, which was not sufficient to rule out the variations caused by the different hemodialysis centers. The positivity rate of the anti-PF4/heparin antibody in MHD patients from a large sample and from multi-center resources in China is currently not available. Thus, in the present study, we prospectively examined the anti-PF4/heparin antibody in 661 MHD patients from nine hemodialysis centers using a two-year follow-up period to ? determine the positivity rate of the anti-PF4/heparin antibody in the Chinese MHD patients; ? resolve its related risk factors; and ? explore the effect of the anti-PF4/heparin antibody on the occurrence of bleeding, thromboembolic events, and the risk of death in the MHD patients.

Methods

Recruitment of the patients and healthy controls

This study was approved by the Ethics Committee of the Chinese People's Liberation Army (PLA) General Hospital and involved the hemodialysis centers of nine hospitals in three cities in northern China; 913 patients were recruited from December 2009 to January 2010. The patient inclusion criteria included the following: (1) maintenance hemodialysis for three months or longer; (2) age greater than 14 years, whether male or female; (3) use of heparin or low-molecular-weight heparin (LMWH) as an anticoagulant; and (4) provision of signed, informed consent. Consequently, 661 patients fulfilled these criteria and were included in this study. (Figure 1)

Concurrently, 62 healthy subjects with ages ranging from 18 – 80 years were selected as the control group. Based on the standardized definition of health from on the SENIEUR protocol [16], the subjects who met all of the following criteria were included in the study: (1) serum liver enzyme level (both serum glutamate oxaloacetate transaminase, GOT, and serum glutamate pyruvate transaminase, GPT) <40 U/L, fasting blood glucose (FBG) <7.1 mmol/L; serum urea nitrogen (UN) 1.8 – 7.5 mmol/L, and serum creatinine (SCr) 50 – 133 μmol/L; (2) hemoglobin (Hb) 110 – 176 g/L, hematocrit (HCT) 0.40 – 0.52 for men and 0.37 – 0.47 for women; (3) normal routine urine test results; (4) absence of any clinical history of visceral (including heart, brain, lung, kidney, and liver) disease, malignancy, rheumatic disease, and chronic infectious disease; (5) no history of exposure to heparin drugs; (6) normal electrocardiogram, chest radiograph, echocardiography, and abdominal ultrasound; and (7) sound character, stable emotions, absence of mental disorders, teachability, and ability to adapt to the environment and to engage in appropriate social interactions and interpersonal relationships.

The heparin group was defined as patients who used heparin as a hemodialysis anticoagulant or to pre-rinse the dialyzer and had used heparin as a long-term central venous catheter anticoagulant. The LMWH group was defined as patients who used LMWH as the hemodialysis anticoagulant and had never been exposed to heparin.

Collecting the clinical data from the research subjects

The clinical data from the MHD patients were collected by the physicians in each hemodialysis center. The recorded contents

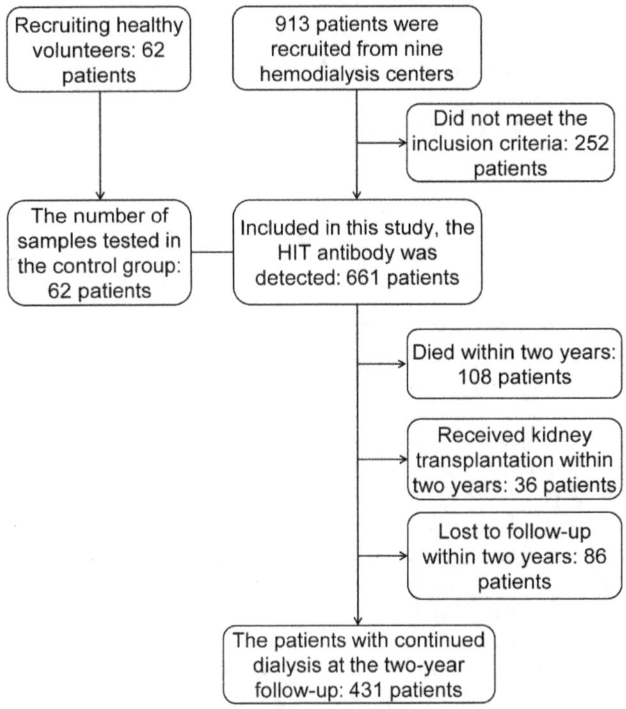

Figure 1. Diagram of MHD patients and healthy controls. The diagram shows the numbers of MHD patients and healthy controls who met the criteria of inclusion in or exclusion from the study and the follow-up of the MHD patients.

included general information (i.e., age, sex, and dry weight), general clinical information (i.e., primary disease of renal failure, drug application, bleeding, and thromboembolic adverse events within the past three months), dialysis-related information (i.e., the dialysis duration in months, the number of weekly dialyses, and the type and amount of anticoagulant), and related laboratory tests (i.e., platelet count, routine blood test, routine urine test, and biochemical indicators). For the healthy controls, data regarding age, sex, weight, blood pressure, and laboratory indicators were determined and recorded. Written informed consent was obtained from each participant. Volunteers who did not meet the inclusion criteria or did not sign the informed consent were excluded from the study.

Definition of previous bleeding and thromboembolic events

Within three months prior to the collection of the clinical information, the clinical bleeding events included conjunctival hemorrhage, bleeding due to the puncture needle, gastrointestinal bleeding, skin ecchymosis, and cerebral hemorrhage. The thromboembolic events included peripheral venous thrombosis, peripheral arterial thrombosis, vascular access occlusion, pulmonary embolism, cerebral infarction, and myocardial infarction. All records of bleeding and thromboembolic events were based on the medical records, laboratory tests, and imaging studies.

Follow-up of the MHD patients

Two years after the detection of the anti-PF4/heparin antibody, follow-up was performed in the 661 patients in the study, of which 431 patients (65.20%) continued dialysis, 108 patients (16.34%) died, 36 patients (5.45%) received renal transplantation within two years, and 86 patients (13.01%) were lost to follow-up because they decided to discontinue the hemodialysis or their addresses were changed due to relocation. All of the above mentioned data were collected again from the 431 patients with continued dialysis and a complete two-year follow-up. The bleeding and/or thromboembolic events that occurred between two years from the first data collection and the time of follow-up were also recorded. For the patients who died within two years, the reasons for their bleeding, thromboembolic events, and deaths were ascertained from the medical records.

Collection of blood samples and detection of the serum anti-PF4/heparin antibody

For the 661 MHD patients included in this study, the predialysis blood samples were collected at various hemodialysis centers between December 2009 and January 2010, and the sera were isolated and transported in aliquots to the State Key Laboratory of Kidney Disease. The State Key Laboratory of Kidney Disease selected the volunteers for the healthy control group, collected their blood samples, and isolated and stored the sera in aliquots. All of the serum samples were stored at –80°C in the State Key Laboratory of Kidney Disease until the unified testing.

The serum anti-PF4/heparin antibody was detected using a heparin/PF4 ELISA kit (PF4 IgG^{TM}, HAT45G, GTI Diagnostics, Waukesha, WI, USA) [17]. The unified testing was conducted by certain technical staff members in strict accordance with the kit's instruction guide. The positive control yielded OD405 nm >1.8, and the negative control yielded OD405 nm <0.3 with a difference between the duplicate wells of <20% [18]. To avoid false positives and improve the detection specificity [19,20], the high-dose heparin confirmatory tests were performed for all of the samples with OD405 nm >0.4. The samples with OD405 nm >0.4 and an inhibition test result >50% were defined as positive for the anti-PF4/heparin antibody.

Data analysis

The chi-square test was used to compare the categorical variables. The t-test or Mann-Whitney U test was used for the continuous variables. Multivariate logistic regression was applied to analyze the correlation between positivity for the anti-PF4/heparin antibody and the risk factors of death in the MHD patients, as well as the correlation between positivity for the anti-PF4/heparin antibody and the occurrence of bleeding and thromboembolic events within two years. P value <0.05 was considered statistically significant. The statistical software SPSS version 17.0 was used in this study.

Results

General clinical data from the research subjects

In total, 62 healthy controls and 661 MHD patients met the inclusion criteria for this study, and their clinical data are presented in Table 1.

The positivity rate of the serum anti-PF4/heparin antibody and its risk factors in the research subjects

The detection of the serum anti-PF4/heparin antibody in the 62 healthy subjects was negative. Among the 661 MHD patients, 37 subjects tested positive for the anti-PF4/heparin antibody (positivity rate of 5.6%), of which 33 individuals had a history of heparin exposure, and the remaining four cases had a history of exposure to LMWH only. Moreover, the 37 patients who tested positive for the anti-PF4/heparin antibody had no clinical diagnosis of HIT. The positivity rate of the anti-PF4/heparin antibody in the MHD patients did not significantly differ among the nine hemodialysis centers. The univariate analysis revealed that the positivity rate of the serum anti-PF4/heparin antibody was significantly increased in the MHD patients whose primary diseases were diabetes and elevated diastolic blood pressures (DBPs). No significant difference between the groups testing positive versus negative for the serum anti-PF4/heparin antibody was found in age, sex, dry weight, body mass index (BMI), systolic blood pressure (SBP), hemoglobin, platelet count and thrombocytopenia (defined as PLT $<100\times10^9$/L), serum creatinine, albumin, bleeding events within the past three months, thromboembolic events within the past three months, dialysis duration in months, number of weekly dialyses, dialysis membrane, dialyzer, anticoagulant, and Kt/v (Table 2).

The multivariate logistic regression analysis revealed that diabetes (OR =4.405, 95% CI [1.573 – 12.334], P=0.005) significantly increased the positivity rate of the serum anti-PF4/heparin antibody in the MHD patients, and the number of weekly dialyses (≥3 times) reduced the positivity rate of the serum anti-PF4/heparin antibody (OR =0.324, 95% CI [0.114 – 0.925], P=0.035). The positivity rate of the serum anti-PF4/heparin antibody was not significantly correlated with age, sex, body weight, BMI, SBP, DBP, hemoglobin, platelet count and thrombocytopenia, serum creatinine, albumin, bleeding events within the past three months, thromboembolic events within the past three months, the dialysis duration in months, the number of weekly dialyses, dialysis membrane, dialyzer, anticoagulant, and Kt/v (Table 3).

The risk factors for death in the MHD patients

At the two-year follow-up, among the 661 MHD patients, there were 431 cases with continued dialysis, 108 cases of death, 36 cases of kidney transplant or peritoneal dialysis, and 86 cases lost to follow-up. The 37 patients who tested positive for the anti-PF4/heparin antibody included 21 cases with continued dialysis, six cases of death, two cases of kidney transplantation or peritoneal dialysis, and eight cases lost to follow-up. Among the 539 patients with complete follow-up data (431 cases with continued dialysis and 108 cases of death), the two-year cumulative mortality rate for the MHD patients was 20.0% with an average annual mortality rate of 10.6%. The multivariate logistic regression analysis revealed that advanced age and diabetes mellitus significantly increased the risk of death in the patients undergoing maintenance hemodialysis, whereas utilizing a synthetic membrane dialyzer significantly reduced the patient's risk of death. The death of the patients was not significantly associated with the sex, body weight, SBP, DBP, anti-PF4/heparin antibody, hemoglobin, platelet count and thrombocytopenia, serum creatinine, albumin, bleeding events within the past three months, thromboembolic events within the past three months, dialysis duration in months, number of weekly dialyses (≥3), dialyzer, anticoagulant, and Kt/v (P>0.05). (Table 4)

Prediction of bleeding and thromboembolic events in the MHD patients based on the serum anti-PF4/heparin antibody combined with either thrombocytopenia or the administration of antiplatelet drugs

Of the 431 patients with continued hemodialysis after two years of follow-up, 159 patients experienced new bleeding events within the two years with an incidence of 36.9% for the two-year cumulative bleeding events and an average annual incidence of 20.6%; 91 patients experienced new thromboembolic events with

Table 1. MHD patients and healthy controls characteristics according to baseline status.

	MHD patients		healthy controls	
Sex (female;n [%])	287	(43%)	39	(63%)
Age (years;median [25th to 75th percentiles])	57	(44–70)	60	(55–69)
Dry Weight(kg;median [25th to 75th percentiles])	62	(54–71)	65	(55–70)
BMI (mean [SD])	22.6±4.0		24.3±3.0	
SBP(mmHg;median [25th to 75th percentiles])	140	(130–155)	130	(120–135)
DBP(mmHg;median [25th to 75th percentiles])	80	(70–90)	78	(70–80)
Hb(g/L; median [25th to 75th percentiles])	105	(94–115)	143	(135–147)
Platelet count (10̂9/L; mean [SD])	167±58		222±53	
Thrombocytopenia (n [%])	80	(12%)	0	(0%)
SCr(μmol/L; mean [SD])	883±313		67±12	
ALB(g/L;median [25th to 75th percentiles])	40	(37–42)	46	(44–48)
Diabetes(n [%])	127	(19%)	0	(0%)
Bleeding events within the past three months (n [%])	83	(13%)	0	(0%)
Thromboembolic events within the past three months (n [%])	66	(10%)	0	(0%)
Dialysis duration (months ;n [%])				
3~6	73	(11%)	-	
7~12	69	(10%)	-	
13~36	205	(31%)	-	
37~60	149	(23%)	-	
>=60	165	(25%)	-	
Number of weekly dialyses (n [%])				
<3	209	(32%)	-	
>=3	452	(68%)	-	
Dialysis membrane (n [%])				
Non-synthetic membrane	71	(11%)	-	
synthetic membrane	590	(89%)	-	
Dialyzer (n [%])				
Low-flux	307	(46%)	-	
Middle-flux	238	(36%)	-	
High-flux	116	(18%)	-	
Anticoagulant (n [%])				
heparin	578	(87%)	-	
LMWH	83	(13%)	-	
Kt/v(;median [25th to 75th percentiles])	1.421	(1.245–1.619)	-	

BMI: body mass index; SBP: systolic blood pressure; DBP: diastolic blood pressure; Hb:hemoglobin; SCr: serum creatinine; ALB: albumin.

an incidence of 21.1% for the two-year cumulative thromboembolic events and an average annual incidence of 11.2%. According to the baselines of the anti-PF4/heparin antibody and platelet count or the anti-PF4/heparin antibody and antiplatelet drugs, the patients with continued MHD after two years of follow-up were divided into four groups: antibody negative + normal platelets, antibody negative + reduced platelets, antibody positive + normal platelets, and antibody positive + reduced platelets. In addition, there were four groups, as follows: antibody negative without antiplatelet drug administration, antibody negative with antiplatelet drug administration, antibody positive without antiplatelet drug administration, and antibody positive with antiplatelet drug administration. Respectively taking the group of antibody negative + normal platelets or the group of antibody negative without antiplatelet drug administration as the standard group (the OR value was set to 1), the risk of the occurrence of bleeding events and thromboembolic events during the two-year follow-up was analyzed for the patients in the other groups. The results revealed that the group of antibody negative + reduced platelets (OR = 1.890, 95% CI [1.014 – 3.522], $P=0.045$) and the group of antibody negative with antiplatelet drug administration (OR = 1.586, 95% CI [1.034 – 2.432], $P=0.034$) had a significantly increased risk of occurrence of bleeding events. The risks of bleeding events in the other groups were not significantly different from those in the standard groups. No significant difference was found in the risk of clinical thromboembolic events between the groups (Table 5).

Table 2. Results of univariate analysis.

	Anti-PF4/heparin antibody				
	Positive (n = 37)		Negative (n = 624)		*P* value
Age(years;mean [SD])	56±17		56±16		0.944
Sex (female;n [%])	15	(41%)	272	(44%)	0.737
Dry Weight(kg;median [25th to 75th percentiles])	61.5	(54–71)	62.8	(55–70)	0.706
BMI (mean [SD])	23.4±5.5		22.6±3.9		0.236
SBP(mmHg; mean [SD])	148±19		141±21		0.066
DBP(mmHg; mean [SD])	86±13		80±13		0.032
Hb(g/L; median [25th to 75th percentiles])	105	(94–115)	105	(90–118)	0.904
Platelet count (1Ô9/L; mean [SD])	166±58		178±53		0.144
Thrombocytopenia (n [%])	4	(11%)	76	(12%)	0.804
SCr(μmol/L; mean [SD])	885±314		838±279		0.493
ALB(g/L;median [25th to 75th percentiles])	40	(37–42)	40	(38–42)	0.811
Diabetes(n [%])	13	(35%)	114	(18%)	0.017
Bleeding events within the past three months (n [%])	4	(11%)	79	(13%)	0.941
Thromboembolic events within the past three months (n [%])	3	(8%)	63	(10%)	0.913
Dialysis duration (months ;n [%])					
3~6	7	(19%)	66	(11%)	0.305
7~12	6	(16%)	63	(10%)	
13~36	11	(30%)	194	(31%)	
37~60	6	(16%)	143	(23%)	
>=60	7	(19%)	158	(25%)	
Number of weekly dialyses (>=3 times; n [%])	20	(54%)	432	(69%)	0.095
Dialysis membrane (synthetic membrane; n [%])	32	(86%)	558	(89%)	0.582
Dialyzer (n [%])					
Low-flux	19	(51%)	288	(46%)	0.855
Middle-flux	12	(33%)	226	(36%)	
High-flux	6	(16%)	110	(18%)	
Anticoagulant (heparin; n [%])	33	(89%)	545	(87%)	0.809
Kt/v(;median [25th to 75th percentiles])	1.295	(1.097–1.492)	1.430	(1.250–1.620)	0.104

BMI: body mass index; SBP: systolic blood pressure; DBP: diastolic blood pressure; Hb:hemoglobin; SCr: serum creatinine; ALB: albumin.

Discussion

In this study, we first investigated the serum anti-PF4/heparin antibody levels in 661 MHD patients from nine hemodialysis centers in three cities of northern China, in which 37 patients tested positive for the anti-PF4/heparin antibody, with a positivity rate of 5.6% being observed for the serum anti-PF4/heparin antibody. According to the diagnosis criteria[6], clinicians make a diagnosis of HIT when any of the following events occurs in association with the presence of "HIT antibodies" detected by in vitro assays: (1) an unexplained platelet count fall; (2) venous or arterial thrombosis; (3) skin lesions at heparin injection sites; or (4) acute systemic (anaphylactoid) reactions that occur after IV heparin bolus administration. Although some of the patients tested positive for the antibody also had thrombocytopenia, bleeding or thromboembolic events within the past three months, not a single patient was clinically diagnosed with HIT. The main reason for the low diagnosis rate is that the detection of anti-PF4/heparin antibodies is not a routine clinical test in China. In addition, few publications regarding HIT-related research on hemodialysis patients are available. Therefore, it is necessary to improve the clinical detection of anti-PF4/heparin antibodies in China.

Nearly a decade of research on HIT has revealed positivity rates of the anti-PF4/heparin antibody that are mostly within the range of 1.2% to 10.3% [8–12]; however, it has also been reported that the positivity rate of the anti-PF4/heparin antibody in maintenance dialysis patients is as high as 17.9% [21], and even up to 47% [13]. One of the reasons for the difference between the results of the individual reports is that most of the studies were based on a single-center resource; thus, the results are not representative. A study of 305 MHD patients from four centers in Japan revealed a 2.3% positivity rate of the anti-PF4/heparin antibody [11]. The CHOICE Cohort Study in the USA showed that the positivity rate of the anti-PF4/heparin antibody was 10.6% among 596 selected MHD patients [10]. Our present study demonstrated a serum anti-PF4/heparin antibody positivity rate of 5.6% among 661 MHD patients from nine centers in China, indicating that the positivity rate of the anti-PF4/heparin antibody might differ in MHD patients of various nationalities and ethnicities. However, the positivity of HIT antibody is also largely influenced by the kit and detection method used in a study [19]. The kit and detection

Table 3. Results of multivariate analysis.

	OR	95% C.I.	P value
Age	1.002	0.969–1.037	0.888
Sex (female])	0.877	0.411–1.870	0.733
Dry Weight	0.968	0.926–1.011	0.144
BMI	0.992	0.867–1.136	0.911
SBP	0.999	0.973–1.026	0.948
DBP	1.041	0.993–1.092	0.094
Hb	1.006	0.980–1.033	0.640
Platelet count	1.000	0.990–1.011	0.971
Thrombocytopenia	0.796	0.116–5.463	0.817
SCr	1.000	0.998–1.001	0.626
ALB	1.030	0.946–1.122	0.498
Diabetes	4.405	1.573–12.334	0.005
Bleeding events within the past three months	0.535	0.062–4.576	0.568
Thromboembolic events within the past three months	0.838	0.167–4.206	0.830
Dialysis duration (months)			
7~12	0.509	0.085–3.049	0.460
13~36	0.452	0.111–1.850	0.270
37~60	0.478	0.100–2.293	0.356
>=60	0.671	0.139–3.233	0.619
Number of weekly dialyses (>=3 times)	0.324	0.114–0.925	0.035
Dialysis membrane (synthetic membrane)	1.204	0.088–16.418	0.889
Anticoagulant (heparin)	0.654	0.188–2.281	0.505
Kt/v	0.283	0.041–1.931	0.197

OR: odds ratio; CI: confidence interval; BMI: body mass index; SBP: systolic blood pressure; DBP: diastolic blood pressures; Hb:hemoglobin; SCr: serum creatinine; ALB: albumin.

method used in the previous studies were varied, and this variety can not be excluded from the reasons for the difference of anti-PF4/heparin antibody positivity rate in these studies. Currently, the major method of detection of anti-PF4/heparin antibodies is ELISA, in which the sensitivity can be as high as 80% – 100%. However, the specificity is low because of the simultaneous detection of non-specific antibodies [22,23]. Studies have shown that only the IgG class of anti-PF4/heparin antibodies are platelet-activating and thus have the potential to cause heparin-induced thrombocytopenia [19,24–26]. Therefore, in this study, we only detected the IgG anti-PF4/heparin antibody. Additionally, to improve the specificity of detection of the anti-PF4/heparin antibody, the high-dose heparin confirmatory tests were performed [19,20,27] to set the positive standard of OD405 nm >0.4 and the inhibition test >50% for the anti-PF4/heparin antibody. This step ensured the reliability of the results in the present study, and the negative result for the serum anti-PF4/heparin antibody using the same detection method in the 62 healthy controls also confirmed the accuracy of the method applied in our study.

Moreover, the frequency of antibody formation depends on a variety of factors, including the chain length of the heparin molecule and degree of sulfation, amount and frequency of heparin administration, clinical setting, and degree of nonimmune platelet activation [28]. The results of this study indicates that ① the positivity rate of the anti-PF4/heparin antibody in MHD patients is not associated with their age, sex, and dialysis duration, which is similar to previous findings [13,21]. ② The positivity rate of the anti-PF4/heparin antibody is unrelated to the occurrence of thrombocytopenia, which is also consistent with previously reported results [21]. ③ The positivity rate of the anti-PF4/heparin antibody in MHD patients undergoing three or more dialyses per week was significantly lower than that in patients undergoing less than three dialyses per week. Although a high frequency of dialyses could lead to an increased dose and frequency of heparin use (as well as increase the levels of heparin exposure in the patients), whether long-term and high-frequency exposure to heparin can induce immune tolerance in patients remains to be studied. ④ Although the diabetic MHD patients in this study were significantly more likely than the non-diabetic patients to undergo more than three dialyses per week (97/127 cases, 76.4% *vs* 355/530 cases, 67.0%, respectively; $P=0.043$), the positivity rate of the anti-PF4/heparin antibody was significantly increased in the diabetic patients with MHD, which differs from the conclusion of Diaz J *et al.* [29] that diabetes does not increase the positivity rate of the anti-PF4/heparin antibody. The reason for the increased positivity rate of the anti-PF4/heparin antibody in the MHD patients remains unclear. ⑤ The result of this study revealed no significant difference in the positivity rate of the HIT antibody between the patients using heparin and LMWH. Although it is widely accepted that the frequency of HIT is greater in non-hemodialysis populations treated with unfractionated heparin compared with LMWH [30], it has also been reported that no significant difference in the positivity rate of the antibody in MHD patients was found between these two types of heparin[11].In this study, the patients in the heparin group included the patients using heparin as the hemodialysis anticoag-

Table 4. The baseline-factor analysis between the patients with continued dialysis and death.

	Continued dialysis (n = 431)		Death (n = 108)		OR	95% C.I.	*P* value
Age (years;median [25th to 75th percentiles])	55	(27–77)	67	(43–85)	1.069	(1.039–1.099)	<0.001
Sex (female;n [%])	201	(47%)	45	(42%)	0.564	(0.292–1.089)	0.088
Dry Weight	60.8	(54–68)	61.1	(55–69)	1.002	(0.971–1.033)	0.922
BMI	22.5±3.8		22.5±4.0		1.047	(0.968–1.131)	0.250
SBP(mmHg; mean [SD])	141±21		142±22		1.003	(0.988–1.019)	0.681
DBP(mmHg; mean [SD])	81±12		76±14		1.002	(0.973–1.032)	0.880
Anti-PF4/heparin antibody(positive;n [%])	21	(5%)	6	(6%)	1.267	(0.336–4.780)	0.727
Hb(g/L; median [25th to 75th percentiles])	107	(96–116)	102	(91–115)	0.994	(0.977–1.011)	0.506
PLT(10^9/L; mean [SD])	167±57		163±59		0.998	(0.992–1.005)	0.607
thrombocytopenia (n [%])	47	(11%)	13	(12%)	0.451	(0.139–1.464)	0.185
SCr(μmol/L; mean [SD])	908	(344–1392)	705	(208–1301)	1.000	(0.999–1.001)	0.750
ALB(g/L;median [25th to 75th percentiles])	40	(32–45)	37	(29–45)	0.966	(0.911–1.025)	0.253
diabetes(n [%])	68	(16%)	41	(38%)	2.061	(1.062–4.000)	0.033
Bleeding events within the past three months (n [%])	60	(14%)	14	(13%)	0.963	(0.396–2.340)	0.934
Thromboembolic events within the past three months (n [%])	39	(9%)	17	(16%)	1.624	(0.724–3.641)	0.239
Time on dialysis (months ;n [%])							
3~6	27	(6%)	13	(12%)	1.000	-	-
7~12	50	(12%)	10	(9%)	0.835	(0.189–3.683)	0.812
13~36	127	(29%)	41	(38%)	2.118	(0.617–7.271)	0.233
37~60	104	(24%)	25	(23%)	1.321	(0.365–4.779)	0.671
>=60	123	(29%)	19	(18%)	1.175	(0.309–4.472)	0.813
Number of weekly dialyses (>=3 times; n [%])	281	(65%)	85	(79%)	1.792	(0.805–3.991)	0.153
Dialysis membrane (synthetic membrane;n [%])	388	(90%)	96	(89%)	0.145	(0.024–0.885)	0.036
Dialyzer (n [%])							
Low-flux	199	(46%)	59	(55%)	1.000	-	-
Middle-flux	158	(37%)	32	(30%)	0.879	(0.400–1.935)	0.749
High-flux	74	(17%)	17	(16%)	1.130	(0.453–2.818)	0.794
Anticoagulant (heparin; n [%])	381	(88%)	88	(81%)	0.693	(0.323–1.485)	0.345
Kt/v(;median [25th to 75th percentiles])	1.430	(1.266–1.640)	1.462	(1.230–1.599)	0.681	(0.285–1.623)	0.386

OR: odds ratio; CI: confidence interval; BMI: body mass index; SBP: systolic blood pressure; DBP: diastolic blood pressures; Hb:hemoglobin; SCr: serum creatinine; ALB: albumin.

ulant or to pre-rinse the dialyzer, as well as the patients using heparin for long-term anticoagulation of the central venous catheter; furthermore, the patients who used LMWH as the hemodialysis anticoagulant and had never been exposed to heparin were defined as the LMWH group. Because the patients in the heparin group were significantly more numerous than the patients in the LMWH group (578/83 cases), the difference in the number of cases between the groups may reflect the difference in the positivity rate of the anti-PF4/heparin antibody between the two anticoagulants. ⑥ It was confirmed that the unified detection of the PF4/heparin antibody demonstrated no significant differences in the positivity rate of the anti-PF4/heparin antibody between the patients from the different hemodialysis centers in the same region of the same country. This finding might be related to the similar qualities and methods of applications of the heparin drugs used by hemodialysis patients in the same region of the same country.

The occurrence of HIT leads to platelet activation, thereby increasing the risk of occurrence of thromboembolic events in patients [31–34] and most likely increasing the mortality in MHD patients [9]. However, it has also been reported that an increase in anti-PF4/heparin antibody levels does not increase the incidence of thromboembolic events [8,21] and the anti-PF4/heparin antibody had no effect on the overall mortality or cardiovascular events in the absence of thrombocytopenia[10]. Tsai YF et al. [34] reported that the anti-PF4/heparin antibody increases the risk of thromboembolic events, but they also determined that the anti-PF4/heparin antibody is not correlated with peripheral arterial disease (PAD) and coronary heart disease (CHD). In this study, a two-year follow-up was conducted for detection of the anti-PF4/heparin antibody in 661 MHD patients from nine centers, of which 431 patients (65.20%) were on continued dialysis and 108 patients (16.34%) died. The results further confirmed that the occurrence of thromboembolic events was not significantly associated with the anti-PF4/heparin antibody in the MHD patients, and testing positive for the anti-PF4/heparin antibody was not correlated with the two-year mortality of the patients. Further analysis of risk factors in the MHD patients who died

Table 5. Analysis of clinical bleeding & thromboembolic events within the two years.

	Bleeding events within the two years					Thromboembolic events within the two years				
	n/n, (percentage)		OR	95% C.I.	*P* value	n/n, (percentage)		OR	95% C.I.	*P* value
antibody negative + normal platelets	130/365	(36%)	1.000	—	0.155	71/365	(19%)	1.000	—	0.220
antibody negative + reduced platelets	23/45	(51%)	1.890	1.014–3.522	0.045	13/45	(29%)	1.682	0.840–3.370	0.142
antibody positive + normal platelets	5/20	(25%)	0.603	0.214–1.696	0.337	7/20	(35%)	2.230	0.858–5.792	0.100
antibody negative + reduced platelets	1/1	(100%)	—	—	>0.999	0/1	(0%)	—	—	>0.999
antibody negative without antiplatelet drug administration	96/283	(34%)	1.000	—	0.153	59/283	(21%)	1.000	—	0.401
antibody negative with antiplatelet drug administration	57/127	(45%)	1.586	1.034–2.432	0.034	25/127	(20%)	0.931	0.552–1.570	0.787
antibody positive without antiplatelet drug administration	3/12	(25%)	0.649	0.172–2.454	0.524	3/12	(25%)	1.266	0.332–4.822	0.730
antibody positive with antiplatelet drug administration	3/9	(33%)	0.974	0.238–3.980	0.971	4/9	(44%)	3.037	0.791–11.666	0.106

Values are shown as the Number of bleeding (or thromboembolic) events/the number of the patients of the group, (percentage). OR: odds ratio; CI: confidence interval.

revealed that advanced age and diabetes increased the risk of death, and dialysis with a synthetic membrane reduced the risk of death, which is consistent with findings of DOPPS [35–37]. However, no impact of the anti-PF4/heparin antibody on patient mortality was determined.

Based on the fundamental *in vitro* and *in vivo* experiments, antiplatelet drugs might prevent the occurrence of HIT [38,39]; by contrast, several clinical trials have confirmed that antiplatelet drugs do not effectively suppress the occurrence of HIT [40], and antiplatelet drugs do not reduce the occurrence and degree of thrombocytopenia [41]. However, these studies were limited to case reports or research using a small sample size. Because the proportion of elderly patients and patients with diabetes and other cardiovascular complications (such as hypertension in MHD patients) has increased annually, the number of MHD patients taking antiplatelet drugs is also gradually increasing. In this study, the use of antiplatelet agents was an observational indicator, rather than an intervention. In the MHD patients who were using antiplatelet drugs, combined predictive effects were mainly observed for the presence of serum anti-PF4/heparin antibodies and the administration of antiplatelet drugs for bleeding and thromboembolic events. According to the baseline level of the anti-PF4/heparin antibody and antiplatelet drugs, the patients with continued MHD after the two years of follow-up were divided into four groups: antibody negative without antiplatelet drug administration, antibody negative with antiplatelet drug administration, antibody positive without antiplatelet drug administration, and antibody positive with antiplatelet drug administration. The results showed that the patients in the group of antibody negative with antiplatelet drug administration had a significantly increased risk for the occurrence of bleeding events during the two years of follow-up compared with the patients in the other three groups; whether the anti-PF4/heparin antibody was present and whether the patient was taking antiplatelet drugs had no significant effect on the occurrence of thromboembolic events during the two years of follow-up. In addition, the combined predictive effects of the serum anti-PF4/heparin antibody and the platelet count in MHD patients on the clinical bleeding and thromboembolic events were also observed. According to the baseline level of the anti-PF4/heparin antibody and platelet count, the patients with continued MHD after the two years of follow-up were divided into four groups: antibody negative + normal platelets, antibody negative + reduced platelets, antibody positive + normal platelets, and antibody positive + reduced platelets. The results showed that the patients in the antibody negative + reduced platelet group had a significantly increased incidence of bleeding events during the two-year follow-up compared with the patients in the other three groups, whereas neither the level of serum anti-PF4/heparin antibody nor the platelet count predicted the incidence of thromboembolic events. The pathogenesis of HIT by now are mainly regarded as HIT antibodies activate platelets intravascularly, causing the release of platelet microparticles and increased thrombin generation[42,43]. Therefore, we consider that the activations of platelets by anti-PF4/heparin antibody, are likely to offset the risk of bleeding due to antiplatelet drugs and the decreased number of platelets. Although the majority of studies have reported an increased incidence of heparin-PF4 antibodies in patients with thromboembolic events, this has not been universal[8,10,13]. Therefore, we think that anti-PF4/heparin antibody or the activations of platelets are inadequate to cause thromboembolic events. Our data also showed that even considering the impact of the platelet count and antiplatelet drugs, the positive serum anti-PF4/heparin antibody can not predict the risk of occurrence of thromboembolic events in the MHD patients. In addition, the small number of patients tested positive for the serum anti-PF4/heparin antibody might potentially cause a deviation in the analysis.

The advantages of this study are as follows: ① A standard detection method for the anti-PF4/heparin antibody was applied, which was verified by the healthy control. ② As a prospective and multi-center clinical cohort study with a large sample size, the present investigation should be more representative. ③ This study is the first multi-center investigation that addresses the anti-PF4/heparin antibody and its risk factors in Chinese MHD patients, at the level of clinical significance. The limitations of this study include the following: ① lack of dynamic monitoring and recording during the two years of follow-up (with the indicators being observed at multiple time points); ② failure to redetect the serum anti-PF4/heparin antibody after the two years of observation; ③ use of antiplatelet drugs as an observational indicator, rather than an intervention; ④ the smaller number of patients who tested positive for the serum anti-PF4/heparin antibody, which might have potentially caused a deviation in the analysis.

In summary, this study is the first to indicate that the positivity rate of the anti-PF4/heparin antibody in Chinese MHD patients was 5.6% using a prospective and multi-center clinical cohort study with a large sample size. We further verified that a single detection of anti-PF4/heparin antibody did not predict the occurrence of bleeding, thromboembolic events, and risk of death in the MHD patients. Finally, we demonstrated that the patients who tested negative for the anti-PF4/heparin antibody and who also exhibited a thrombocytopenia or underwent administration of antiplatelet drugs were at significantly increased risk for clinical bleeding.

Acknowledgments

We thank all the staff and participants of the hemodialysis centers of the nine hospitals for their important contributions.

Author Contributions

Conceived and designed the experiments: XS XC. Performed the experiments: QH. Analyzed the data: DZ XS. Contributed reagents/materials/analysis tools: LY HL JL J. Zhao ZZ LL J. Zhang ML YY SJ YW HZ. Wrote the paper: DZ XS.

References

1. Shen JI, Winkelmayer WC (2012) Use and Safety of Unfractionated Heparin for Anticoagulation During Maintenance Hemodialysis. American Journal of Kidney Diseases 60: 473–486.
2. Aster RH (1999) Drug-induced immune thrombocytopenia: An overview of pathogenesis. Seminars in Hematology 36: 2–6.
3. Haase M, Bellomo I, Rocktaeschel J, Ziemer S, Kiesewetter H, et al. (2005) Use of fondaparinux (ARIXTRA((R))) in a dialysis patient with symptomatic heparin-induced thrombocytopaenia type II. Nephrology Dialysis Transplantation 20: 444–446.
4. Warkentin TE (2004) An overview of the heparin-induced thrombocytopenia syndrome. Semin Thromb Hemost 30: 273–283.
5. Hirsh J, Heddle N, Kelton JG (2004) Treatment of heparin-induced thrombocytopenia: a critical review. Arch Intern Med 164: 361–369.
6. Warkentin TE, Greinacher A, Koster A, Lincoff AM (2008) Treatment and prevention of heparin-induced thrombocytopenia: American College of Chest Physicians Evidence-Based Clinical Practice Guidelines (8th Edition). Chest 133: 340S–380S.
7. Kato S, Takahashi K, Ayabe K, Samad R, Fukaya E, et al. (2011) Heparin-induced thrombocytopenia: analysis of risk factors in medical inpatients. Br J Haematol 154: 373–377.
8. O'Shea SI, Sands JJ, Nudo SA, Ortel TL (2002) Frequency of anti-heparin-platelet factor 4 antibodies in hemodialysis patients and correlation with recurrent vascular access thrombosis. Am J Hematol 69: 72–73.
9. Pena de la Vega L, Miller RS, Benda MM, Grill DE, Johnson MG, et al. (2005) Association of heparin-dependent antibodies and adverse outcomes in hemodialysis patients: a population-based study. Mayo Clin Proc 80: 995–1000.
10. Asmis LM, Segal JB, Plantinga LC, Fink NE, Kerman JS, et al. (2008) Heparin-induced antibodies and cardiovascular risk in patients on dialysis. Thromb Haemost 100: 498–504.
11. Matsuo T, Kobayashi H, Matsuo M, Wanaka K, Nakamoto H, et al. (2006) Frequency of anti-heparin-PF4 complex antibodies (HIT antibodies) in uremic patients on chronic intermittent hemodialysis. Pathophysiol Haemost Thromb 35: 445–450.
12. Hutchison CA, Dasgupta I (2007) National survey of heparin-induced thrombocytopenia in the haemodialysis population of the UK population. Nephrol Dial Transplant 22: 1680–1684.
13. Benjamin J, Moldavsky S, Lee J, Rubin R (2009) Prevalence of heparin-induced antibody in African-American hemodialysis patients—comparison to non-dialysis patients. Clin Nephrol 71: 263–266.
14. Nakamoto H, Shimada Y, Kanno T, Wanaka K, Matsuo T, et al. (2005) Role of platelet factor 4-heparin complex antibody (HIT antibody) in the pathogenesis of thrombotic episodes in patients on hemodialysis. Hemodial Int 9 Suppl 1: S2–7.
15. O'Shea S I, Lawson JH, Reddan D, Murphy M, Ortel TL (2003) Hypercoagulable states and antithrombotic strategies in recurrent vascular access site thrombosis. J Vasc Surg 38: 541–548.
16. Ligthart GJ, Corberand JX, Fournier C, Galanaud P, Hijmans W, et al. (1984) Admission criteria for immunogerontological studies in man: the SENIEUR protocol. Mech Ageing Dev 28: 47–55.
17. Warkentin TE, Sheppard JI, Moore JC, Kelton JG (2010) The use of well-characterized sera for the assessment of new diagnostic enzyme-immunoassays for the diagnosis of heparin-induced thrombocytopenia. J Thromb Haemost 8: 216–218.
18. Warkentin TE, Sheppard JI, Moore JC, Sigouin CS, Kelton JG (2008) Quantitative interpretation of optical density measurements using PF4-dependent enzyme-immunoassays. J Thromb Haemost 6: 1304–1312.
19. McFarland J, Lochowicz A, Aster R, Chappell B, Curtis B (2012) Improving the specificity of the PF4 ELISA in diagnosing heparin-induced thrombocytopenia. Am J Hematol 87: 776–781.
20. Aster RH (2010) Improving specificity in HIT testing. blood 116.
21. Palomo I, Pereira J, Alarcon M, Diaz G, Hidalgo P, et al. (2005) Prevalence of heparin-induced antibodies in patients with chronic renal failure undergoing hemodialysis. J Clin Lab Anal 19: 189–195.
22. Arepally GM, Ortel TL (2006) Clinical practice. Heparin-induced thrombocytopenia. N Engl J Med 355: 809–817.
23. Warkentin TE, Sheppard JAI, Moore JC, Moore KM, Sigouin CS, et al. (2005) Laboratory testing for the antibodies that cause heparin-induced thrombocytopenia: How much class do we need? Journal of Laboratory and Clinical Medicine 146: 341–346.
24. Greinacher A, Juhl D, Strobel U, Wessel A, Lubenow N, et al. (2007) Heparin-induced thrombocytopenia: a prospective study on the incidence, platelet-activating capacity and clinical significance of antiplatelet factor 4/heparin antibodies of the IgG, IgM, and IgA classes. J Thromb Haemost 5: 1666–1673.
25. Warkentin TE, Sheppard JA (2006) Testing for heparin-induced thrombocytopenia antibodies. Transfus Med Rev 20: 259–272.
26. Pouplard C, Leroux D, Regina S, Rollin J, Gruel Y (2010) Effectiveness of a new immunoassay for the diagnosis of heparin-induced thrombocytopenia and improved specificity when detecting IgG antibodies. Thromb Haemost 103: 145–150.
27. Whitlatch NL, Kong DF, Metjian AD, Arepally GM, Ortel TL (2010) Validation of the high-dose heparin confirmatory step for the diagnosis of heparin-induced thrombocytopenia. Blood 116: 1761–1766.
28. Davenport A (2009) Antibodies to heparin-platelet factor 4 complex: pathogenesis, epidemiology, and management of heparin-induced thrombocytopenia in hemodialysis. Am J Kidney Dis 54: 361–374.
29. Diaz J, Prechel M, Emanuele M, Emanuele N, Walenga JM (2010) Profiling of heparin-induced thrombocytopenia antibody levels in patients with and without diabetes. Clin Appl Thromb Hemost 16: 121–125.
30. Martel N, Lee J, Wells PS (2005) Risk for heparin-induced thrombocytopenia with unfractionated and low-molecular-weight heparin thromboprophylaxis: a meta-analysis. Blood 106: 2710–2715.
31. Matsuo T, Wanaka K (2008) Management of uremic patients with heparin-induced thrombocytopenia requiring hemodialysis. Clin Appl Thromb Hemost 14: 459–464.
32. Ban-Hoefen M, Francis C (2009) Heparin induced thrombocytopenia and thrombosis in a tertiary care hospital. Thromb Res 124: 189–192.
33. Yu A, Jacobson SH, Bygden A, Egberg N (2002) The presence of heparin-platelet factor 4 antibodies as a marker of hypercoagulability during hemodialysis. Clin Chem Lab Med 40: 21–26.
34. Tsai YF, Chen CA, Kuo C, Lin KC (2012) Anti-PF4/heparin antibodies are associated with arteriovenous fistula thrombosis in non-diabetic hemodialysis patients. Clin Exp Nephrol 16: 300–305.
35. Inaba M, Hayashino Y, Shoji T, Akiba T, Akizawa T, et al. (2012) Disappearance of association in diabetic patients on hemodialysis between anemia and mortality risk: the Japan dialysis outcomes and practice pattern study. Nephron Clin Pract 120: c91–c100.
36. Canaud B, Tong L, Tentori F, Akiba T, Karaboyas A, et al. (2011) Clinical practices and outcomes in elderly hemodialysis patients: results from the Dialysis Outcomes and Practice Patterns Study (DOPPS). Clin J Am Soc Nephrol 6: 1651–1662.
37. Chauveau P, Nguyen H, Combe C, Chene G, Azar R, et al. (2005) Dialyzer membrane permeability and survival in hemodialysis patients. Am J Kidney Dis 45: 565–571.
38. Gruel Y, Lermusiaux P, Lang M, Darnige L, Rupin A, et al. (1991) Usefulness of antiplatelet drugs in the management of heparin-associated thrombocytopenia and thrombosis. Ann Vasc Surg 5: 552–555.
39. Kappa JR, Fisher CA, Addonizio VP Jr (1989) Heparin-induced platelet activation: the role of thromboxane A2 synthesis and the extent of platelet granule release in two patients. J Vasc Surg 9: 574–579.
40. Greinacher A, Warkentin TE (2004) Treatment of heparin-induced thrombocytopenia: an overview. Heparin-induced thrombocytopenia, 3rd ed New York:Marcel Dekker: 335–370.
41. Bream-Rouwenhorst HR, Hobbs RA, Horwitz PA (2008) Thrombocytopenia in patients treated with heparin, combination antiplatelet therapy, and intra-aortic balloon pump counterpulsation. J Interv Cardiol 21: 350–356.
42. Poncz M (2005) Mechanistic basis of heparin-induced thrombocytopenia. Semin Thorac Cardiovasc Surg 17: 73–79.
43. Kelton JG (2005) The pathophysiology of heparin-induced thrombocytopenia: biological basis for treatment. Chest 127: 9S–20S.

Aldosterone and Mortality in Hemodialysis Patients: Role of Volume Overload

Szu-Chun Hung[1]☯, Yao-Ping Lin[2]☯, Hsin-Lei Huang[3], Hsiao-Fung Pu[3], Der-Cherng Tarng[2,3]*

1 Division of Nephrology, Buddhist Tzu Chi General Hospital, Taipei Branch, Taipei, Taiwan, **2** Division of Nephrology, Department of Medicine, and Immunology Research Center, Taipei Veterans General Hospital, Taipei, Taiwan, **3** Department and Institute of Physiology, School of Medicine, National Yang-Ming University, Taipei, Taiwan

Abstract

Background: Elevated aldosterone is associated with increased mortality in the general population. In patients on dialysis, however, the association is reversed. This paradox may be explained by volume overload, which is associated with lower aldosterone and higher mortality.

Methods: We evaluated the relationship between aldosterone and outcomes in a prospective cohort of 328 hemodialysis patients stratified by the presence or absence of volume overload (defined as extracellular water/total body water >48%, as measured with bioimpedance). Baseline plasma aldosterone was measured before dialysis and categorized as low (<140 pg/mL), middle (140 to 280 pg/mL) and high (>280 pg/mL).

Results: Overall, 36% (n = 119) of the hemodialysis patients had evidence of volume overload. Baseline aldosterone was significantly lower in the presence of volume overload than in its absence. During a median follow-up of 54 months, 83 deaths and 70 cardiovascular events occurred. Cox multivariate analysis showed that by using the low aldosterone as the reference, high aldosterone was inversely associated with decreased hazard ratios for mortality (0.49; 95% confidence interval, 0.25–0.76) and first cardiovascular event (0.70; 95% confidence interval, 0.33−0.78) in the presence of volume overload. In contrast, high aldosterone was associated with an increased risk for mortality (1.97; 95% confidence interval, 1.69–3.75) and first cardiovascular event (2.01; 95% confidence interval, 1.28−4.15) in the absence of volume overload.

Conclusions: The inverse association of aldosterone with adverse outcomes in hemodialysis patients is due to the confounding effect of volume overload. These findings support treatment of hyperaldosteronemia in hemodialysis patients who have achieved strict volume control.

Editor: Leighton R James, University of Florida, United States of America

Funding: This study was supported by grants from the National Science Council (NSC 96-2628-B-010-001-MY3 and 99-2314-B-010-004-MY3), Taipei City Hospital (97001-62-002), National Yang-Ming University Hospital (RD2011-025), and Ministry of Education's aim for the Top University Plan. The funders had no role in study design, data collection and analysis, decision to publish, or preparation of the manuscript.

Competing Interests: The authors have declared that no competing interests exist.

* E-mail: dctarng@vghtpe.gov.tw

☯ These authors contributed equally to this work.

Introduction

Cardiovascular disease (CVD) is the leading cause of death in patients with end-stage renal disease (ESRD) [1]. There is accumulating evidence that aldosterone, in addition to its classical role in regulating fluid and electrolyte balance, plays a significant role in the pathogenesis of CVD [2]. Patients with chronic kidney disease (CKD) have higher aldosterone concentrations than the general population [3], suggesting that aldosterone might modulate the development of CVD in CKD. However, higher aldosterone levels are associated with lower mortality in CKD patients on hemodialysis [4,5], which is in marked contrast to findings from prospective studies in the general population and in early CKD [6,7]. A similar inverse association of serum cholesterol levels with mortality has been previously documented in dialysis patients [8–10]. It has been suggested that this paradoxical association results from a confounding effect of inflammation and/or malnutrition, which leads to lower cholesterol levels and higher mortality (the so called reverse epidemiology).

Volume overload is a common finding in dialysis patients and has been recognized as an important contributor to an adverse prognosis [11,12]. This factor may explain the inverse association between aldosterone level and mortality because volume overload is strongly associated with lower aldosterone levels and higher mortality [13]. In view of the particularly high incidence of CVD in dialysis patients, a better understanding of the diagnostic implications of aldosterone levels in these patients is needed. Therefore, we investigated whether the association between aldosterone levels and mortality would be modified by the presence of volume overload.

Materials and Methods

Ethics Statement

The study complied with the Declaration of Helsinki and was approved by the institutional review board of National Yang-Ming University Hospital. All participants gave their written informed consent before inclusion.

Patient Population

This prospective cohort study was conducted at the dialysis centers of affiliated hospitals of National Yang-Ming University, Taipei. The study subjects were recruited from November 1 to December 31, 2004. Initially, all patients (n = 418) undergoing hemodialysis were screened, and 366 clinically stable patients aged older than 20 years, who had been on hemodialysis for more than 6 months, were included. Exclusion criteria were dialysis for less than 12 h per week; inadequacy of dialysis, defined as Kt/V urea <1.2; conditions of malignancy, infectious disease, sepsis, or hepatobiliary disease; and unwillingness to participate in this study. Finally, the study population of 328 patients (188 men and 140 women; mean age of 59 years) was followed up until June 30, 2009. All the patients were subjected to a standard bicarbonate dialysis session with use of 137 mEq/L sodium and 2.0 mEq/L potassium dialysate. Hemodialysis was performed three times weekly using single-use dialyzers with a membrane surface area of 1.6–1.7 m^2.

Laboratory Investigations

Blood samples were drawn from patients who had fasted overnight before the start of a mid-week dialysis session, and heparin was then administered. Plasma and serum were separated and kept frozen at −70°C when not analyzed immediately. Plasma aldosterone levels were measured according to the manufacturer's instructions using a commercially available radioimmunoassay kit (Diagnostic Systems Laboratories, Webster, TX). The intra- and inter-assay coefficients of variation were 3.4% and 8.9%, respectively, at an aldosterone level of 60 pg/mL, 4.7% and 7.6%, respectively, at a level of 250 pg/mL, and 4.0% and 5.2%, respectively, at a level of 500 pg/mL. Albumin, urea, creatinine, calcium, phosphate, iron, and total iron-binding capacity (TIBC) in serum were determined with a Hitachi 7600 autoanalyzer (Roche Modular; Hitachi Ltd, Tokyo, Japan) using commercial kits. Serum high-sensitivity C-reactive protein (hs-CRP) levels were measured using an immunoturbidimetric assay and rate nephelometry (IMMAGE; Beckman Coulter, Galway, Ireland). The adequacy of dialysis was estimated by measuring mid-week urea clearance (Kt/V urea) using the standard method [14]. Blood pressure (BP) was measured and recorded by an automated sphygmomanometer. Pre-dialysis BP (before placement of a dialysis needle) was measured in the nonaccess arm after a 5-minute rest while the patient was seated with both feet on the floor.

Bioimpedance Study

Multifrequency bioimpedance method (Model 310 Bioimpedance Analyzer; Biodynamics, Seattle, WA) was performed within 30 minutes after a dialysis session at presumed dry weight. The ratio of extracellular water to total body water (ECW/TBW) was then taken as a measure of volume status. To avoid inter-observer variation, a single well-trained dietitian was involved in the measurement of bioimpedance.

Outcomes

In all patients, a thorough medical history was taken at the time of study enrollment. Presence of CVD was defined as a medical history and clinical findings of congestive heart failure, coronary artery disease, cerebrovascular disease, and/or peripheral vascular disease. No major modifications were made in dialysis treatments during the follow-up period. The primary outcome measures were death from any cause and CV events from the time of inclusion in the study. CV events included fatal and nonfatal myocardial infarction, stroke and congestive heart failure, as well as complicated peripheral vascular disease and sudden death. A trained physician who had no knowledge of the results of plasma aldosterone measurements independently reviewed all suspected CV events by examining each medical chart.

Statistical Analysis

All variables were expressed as percentages for categorical data and as means ± SDs or medians and interquartile ranges (IQRs) for continuous data with or without a normal distribution, respectively. The baseline characteristics of the 2 study subgroups with ECW/TBW ≤48% and >48% were compared using a *t*-test, x^2 statistics, and Mann-Whitney U test as appropriate. Potential differences among the 3 patient groups for each baseline plasma aldosterone tertile were assessed by an analysis of variance (ANOVA), x^2 statistics, or the Kruskal-Wallis test, as appropriate. Receiver operating characteristic (ROC) curves were constructed for prediction of mortality using ECW/TBW at baseline. The optimal cutoff point for volume overload (ECW/TBW >48%) is listed in Figure 1, along with the sensitivity, specificity and accuracy for predicting mortality at the end of the follow-up period. Confidence intervals (CI) for the area under the ROC curves were calculated using nonparametric assumptions. Univariate correlations between ECW/TBW or plasma aldosterone and potentially explanatory variables were assessed by Pearson correlation analyses.

The Kaplan-Meier method was used to describe survival curves. Individuals were censored at the time of kidney transplantation, peritoneal dialysis, and withdrawal from the study, or at the end of the follow-up period on June 30, 2009. Cox proportional hazards models were used to investigate the role of volume overload as a potential effect modifier for relationships between diverse independent variables and either all-cause mortality or first CV event. For all multivariate survival analyses, clinically relevant variables with a P value ≤0.1 in the univariate analysis were fitted and the backward selection procedure was used for model selection [15]. The aldosterone variables were modeled as categorical variables (<140, 140–280, and >280 pg/mL) or continuous variables (per 100 pg/mL). Adjusted hazard ratios with 95% CI were reported. P values less than 0.05 were considered statistically significant. P values for interactions between the volume indicators and the aldosterone levels were computed using likelihood ratio tests. All statistical analyses were performed using the computer software Statistical Package for the Social Science, version 16.0 (SPSS Inc., Chicago, IL).

Results

Clinical Characteristics

The mean baseline age of the 328 patients was 59±13 years, 57.3% were male, and 29.3% had diabetes. The baseline characteristics for the patient groups divided by the absence or presence of volume overload [defined as ECW/TBW >48%] are presented in Table 1. Overall, 36% (n = 119) of the dialysis patients had evidence of volume overload. The presence of volume overload was associated with older age, diabetes, prior CVD, hypertension, higher inflammatory markers, and lower aldosterone, albumin, calcium, phosphate, and hemoglobin levels. There

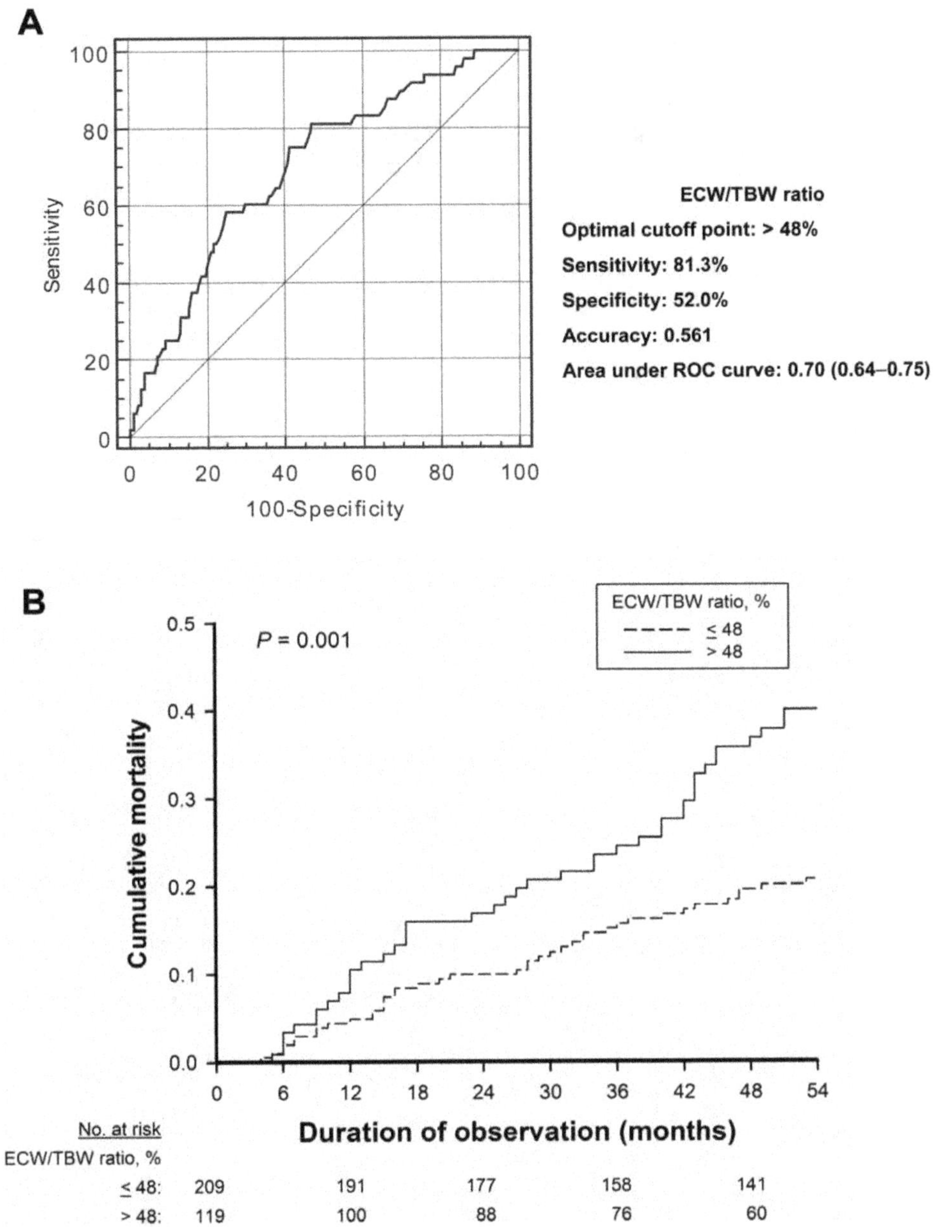

Figure 1. Volume status for predicting mortality. The receiver operating characteristic (ROC) curve for prediction of all-cause mortality constructed using the ratio of extracellular water to total body water (ECW/TBW) at baseline (A). The optimal cutoff point for ECW/TBW is listed in the attached table, along with the sensitivity, specificity and accuracy for predicting mortality at the end of the follow-up period. The area under ROC curve is significantly larger than 0.5. Kaplan-Meier analysis curve for all-cause mortality in relation to the ECW/TBW at baseline, stratified by the cutoff point among hemodialysis patients (B).

were no significant differences between groups regarding the type of antihypertensive medications, dialysis prescription, and serum potassium levels. The median plasma aldosterone concentration was 184 pg/mL (IQR: 97–484 pg/mL), which is above the 75th percentile for aldosterone in a large cohort of non-CKD patients referred for coronary angiography [3]. Table 2 shows the baseline characteristics stratified by both volume status and plasma aldosterone categories. In patients without volume overload, hs-CRP and interleukin-6 (IL-6) levels were significantly higher in patients in the >280 pg/mL aldosterone category than in patients in the <140 pg/mL aldosterone category ($P<0.05$). This relationship was inversed in patients with volume overload. The number of antihypertensive medication was positively and significantly associated with the aldosterone categories for patients without volume overload, but the trend was reversed for patients with volume overload.

Table 3 shows univariate correlations between ECW/TBW or plasma aldosterone levels and potentially explanatory variables. The ECW/TBW was negatively correlated with plasma aldosterone, hemoglobin, albumin, calcium, and phosphate levels and was positively correlated with age, hs-CRP, IL-6, ferritin levels, and systolic BP. In contrast, plasma aldosterone was positively associated with albumin and phosphate levels and was negatively associated with age, ECW/TBW, ferritin and systolic BP.

Table 1. Baseline characteristics of the study participants by categories of ECW/TBW.

Baseline values	Total patients (n = 328)	ECW/TBW ≤48% (n = 209)	ECW/TBW >48% (n = 119)	P-value[a]
Age (years)	59±13	55±12	65±11	<0.001[b]
Male (%)	57.3	59.8	52.9	0.23[c]
Smoking history (%)	31.7	32.1	31.1	0.86[c]
Diabetes mellitus (%)	29.3	19.1	47.1	<0.001[c]
Prior CVD (%)	23.4	18.2	32.8	0.002[c]
Hypertension (%)	48.2	40.6	61.3	<0.001[c]
Systolic BP (mmHg)	136±24	134±22	140±26	0.04[b]
Diastolic BP (mmHg)	76±12	76±11	76±14	0.99[b]
RAAS blockade (%)	27.1	24.9	31.1	0.22[c]
Calcium channel blocker (%)	62.2	59.8	66.4	0.31[c]
β-blocker (%)	32.6	32.0	33.6	0.53[c]
No. of antihypertensives	2.0±1.3	2.0±1.1	2.1±1.5	0.72[b]
Statin use (%)	15.9	16.3	15.1	0.79[c]
HD duration (months)	66±54	67±53	65±56	0.84[b]
Kt/V urea	2.0±0.6	2.0±0.5	2.1±0.7	0.11[b]
Intradialytic UF (L)	2.9±0.6	2.9±0.7	2.8±0.5	0.87[b]
BMI (kg/m²)	22.6±3.5	22.0±3.1	23.3±4.1	0.02[b]
ECW (L)	13.0±2.1	12.5±2.1	13.7±2.0	<0.001[b]
TBW (L)	28.4±4.6	29.3±4.8	26.9±3.9	<0.001[b]
ECW/TBW (%)	45.8±5.0	42.9±3.4	50.9±2.8	<0.001[b]
Aldosterone (pg/mL)	184 (97–484)	215 (99–768)	166 (95–263)	0.02[d]
hs-CRP (mg/L)	3.94 (1.29–7.86)	3.74 (1.55–6.74)	4.10 (1.24–8.09)	0.04[d]
IL-6 (pg/mL)	2.92 (2.21–7.87)	2.80 (1.78–5.53)	4.59 (2.66–9.67)	<0.001[d]
Albumin (g/L)	39.3±3.5	39.9±3.2	38.2±3.7	<0.001[b]
Total cholesterol (mg/dL)	186±33	188±32	180±35	0.16[b]
Triglyceride (mg/dL)	127±61	130±64	121±57	0.18[b]
Potassium (mmol/L)	4.01±0.36	4.02±0.37	3.98±0.37	0.28[b]
Calcium (mg/dL)	9.7±0.7	9.8±0.7	9.6±0.8	0.03[b]
Phosphate (mg/dL)	5.0±1.4	5.2±1.4	4.8±1.3	0.002[b]
Hemoglobin (g/dL)	10.5±1.5	10.8±1.5	9.8±1.4	<0.001[b]
EPO dose (u/kg/wk)	66±46	55±47	87±36	<0.001[b]
Ferritin (μg/L)	344 (201–538)	291 (129–439)	361 (255–606)	0.001[d]
Transferrin saturation (%)	27±13	27±13	27±14	0.77[b]

Abbreviations: BMI denotes body mass index; BP, blood pressure; CVD, cardiovascular disease; ECW, extracellular water; ECW/TBW, ratio of extracellular water to total body water; EPO, erythropoietin; HD, hemodialysis; hs-CRP, high-sensitivity C-reactive protein; IL-6, inerleukin-6; RAAS, renin-angiotensin-aldosterone system; TBW, total body water; UF, ultrafiltration.

[a]Comparison between two groups of patients with ECW/TBW ≤48% and >48%.

Statistical analysis by [b]Student *t*-test, [c]Pearson x^2 test, and [d]Mann-Whitney U test.

Prior CVD category consisted of congestive heart failure, coronary artery disease, cerebrovascular disease, and peripheral arterial disease.

Follow-up Data

During the follow-up period, 16 patients received kidney transplants, and 4 patients transitioned to peritoneal dialysis. Thirty-three patients who were transferred to other dialysis units were followed up using questionnaire forms completed by the attending physicians at the units. At the end of the follow-up period, 225 patients were confirmed to be alive on hemodialysis treatment, and 83 patients died while being treated; 37 (44.6%) of these deaths were due to CVD-related causes. There were 70 CV events in the median follow-up period of 54 months (IQR: 27–107 months). In unadjusted analysis, lower aldosterone levels were associated with higher mortality in the overall cohort (P for trend = 0.006) (Fig. 2) and in the presence of volume overload (P for trend = 0.001) (Fig. 3A), respectively. However, in the absence of volume overload, the association was reversed, with higher aldosterone levels associated with higher mortality (P for trend = 0.042) (Fig. 3B).

Multivariate analysis with plasma aldosterone, age, gender, prior CVD, presence of diabetes mellitus, smoking status, body mass index, systolic blood pressure, dialysis vintage, baseline levels of serum albumin, total cholesterol, hemoglobin, ferritin, calcium×phosphate, Kt/V urea, and IL-6 as the independent

Table 2. Baseline characteristics of the study participants by categories of ECW/TBW and plasma aldosterone.

	ECW/TBW ≤48%			**ECW/TBW >48%**		
	Plasma aldoterone, pg/mL			**Plasma aldoterone, pg/mL**		
	<140	**140–280**	**>280**	**<140**	**140–280**	**>280**
Baseline values	(n = 69)	(n = 53)	(n = 87)	(n = 39)	(n = 56)	(n = 24)
Age (years)	55±12	57±11	54±11	67±9	66±13	64±9
Male (%)	63.8	54.7	59.8	51.3	53.6	54.2
Smoking history (%)	34.8	32.1	29.9	30.8	28.6	37.5
Diabetes mellitus (%)	23.2	24.5	12.6	38.5	51.8	50.0
Prior CVD (%)	20.3	22.6	13.8	38.5	30.4	29.2
Hypertension (%)	39.4	41.8	41.3	67.9	66.7	41.6[b,c]
Systolic BP (mmHg)	132±19	134±24	135±24	143±27	140±25	135±26[b,c]
Diastolic BP (mmHg)	76±9	76±11	75±11	74±12	77±18	76±7
RAAS blockade (%)	15.9	28.3	29.9	28.2	30.4	37.5
No. of antihypertensives	1.5±1.0	2.0±1.0	2.4±1.5[b]	2.5±1.5	2.4±1.5	1.4±1.0[b,c]
Statin use (%)	11.6	17.0	19.5	17.9	14.3	12.5
HD duration (months)	67±49	65±53	68±56	59±47	67±52	74±74
Kt/V urea	2.0±0.6	2.0±0.3	2.0±0.4	2.0±0.4	2.3±0.9	2.0±0.3
BMI (kg/m^2)	21.8±3.1	21.7±2.8	22.6±3.1	23.1±5.2	23.5±3.4	22.5±4.8
ECW (L)	12.4±1.5	12.3±2.2	12.8±2.2	13.9±2.2	13.0±1.9	13.6±2.1
TBW (L)	28.2±3.7	28. ±9 4.8	30.1±5.1	27.1±4.6	26.7±3.4	27.3±4.4
ECW/TBW (%)	44.2±2.9	42.7±4.1[b]	42.7±3.1[b]	51.4±2.9	50.9±2.8	49.9±2.0[b,c]
hs-CRP (mg/L)	2.53 (1.09–4.99)	3.85 (1.26–5.79)	4.76 (1.62–7.55)[b]	6.12 (2.28–8.63)	4.70 (0.94–8.06)	1.53 (0.59–5.82)[b]
IL-6 (pg/mL)	2.42 (1.62–4.44)	3.10 (1.87–5.84)	3.85 (2.19–6.04)[b]	5.42 (2.52–11.57)	4.86 (3.04–12.36)	3.62 (2.55–6.43)[b]
Albumin (g/L)	39.5±3.1	39.9±3.4	40.0±3.2	36.8±1.3	38.9±3.5	39.3±4.0[b]
Total cholesterol (mg/dL)	193±45	189±40	183±30	177±32	180±34	185±38
Triglyceride (mg/dL)	133±68	130±60	128±48	122±53	120±47	121±49
Potassium (mmol/L)	4.03±0.37	4.02±0.37	4.01±0.37	4.00±0.36	3.99±0.37	3.98±0.37
Calcium (mg/dL)	9.8±0.7	9.6±0.7	9.8±0.7	9.4±0.9	9.7±0.8	9.4±0.6
Phosphate (mg/dL)	4.8±1.2	5.1±1.4	5.5±1.5	4.5±1.2	4.8±1.3	4.8±1.2
Hemoglobin (g/dL)	10.8±1.2	10.6±1.6	10.8±1.6	9.7±1.3	9.8±1.4	10.0±1.2
EPO dose (u/kg/wk)	51±44	72±50[b]	52±45[c]	89±31	87±41	77±36
Ferritin (μg/L)	323 (157–407)	277 (142–541)	271 (101–466)	370 (272–675)	393 (264–593)	278 (239–514)
Transferrin saturation (%)	29±12	24±10	28±14	27±14	27±14	26±15

For abbreviations see Table 1.
[a]Comparisons among three groups in patients with ECW/TBW ≤48% and >48%, respectively. Statistical analysis by one-way ANOVA test, Pearson x^2 test, and Kruskal-Wallis test as appropriate.
[b]P<0.05 versus patients with plasma aldosterone of <140 pg/mL.
[c]P<0.05 versus patients with plasma aldosterone of 140–280 pg/mL.
Prior CVD category consisted of congestive heart failure, coronary artery disease, cerebrovascular disease, and peripheral arterial disease.

variables demonstrated that plasma aldosterone, age, prior CVD, serum albumin, and IL-6 were independently related to mortality and first CV event. The inverse association of aldosterone level with mortality, both in the entire patient population and in the presence of volume overload (ECW/TBW >48%), was also seen in adjusted analysis (Table 4). Furthermore, volume overload was found to modify the risk relationship between aldosterone and first CV event in the Cox regressions with plasma aldosterone level as a categorical (interaction, P = 0.02) or a continuous measure (interaction, P = 0.03). In the absence of volume overload (ECW/TBW ≤48%), the aldosterone category was positively associated with all-cause mortality and first CV event. Analyzing aldosterone as a continuous variable also showed the similar association of aldosterone with all-cause mortality and first CV event.

Discussion

This study demonstrates an inverse association of aldosterone levels with all-cause mortality and CV event rates in the presence of volume overload. This represents a paradoxical effect of volume status on mortality. In contrast, there was a significant, graded, and positive association of aldosterone levels with all-cause mortality and CV event rates in the 64% of participants without volume overload. Accordingly, some ESRD patients with low aldosterone levels have a low risk of adverse outcomes, as in the general population, whereas others have a high risk because they

Table 3. Univariate correlations between ECW/TBW or plasma aldosterone and potentially explanatory variables.

	ECW/TBW		Aldosterone	
Variables	*r*	P-value	*r*	P-value
Age (years)	−0.555	<0.001	−0.286	<0.001
Body mass index (kg/m^2)	−0.136	0.02	−0.038	0.54
ECW/TBW (%)	–	–	−0.200	0.001
Aldosterone (pg/mL)	−0.200	0.001	–	–
hs-CRP (mg/L)	−0.180	0.002	−0.013	0.81
IL-6 (pg/mL)	−0.310	<0.001	−0.069	0.22
Hemoglobin (g/dL)	−0.368	<0.001	−0.067	0.24
Serum ferritin (μg/L)	−0.208	<0.001	−0.169	0.003
Transferrin saturation (%)	−0.092	0.10	−0.029	0.61
Albumin (g/L)	−0.337	<0.001	−0.189	0.001
Calcium (mg/dL)	−0.123	0.03	−0.082	0.15
Phosphate (mg/dL)	−0.177	0.001	−0.222	<0.001
Potassium (mmol/L)	−0.080	0.19	−0.024	0.69
Systolic BP (mmHg)	−0.123	0.03	−0.135	0.02
Diastolic BP (mmHg)	−0.032	0.57	−0.081	0.16
Kt/V urea	−0.089	0.06	−0.028	0.63

For abbreviations see Table 1.

are in a state of volume overload, which lowers aldosterone levels and increases the risk of mortality and CV events. These findings underline the importance of hyperaldosteronemia as a risk factor for adverse long-term outcomes among patients with ESRD, and of the masking of this association among individuals with volume overload.

A growing body of evidence has linked aldosterone excess to the development and progression of different CVD processes, including hypertension, congestive heart failure, and coronary artery disease [16,17]. Plasma aldosterone levels are markedly elevated among patients with CKD [3–5] which is similar to the remnant kidney model in the rat [18]. In a study of 28 selected patients with varying degrees of CKD and normal serum potassium levels and plasma renin activity, Hene et al. showed that aldosterone levels were elevated when creatinine clearance was less than 50% of normal, increasing three- to four-fold above normal levels as clearance values decreased [3]. Therefore, aldosterone-mediated CV damage might be amplified by decreased kidney function, which by itself is a potent CV risk factor [7].

Plasma aldosterone levels are influenced by a number of factors, including potassium and volume status. Our results showed that a relatively lower aldosterone level was in fact a surrogate marker of volume overload in hemodialysis patients. In healthy volunteers with salt loading and in hemodialysis patients with increased interdialytic weight gain, expansions of ECW led to reciprocal declines in plasma aldosterone concentrations. The relationship was more profound in healthy volunteers than in hemodialysis patients. As a result, the shift of the volume-aldosterone curve in hemodialysis patients suggests that ESRD is a state of high volume and

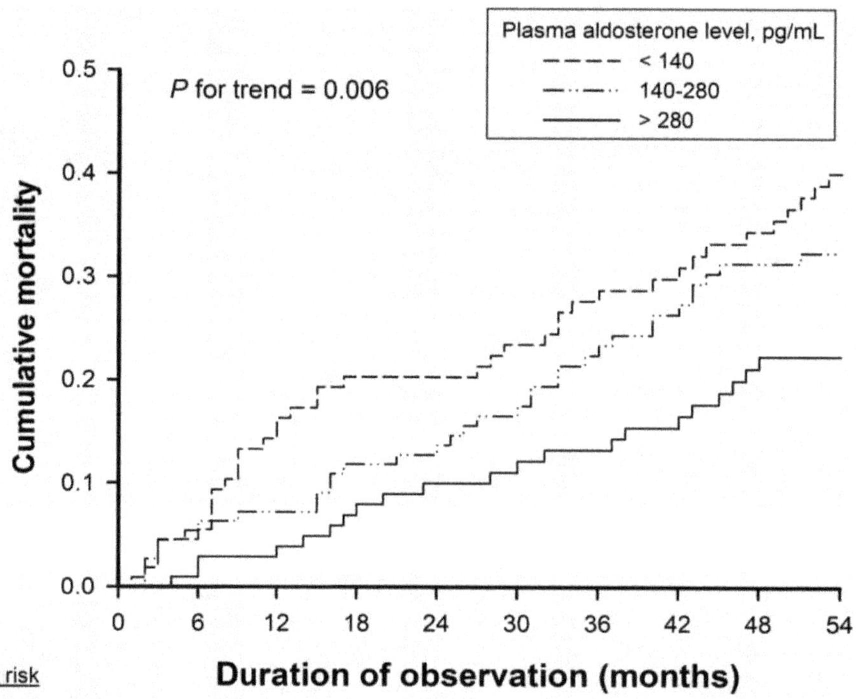

No. at risk Aldosterone level, pg/mL					
< 140:	108	98	90	77	70
140-280:	109	92	87	76	67
> 280:	111	101	88	80	63

Figure 2. Kaplan-Meier mortality curves according to aldosterone tertile. All-cause mortality in relation to plasma aldosterone levels at baseline among hemodialysis patients.

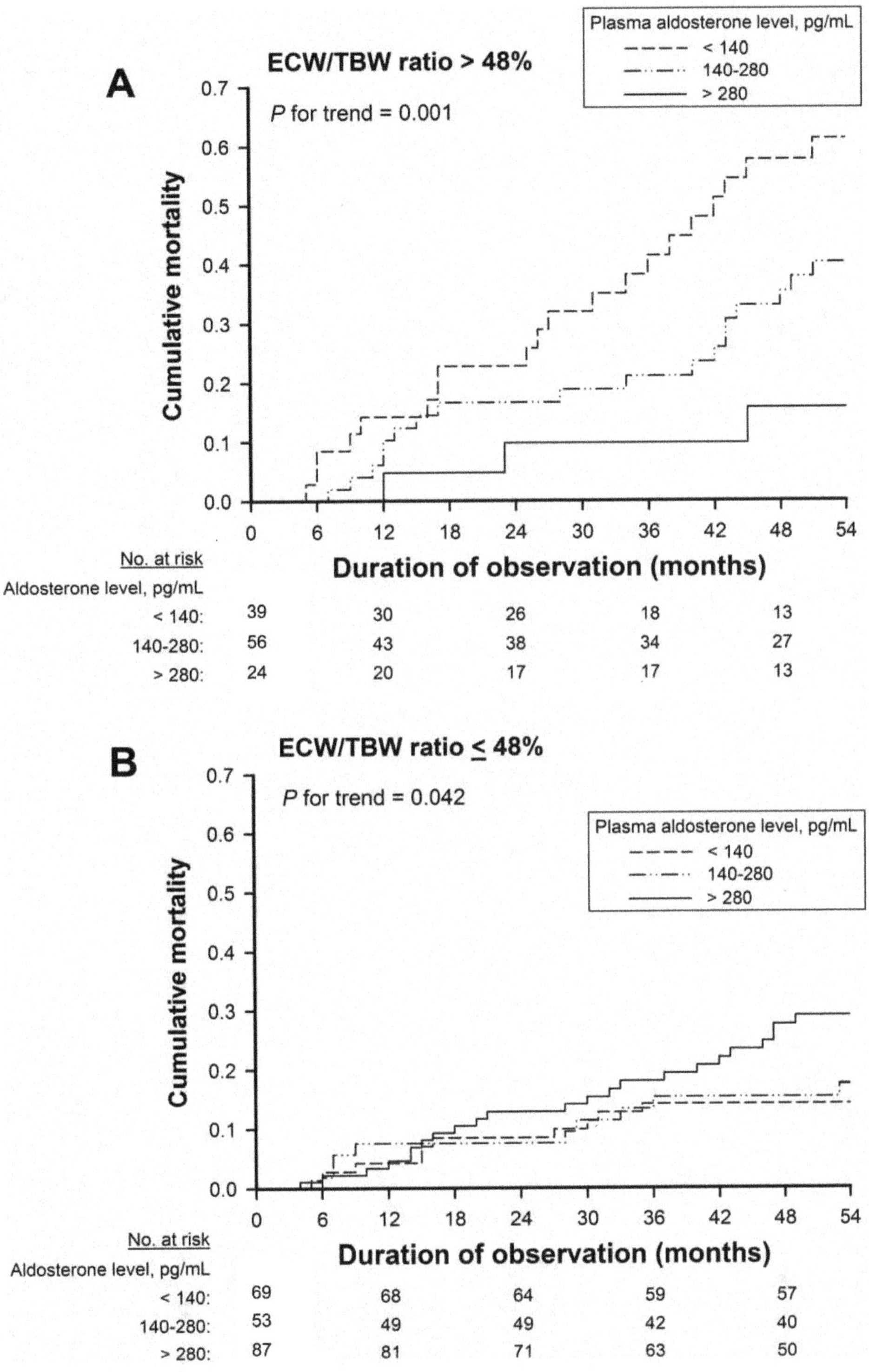

Figure 3. Kaplan-Meier mortality curves according to aldosterone tertile, modified by volume status. All-cause mortality in relation to plasma aldosterone levels at baseline modified by the ratio of extracellular water to total body water (ECW/TBW) >48% (A) and ≤48% (B) among hemodialysis patients.

inappropriately high aldosterone levels [19]. ESRD patients are particularly vulnerable to sudden cardiac death resulting from left ventricular hypertrophy (LVH) and fibrosis [20]. Cumulative evidence has indicated that aldosterone, beyond its classical actions on epithelial cells with BP-dependent organ damage, exerts non-classical effects on interstitial tissues, which are involved in cardiac and renal fibrosis [21–24]. These non-epithelial effects of aldosterone are exaggerated in conditions of elevated aldosterone levels and expanded ECW, such as ESRD [25].

In a large cohort of non-CKD patients scheduled for coronary angiography, variations in aldosterone concentrations within the normal range were associated with increased all-cause and CV

Table 4. Hazard ratios for mortality and first cardiovascular event by categorical or continuous measure of plasma aldosterone modified by ECW/TBW.

	Overall (n = 328)	ECW/TBW >48% (n = 119)	ECW/TBW ≤48% (n = 209)	P-value[a]
All-cause Mortality, Adjusted HR (95% Confidence Interval)				
Categorical measure				
Aldosterone <140 pg/mL	1.00	1.00	1.00	0.01
Aldosterone 140–280 pg/mL	0.87 (0.58−1.31)	0.82 (0.43−1.45)	1.15 (0.91−2.23)	
Aldosterone >280 pg/mL	0.65 (0.48-0.91)	0.49 (0.25−0.76)	1.97 (1.69−3.75)	
Age, per 1 year	1.05 (1.03−1.07)	1.03 (1.00−1.08)	1.07 (1.02−1.12)	
Prior CVD	2.54 (1.54−4.17)	5.29 (2.44−11.49)	2.35 (1.87−6.36)	
Albumin, per 1 g/L	0.92 (0.85−0.98)	0.87 (0.75−0.91)	0.91 (0.79−0.92)	
IL-6, per 1 pg/mL	1.07 (1.01−1.14)	1.11 (1.01−1.23)	1.08 (1.04−1.12)	
Continuous measure				
Aldosterone, per 100 pg/mL	0.75 (0.60−0.91)	0.84 (0.67−0.96)	1.61 (1.20−2.73)	0.03
Age, per 1 year	1.05 (1.03−1.08)	1.03 (0.99−1.07)	1.07 (1.02−1.12)	
Prior CVD	2.58 (1.40−4.76)	5.52 (2.53−12.07)	2.14 (1.80−5.67)	
Albumin, per 1 g/L	0.92 (0.85−0.99)	0.85 (0.77−0.94)	0.93 (0.89−0.97)	
IL-6, per 1 pg/mL	1.05 (1.02−1.13)	1.11 (1.02−1.27)	1.07 (1.03−1.11)	
First CV Event, Adjusted HR (95% Confidence Interval)				
Categorical measure				
Aldosterone <140 pg/mL	1.00	1.00	1.00	0.02
Aldosterone140–280 pg/mL	0.89 (0.65−1.41)	0.81 (0.51−1.89)	1.21 (0.92−2.43)	
Aldosterone >280 pg/mL	0.79 (0.41−0.81)	0.70 (0.33−0.78)	2.01 (1.28−4.15)	
Age, per 1 year	1.03 (1.02−1.06)	1.02 (0.97−1.08)	1.04 (0.99−1.10)	
Prior CVD	5.08 (2.57−10.09)	6.45 (2.52−16.52)	3.41 (1.24−9.39)	
Albumin, per 1 g/L	0.89 (0.80−0.99)	0.80 (0.65−0.98)	0.82 (0.68−0.98)	
IL-6, per 1 pg/mL	1.14 (1.04−1.25)	1.14 (1.02−1.29)	1.21 (1.01−1.45)	
Continuous measure				
Aldosterone, per 100 pg/mL	0.80 (0.69−0.95)	0.69 (0.57−0.90)	1.67 (1.12−2.89)	0.03
Age, per 1 year	1.04 (1.01−1.08)	1.03 (0.97−1.09)	1.05 (0.99−1.12)	
Prior CVD	5.10 (2.26−11.56)	6.45 (2.52−16.52)	3.42 (1.24−9.39)	
Albumin, per 1 g/L	0.89 (0.79−0.96)	0.81 (0.65−0.99)	0.82 (0.68−0.98)	
IL-6, per 1 pg/mL	1.13 (1.02−1.25)	1.15 (1.02−1.29)	1.21 (1.01−1.45)	

Abbreviations: CI denotes confidence interval; CV, cardiovascular; CVD, cardiovascular disease; ECW/TBW, ratio of extracellular water to total body water; HR, hazard ratio; IL-6, inerleukin-6.

[a]The interaction P values assessed the modifying effect of volume overload (ECW/TBW >48%) on the risk relationship between plasma aldosterone and overall mortality and CV events.

mortality independent of major established CV risk factors [6]. In the same cohort, the association of higher plasma aldosterone concentrations with overall CV mortality and sudden cardiac death was stronger for patients with decreased kidney function [7]. Furthermore, a recent study by Edwards et al. also showed that the use of spironolactone reduced left ventricular (LV) mass and improved arterial stiffness in early-stage CKD [26]. Unfortunately, the largest trials to date that used mineralocorticoid receptor antagonists and demonstrated a mortality benefit in patients with severe heart failure due to systolic LV dysfunction or acute myocardial infarction [27,28], excluded patients with moderate to advanced CKD. Once CKD patients have progressed to ESRD, aldosterone levels may remain elevated [29–31]. The markedly elevated levels of aldosterone levels seen in ESRD suggest that mineralocorticoid receptor blockade could emerge as a crucial strategy against CVD in this population [32]. Randomized controlled trials are required to confirm our preliminary findings and define the risk of potential hazards, particularly those involving hyperkalemia [33].

The present study has a number of limitations. First, the modifying effect of volume overload on the risk relationship between aldosterone and mortality may still be subject to residual confounding. Furthermore, as with any cohort study, this study cannot establish causality between volume overload or aldosterone levels and mortality, and we caution against translating the results of observational studies into therapeutic practice. Finally, the impact of volume overload on the association between aldosterone and mortality might be different at different stages of CKD. It is unclear whether findings from our study of patients on dialysis can be extrapolated to patients who have moderate to advanced CKD and are not yet on dialysis.

Our study has biological plausibility and important therapeutic implications. In CKD patients, a progressive decline in glomerular filtration rate, activation of the renin-angiotensin-aldosterone system (RAAS), and superimposed CV comorbidities contribute to salt and water retention. Volume overload and inappropriately high aldosterone levels in CKD patients resulted in more severe LVH and increased arterial stiffness [34,35], both of which are independent predictors of CV mortality in dialysis patients [36,37]. Achieving strict volume control appears to be an imperative therapeutic strategy for inducing regression of LVH and arterial compliance, and lowering the CVD risk in dialysis patients. However, our study provides strong evidence that favorable effects of volume correction might be negated by the simultaneous stimulation of RAAS and thus may become apparent only if this response is inhibited [38,39].

In summary, aldosterone level is inversely associated with adverse outcomes in hemodialysis patients. Volume overload underlies this paradox. In the absence of volume overload, aldosterone is an independent risk factor for all-cause mortality and CV events in this population. These data provide evidence for the confounding and effect modification of the association of aldosterone with adverse outcomes by volume overload. Hence, further research is warranted to clarify the pathophysiological mechanisms that link volume overload and hyperaldosteronemia to increased mortality and CV events and whether therapeutic interventions to mitigate volume overload and lower aldosterone concentrations may lead to improved outcomes in dialysis patients.

Acknowledgments

We are deeply indebted to Miss P.C. Lee for her expert secretarial assistance and graphic design.

Author Contributions

Conceived and designed the experiments: DCT. Performed the experiments: HLH HFP. Analyzed the data: SCH YPL. Wrote the paper: SCH.

References

1. Foley RN, Parfrey PS, Sarnak MJ (1998) Clinical epidemiology of cardiovascular disease in chronic kidney disease. Am J Kidney Dis 32: 112–119.
2. Rossignol P, Ménard J, Fay R, Gustafsson F, Pitt B, et al. (2011) Eplerenone survival benefits in heart failure patients post-myocardial infarction are independent from its diuretic and potassium-sparing effects: Insights from an EPHESUS (Eplerenone Post-Acute Myocardial Infarction Heart Failure Efficacy and Survival Study) Substudy. J Am Coll Cardiol 58: 1958–1966.
3. Hene R, Boer P, Koomans H, Mees E (1982) Plasma aldosterone concentrations in chronic renal disease. Kidney Int 21: 98–101.
4. Diskin CJ, Stokes TJ, Dansby LM, Carter TB, Radcliff L (2004) The clinical significance of aldosterone in ESRD: Part II. Nephrol Dial Transplant 19: 1331–1332.
5. Kohagura K, Higashiuesato Y, Ishiki T, Yoshi S, Ohya Y, et al. (2006) Plasma aldosterone in hypertensive patients on chronic hemodialysis: distribution, determinants and impact on survival. Hypertens Res 29: 597–604.
6. Tomaschitz A, Pilz S, Ritz E, Meinitzer A, Boehm BO, et al. (2010) Plasma aldosterone levels are associated with increased cardiovascular mortality: the Ludwigshafen Risk and Cardiovascular Health (LURIC) Study. Eur Heart J 31: 1237–1247.
7. Tomaschitz A, Pilz S, Ritz E, Grammer T, Drechsler C, et al. (2011) Association of plasma aldosterone with cardiovascular mortality in patients with low estimated GFR: the Ludwigshafen Risk and Cardiovascular Health (LURIC) Study. Am J Kidney Dis 57: 403–414.
8. Lowrie EG, Lew NL (1990) Death risk in hemodialysis patients: the predictive value of commonly measured variables and an evaluation of death rate differences between facilities. Am J Kidney Dis 15: 458–482.
9. Liu Y, Coresh J, Eustace JA, Longenecker JC, Jaar B, et al. (2004) Association between cholesterol level and mortality in dialysis patients: Role of inflammation and malnutrition. JAMA 291: 451–459.
10. Contreras G, Hu B, Astor BC, Greene T, Erlinger T, et al. (2010) Malnutrition-Inflammation modifies the relationship of cholesterol with cardiovascular disease. J Am Soc Nephrol 21: 2131–2142.
11. Kalantar-Zadeh K, Regidor DL, Kovesdy CP, Van Wyck D, Bunnapradist S, et al. (2009) Fluid retention is associated with cardiovascular mortality in patients undergoing long-term hemodialysis. Circulation 119: 671–679.
12. Agarwal R (2010) Hypervolemia is associated with increased mortality among hemodialysis patients. Hypertension 56: 512–517.
13. Klemmer PJ, Bomback AS (2009) Extracellular volume and aldosterone interaction in chronic kidney disease. Blood Purif 27: 92–98.
14. Daugirdas JT (1993) Second generation logarithmic estimates of single-pool variable volume Kt/V: an analysis of errors. J Am Soc Nephrol 4: 1205–1213.
15. Parmar MKB, Machin D (1995) Survival Analysis. A Practical Approach. New York, John Wiley & Sons.
16. Guder G, Bauersachs J, Frantz S, Weismann D, Allolio B, et al. (2007) Complementary and incremental mortality risk prediction by cortisol and aldosterone in chronic heart failure. Circulation 115: 1754–1761.
17. Beygui F, Collet JP, Benoliel JJ, Vignolles N, Dumaine R, et al. (2006) High plasma aldosterone levels on admission are associated with death in patients presenting with acute ST-elevation myocardial infarction. Circulation 114: 2604–2610.
18. Ibrahim HN, Hostetter TH (1998) The renin-aldosterone axis in two models of reduced renal mass in the rat. J Am Soc Nephrol 9: 72–76.
19. Bomback AS, Kshirsagar AV, Ferris ME, Klemmer PJ (2009) Disordered aldosterone-volume relationship in end-stage kidney disease. J Renin Angiotensin Aldosterone Syst 10: 230–236.
20. Green D, Roberts PR, New DI, Kalra PA (2011) Sudden cardiac death in hemodialysis patients: an in-depth review. Am J Kidney Dis 57: 921–929.
21. Hostetter TH, Ibrahim HN (2003) Aldosterone in chronic kidney and cardiac disease. J Am Soc Nephrol 14: 2395–2401.
22. Weber KT, Brilla CG (1991) Pathological hypertrophy and cardiac interstitium. Fibrosis and renin-angiotensin-aldosterone system. Circulation 83: 1849–1865.
23. Young M, Funder JW (2004) Eplerenone, but not steroid withdrawal, reverses cardiac fibrosis in deoxycorticosterone/salt-treated rats. Endocrinology 145: 3153–3157.
24. Juknevicius I, Segal Y, Kren S, Lee R, Hostetter TH (2004) Effect of aldosterone on renal transforming growth factor-beta. Am J Physiol Renal Physiol 286: F1059–F1062.
25. Sato A, Saruta T (2004) Aldosterone-induced organ damage: plasma aldosterone level and inappropriate salt status. Hypertens Res 27: 303–310.
26. Edwards NC, Steeds RP, Stewart PM, Ferro CJ, Townend JN (2009) Effect of spironolactone on left ventricular mass and aortic stiffness in early-stage chronic kidney disease: a randomized controlled trial. J Am Coll Cardiol 54: 505–512.
27. Pitt B, Zannad F, Remme WJ, Cody R, Castaigne A, et al. (1999) The effect of spironolactone on morbidity and mortality in patients with severe heart failure. Randomized Aldactone Evaluation Study Investigators. N Engl J Med 341: 709–717.
28. Pitt B, Remme W, Zannad F, Neaton J, Martinez F, et al. (2003) Eplerenone, a selective aldosterone blocker, in patients with left ventricular dysfunction after myocardial infarction. N Engl J Med 348: 1309–1321.
29. Berl T, Katz FH, Henrich WL, de Torrente A, Schrier RW (1978) Role of aldosterone in the control of sodium excretion in patients with advanced chronic renal failure. Kidney Int 14: 228–235.
30. Ratge D, Augustin R, Wisser H (1983) Catecholamines, renin, aldosterone and arterial pressure in patients on chronic hemodialysis treatment. Int J Artif Organs 6: 255–260.
31. McLaughlin N, Gehr TW, Sica DA (2004) Aldosterone-receptor antagonism and end-stage renal disease. Curr Hypertens Rep 6: 327–330.
32. Covic A, Gusbeth-Tatomir P, Goldsmith DJ (2006) Is it time for spironolactone therapy in dialysis patients? Nephrol Dial Transplant 21: 854–858.
33. Ritz E, Koleganova N (2010) Aldosterone in uremia–beyond blood pressure. Blood Purif 29: 111–113.
34. Barenbrock M, Spieker C, Laske V, Heidenreich S, Hohage H, et al. (1994) Studies of the vessel wall properties in hemodialysis patients. Kidney Int 45: 1397–1400.
35. London GM, Pannier B, Vicaut E, Guerin A, Marchais SJ, et al. (1996) Antihypertensive effects and arterial haemodynamic alterations during angiotensin converting enzyme inhibition. J Hypertens 14: 1139–1146.
36. London GM, Pannier B, Guerin AP, Blacher J, Marchais SJ, et al. (2001) Alterations of left ventricular hypertrophy in and survival of patients receiving hemodialysis: follow-up of an interventional study. J Am Soc Nephrol 12: 2759–2767.
37. Blacher J, Guerin AP, Pannier B, Marchais SJ, Safar ME, et al. (1999) Impact of aortic stiffness on survival in end-stage renal disease. Circulation 99: 2434–2439.
38. Tycho Vuurmans JL, Boer WH, Bos WJ, Blankestijn PJ, Koomans HA (2002) Contribution of volume overload and angiotensin II to the increased pulse wave velocity of hemodialysis patients. J Am Soc Nephrol 13: 177–183.
39. Cice G, Di Benedetto A, D'Isa S, D'Andrea A, Marcelli D, et al. (2010) Effects of telmisartan added to angiotensin-converting enzyme inhibitors on mortality and morbidity in hemodialysis patients with chronic heart failure: A double-blind, placebo-controlled trial. J Am Coll Cardiol 56: 1701–1708.

27

Evidence that p-Cresol and IL-6 are Adsorbed by the HFR Cartridge: Towards a new Strategy to Decrease Systemic Inflammation in Dialyzed Patients?

Eleonora Riccio[1], Mauro Cataldi[2], Maristella Minco[1], Gennaro Argentino[1], Roberta Russo[1], Stefania Brancaccio[1], Andrea Memoli[1], Lucia Grumetto[3], Loredana Postiglione[4], Bruna Guida[5], Bruno Memoli[1]*

1 Department of Public Health, Section of Nephrology, Federico II University of Naples, Naples, Italy, **2** Department of Neuroscience, Reproductive and Odontostomatologic Sciences, Section of Pharmacology, Federico II University of Naples, Naples, Italy, **3** Department of Pharmaceutical and Toxicological Chemistry, Federico II University of Naples, Naples, Italy, **4** Department of Cellular and Molecular Biology and Pathology, Federico II University of Naples, Naples, Italy, **5** Department of Clinical Medicine and Surgery, Federico II University of Naples, Naples, Italy

Abstract

Introduction: Hemodialysis (HD) and hemodiafiltration clear only with a low efficiency the plasma from interleukin-6 and p-cresol, two protein-bound uremic toxins associated with high cardiovascular risk in end stage renal disease. HFR Supra is a double-chamber hemodiafiltration system in which the ultrafiltrate returns to the patient after its regeneration through a resin cartridge that binds hydrophobic and protein-bound solutes. In the present study, we evaluated whether the HFR cartridge can also bind total p-cresol and IL-6 and remove them from the ultrafiltrate.

Methods: We compared the levels of IL-6 and p-cresol in ultrafiltrate samples collected at the inlet (UF_{in}) and at the outlet (UF_{out}) of the cartridge at the start or at the end of a 240 min HFR session in 12 inflamed chronic HD patients. The pro-inflammatory activity of the ultrafiltrate samples was also determined by evaluating the changes that they induced in IL-6 mRNA expression and protein release in peripheral blood mononuclear cells from 12 healthy volunteers. IL-6 and p-cresol circulating levels were also assessed in peripheral plasma blood samples collected before and after HFR and, for comparison, a control HD.

Results: p-Cresol and IL-6 were lower in UF_{out} than in UF_{in} both at the start and at the end of the HFR session, suggesting that they were retained by the cartridge. IL-6 mRNA expression and release were lower in PBMC incubated with UF_{out} collected at the end than with UF_{in} collected at the start of HFR, suggesting that passage through the cartridge reduced UF pro-inflammatory activity. Plasma total p-cresol decreased by about 53% after HFR, and 37% after HD. IL-6 circulating values were unmodified by either these dialysis procedures.

Conclusions: This study shows that the HFR-Supra cartridge retains total p-cresol and IL-6 in the ultrafiltrate and lowers plasma total p cresol but not IL-6 levels.

Editor: Emmanuel A. Burdmann, University of Sao Paulo Medical School, Brazil

Funding: The authors have no support or funding to report.

Competing Interests: The authors have declared that no competing interests exist.

* E-mail: memoli@unina.it

Introduction

Cardiovascular disease (CVD) is the primary cause of morbidity and mortality in End Stage Renal Disease (ESRD): approximately 50% of ESRD patients die because of CVD, and cardiovascular mortality is 15–30 times higher in ESRD than in age-adjusted general population [1,2]. This excess in morbidity and mortality cannot be explained only by the high prevalence of the traditional Framingham risk factors in these patients [3,4]. It seems, instead, to be also dependent on Chronic Kidney Disease (CKD)-specific, non-classical factors, such as inflammation [5], vascular calcification [6], anemia and left ventricular hypertrophy [7]. A wealth of data points to the retention of organic waste solutes as one of the mechanisms leading to the development of these non-traditional risk factors in CKD. In particular, a major role has been recently attributed to p-cresol and to its metabolites. This aromatic compound is generated in the gut through the bacterial degradation of tyrosine and phenylalanine [8,9]. Once absorbed from the intestinal mucosa, p-cresol is almost completely converted in two main metabolites, p-cresylsulfate and p-cresylglucuronide that are efficiently removed by the kidney [10]. Observational studies showed that the metabolites of p-cresol accumulate in the plasma of patients affected with CKD. It was also shown that high plasma concentrations of total p-cresol and, specifically, of its p-cresylsulfate metabolite, are independently associated with CVD and mortality, even after adjustment for known risk factors [10–12]. Available data suggest that p-cresylsulfate may cause a diffuse endothelial damage [13–15] and increase the percentage of leucocytes displaying oxidative burst activity [16]. Therefore a role has been posited for p-cresol and its metabolites as a factor contributing to the systemic inflammation that is commonly observed in dialysis patients [17,18].

In ESRD, there is also a strong association between elevated circulating levels of markers of inflammations such as C-reactive protein (CRP) and interleukin-6 (IL-6) and cardiovascular morbidity and mortality, suggesting that systemic inflammation could have a pathogenic role in CVD in these patients [19–23]. This could in part be due to the ability of circulating cytokines, like IL-6, to exert a direct pro-aterogenic effect or to regulate the release of acute phase reactants [24].

Combined, these data suggest that cardiovascular prognosis in ESRD patients could be improved by decreasing the circulating concentration of p-cresol and its metabolites and/or of IL-6. Unfortunately, both conventional bicarbonate hemodialysis (HD) and hemodiafiltration (HDF) may remove p-cresol only with a low efficiency and they are unable to clear the plasma from IL-6 [25–27]. Indeed, although the molecular weight of p-cresol and its metabolites is very low, ranging around 100 Da, these compounds cannot cross the dialysis membrane because they circulate in plasma mostly bound to albumin being their free percentage less than 1% [28]. Conversely, IL-6, also in its free form (MW 24.5 kDa), is a large, difficult to dialyze solute [29]. Moreover, only about 30% of circulating IL-6 is free and the remaining 70% circulates bound to its two soluble receptors, sIL-6R (MW 55 kDa) and sgp80 (100 kDa), forming very high molecular weight complexes [30].

Alternative dialysis strategies have been developed with the aim of improving the efficiency of protein-bound compounds removal from plasma. They are based either on the adsorption of these compounds on resin cartridges [31,32], or on strategies that could lower the binding of uremic toxins to plasma proteins [33]. One of the most promising among the former is Hemo-Filtrate-Reinfusion (HFR), a new dialysis technique that combines the processes of diffusion, convection and adsorption [34]. In this double chamber hemodiafiltration system, the UF is reinfused into the blood of the patient after its passage through a resin cartridge that binds many medium-high molecular weight solutes including some pro-inflammatory cytokines [35]. No data are available on the ability of this dialysis system to clear the blood of IL-6 and p-cresol or its metabolites. Therefore, we designed the present study to evaluate whether, during a single dialysis session, the HFR sorbent cartridge may efficiently bind and remove from the UF either p-cresol and its metabolites or IL-6 or both of them. To address this question we measured total p-cresol and IL-6 concentrations in the UF produced in the first filter of HFR system, before and after its passage through the sorbent cartridge. We also evaluated whether the pro-inflammatory activity exerted by the UF on peripheral blood mononuclear cells (PBMC), harvested from healthy subjects and cultured *in vitro*, was lowered by the passage through the sorbent cartridge.

Patients and Methods

Patient selection and study protocol

This study was performed in 2011 in the Dialysis Unit of Federico II University of Naples. We obtained approval by our ethic committee "Carlo Romano" of the Federico II University and written informed consent from all subjects, according to the Helsinki declaration as revised in 1996. The protocol for this trial and supporting TREND checklist are available as supporting information; see Checklist S1 and Protocol S1.

Inclusion criteria were: the diagnosis of ESRD, the inclusion in a regular three times weekly hemodialysis program and the evidence of ongoing systemic inflammation, as stated by high-sensitivity CRP (hsCRP) concentrations higher than 3 mg/L. We chose to perform the study in patients with high circulating values of hsCRP because they are expected to also have high IL-6 concentrations both in plasma and in the UF.

Exclusion criteria were: malignancies, systemic autoimmune and/or infectious diseases, severe malnutrition or conditions making necessary to artificially feed the patient.

Twelve patients (6 male/6 female) were recruited for the study. Their mean age was 60.1 ± 11.5 years; mean dialysis vintage was 80 ± 39 months. Plasma high-sensitivity CRP was above the upper normal limit in all patients (mean $\pm$ SD values: 44.01 ± 22.18 mg/l, normal values <3.0 mg/l).

The primary endpoint of the study was to establish whether IL-6 and p-cresol were retained on the HFR cartridge during a single dialysis session. To assess this point, we compared the concentrations of these uremic toxins in UF entering (UF_{in}) and UF exiting (UF_{out}) from the cartridge, collected 15 minutes after the start (start-15 min) and 15 minutes before the end (end-225 min) of the HFR session.

Secondary endpoints were: 1) to assess whether the pro-inflammatory activity of the ultrafiltrate (UF) was lowered after the passage through the HFR cartridge and 2) whether a single HFR session decreased the circulating concentrations of total p-cresol and IL-6 more efficiently than HD. To address the first point, we compared the ability of UF samples collected at the beginning and at the end of the HFR session to induce an inflammatory response in peripheral blood mononuclear cells (PBMCs) drawn from healthy subjects in vitro, as indicated by an increase in IL-6 gene expression and release. To establish whether HFR is more effective than HD in lowering IL-6 and p-cresol serum concentrations, we compared the circulating levels of these uremic toxins in blood samples collected before and after a single session of either HFR or HD performed at different times in the same patients.

HFR treatment

HFR was performed using a commercial HFR Supra Bellco filter system (Mirandola, Italy). This system consists of a convective stage, of a sorbent cartridge and of a diffusive stage (Fig. 1). Therefore, in the HFR apparatus, the processes of convection, diffusion and adsorption are physically separated. During HFR, the blood first goes through the 0.7 m^2 high-flux polyethersulfone (polyphenylene) membrane of the convective stage. This highly biocompatible membrane [36] has a sieving coefficient (i.e. the ratio between solute concentrations in ultrafiltrate and plasma) for albumin of 0.02 and, therefore, it generates an ultrafiltrate (UF) containing small amounts of albumin. The UF generated in the convective stage then goes through a sorbent cartridge containing 40 ml of a hydrophobic styrene resin (Selecta; Bellco, Mirandola, Italy) that, because of its high porosity, has a very large adsorption surface area ($\sim$700 m^2/g). The cartridge adsorbs by hydrophobic interaction a number of waste solutes contained in the UF that is, thus, cleaned. Thereafter, this "regenerated" UF is reinfused into the blood stream being mixed with the blood coming from the convection stage into a chamber located at the bottom of the convection stage before the diffusive section of the filter. The

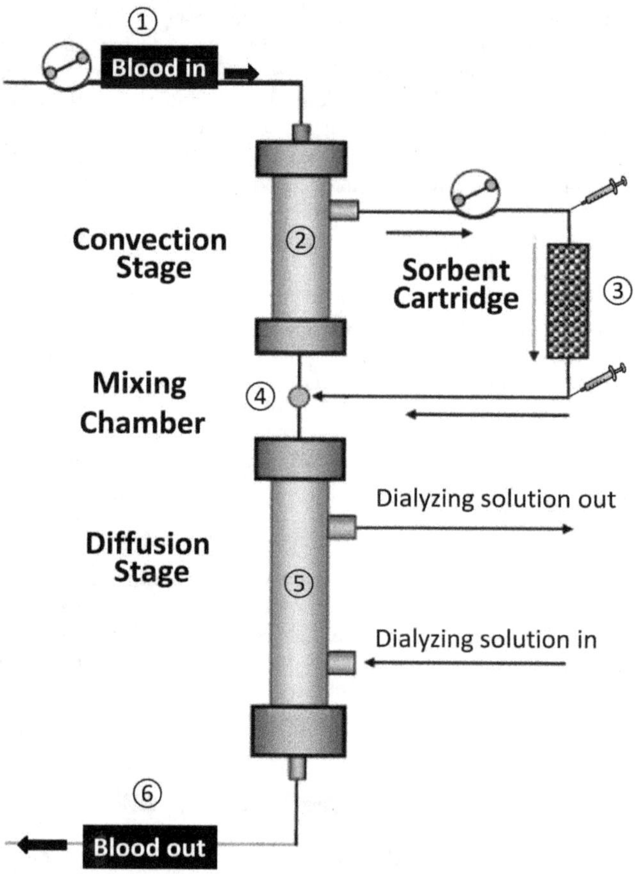

Figure 1. Schematic representation of the HFR apparatus. The figure shows the main components of the HFR Supra system (Bellco, Mirandola, Italy) used in the study. 1-The blood of the patient is pumped into the top filter (the convection stage). 2-In this stage of the HFR apparatus, the blood is filtered by a high flux polyethersulfone membrane. 3-The ultrafiltrate produced in the convection stage is pumped by a second pump through a sorbent cartridge where hydrophobic waste solutes are retained. The small syringes indicate the points of the systems where rubber stopper for UF sample collection are located. 4-The blood coming from the convection stage and the UF coming from the cartridge are mixed in a chamber located between the two filters 5-This "reconstituted" blood enters the bottom filter (the diffusion stage) where it is undergoes dialytic treatment (both diffusion and ultrafiltration for weight loss) with a low flux polyethersulfone membrane. 6-The cleared blood is returned to the patient. (Modified form an original image kindly provided by Dr. G. Palladino, Bellco, Mirandola, Italy).

second filter, the diffusive stage of the HFR apparatus, contains a 1.7 m^2 low-flux polyethersulfone (polyphenylene) membrane (Figure 1). It mostly operates by diffusion and is also responsible for the removal of excess water and patient's weight loss.

The HFR dialysis system was controlled by a Formula Plus monitor (Bellco, Mirandola, Italy) equipped with a software that automatically determines the best ultrafiltration flow rate (Q_{uf}) [37–39]. Mean blood and dialysate flows were 330±20 ml/min and 545±85 ml/min, respectively. The Q_{uf} from the convective section and the ultrafiltrate-reinfusion rate were kept at 50–60 ml/min. Mean dialytic time was 240±15 min. Weight loss, that was obtained only in the diffusive section of the system, was 800±100 g/h.

The sterility of the tap water, of the water obtained after reverse osmosis and of the dialysate was periodically checked by colony forming unit (CFU) testing and by performing the limulus amebocyte test (LAL) test (gel clot test) for endotoxin (PBI, Milan, Italy). These tests gave negative results during the entire duration of the study.

Control hemodialysis

Because both the convective and the diffusive stages of the HFR apparatus can remove waste solutes, they could both contribute to HFR effect on plasma p-cresol or IL-6. Therefore, in order to dissect their respective roles, we also measured the changes of total p-cresol and IL-6 plasma levels after a pure diffusive hemodialysis session performed using only the second stage of the HFR system. This represented an internal control for the HFR experiment and gave an estimate of the HFR cartridge-independent effects. Hemodialysis (HD) was performed with the same monitor (Bellco Formula) and the same low flux (1.7 m^2) polyethersulfone membrane (Diapes, Bellco, Italy) and the same conditions (dialysate and dialysis parameters including dialysate and blood flow rates, weight loss and dialysis efficiency, as KT/V) of HFR.

Ultrafiltrate and blood samples

Four 60 ml UF samples were collected through specific rubber stoppers located at the inlet and at the outlet of the sorbent cartridge, using sterile disposable syringes (Fig. 1). Two of these samples were collected 15 minutes after the beginning of the HFR session (15 min-start), the first (UF_{in}-15) before and the second (UF_{out}-15) after the passage through the adsorbent cartridge. The other two samples were collected 225 min after the beginning of the treatment (i.e. 15 minutes before its end, 225 min-end), also in this case one before and the other after the passage through the cartridge, (UF_{in}-225 and UF_{out}-225, respectively). Immediately after collection, the UF samples were transferred in sterile disposable polypropylene tubes (BD-Falcon, Milan, Italy), stored in ice and transferred into −80° refrigerator where they were kept until assayed for p-cresol and IL-6 determinations or used for the experiments in vitro with human PBMC, as described below.

In all patients, 10 ml blood samples were collected from A-V fistula 15 minutes before the beginning and 15 min after the end of both the HFR and of the HD session. Sera were separated immediately after centrifugation and stored at −20° until assayed.

Albumin concentrations both in serum and UF samples were measured by nephelometry. p-Cresol and IL-6 serum concentrations were measured using the techniques detailed in the next paragraph, whereas high-sensitivity C-reactive protein (hsCRP) was evaluated by a modified high-sensitivity laser nephelometry technique (Berhing Diagnostics, GmbH, Marburg, Germany).

p-cresol assay

Total p-cresol (i.e. the sum of its free and protein-bound fractions) was measured in serum and UF samples with HPLC, as previously described [40,41]. Briefly, after heat-acid denaturation of the binding proteins, p-cresol was extracted in ethyl acetate and injected on the HPLC column. The UF samples (50 ml) were vacuum dried and the obtained pellets were resuspended in 3 ml saline solution before being denaturated and extracted. The preliminary acidification of the samples was performed to release bound p-cresol conjugates from plasma proteins, to make total (bound + free) p-cresol-conjugates available for further HPLC analysis. Plasma acidification also caused the hydrolysis of both p-cresylsulphate and p-cresylglucuronide that were converted in p-cresol. Therefore, this method mainly measured p-cresylsulfate that represents the most prevalent form of p-cresol in plasma [10]. The limits of quantification (LOQ) and of detection (LOD) were

0.150 ng/mL and 0.017 ng/ml, respectively. Calibration procedures were repeated every two weeks (coefficient of variation <0.5%).

Correction for hemoconcentration

The values of the concentrations of the two protein bound solutes total p-cresol and IL-6 were corrected, in the samples drawn at the end of the treatment, for the hemoconcentration that occurs during dialysis by using the method proposed by Lesaffer et al. with modifications [42]. Briefly, the concentrations measured in blood samples collected at the end of the dialysis session were multiplied by a correction factor (CF) consisting in the ratio between total serum albumin concentration at the beginning (Alb_{t0}) and at the end of dialysis (Alb_{t240}): $CF = Alb_{t0}/Alb_{t240}$.

IL-6 gene expression and release

To assess the pro-inflammatory activity of the different UF samples, collected as described in the previous section, we evaluated their ability to induce IL-6 gene expression and IL-6 release in cultured PBMCs.

PBMC were isolated from 12 healthy subjects with normal hsCRP concentrations (1.15±0.8 mg/l) by Ficoll-Hypaque (Flow Laboratories, Irvine, UK) gradient density centrifugation (400×g for 30 min). Cell viability, assessed by trypan blue dye exclusion, was higher than 95%. PBMCs were resuspended in RPMI culture medium (Sigma, Milano, Italy) supplemented with 1% heat-inactivated FCS (Sigma) and antibiotics (penicillin and streptomycin) at a density of 1×10^6/ml, subdivided in three different aliquots in plastic culture tubes (BD-Falcon, Milan, Italy) and cultured for 24 h at 37°C in a 5% CO_2 saturated humidity incubator after the addition of 20% v/v NaCl (0.9%) to the first aliquot, 20% v/v UF_{in-15} to the second aliquot and 20% v/v $UF_{out-225}$ to the third. At the end of the 24 incubation period, cell-free supernatants were collected by centrifugation and stored at −80°C until assayed for IL-6 levels whereas the cell pellets were lysed with Trizol reagent (Life Technologies, Grand Island, NY) for total RNA extraction, as described elsewhere [30]). The concentration and the purity of RNA were evaluated by measuring the absorbance at 260 nm and by calculating the ratio of absorbance at 260–280 nm using a UV spectrophotometer (DU-800 spectrophotometer; Beckman Instruments). Five micrograms of total RNA were retro-transcribed and Real-Time quantitative PCR analysis was performed with an ABI prism 7500 (Applied Biosystems, Foster City, CA) apparatus and the TaqMan system using primers specific for IL-6 mRNA and β-actin (sequence reported in Table 1). IL-6 mRNA levels were normalized to those of β-actin and converted into fold changes based on the doubling of PCR product in each PCR cycle according to the manufacturer's guidelines, as previously described [43].

Statistical analysis

Data are expressed as mean ± standard deviation. They were analyzed using SPSS 12.0 (SPSS Inc, Chicago, IL) setting the threshold for statistical significance at p values <0.05. The Shapiro-Wilk test was performed to assess whether the different sets of data were normally distributed or not. To evaluate percent decrease of IL-6 and total p-cresol plasma concentrations we calculated their *reduction ratios* according to the formula $RR = (C_{before}-C_{after})/C_{before}$, where C_{before} and C_{after} indicate the sera concentrations in blood samples collected 15 min before and 15 after either the HFR or the HD session. Statistical comparisons of two group variables were performed using Student's t-test for normally distributed data and Mann-Whitney test for not-normally distributed data. Multiple group comparisons were performed with one way repeated measure ANOVA followed by the Student-Newman-Keuls post hoc test.

Results

IL-6, p-cresol and albumin concentrations in UF samples

We found measurable concentrations of both total p-cresol and IL-6 in UF_{in}-15 that is produced by the ultrafiltration of plasma through the polyethersulfone membrane of the first stage convection filter. In UF_{in}-15, the concentration of p-cresol was about 30 times lower (0.39±0.2 vs 11.6±6.3 mg/l) and that of IL-6 was 5.6 times lower than in plasma (10.30±10.2 vs 57.6±58.3 pg/ml) (Tables 2 & 3). To assess whether a significant amount of albumin crossed the polyethersulfone membrane of the convection filter, we measured this protein in the UF_{in}-15. The concentration that we found ranged around $1/40^{th}$ of plasma values (0.1±0.03 vs 3.6±0.2 g/dl) in agreement with the value of 0.02 of albumin sieving reported by the manufacturer of these dialysis membranes. Intriguingly, these albumin concentration values are consistent with the hypothesis that most of the filtered p-cresol actually crosses the dialysis membrane as protein-bound forms. Conversely, the percent values of IL-6 concentration was close to that of free IL-6 in plasma suggesting that only free IL-6 could cross the dialysis membrane.

To establish whether p-cresol and IL-6 in the UF_{in} could be adsorbed by the sorbent cartridge of the HFR system we compared the concentrations of these uremic toxins in UF_{in} and UF_{out}. As reported in Table 2, in samples collected 15 min after the beginning of the HFR session both total p-cresol and IL-6 concentrations were significantly lower in UF_{out} than in UF_{in}. Also albumin concentration was lower in UF_{out} than in UF_{in} (Table 2). These findings suggested that the sorbent cartridge could retain p-cresol, IL-6 and a small amount of albumin. To assess whether the ability of the cartridge to adsorb these substances was maintained till the end of the HFR session, we also measured their concentrations in UF_{in}-225 and UF_{out}-225. Total cresol concentration in UF_{in}-225 was lower than in UF_{in}-15, and it was further lowered by the passage through the cartridge, suggesting that the binding capacity of the cartridge was not saturated. In keeping with this hypothesis, albumin concentration in UF_{in}-225 was also significantly lowered upon passage through the cartridge. Also IL-6 concentration was significantly higher in UF_{in}-225 than in UF_{out}-225. However, the concentration of this cytokine in UF_{in}-225 was not different from that in UF_{in}-15 (Table 2).

Table 1. Sequence of the IL-6 and β-actin primers used in the study.

	Forward	Reverse	Reference
IL-6	ATG AAC TCC TTC TCC ACA AGC GC	GAA GAG CCC TCA GGC TGG ACT G	30
β-actin	CACCATGGATGATGATATCG	TGGATAGCAACGTACATGG	51

Table 2. Albumin, total-cresol and IL-6 concentrations in ultrafiltrate samples collected before and after the HFR sorbent cartridge at the beginning and at the end of the dialysis session.

	15 min Pre-cartridge	15 min Post-cartridge	225 min Pre-cartridge	225 min Post-cartridge
Albumin (g/dl)	0.1±0.03	0.08±0.02*	0.09±0.01	0.07±0.01†
Total-Cresol (mg/l)	0.39±0.2	0.14±0.09*	0.25±0.09*	0.04±0.03*
IL-6 (pg/ml)	10.30±10.2	0*	11.68±11.15	0.91±1.01*

The data shown in the Table are the mean ± standard deviation of albumin, total cresol and IL-6 measured in samples of the UF collected before and after being adsorbed by the sorbent cartridge of the convection stage of the HFR Supra apparatus. Note the very low concentrations of albumin in pre-sorbent UF samples that is consistent with the low sieving coefficient (about 0.02 for albumin) of the polyphenylene membrane of the system. The values of total cresol concentration shown are the sum of p-cresol and p-cresol metabolite concentrations because, as we detail in the methods section, the acidic extraction method that we used converts all p-cresol derivatives in p-cresol.
*$p<0.05$ vs 15 min pre-cartridge and †$p<0.05$ vs 225 min pre-cartridge, at repeated measure ANOVA followed by the Student-Newman-Keuls post-hoc test.

Effect of the passage through the sorbent cartridge on IL-6 mRNA expression and protein release induced by the ultrafiltrate in PBMC from healthy subjects

To establish whether the passage through the HFR cartridge could also decrease UF pro-inflammatory activity, we compared IL-6 gene expression in PBMC from healthy subjects cultured in the absence (Control) or in the presence of the UF collected either at the beginning (UF_{in}-15) or at the end of the HFR session (UF_{out}-225). In addition, we compared IL-6 concentrations in the culture media obtained by the same PMBC cultures. As expected, in the presence of UF_{in}-15 normal PBMCs became activated and we observed a significant increase respect to control cultures both in IL-6 mRNA expression (15.76±10.9 fold the basal expression, $p<0.02$) and IL-6 concentrations in the culture medium (1850.92±938.43 vs 462.96±307.28 pg/ml, $p<0.01$) (Fig. 2). In PBMCs exposed to UF_{out}-225 IL-6 mRNA levels were significantly higher than in control cultures but significantly lower than in cultures treated with UF_{in}-15 (4.10±3.99 fold the basal expression, $p<0.05$). Similarly, IL-6 release was higher than in controls but lower than in PBMCs incubated withUF_{in}-15 (462.96±307.28 vs 908.5±623.59 pg/ml $p<0.05$) (Fig. 2).

Effect of HFR and HD on plasma of IL-6 and total p-cresol

To assess whether the HFR session could also modify the circulating levels of either total p-cresol or IL-6, we compared the plasma concentrations of these uremic toxins in blood samples collected from the AV fistula 15 min before the beginning and 15 min after the end of the HFR. Because a significant hemoconcentration occurred during the dialysis, as expected [39] and as indicated by the higher albumin concentration at the end of HFR than at its beginning (Table 3), total p-cresol and IL-6 concentrations were corrected for this factor (see the methods section for details). Total p-cresol plasma concentration was significantly lower after HFR than before, whereas IL-6 level did not change (Table 2). To evaluate whether HFR was more effective than HD in lowering total p-cresol plasma concentrations, we also measured the concentrations of this toxin in blood samples collected in the same patients before and after a standard HD session. Total p-cresol reduction ratio was significantly higher after HFR than after HD (53.6±12.5% vs 37.1±20.2%, n = 12; $p<0.05$ at Student's t-test for paired data) (Table 3). Conversely, even after HD, IL-6 concentrations were not significantly modified by the treatment (Table 2).

Discussion

Because uremic protein-bound toxins are suspected to have a role in worsening the cardiovascular prognosis in patients on dialysis, there is a growing interest in developing therapeutic strategies more effective than those currently available in removing these compounds. In the present study we explored whether the HFR Supra dialysis system could have a role in this context. Specifically, we reported evidence that its sorbent cartridge removed both IL-6 and p-cresol and its metabolites from the UF and significantly lowered the UF pro-inflammatory activity in vitro. Parallel to these effects, we observed a significantly stronger decrease in circulating levels of total cresol, but not of IL-6, after HFR than after HD.

Schematically the HFR apparatus may be considered as composed by two different systems both taking part to waste removal. The first one is a convective stage that operates an

Table 3. Serum albumin, and plasma total cresol and Il-6 concentrations before and after either HFR or HD.

	Before HFR	After HFR	Reduction Ratio (%)	Before HD	After HD	Reduction Ratio (%)
Albumin (g/dl)	3.6±0.2	4.2±0.3	-	3.8±0.3	4.2±0.2	-
Total Cresol (mg/l)	11.6±6.3	5.8±2.7*	53.6±12.5	8.6±5.3	5.4±3.0‖	37.1±20.2°
IL-6 (pg/ml)	57.6±58.3	48.4±53.1	4.3±34.5	48.7±33.6	53.9±48.3	-

The Table reports the mean ± standard deviation of the values of serum albumin, plasma total cresol and IL-6 concentrations obtained in the same 12 ESRD patients before and after two different dialysis sessions performed with standard bicarbonate hemodialysis (HD) or with HFR supra, as indicated. The Table also reports the Reduction Ratio of p-cresol and IL-6 obtained with both HFR and HD. As described in the legend to Table 2, total cresol concentration is the sum of the concentration of p-cresol and of its metabolites. The post-dialysis data shown in the table have been corrected for hemoconcentration as reported in the Methods section.
*$p<0.005$ vs preHFR,
‖$p<0.005$ vs preHD at Mann-Whitney test;
°$p<0.05$ vs RR HFR at Student's t test for paired data.

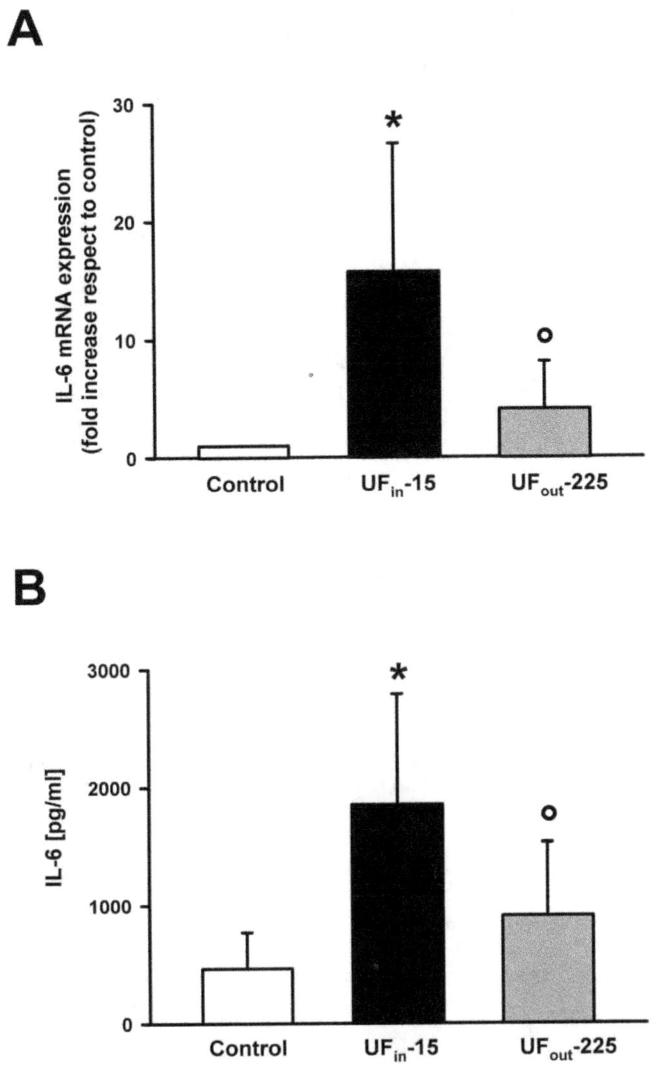

Figure 2. Effect of UF_{in}-15 and UF_{out}-225 on IL-6 gene expression and on IL-6 release in PBMC cultures from healthy subjects. A Mean ± SD of the fold increase in IL-6 gene expression respect to controls observed in PBMC cultures from 12 healthy volunteers, exposed to UF_{in}-15 (black) and UF_{out}-225 (dark gray). Data were normalized to β-actin mRNA expression and expressed as percent increase respect to those obtained in control cultures, set at 1, in which no UF was added. B, Mean ± SD of immunoreactive IL-6 concentrations in culture media of PBMCs from twelve healthy volunteers after a 24 h incubation with saline (basal condition, white), UF_{in}-15 (black), or and UF_{out}-225 (dark gray). *$p<0.05$vs control; °$p<0.05$ vscontrol and UF_{in}-15, at Kruskal-Wallis one way analysis of variance on ranks followed by Student-Newman-Keuls post hoc test.

ultrafiltration process and is coupled with a sorbent cartridge. The second is a diffusive stage essentially similar to conventional HD. As far as the first stage of HFR is concerned, the only mechanism that contributes to the removal of toxins and waste compounds is binding and retention on the HFR cartridge. The UF generated by blood ultrafiltration at this HFR stage is, indeed, entirely reinfused in patient's general circulation after being passed through the sorbent cartridge. Therefore, all the compounds that are not sequestered into the cartridge are actually returned to patient's blood. The results of our study are consistent with the hypothesis that both IL-6 and p-cresol and its derivatives were actually adsorbed by the HFR cartridge in our patients. This is mainly indicated by the evidence that the concentrations in the UF of these uremic toxins were significantly lowered after the passage through the cartridge. The hypothesis that the sorbent cartridge could bind and retain IL-6 and/or p-cresol and its metabolites is consistent with the chemical-physical characteristics of its styrene resin that can establish strong non-covalent interactions with hydrophobic molecules and with albumin [35].

A relevant question arises about the forms in which either p-cresol or IL-6 bind to the resin. Both these molecules circulate, indeed, in the plasma both as protein-bound and as free forms. Specifically, p-Cresol and its derivatives are more than 90% bound to albumin whereas almost 70% of IL-6 circulates as a very high molecular complex with its soluble receptors (sIL-6R and sgp130) [30,44]. The filtering membrane of the convection stage of the HFR Supra apparatus (Fig. 1) has a low but measurable permeability to albumin with an albumin sieving coefficient of 0.02. Therefore, it lets an amount of albumin ranging around $1/40^{th}$ of its plasma concentration cross the membrane and appear into the UF. This implies that uremic toxins, like p-cresol, can be transferred in the UF also in their protein bound forms. In addition, the free forms of p-cresol and of its metabolites are small enough to freely permeate through the convection stage filter. Therefore, both protein-bound and free p-cresol presumably passed through the dialysis membrane into the UF and become available for binding to the cartridge. Conversely, because of the very high molecular weight of its complex with soluble IL-6 receptors, it is likely that IL-6 passed into the UF only as a free molecule. This is consistent with the evidence that IL-6 concentration in the UF averaged $1/5^{th}$ of the plasma concentration, the value expected for free IL-6 (MW 24.5 kDa) crossing through a membrane with IL-6 sieving coefficient of about 0.3. The evidence that we found low or undetectable IL-6 concentrations in the effluent from the cartridge suggests that the IL-6 that crossed the dialysis membrane of the first HFR stage to move into the UF was virtually all retained by the cartridge itself. In keeping with this result is the evidence that the ability of the UF incubation to trigger IL-6 gene expression and release in PBMC from healthy subjects was greatly reduced after its passage through the HFR cartridge sorbent bed.

While the evidence discussed above suggests that HFR cartridge contributed to clear the plasma of our patients from uremic toxins, a role could have been played also by the second, diffusive stage of the HFR apparatus [26]. As mentioned above, this portion of the HFR system operates as a conventional HD system in which diffusion represents the main mechanism of solute removal. However, the removal of p-cresol by this mechanism is expected to be small (regarding only its free form) and that of IL-6 null. Indeed, less than 1% of total p-cresol circulates as free form whereas free IL-6 is still too large to cross the low flux membrane of the second HFR stage. As a whole these considerations suggest that a significant amount of p-cresol and all of IL-6 removal actually took place in the first HFR stage. This can probably account for the significantly higher decrease of plasma p-cresol level that we observed in our patients when they underwent HFR as compared to HD (53.6% vs 37.1%). Interestingly, similar values of percent decrease in plasma p-cresol concentration after HD were recently reported by Meert et al. [45]. Therefore, our data suggest that HFR could perform better than HD in p-cresol removal though this conclusion remains to be confirmed in larger studies specifically designed to address this point. Finally, regarding classical hemodiafiltration (HDF), a previous work showed that total p-cresol concentration decreases by 40% after post-dilution and 42% after pre-dilution HDF [46] but no comparative study with HFR has ever been performed.

Although the HFR cartridge retained IL-6, we did not observe any significant change in serum concentrations of this cytokine when we compared blood samples collected before and following a single HFR session. This finding could be explained considering that the actual amount of IL-6 removed during a single HFR is presumably small. Based on concentration in UF and on the value of Q_{uf} in the HFR system, we estimated that less than 10% of circulating IL-6 could be removed by the cartridge. Remarkably, no additional IL-6 removal can occur in the diffusive stage of the HFR apparatus because free IL-6 cannot be dialyzed by the low flux membrane of its filter. It is likely that the small amount of IL-6 removed by HFR could be entirely replaced either by the new synthesis of this cytokine or by its release from tissues. It has been suggested, indeed, that in inflamed patients, circulating IL-6 remains high despite its very short plasma half-life because it is produced at a very high rate [27]. Under this respect we should consider that all our patients showed a remarkable systemic inflammation as demonstrated by the high serum concentrations of hsCRP. It should be emphasized at this point, however, that such a marked systemic inflammation is not the most typical finding in ESRD patients that, instead, usually present only a moderate inflammatory state known as "microinflammation" [47]. We can speculate, thus, that HFR that was ineffective against the high IL-6 concentration of our markedly inflamed patients could perform better in the average ESRD patient with microinflammation.

Our findings suggest that HFR does not differ from other dialysis systems that have all been shown ineffective in lowering the circulating levels of IL-6 and/or of other cytokines. Specifically, IL-6 levels did not change after a single HD session, as shown by Tarakçioğlu et al. [27] and as also observed by us in the present paper. In addition, continuous hemofiltration was also ineffective in lowering circulating IL-6 levels in patients with systemic inflammatory response syndrome [48]. After measuring the very small amounts of several cytokines such as TNFα and IL-1 that are removed by low-volume HF (Vuf approximately 12 L/day), Van Bommel et al. [49] estimated that a UF volumes of at least 50 L/day should be needed to clear the plasma from these molecules using hemofiltration.

While a single HFR session seems to be ineffective in decreasing plasma IL-6, a substantial lowering of the circulating level of this cytokine has been reported with repeated HFR treatment. Specifically, Panichi et al. [29] showed that IL-6 plasma concentration significantly decreased respect to baseline after 4 months of repeated HFR treatment. This evidence suggests that longer follow up of HFR treatments could slowly decrease plasma IL-6 levels by inducing a decrease in systemic inflammation. A significant decrease of oxidative stress was also reported by Calò et al in patients receiving HFR [50].

In conclusion, our data provided the proof of concept that the HFR system could represent a new method to remove p-cresol and IL-6 from the blood. It would be interesting to evaluate whether HFR efficiency could be increased by the new generation of membranes with a tenfold higher sieving coefficient for albumin (0.2) that are becoming available. These new HFR systems are expected to greatly increase the amount of albumin bound p-cresol and, presumably, of other inflammatory mediators that can be retained by the cartridge and, therefore, to further increase their advantages respect to HD in protein bound solutes removal.

Acknowledgments

Part of this study was presented and published in abstract form at the 50th Congress of ERA-EDTA, Istambul, May 18-21, 2013, and at the World Congress of Nephrology 2013, Hong Kong, May 31–June 4, 2013.

Author Contributions

Conceived and designed the experiments: BM. Performed the experiments: ER MM GA RR SB AM LP LG. Analyzed the data: BM BG MC. Contributed reagents/materials/analysis tools: BM. Wrote the paper: BM MC.

References

1. Shiffer EL, Lipman ML, Mann FE (2007) Chronic kidney disease: effect on the cardiovascular system. Circulation 116: 85–97.
2. Foley RN, Parfrey PS, Sarnak MJ (1998) Epidemiology of cardiovascular disease in chronic renal disease. J Am Soc Nephrol 9: S16–S23.
3. Sarnak M, Coronado B, Greene T (2002) Cardiovascular disease risk factors in chronic renal insufficiency. Clin Nephrol 57: 327–335.
4. Stenvinkel P, Carrero JJ, Axelsson J, Lindholm B, Heimburger O, et al. (2008) Emerging biomarkers for evaluating cardiovascular risk in the chronic kidney disease patient: How do new pieces fit into the uremic puzzle? Clin J Am Soc Nephrol 3: 505–521.
5. Kaysen GA (2001) The microinflammatory state in uremia: causes and potential consequences. J Am Soc Nephrol 12: 1549–1557.
6. Cozzolino M, Brancaccio D, Gallieni M, Slatopolsky E (2005) Pathogenesis of vascular calcification in chronic kidney disease. Kidney Int 68: 429–436.
7. Levin A (2002) Anemia and left ventricular hypertrophy in chronic kidney disease populations: a review of the current state of knowledge. Kidney Int 61 (Suppl. 80): S35–S38.
8. Cummings JH (1983) Fermentation in the human large intestine: evidence and implications for health. Lancet 1: 1206–1209.
9. Evenepoel P, Meijers BKI, Bammens BRM, Verbeke K (2009) Uremic toxins originating from colonic microbial metabolism. Kidney Int 76 (Suppl 114): S12–S19.
10. Vanholder R, Bammens B, de Loor H, Glorieux G, Meijers B, et al. (2011) Warning: The unfortunate end of p-cresol as a uraemic toxin. Nephrol Dial Transplant 26: 1464–1467.
11. Meijers BKI, Bammens B, De Moor B, Verbeke K, Vanrenterghem Y, et al. (2008) Free p-cresol is associated with cardiovascular disease in hemodialysis patients. Kidney Int 73: 1173–1180.
12. Bammens B, Evenepoel P, Keuleers H, Verbeke K, Vanrenterghem Y (2006) Free serum concentrations of the protein-bound retention solute *p*-cresol predict mortality in hemodialysis patients. Kidney Int 69:1081–1087.
13. Cerini C, Dou L, Anfosso F, Sabatier F, Moal V, et al. (2004) P-cresol, a uremic retention solute, alters the endothelial barrier function in vitro. Thromb Haemost 92:140–150.
14. Ying Y, Yang K, Liu Y, Chen QJ, Shen WF, et al. (2011) A uremic solute, P-cresol, inhibits the proliferation of endothelial progenitor cells via the p38 pathway. Circ J 75: 2252–2259.
15. Meijers BK, Van Kerckhoven S, Verbeke K, Dehaen W, Vanrenterghem Y, et al. (2009) The uremic retention solute p-cresylsulfate and markers of endothelial damage. Am J Kidney Dis 54: 891–901.
16. Schepers E, Meert N, Glorieux G, Goeman J, Van der Eycken J, et al. (2007) P-cresylsulphate, the main in vivo metabolite of *p*-cresol, activates leucocyte free radical production. Nephrol Dial Transplant; 22 592–596.
17. Stenvinkel P, Heinburger O, Paultre F, Diczfalusy U, Wang T, et al. (1999) Strong associations between malnutrition, inflammation and atherosclerosis in chronic renal failure. Kidney Int 55: 1899–1911.
18. Zimmermann J, Herrlinger S, Pruy A, Metzger T, Wanner C. (1999) Inflammation enhances cardiovascular risk and mortality in hemodialysis. Kidney Int 55: 648–658
19. Serur D, Stenzel KH, Rubin AL. (1998) Interleukin 6 predicts hypoalbuminemia, hypocholesterolemia, and mortality in hemodialysis patients. Am J Kidney Dis 32: 107–114.

20. Panichi V, Rizza GM, Paoletti S, Bigazzi R, Aloisi M, et al. (2008) Chronic inflammation and mortality in haemodialysis: effect of different renal replacement therapies: Results from the RISCAVID study. Nephrol Dial Transplant 23: 2337–2343.
21. Yeun JY, Levine RA, Mantadilok V, Kaysen GA. (2000) C-reactive protein predicts all-cause and cardiovascular mortality in hemodialysis patients. Am J Kidney Dis 35: 469–476.
22. Rao M, Guo D, Perianayagam MC, Tighiouart H, Jaber BL, et al. (2005) Plasma interleukin-6 predicts cardiovascular mortality in hemodialysis patients. Am J Kidney Dis 45: 324–333.
23. Barreto DV, Barreto FC, Liabeuf S, Temmar M, Lemke HD, et al. (2010) Plasma Interleukin-6 is independently associated with mortality in both hemodialysis and pre-dialysis patients with chronic kidney diasease. Kidney Int 77: 550–556.
24. Stenvinkel P, Ketteler M, Johnson RJ, Lindholm B, Pecoits-Filho R, et al. (2005) IL-10, IL-6, and TNF-alpha: central factors in the altered cytokine network of uremia-the good, the bad, and the ugly. Kidney Int 67: 1216–1233.
25. Jourde-Chiche N, Dou L, Cerini C, Dignat-George F, Vanholder R, et al. (2009) Protein-Bound Toxins-Update in 2009. Seminars in Dialysis 22: 334–339.
26. Martinez AW, Recht NS, Hostetter TH, Meyer TW (2005) Removal of p-cresol sulfate by hemodialysis. J Am Soc Nephrol 16: 3430–3436.
27. Tarakçioğlu M, Erbağci AB, Usalan C, Deveci R, Kocabaş R (2003) Acute effect of hemodialysis on serum levels of the proinflammatory cytokines. Mediators Inflamm 12: 15–19.
28. Meijers BK, De Loor H, Bammens B, Verbeke K, Vanrenterghem Y, et al. (2009) p-Cresyl sulfate and indoxyl sulfate in hemodialysis patients. Clin J Am Soc Nephrol 4: 1932–1938.
29. Vanhoder R, Glorieux G, Lameire N, European Uremic Toxin Work Group (2003) Uraemic toxins and cardiovascular disease.Nephrol Dial Transplant 18: 463–466.
30. Memoli B, Grandaliano G, Soccio M, Postiglione L, Guida B, et al. (2005) In vivo modulation of soluble "antagonistic" IL-6 receptor synthesis and release in ESRD. J Am Soc Nephrol 16:1099–1107.
31. Meyer TW, Peattie JW, Miller JD, Dinh DC, Recht NS, et al. (2007) Increasing the clearance of protein-bound solutes by addition of a sorbent to the dialysis. J Am Soc Nephrol 18: 868–874.
32. Meijers BK, Weber V, Bammens B, Dehaen W, Verbeke K, et al. (2007) Removal of the uremic retention solute p-cresol using fractionated plasma separation and adsorption. Artif Organs 32: 214–219.
33. Krieter DH, Hackl A, Rodriguez A, Chenine L, Moragues HL, et al. (2010) Protein-bound uraemic toxin removal in haemodialysis and post-diluition haemodiafiltration. Nephrol Dial Transplant 25: 212–218.
34. Ghezzi PM, Gervasio R, Tessore V, Sartoris AM, Botella J. (1992) Hemodiafiltration without replacement fluid: an experimental study. ASAIO Journal 38: 61–65.
35. de Francisco ALM, Ghezzi PM, Brendolan A, Fiorini F, La Greca G, et al. (2000) Hemodiafiltration with on-line regeneration of the ultrafiltrate. Kidney Int 58: S66–S71.
36. Memoli B, Bisesti V, Saravo MT, Esposito P, D'Arcangelo R, et al. (2003) Cytokine production in standard hemodialysis with a new polyethersulfone membrane: a cross-over study. Contrib Nephrol 138:80–87.
37. Wratten ML, Sereni L, Lupotti M, Ghezzi PM, Atti M, et al. (2004) Optimization of a HFR sorbent cartridge for high molecular weight uremic toxins. G Ital Nefrol 21: S67–S70.
38. De Nitti C, Giordano R, Gervasio R, Castellano G, Podio V, et al. (2001) Choosing new sorbents for endogenous ultrapure infusion fluid: performances, safety and flow distribution. Int J Artif Organs 24: 765–776.
39. Tetta C, Ghezzi PM, De Nitti C, Fiorenzi A, Cianciavicchia D, et al. (2002) New options for on-line hemodiafiltration. Contrib Nephrol 137: 212–220.
40. Guida B, Cataldi M, Riccio E, Grumetto L, Pota A, et al. (2013) Plasma p-Cresol Lowering Effect of Sevelamer in Peritoneal Dialysis Patients: Evidence from a Cross-Sectional Observational Study. PLoS One 8: e73558.
41. Calaf R, Cerini C, Génovésio C, Verhaeghe P, Jourde-Chiche N, et al. (2011) Determination of uremic solutes in biological fluids of chronic kidney disease patients by HPLC assay. J Chromatogr B Analyt Technol Biomed Life Sci 879:2281–2286.
42. Lesaffer G, De Smet R, Lameire N, Dhondt A, Duym P, et al. (2000) Intradialytic removal of protein-bound uraemic toxins: role of solute characteristics and of dialyser membrane. Nephrol Dial Transplant 15: 50–57.
43. Overbergh L, Giulietti A, Valckx D, Decallonne R, Bouillon R, et al. (2003) The use of real-time reverse transcriptase PCR for the quantification of cytokine gene expression. J Biomol Tech14: 33–43.
44. Memoli B, Postiglione L, Cianciaruso B, Bisesti V, Cimmaruta C, et al. (2000) Role of different dialysis membranes in the release of interleukin-6-soluble receptor in uremic patients. Kidney Int, 58: 417–424.
45. Meert N, Eloot S, Schepers E, Lemke HD, Dhondt A, et al. (2011) Comparison of removal capacity of two consecutive generations of high-flux dialysers during different treatment modalities. Nephrol Dial Transplant 26: 2624–2630.
46. Meert N, Eloot S, Waterloos MA, Van Landschoot M, Dhondt A, et al. (2009) Effective removal of protein-bound uraemic solutes by different convective strategies: a prospective trial. Nephrol Dial Transplant 24: 562–570.
47. Memoli B, Salerno S, Procino A, Postiglione L, Morelli S, et al. (2010) A translational approach to micro-inflammation in end-stage renal disease: molecular effects of low levels of interleukin-6. Clin Sci 119: 163–174.
48. Sander A, Armbruster W, Sander B, Daul AE, Lange R, et al. (1997) Hemofiltration increases IL-6 clearance in early systemic response syndrome but does not alter IL-6 and TNFα plasma concentrations. Intensive Care Med 23: 878–884.
49. van Bommel EF, Hesse CJ, Jutte NH, Zietse R, Bruining HA, et al. (1997) Impact of continuous hemofiltration on cytokines and cytokine inhibitors in oliguric patients suffering from systemic inflammatory response syndrome. Renal Failure 19: 443–454.
50. Calò LA, Naso A, Carraro G, Wratten ML, Pagnin E, et al. (2007) Effect of haemodiafiltration with online regeneration of ultrafiltrate on oxidative stress in dialysis patients. Nephrol Dial Transplant 22: 1413–1419.

Uremic Conditions Drive Human Monocytes to Pro-Atherogenic Differentiation via an Angiotensin-Dependent Mechanism

Bogusz Trojanowicz*, Christof Ulrich, Eric Seibert, Roman Fiedler, Matthias Girndt

Department of Internal Medicine II, Martin-Luther-University Halle-Wittenberg, Germany

Abstract

Aims: Elevated expression levels of monocytic-ACE have been found in haemodialysis patients. They are not only epidemiologically linked with increased mortality and cardiovascular disease, but may also directly participate in the initial steps of atherosclerosis. To further address this question we tested the role of monocytic-ACE in promotion of atherosclerotic events in vitro under conditions mimicking those of chronic renal failure.

Methods and Results: Treatment of human primary monocytes or THP-1 cells with uremic serum as well as PMA-induced differentiation led to significantly up-regulated expression of ACE, further increased by additional treatment with LPS. Functionally, these monocytes revealed significantly increased adhesion and transmigration through endothelial monolayers. Overexpression of ACE in transfected monocytes or THP-1 cells led to development of more differentiated, macrophage-like phenotype with up-regulated expression of Arg1, MCSF, MCP-1 and CCR2. Expression of pro-inflammatory cytokines TNFa and IL-6 were also noticeably up-regulated. ACE overexpression resulted in significantly increased adhesion and transmigration properties. Transcriptional screening of ACE-overexpressing monocytes revealed noticeably increased expression of Angiotensin II receptors and adhesion- as well as atherosclerosis-related ICAM-1 and VCAM1. Inhibition of monocyte ACE or AngII-receptor signalling led to decreased adhesion potential of ACE-overexpressing cells.

Conclusions: Taken together, these data demonstrate that uremia induced expression of monocytic-ACE mediates the development of highly pro-atherogenic cells via an AngII-dependent mechanism.

Editor: Paula A. da Costa Martins, Maastricht University Faculty of Health, Medicine, and Life Sciences, Netherlands

Funding: This work was supported by intramural funding of the University Halle (Saale). The funders had no role in study design, data collection and analysis, decision to publish, or preparation of the manuscript.

Competing Interests: The authors have declared that no competing interests exist.

* Email: bogusz.trojanowicz@uk-halle.de

Introduction

Systemic chronic inflammation plays a crucial role in the initiation and progression of atherosclerosis. Patients with chronic kidney disease (CKD) maintained on intermittent hemodialysis develop progressive atherosclerosis leading to cardiovascular events such as myocardial infarction and stroke [1], [2], [3]. These patients are at higher risk of all-cause mortality [4] and obviously suffer from both atherosclerosis [5] and arteriosclerosis [6]. Recent data suggest that inflammation is predominantly associated with that plaque forming disease of atherosclerosis rather than vascular stiffening [7].

So called "classical" cardiovascular risk factors such as dyslipidemia, hypertension, diabetes or smoking promote initiation and progression of atherosclerosis by recruitment of circulating immune cells to infiltrate the injured vascular endothelium [8], [9]. The monocytes infiltrating in the subendothelial space differentiate into macrophages and dendritic cells which trigger the accumulation of lipids, extracellular matrix components and other cells in the vessel wall. Extensive and prolonged accumulation of lipid-carrying apoptotic cells, cell debris and cholesterol crystals leads to the formation of atherosclerotic plaque [10]. Infiltrating monocytes may differentiate into different macrophage subtypes with either protective or pathogenic activities. Recent studies suggest that classically activated macrophages (M1 or CAMs) may possess pro-atherogenic abilities in contrast to alternatively activated athero-protective macrophages M2 (or AAMs) [11], [12]. However in advanced stages of atherosclerosis, secretion of metalloproteinases, typical for M2-like macrophages, may contribute to matrix degradation and rupture, which may trigger a myocardial infarction or stroke [13], [14], [15], [16].

Angiotensin converting enzyme (ACE) participates in the regulation of blood pressure (arterial vasoconstriction) and sodium and water balance. The circulating exopeptidase catalyzes the conversion of decapeptide angiotensin I (AngI) to octapeptide angiotensin II (AngII), a potent vasoconstrictor. ACE is not only secreted by pulmonary and renal endothelial cells, but is also expressed on the surface of monocytes, macrophages and smooth muscle cells [17]. Furthermore, ACE has also been detected in human atherosclerotic lesions, where it is associated with a subset of macrophages [18], [19], [20] or cells possessing dendritic-like properties [21].

The presence of angiotensinogen (AGT), AngI, AngII and its receptors on human monocytes indicate that this cell type might have a functionally relevant auto- or paracrine angiotensin system potentially involved in the pathogenesis of vascular disease [22]. Inhibition of ACE and/or employment of AngII receptor 1 (AT1R) antagonists has been shown to be effective in decreasing clinical events in patients with atherosclerosis [23]. Little is known about local cellular effects besides systemic blood pressure control, particularly on monocytic ACE (mACE).

In patients with end stage renal disease circulating monocytes are activated and proinflammatory monocytes are expanded. We recently demonstrated that elevated levels of mACE on those cells in hemodialysis patients are associated with increased mortality and cardiovascular morbidity and may also participate in the initial steps of atherosclerosis [7], [24], [25].

In this study we used the primary human monocytes and myelomonocytic cell line THP-1 to investigate the regulation of mACE under conditions of uremia. Furthermore, a potentially causal involvement of ACE upregulation for atherosclerosis initiation was studied.

Materials and Methods

Human serum and isolation of primary human monocytes

Pooled uremic sera (HD) were obtained from chronic hemodialysis patients (n = 10; both males and females) treated at the Dialysis Ward of the University Clinic Halle. All HD patients were treated three times weekly by standard bicarbonate hemodialysis with ultrapure water quality (by reverse osmosis and sterile filters) using high flux polynephron membranes (Nipro Europe). All HD samples were obtained prior to a regular hemodialysis session from the dialysis access and anti-coagulated with heparin. Pooled uremic sera from peritoneal dialysis (PD) were obtained from 5 patients (both males and females). Additionally pooled uremic sera were isolated from 3 CKD5 patients (males) not on dialysis and 10 HD patients (both males and females) prior to (pre-HD) and after (post-HD) a hemodialysis session. HD, PD, CKD 5, pre- and post-HD patients were aged between 40 and 70 years, they were free of acute infectious complications and were not treated by immunosuppressive medication. Normal sera (NS) were obtained from age matched healthy volunteers (n = 8; age range 50 to 67 years; both males and females). Human primary monocytes were isolated from 3 healthy volunteers by employment of Pan Monocyte Isolation Kit (Miltenyi) and AutoMacs cell separator (Miltenyi) according to manufacturer's instructions. All healthy volunteers were normotensive and none was taking any medication. The isolation of the human sera and primary monocytes were performed according to the declaration of Helsinki. This study was approved by the ethical committee of the Martin Luther University, Faculty of Medicine. All patients and persons involved in this study gave written consent.

Cell culture and treatments of primary human monocytes and THP-1 cells

THP-1 monocytes were cultured in RPMI (Sigma) medium, supplemented with 1.125 g/l sodium carbonate, 10% heat inactivated (65°C/30 min) fetal calf serum (FCS) and 100 µg/ml penicillin/streptomycin (Biochrom). THP-1 cells (1×10^6/well) cells were treated with RPMI medium containing 10% HD or NS or 10 ng/ml LPS (Sigma) or combination of LPS and human sera in the presence of 10 ng/ml PMA (Sigma) as differentiating agent for 72 h. Treatment medium was replaced daily.

3×10^5/well primary human monocytes were treated with 10% NS or HD or PD or CKD5 or pre-HD or post-HD sera for 72 h in RPMI medium without FCS. All treatments were performed in hydrophobic 6-well plates (Greiner bio One) in a standard humidified incubator (37 °C, 5% CO2). Total RNA from THP-1 cells and human primary monocytes was isolated at 0 h, 24 h, 48 h and 72 h by employment of Tri Reagent (Sigma) and ZR RNA MiniPrep Kit (Zymo Research), respectively, both according to manufacturer's instructions.

ACE/AngII-receptor inhibition studies were performed with captopril (ACE inhibitor, Santa Cruz Biotechnology) or losartan (Angiotensin II type 1 receptor (AT1R) antagonist, Santa Cruz Biotechnology) or angiotensin II (Sigma). Briefly calcein-labelled (calcein-AM, 1 µM, Cayman Chemical) control or ACE-overexpressing monocytes were tested for their adhesion abilities to endothelial monolayers in the presence or absence of 500 nM captopril or 1 µM losartan for 30 min. Additionally endothelial-adhesion of ACE-negative THP-1 cells was tested in the presence or absence of Angiotensin II (1 µM) or losartan (1 µM). For details see below (adhesion assay) and corresponding figure legends.

HUVEC (Human umbilical vein endothelial cells) cell line was cultured in Medium 200 supplemented with LSGS (Low Serum Growth Supplement, Gibco).

Table 1. Primer sequences employed in this study.

Target	Sequences
RPL37A	S-5′-ATTGAAATCAGCCAGCACGC, AS-5′-AGGAACCACAGTGCCAGATCC
MCSF	S-5′-TAGCCACATGATTGGGAGTG, AS-5′-TATCTCTGAAGCGCATGGTG
AT1R	S-5′-GCACAATGCTTGTAGCCAAA, AS-5′-GGGTTGAATTTTGGGACTCA
AT2R	S-5′-TTCCCTTCCATGTTCTGACC, AS-5′-AAACACACTGCGGAGCTTCT
ICAM-1	S-5′-GGCCTCAGTCAGTGTGA, AS-5′-AACCCCATTCAGCGTCA
VCAM-1	S- 5′-CCGGATTGCTGCTCAGATTGGA, AS- 5′-AGCGTGGAATTGGTCCCCTCA
MCP-1	S-5′-TCGCGAGCTATAGAAGAATCA, AS-5′-TGTTCAAGTCTTCGGAGTTTG
Arg1	S-5′-GGAGACCACAGTTTGGCAAT, AS-5′-CCACTTGTGGTTGTCAGTGG
Arg2	S-5′-TTCCATCCTGAAGAAATCCG, AS-5′-AGAGCCTTTTCATCAAGCCA
iNOS	S-5′-AAAGACCAGGCTGTCGTTGA, AS-5′-ACGGGACCGGTATTCATTCT

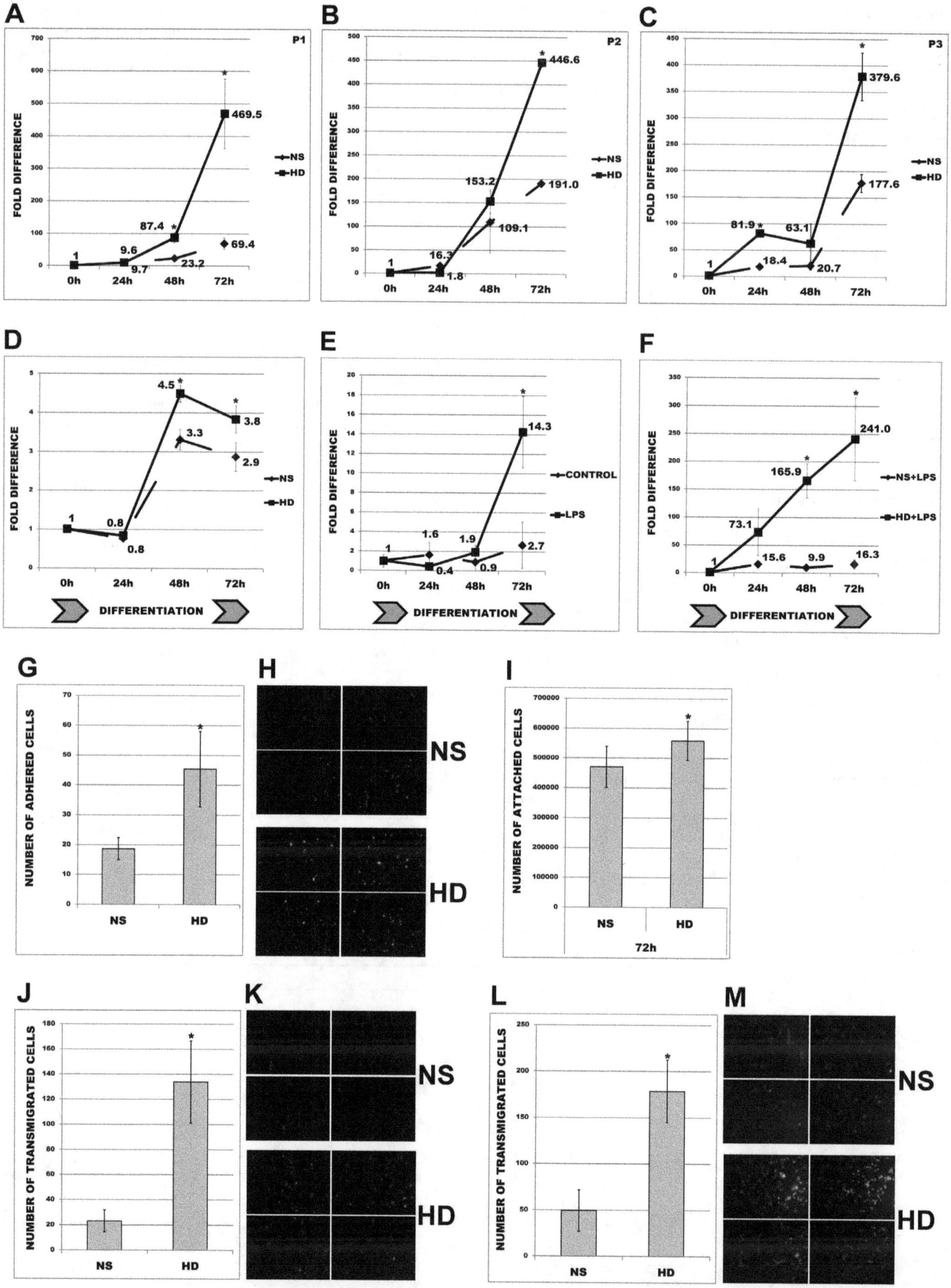
A
P1
FOLD DIFFERENCE
NS
HD
1
9.6
9.7
87.4
23.2
469.5
69.4
0h 24h 48h 72h
B
P2
FOLD DIFFERENCE
NS
HD
1
16.3
1.8
153.2
109.1
446.6
191.0
0h 24h 48h 72h
C
P3
FOLD DIFFERENCE
NS
HD
1
81.9
18.4
63.1
20.7
379.6
177.6
0h 24h 48h 72h
D
FOLD DIFFERENCE
NS
HD
1
0.8
0.8
4.5
3.3
3.8
2.9
0h 24h 48h 72h
DIFFERENTIATION
E
FOLD DIFFERENCE
CONTROL
LPS
1
1.6
0.4
1.9
0.9
14.3
2.7
0h 24h 48h 72h
DIFFERENTIATION
F
FOLD DIFFERENCE
NS+LPS
HD+LPS
1
73.1
15.6
165.9
9.9
241.0
16.3
0h 24h 48h 72h
DIFFERENTIATION
G
NUMBER OF ADHERED CELLS
NS
HD
H
NS
HD
I
NUMBER OF ATTACHED CELLS
NS
HD
72h
J
NUMBER OF TRANSMIGRATED CELLS
NS
HD
K
NS
HD
L
NUMBER OF TRANSMIGRATED CELLS
NS
HD
M
NS
HD

Figure 1. Expression of ACE and behaviour of human monocytes under uremic status I. (A, B, C) Primary human monocytes obtained from healthy volunteers P1, P2, and P3 were treated with 10% NS or HD sera for 72 h and investigated for ACE-mRNA expression. Means ± SD of three independent experiments. (D, E, F) THP-1 monocytes were PMA-differentiated (10 ng/ml) into macrophages in the presence of (D) 10% NS or HD sera or (E) 10 ng/ml LPS or (F) 10 ng/ml LPS and both of them for 72 h. Means ± SD of three independent experiments. (G, H, I) Attachment and adhesion of THP-1 monocytes and primary monocytes treated with NS or HD. Primary human monocytes were incubated in the presence of 10% NS or HD sera for 30 min and investigated for their endothelial-adhesion. The number (G) and corresponding images of endothelial-adhered monocytes (H) are shown. Means ± SD of cell number in 10 microscopic fields in three independent experiments. (I) THP-1 were incubated in the presence of 10% NS or HD sera for 72 h and investigated for their attachment abilities. The number of attached cells (detached prior to counting) was counted by FACS. Means ± SD of four independent experiments. (J, K, L, M) Transmigration of calcein-labelled primary monocytes (J, K) or THP-1 cells (L, M) through endothelial monolayer towards lower chamber filled with RPMI medium supplemented with 10% NS or HD sera. Transmigrated cells were visualized with fluorescent microscopy (K, M) and counted in 10 random fields (J, L). Representative images are shown. Means ± SD of cell number in 10 microscopic fields in three independent experiments. * $p< 0.05$ indicates statistical significance.

Transfection

For generation of THP-1 cells stably overexpressing human ACE, the cells were transfected with pcDNA3.1(-) carrying the full coding sequence of ACE (a gift from Dr. K. Kohlstedt, Goethe-University, Frankfurt am Main, Germany). Control cells received empty plasmid only. Transfection of the cells was performed in 24-well plates in normal growth medium. 1×10^6 THP-1 cells/well were transfected with 1 µg of ACE or empty plasmid in the presence of Lipofectamine 2000 as a carrier. After 24 h the cells were selected with growth medium supplemented with 1000 µg/ml neomycin G-418 (Biochrom) for next 8 weeks. Thereafter, the concentration of neomycin in growth medium was set up to 500 µg/ml. Transient transfection of primary human monocytes was performed with the same plasmids in 24-well plates in RPMI medium without FCS. 1×10^6/well of pooled primary human monocytes, obtained from volunteers were transfected with 1 µg of ACE or empty plasmid and Lipofectamine 2000 in the presence of RPMI medium. Expression of ACE and corresponding assays were performed 24 h after transfection.

RNA isolation and Real Time PCR

Total RNA was isolated using Tri-Reagent (Sigma) or ZR RNA MiniPrep Kit (Zymo Research), both according to manufacturer's instructions. Depending on the experiment 50 ng-1 µg of total RNA was used as a template for first strand cDNA synthesis employing High Capacity cDNA Reverse Transcription Kit according to manufacturer's instructions (Life Technologies). The samples were stored at -20°C.

Amplifications of ACE, TNFa, IL-6, 18S and RPL37A were performed with TaqMan Gene Expression Assays (Life Technologies) and FastStart Universal Probe Master Mix (Roche) in a StepOne plus System. 18S and RPL37A (Ribosomal Protein 37a) were employed for normalization of target mRNA expression. Thermal cycling conditions were as follows: hold 10 min at 95°C, followed by 40 cycles of 10 sec at 95°C and 30 sec at 60°C. Amplifications of, MCSF (Macrophage Colony-Stimulating Factor), AT1R (Angiotensin II Type I Receptor), AT2R (Angiotensin II Type II Receptor), ICAM-1 (Intercellular Adhesion Molecule 1), VCAM-1 (Vascular Cell Adhesion Molecule 1), MCP-1/CCL2 (Monocyte Chemotactic Protein-1), Arg1 (Arginase-1), Arg2 (Arginase-2), iNOS (inducible nitric oxide synthase) and RPL37A were performed with sequences presented in Table 1 and Maxima SYBR Green-qPCR Master Mix (Thermo Scientific). RPL37A was employed for normalization. Thermal cycling conditions were as follows: hold 10 min at 95°C, followed by 40 cycles of 15 sec at 95°C, 30 sec at 60°C and 30 sec at 72°C. Data evaluation was performed with DataAssist Software (Life Technologies).

MTT

In 96-well plates, 3000 THP-1 cells/well were seeded and cultured in growth medium for 24h, 48h and 72 h. For MTT assay, cells were then stained with MTT (3-[4,5-dimethylthiazol-2-yl]-2,5-diphenyltetrazolium bromide, Sigma) for 4 h at 37 °C and shortly incubated with dimethyl sulfoxide (DMSO, Roth). Thereby, a coloured formazan salt develops depending on the availability of mitochondrial NADH2 only in living, but not dead cells. Optical density was measured with BioRad ELISA reader at 550 nm. Experiment was repeated at least three times.

Attachment assay

In 96-well plates, 3000 THP-1 cells/well were seeded and cultured in growth medium in the presence of 10 ng/ml PMA for 72 h. Thereafter the cells were fixed with 4% PFA/PBS for 30 min and vigorously washed with PBS. Remaining cells were stained with 0.2% crystal violet (CV, dissolved in water and filtered before use, Roth) for 30 min at RT. The excess of CV was removed by washing with deionized water until no violet colour release from culture plate was observed. Cellular CV was solubilized by addition of 0.1% SDS (Roth). The absorbance was measured after 15 min. incubation at RT at 550 nm. In long time attachment experiments 1×10^6 THP-1 cells were incubated in the presence of 10% NS or HD sera for 72 h. After two times washing with PBS, adhered cells were detached with Accutase and counted with FACS. Experiment was repeated at least three times.

Adhesion assay

Adhesion of primary human monocytes or THP-1 cells to endothelial HUVEC monolayers was investigated in 24-well plates. Briefly, HUVEC cells were cultured in growth medium until they created monolayer on the bottom of 24-well plate. For labelling, primary monocytes or THP-1 cells were incubated in RPMI containing 1 µM calcein-AM at 37 °C for 60 min. The cells were washed with RPMI twice. Depending on the experiment fluorescence-labelled cells were re-suspended in 2 ml RPMI medium or RPMI medium containing 10% NS or HD or PD or CKD5 sera. HUVEC monolayers were washed twice with RPMI medium before addition of 2 ml labelled primary monocytes (3×10^5 cells/well) or THP-1 cells (1×10^6 cells/well) per well. The plates were incubated for 30 min at 37 °C. After incubation, the monolayer was gently washed three times with RPMI. Adherent monocytes were photographed using a Biozero BZ-9000 fluorescence microscope (Keyence). The number of the adherent cells was evaluated in 10 microscopic fields for each situation by employment of ImageJ software (Wayne Rasband, National Institutes of Health, USA). All experiments were repeated at least three times.

Transmigration assay

All transmigration assays were performed by employment of Millicell Cell Culture Inserts (Millipore, 8 µM pore size, 12 mm diameter). Primary monocytes or THP-1 cells were incubated in RPMI medium containing 1 µM calcein-AM at 37 °C for 60 min.

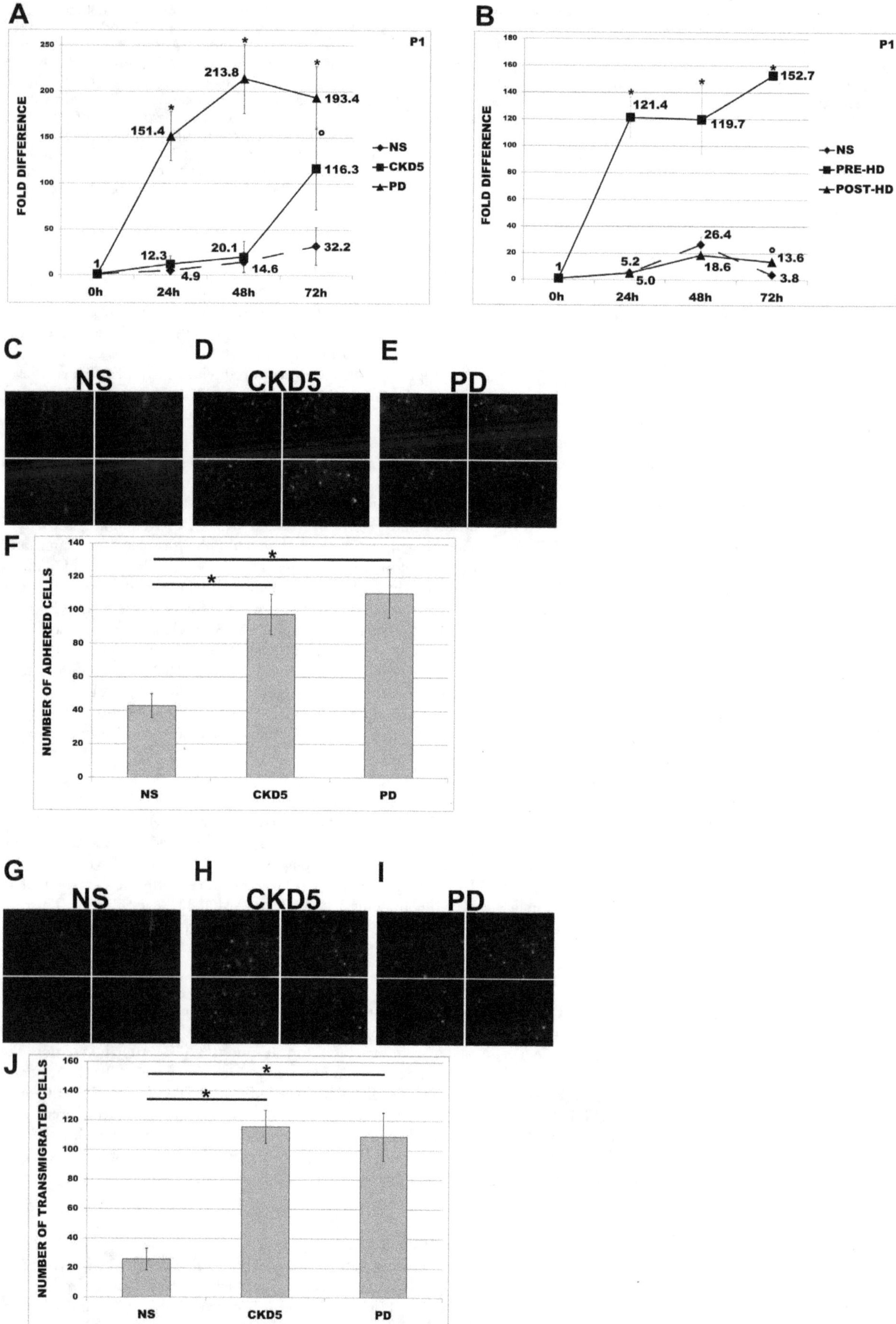
A
P1
FOLD DIFFERENCE
0h
24h
48h
72h
NS
CKD5
PD
213.8
193.4
151.4
116.3
12.3
20.1
32.2
14.6
4.9
B
P1
FOLD DIFFERENCE
NS
PRE-HD
POST-HD
121.4
119.7
152.7
26.4
13.6
18.6
5.2
5.0
3.8
C
D
E
NS
CKD5
PD
F
NUMBER OF ADHERED CELLS
NS
CKD5
PD
G
H
I
NS
CKD5
PD
J
NUMBER OF TRANSMIGRATED CELLS
NS
CKD5
PD

Figure 2. Expression of ACE and behaviour of human monocytes under uremic status II. (A, B) Primary human monocytes obtained from healthy volunteer P1 were treated with (A) 10% NS or PD or CKD5 or (B) 10% NS or pre- or post-HD sera for 72 h and investigated for ACE-mRNA expression. Means ± SD of three independent experiments. * $p < 0.05$ (PD vs. NS; pre-HD vs. NS; pre-HD vs. post-HD) and °$p < 0.05$ (CKD5 vs. NS; post-HD vs. NS) indicate statistical significance. (C, D, E, F) Adhesion of primary monocytes treated with NS or PD or CKD5 sera. Primary human monocytes were incubated in the presence of 10% NS or PD or CKD5 sera for 30 min and investigated for their endothelial-adhesion. The number (F) and corresponding images of endothelial-adhered monocytes (C, D, E) are shown. Means ± SD of cell number in 10 microscopic fields in three independent experiments. (G, H, I, J) Transmigration of calcein-labelled primary monocytes through endothelial monolayer towards lower chamber filled with RPMI medium supplemented with 10% NS or PD or CKD5 sera. Transmigrated cells were visualized with fluorescent microscopy (G, H, I) and counted in 10 random fields (J). Representative images are shown. Means ± SD of cell number in 10 microscopic fields in three independent experiments. * $p < 0.05$ indicates statistical significance.

The cells were washed with RPMI twice. 3×10^5 primary monocytes or 5×10^5 calcein-labelled THP-1 cells were re-suspended in 400 µl RPMI medium and seeded into upper transmigration chamber. Depending on the experiment, the cells transmigrated through uncoated or HUVEC monolayers coated membranes towards lower chamber filled with 600 µl RPMI medium supplemented with 50 ng/ml MCP-1 (Miltenyi) or 10% NS or HD or PD or CKD5 sera. In some experiments, THP-1 cells transmigrated towards HUVEC monolayers created on the bottom of lower chamber in the presence of RPMI only in both chambers. All transmigrations were performed at 37 °C for 60 min in the absence of FCS. Transmigrated cells were visualized by fluorescence microscopy (Biozero BZ-9000, Keyence) and counted in 10 microscopic fields for each situation by employment of ImageJ software (Wayne Rasband, National Institutes of Health, USA). In some experiments transmigrated cells were counted by FACS. Experiment was repeated at least three times.

Immunocytochemistry

1×10^5 THP-1 cells were seeded in chamber slides and let grown in normal medium for 24 h. The cells were gently washed with PBS and fixed in 4% PFA/PBS mixture for 10 min at RT. After washing twice with PBS, cells were incubated overnight with FITC-labelled mouse anti-human ACE antibody (AbD Serotec, clone 9B9, diluted 1.100 with PBS) at 4°C in the dark. Negative control was exposed to FITC-labelled IgG2a mouse anti-human antibody (BD Pharmingen) and processed as described above. After 3×10 min washing in PBS, the slides were covered with mounting medium containing a DAPI dye (Vectashield, Vector Laboratories) and dried 1 hour at RT in the dark. Microscopic investigations were performed with fluorescence microscope (Biozero BZ-9000, Keyence). Additionally the living cells were photographed in a phase contrast modus with the same microscope.

FACS

5×10^4 cells were washed twice with MACS buffer (1× PBS supplemented with 0.5%BSA 2 mM EDTA and 0.07% NaN3) and incubated with FITC-conjugated mouse anti-human ACE (AbD Serotec, clone 9B9) and PE-conjugated mouse anti-human CCR2 (R&D, clone 48607) for 30 min at RT in the dark. Measurements were performed with MacsQuant (Miltenyi) flow cytometer. Expression data (Isotype corrected) were presented as mean fluorescence intensity (MFI).

Statistics

Each experiment was repeated at least three times. Data are presented as mean ±SD. Statistical significance was calculated by employment of two-sided Student-t-test. The values of $p < 0.05$ were considered statistically significant. Bonferroni correction was applied for multiply comparisons dividing the significance level by the number of tested variables.

Results

Uremic serum or LPS increase the expression of ACE

To test whether uremic serum or inflammatory conditions are able to regulate the expression of ACE we subjected primary human monocytes or undifferentiated THP-1 cells to 72 h treatment with normal (NS) or uremic (HD) serum or LPS. As shown in Fig. 1A–C primary human monocytes (P1, P2, P3) treated with HD revealed dramatically increased expression of ACE resulting after 72 h in an up-regulation range of 379.6–469.5 fold in all investigated samples. In order to investigate the uremic regulation of ACE during PMA-mediated differentiation into macrophages in the presence of HD or inflammatory conditions, THP-1 were incubated with 10 ng/ml PMA and corresponding sera or 10 ng/ml LPS or both of them for 72 h. As demonstrated in Fig. 1D, the cells differentiated in uremic conditions revealed significantly increased ACE after 72 h as compared to monocytes treated with NS. Further, HD serum potentiated the up-regulation of ACE by LPS (Fig. 1E, F).

Uremia-mediated increase in ACE expression coincided with elevated adhesion and transmigration

In further investigations we tested whether uremic stimulus is able to affect the adhesion and transmigration of primary human monocytes and undifferentiated THP-1 cells. As shown in Fig. 1G, H primary monocytes reacted on HD stimulus with significantly increased number of the cells adhered to endothelial monolayers. Similarly, THP-1 treatment with HD for 72 h led to significantly stronger attachment abilities when compared to NS (Fig. 1I). Additionally HD-stimulus led to development of higher number of more differentiated cells than NS treatment (data not shown). Also under HD both cell-types transmigrated significantly faster through endothelial monolayers than corresponding controls (Fig. 1J, K, L, M).

In order to test whether observed effects on primary monocytes may also be induced with sera coming from non-dialysed CKD patients or patients on other type of dialysis, we subjected P1-monocytes to the treatment with NS or PD or CKD5 sera. Additionally, to examine the pre- and post-dialysis effects of HD-sera on the regulation of ACE, the same cells were preconditioned in the presence of NS or sera obtained prior to (pre-HD) and after (post-HD) dialysis sessions. As demonstrated in Fig. 2A, treatment with PD or CKD5 sera for 72 h, exerted significantly up-regulated ACE expression pattern, similar to those observed under HD treatment. Furthermore, PD or CKD5 conditions led to significantly increased transmigration and endothelial adhesion of the monocytes when compared to corresponding controls (Fig. 2C, D, E, F, G, H, I, J). Treatment of the primary monocytes with pre- or post-HD sera for 72 h revealed significantly up-regulated ACE expression as compared to NS treatments. However, increase in ACE level in pre- HD treatments was significantly and noticeably higher as compared to post-HD or NS (Fig. 2B).

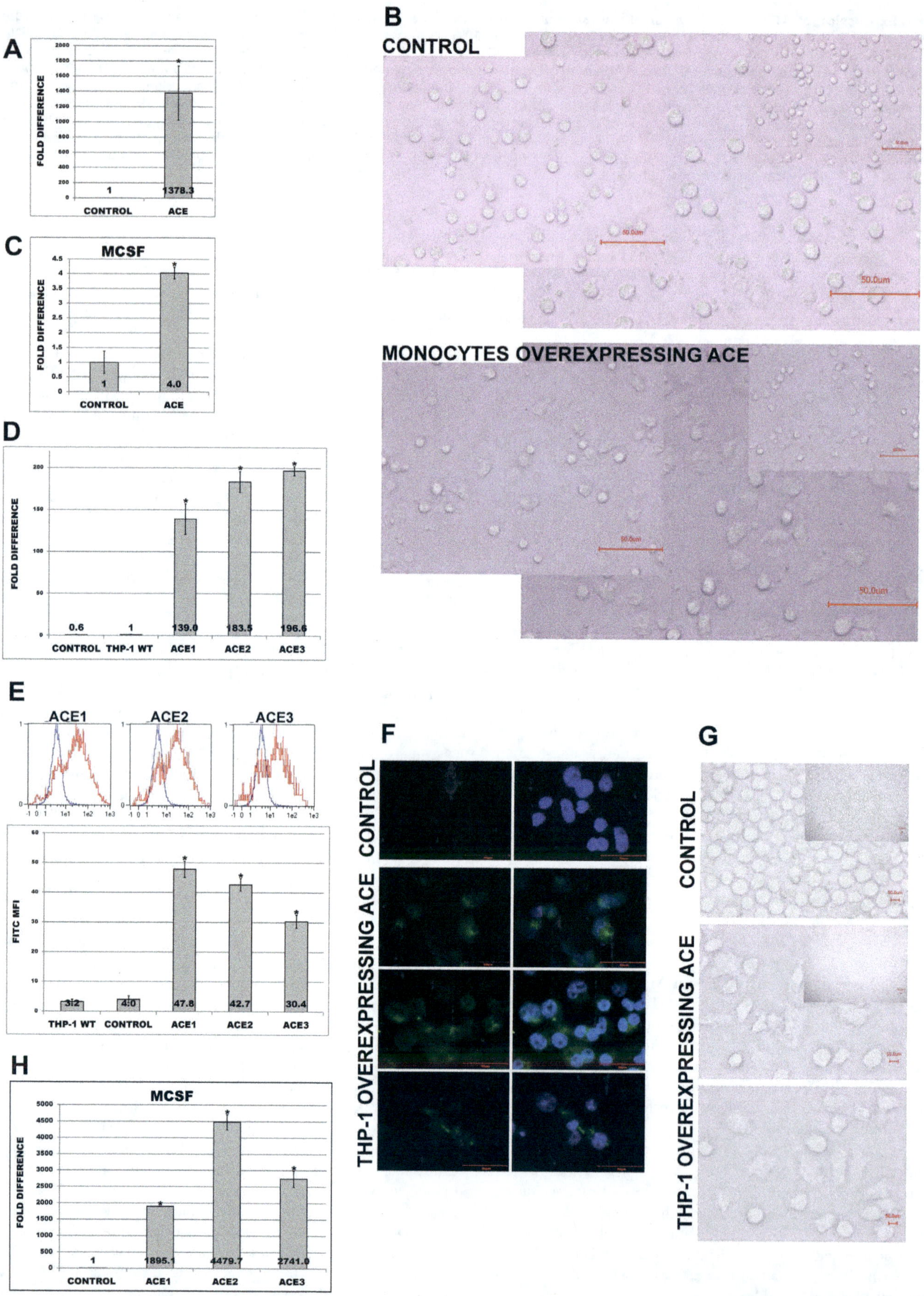
A
FOLD DIFFERENCE
2000
1800
1600
1400
1200
1000
800
600
400
200
0
1
1378.3
CONTROL
ACE
B
CONTROL
50.0um
MONOCYTES OVEREXPRESSING ACE
50.0um
C
MCSF
FOLD DIFFERENCE
4.5
4
3.5
3
2.5
2
1.5
1
0.5
0
1
4.0
CONTROL
ACE
D
FOLD DIFFERENCE
200
150
100
50
0
0.6
1
139.0
183.5
196.6
CONTROL
THP-1 WT
ACE1
ACE2
ACE3
E
ACE1
ACE2
ACE3
FITC MFI
60
50
40
30
20
10
0
3.2
4.0
47.8
42.7
30.4
THP-1 WT
CONTROL
ACE1
ACE2
ACE3
F
CONTROL
THP-1 OVEREXPRESSING ACE
G
CONTROL
THP-1 OVEREXPRESSING ACE
H
MCSF
FOLD DIFFERENCE
5000
4500
4000
3500
3000
2500
2000
1500
1000
500
0
1
1895.1
4479.7
2741.0
CONTROL
ACE1
ACE2
ACE3

Figure 3. Expression of ACE and morphology of human monocytes overexpressing ACE. (A, B, C) Human primary monocytes were transiently transfected with empty or pcDNA3.1(-) plasmid carrying full coding sequence of ACE. Investigations of (A) ACE-expression, (B) cell morphology and (C) MCSF-expression were performed 24 h after transfection. Note differentiated, macrophage-like phenotype of primary monocytes overexpressing ACE. (D, E, F, G, H) Wild type (THP-1 WT), empty plasmid (Control) and ACE-overexpressing cells (ACE1, ACE2, ACE3) were investigated for (D) ACE transcript or (E) protein levels by employment of specific TaqMan probes or FACS analysis. (F) Representative immunofluorescence of control and ACE1 cells stained with FITC-ACE antibody (green) and DAPI staining (blue, nuclear). Note that left panel represents ACE staining only; right panel- ACE expression merged with DAPI; note mostly membrane-cytoplasmic localization of ACE. (G) Representative microscopic analysis of control and ACE1 cells under different magnifications. Note differentiated, macrophage-like phenotype of ACE1 cells. (H) RT-PCR analysis of MCSF expression in control and ACE-overexpressing cells (ACE1, ACE2, ACE3). Means ± SD of three independent experiments. * $p < 0.05$ indicates statistical significance.

Phenotype, attachment and adhesion of monocytes are affected by ACE

To demonstrate a functional correlation between ACE expression and adhesive properties of the monocytes, we transfected primary human monocytes or THP-1 cells with plasmid carrying full coding sequence of human ACE. As demonstrated in Fig. 3A, transient transfection of primary monocytes resulted not only in significantly increased overexpression of ACE, but also led to development of more differentiated, macrophage-like phenotype (Fig. 3B). In addition these cells showed higher expression of MCSF (Fig. 3C).

Due to the limited nature of transient transfection and very short life-span of primary monocytes, we generated THP-1 monocytes stably overexpressing ACE. For further experiments we selected three clones demonstrating the highest ACE levels (designated as ACE1, ACE2 and ACE3). Control cells were transfected with empty plasmid. The overexpression of ACE in THP-1 was verified by RT-PCR, FACS analysis and immunofluorescence microscopy (Fig. 3D, E, F). Similar to primary monocytes, ACE-clones revealed also a macrophage-like phenotype and significantly increased expression of MCSF (Fig. 3G, H). Further analysis of macrophage markers demonstrated noticeably elevated expression of Arg1; however no significant changes for Arg2 or iNOS were observed (Fig. 4A, B, C). Investigations of inflammation markers demonstrated a marked up-regulation of TNFa and IL-6 (Fig. 4D, E). These observations suggest that ACE may promote an alternative activation of the macrophages, leading to M2-phenotype with pro-inflammatory and pro-atherosclerotic properties.

Fig. 5A shows that these more differentiated, ACE-overexpressing cells revealed significantly decreased proliferation rates than corresponding controls. Furthermore, these cells demonstrated not only increased attachment to plastic surface (Fig. 5B), but also to endothelial human monolayers as compared to corresponding controls (Fig. 5C, D, E). To test whether uremia-mimicked conditions add to the transfection related effects we subjected wild type, empty plasmid and ACE1 cells to adhesion assays in the presence of HD or NS. As demonstrated in Fig. 5F, G treatment with HD not only led to significantly increased adhesion of control THP-1, but further amplified the adhesion of ACE1 cells.

Overexpression of ACE led to increased transmigratory potential

We observed that ACE-overexpressing cells possess stronger adhesion properties than corresponding controls. In order to investigate whether these cells are able to transmigrate faster through the endothelial barrier, we subjected wild type, control and ACE clones to transmigration assays. As demonstrated in Fig. 6A, the number of cells transmigrating through the membrane upon MCP-1 was significantly higher with ACE transfectants than corresponding controls. Significantly increased transmigratory potential of ACE clones was also demonstrated when the cells were transmigrated without MCP-1 towards an endothelial-monolayer seeded on the bottom of the chamber (Fig. 6B) or through an endothelial-barrier in the presence of MCP-1 (Fig. 6C, D, E).

We speculated that increased transmigration potential may be due to altered chemotactic signalling towards these cells. In order to prove this hypothesis, we investigated ACE-clones and control cells for the expression of MCP-1/CCL2 and its receptor CCR2. As demonstrated in Fig. 6F expression of MCP-1/CCL2 was noticeably increased in ACE-overexpressing cells than in empty plasmid cells and resulted in an up-regulation range of 13.7–15.4 fold. Similar results were obtained for CCR2 where FACS analysis revealed a 7.8–9.0 times increase in MFI as compared to corresponding control (Fig. 6G).

Increased ACE levels affect the expression of adhesion-related genes and the status of Angiotensin II receptors

The effect of ACE-overexpression on adhesion-related genes was tested by qPCR. As demonstrated in Fig. 7A, expression of ICAM-1 and VCAM-1 was noticeably increased in primary monocytes transiently overexpressing ACE (4.3 and 16.5 fold increase respectively). ACE overexpression also led to a strong increase in the expression of AT1R (increase by factor 11.8) and AT2R (13.3). Investigations on THP-1 monocytes stably overexpressing ACE revealed similar expression patterns to those observed in primary monocytes (Fig. 7B). Expression of ICAM-1 and VCAM-1 was strongly up-regulated in all ACE-clones when compared to control cells (increase 189.9–712.6 fold and 17.8–53.5 fold respectively). Further ACE-mediated up-regulations were also observed for two AngII-receptors AT1R (increase by factor 184.8–809.2) and AT2R (86.9–257.0).

Inhibition of ACE/AngII-receptor signalling and AT1R-blockage in AngII-treated THP-1 monocytes led to decreased adhesion to endothelial monolayers

To test whether inhibition of ACE/AngII-receptor signalling could affect the adhesive abilities of ACE-monocytes, the effects of ACE-inhibitor Captopril or AT1R-blocker Losartan were tested. As demonstrated in Fig. 8A, B, both drugs were effective in decreasing the endothelial adhesion of ACE-overexpressing monocytes significantly. These results suggest that higher endothelial-adhesion of ACE-overexpressing monocytes may be mediated by increased generation of local AngII and its receptor. To finally confirm these observations we subjected ACE-negative THP-1 wild type cells to adhesion assay with AngII and/or losartan. As demonstrated in Fig. 8C, adhesion of THP-1 is dramatically increased in the presence of AngII and almost totally abolished by AT1R-blockage (co-incubation with losartan).

Discussion

This study clearly demonstrates a role of mACE for the uremia-associated atherogenic potential of monocytes and suggests an

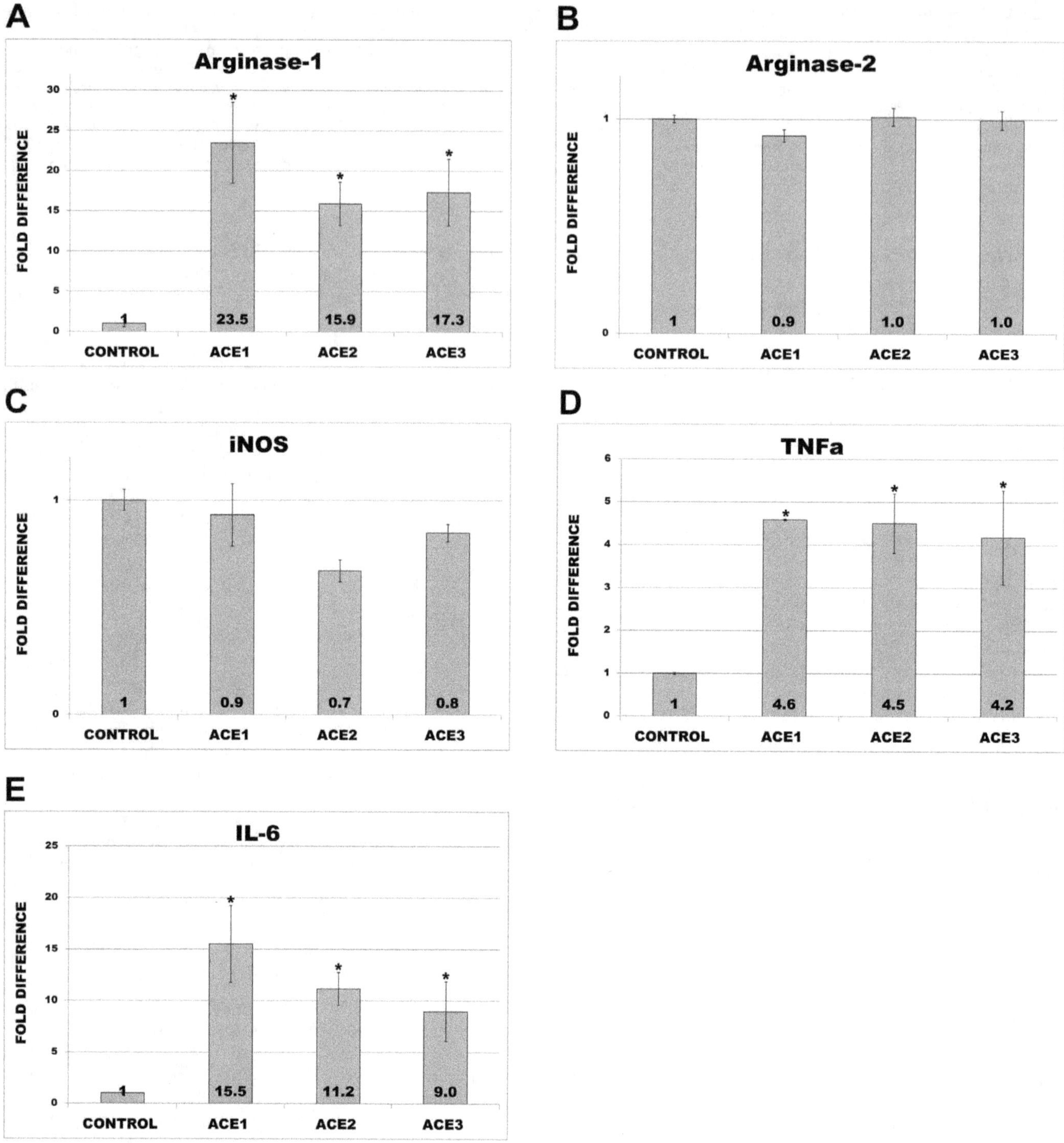

Figure 4. RT-PCR analysis of macrophage markers in control and THP-1 cells overexpressing ACE (ACE1, ACE2 and ACE3). Analyses were performed with primers specific for Arg1 (A), Arg2 (B), and iNOS (C), and TaqMan probes for TNFa (D) and IL6 (E). * $p < 0.05$ indicates statistical significance. Means ± SD of three independent experiments.

autocrine/paracrine mechanism of activation of these pro-atherogenic cells.

We found that both uremic and inflammatory conditions affect and regulate the expression of mACE. Our studies revealed that either treatment or prolonged monocyte differentiation in the presence of uremic or inflammatory conditions led to up-regulation of ACE. Furthermore, we were able to show that elevation of mACE coincided with increased transmigration and adhesion of these cells. To our knowledge, this is the first report demonstrating uremic elevation of mACE-expression in relation to pro-atherogenic behaviour of primary human monocytes or THP-1 cells. Such a potential of ACE was previously reported in animal and cell culture models but was not directly correlated with influences of uremia on human monocytes in vitro [26], [27], [28],

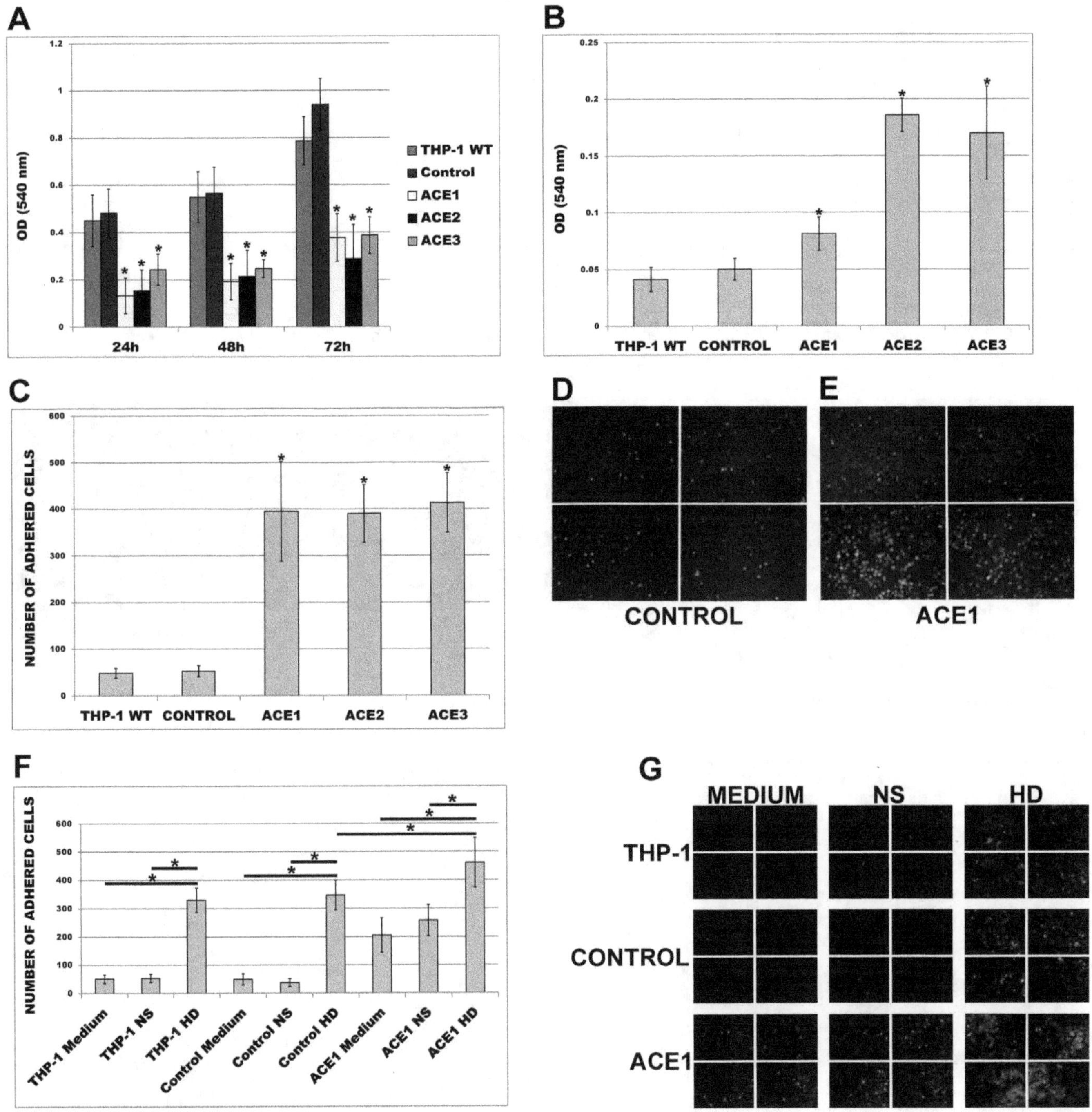

Figure 5. Proliferation, attachment and adhesion of ACE-overexpressing THP-1 monocytes investigated on wild type (THP-1 WT), empty plasmid (Control) and ACE-overexpressing cells (ACE1, ACE2, ACE3). (A) MTT-proliferation and (B) attachment of the cells. The cells for (B) were treated with 10 ng/ml PMA for 72 h prior to assay. (C, D, E, F, G) Adhesion of THP-1 to HUVEC endothelial monolayers. Calcein-labelled cells were incubated for 30 min in the presence of endothelial monolayers at the chamber bottom. Means ± SD of three independent experiments. (C) Adhesion under normal conditions (medium only, no FCS). See representative images (D, E). * $p < 0.05$ vs. control indicates statistical significance. (F) Adhesion under normal conditions or medium supplemented with 10% NS or HD sera. See representative images (G). * $p < 0.05$ indicates statistical significance. Note that for F and G one representative ACE-overexpressing clone (ACE1) was used. Analyses of (C, D, E, F, G) were performed in 10 random microscopic fields each. Means ± SD of cell number in 10 microscopic fields in three independent experiments.

[29]. With regards to other cell culture systems, it has been demonstrated that uremic toxins may affect oxidative burst activity of the leukocytes and increase their pro-inflammatory effects. This may contribute to the tendency to vascular damage in CKD [30]. Furthermore, Shimizu et al. reported that indoxyl sulphate (IS), one of the most representative uremic toxins, up-regulated AGT expression in proximal tubular cells [31]. In studies by Sun et al. IS and p-cresol sulphate up-regulated in addition to elevated AGT expression, other renin–angiotensin–aldosterone system (RAAS) components such as renin and AT1R [32]. Up-regulation of these

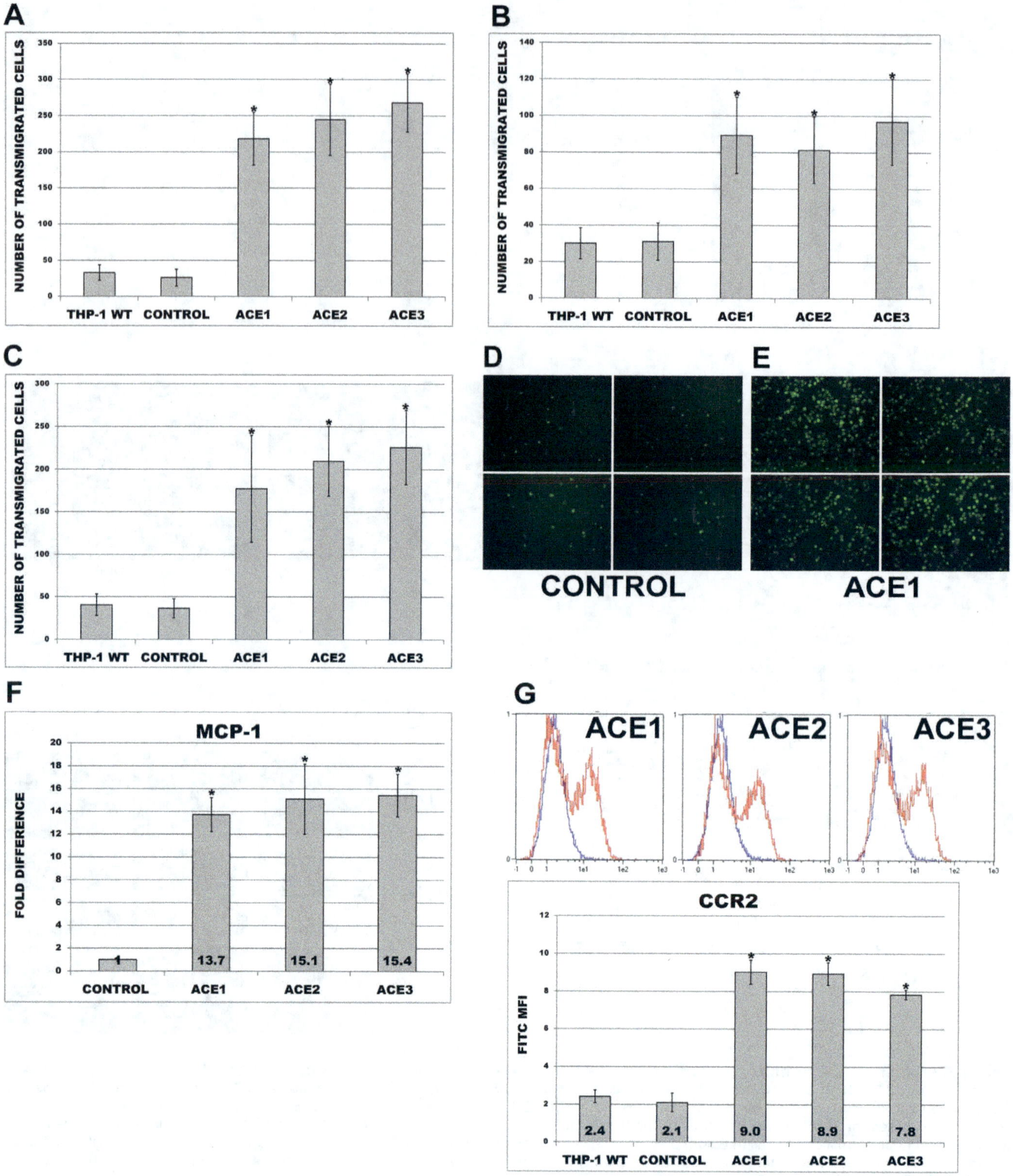

Figure 6. Transmigration of wild type (THP-1 WT), empty plasmid (Control) and ACE-overexpressing THP-1 monocytes (ACE1, ACE2, ACE3). (A) Transmigration of calcein-labelled cells through membrane towards (A) medium supplemented with MCP-1 or (B) HUVEC monolayers in the presence of medium only. (C, D, E) Transmigration of the cells through endothelial monolayers under MCP-1. See representative images (D, E). Analyses were performed in 10 random microscopic fields each. Means ± SD of cell number in 10 microscopic fields in three independent experiments. (F, G) Expression of MCP1 and CCR2 by RT-PCR and FACS analysis respectively. * $p < 0.05$ vs. control indicates statistical significance. Means ± SD of three independent experiments.

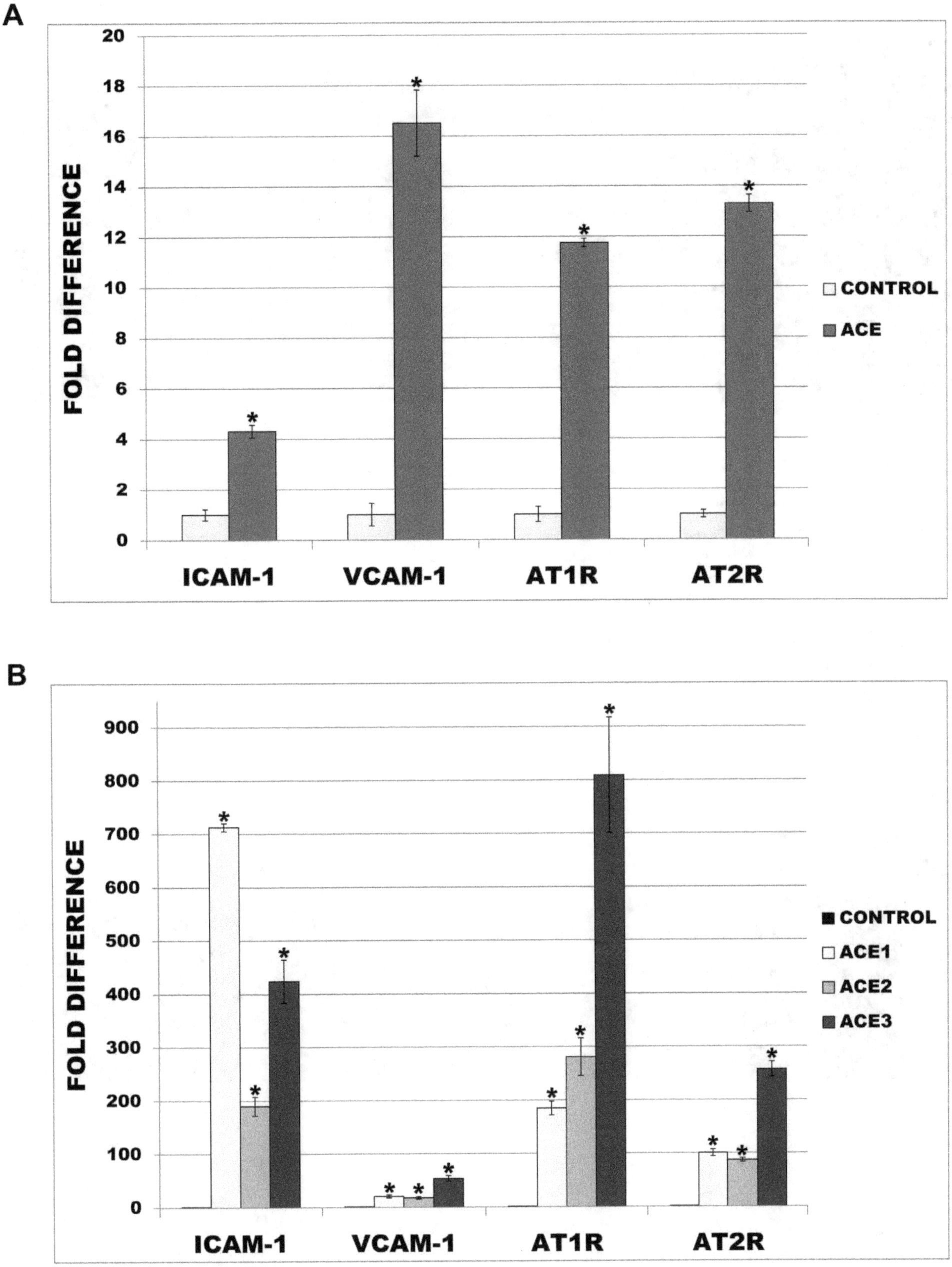

Figure 7. RT-PCR analysis of human primary monocytes and THP-1 cells overexpressing ACE. (A) Primary monocytes were transiently transfected with empty (Control) or ACE-plasmid and subjected to qPCR with primers specific for ICAM-1, VCAM-1, AT1R and AT2R. (B) Analysis of empty plasmid (Control) and ACE-overexpressing THP-1 monocytes (ACE1, ACE2, ACE3) were performed for the same transcripts. * $p < 0.05$ indicates statistical significance. Means ± SD of three independent experiments.

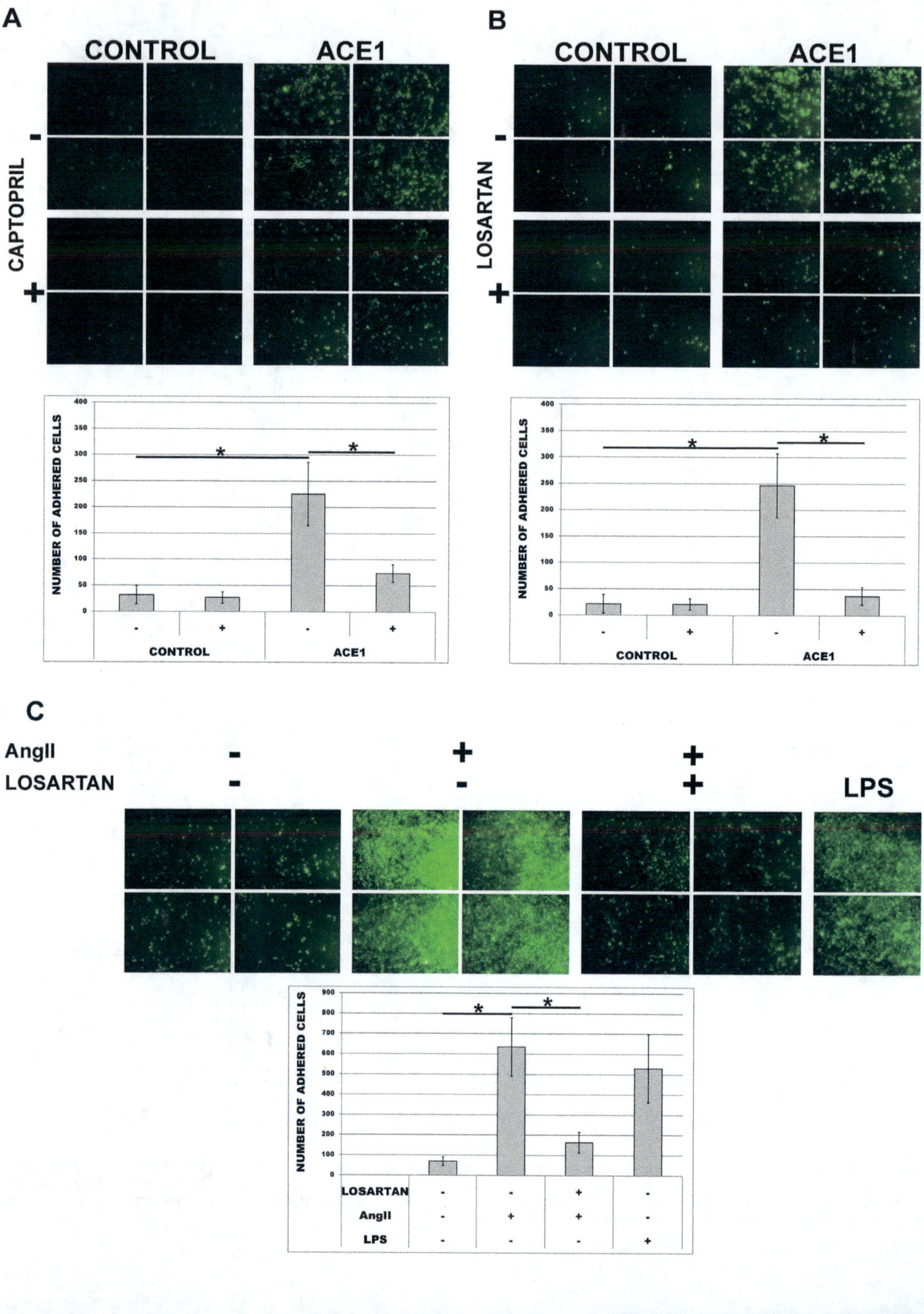
A
CONTROL
ACE1
CAPTOPRIL
-
+
NUMBER OF ADHERED CELLS
400
350
300
250
200
150
100
50
0
-
+
-
+
CONTROL
ACE1
B
CONTROL
ACE1
LOSARTAN
-
+
NUMBER OF ADHERED CELLS
CONTROL
ACE1
C
AngII
LOSARTAN
LPS
NUMBER OF ADHERED CELLS
900
800
700
600
500
400
300
200
100
0
LOSARTAN
AngII
LPS

Figure 8. Effect of the ACE-inhibitor Captopril, the AngII-receptor blocker Losartan and AngII on adhesion of wild type (THP-1 WT), empty plasmid (Control) and ACE-overexpressing cells (ACE1). Calcein-labelled cells were incubated in the presence or absence of (A) 500 nM captopril or (B) 1 μM losartan for 30 min and tested for their adhesion abilities to endothelial HUVEC monolayers. (C) Endothelial-adhesion of ACE-negative wild type THP-1 cells in the presence of 1 μM AngII only or co-incubation with 1 μM losartan investigated for 30 min. Representative images for (A, B, C) are shown. Analyses for (A, B, C) were performed in 10 random microscopic fields each. * $p < 0.05$ indicates statistical significance. Means ± SD of cell number in 10 microscopic fields in three independent experiments.

RAAS components may subsequently exert, as observed in our study, increased expression of mACE and facilitate behavioural and morphological changes of the monocytes under uremia. Indeed, previous studies reported a possible link between uremic toxins and cardiovascular diseases. The authors demonstrated that uremia-mediated increase in leukocyte-endothelial adhesion occurs through elevation of E-selectin in HUVEC cells and is mediated via the JNK- and NF-κB-dependent pathway [33]. Furthermore, the studies by Vanholder et al. and Pletinck et al. showed clearly that proinflammatory effects exerted by protein-bound uremic toxins contribute to vascular damage and renal disease progression by stimulating crosstalk between leukocytes and vessels [34,35]. On the other hand the existence of lipid or smooth muscle-derived serum factor which could be responsible for such alterations had been previously speculated [16], [36]. The levels of oxidized LDL are generally increased in hemodialysis patients and previous reports demonstrated that local AngII production increases as macrophages become activated by ox-LDL [37], [38]. Also the levels of MCP-1 and its receptor in uremic serum and atherosclerotic plaques were reported to be significantly higher than in healthy controls and could be the reason of increased transmigration [39].

What are the consequences of ACE-overexpression in human monocytes? Microscopic investigations revealed noticeable alterations in cell morphology. Introduction of ACE into monocytes changed not only their structure towards macrophage-like cells, but also dramatically elevated the expression of MCSF. These observations correlate with previous findings demonstrating that accumulation of monocyte-derived macrophages at the sites of endothelial dysfunction is a crucial event in atherogenesis [40]. Our data suggest that ACE mediates an alternative activation of macrophages and may promote M2-phenotype with pro-inflammatory and pro-atherosclerotic properties. ACE-overexpressing cells revealed not only significantly elevated levels of Arg1, but also pro-inflammatory cytokines TNFa and IL-6. It has been demonstrated that such M2 macrophages have a higher capacity to accumulate modified lipids than M1 and upon exposure to ox-LDL the pro-inflammatory responses of M2 cells are increased [41]. Furthermore, M2 cells are present in plaques where surround the lipid core. Arg1, typical for these cells, may promote stabilisation of atherosclerotic plaques and enhance the proliferation of vascular smooth muscle cells [42].

We demonstrated that ACE-overexpressing monocytes transmigrate through endothelial barrier significantly faster than corresponding controls as they express not only more MCP-1 but also its ligand CCR2. These novel findings are extremely important because the motility of these cells may be boosted in an autocrine manner independently from endothelial function. The fact that MCP-1 is up-regulated in atherosclerotic plaques and arteries of animals fed a high cholesterol diet and that disruption of CCR2 in mouse models is related to anti-atherosclerotic actions [43], [44], [45], [46], [47], allows us to designate ACE-overexpressing monocytes as highly pro-atherogenic.

Studies in mice revealed that infusion of AngII led not only to increased plaque size, but also induced the expression of inflammatory TNFa, IL-6, and migration-related MCP-1, CCR2 in aortic roots. In that study disruption of MCP-1 led to decrease in AngII-mediated pro-atherosclerotic events [48]. Interestingly, in CCR2 knock-out mice or mice bearing specific leukocyte CCR2-deficiency, AngII was not able to induce previously described vascular remodelling but promoted the development of left ventricular hypertrophy instead [49]. In studies by Chen at al. the authors demonstrated that ACE deficiency in bone marrow–derived cells decreased hypercholesterolemia-induced atherosclerosis and correlated with reduced levels of MCP-1[17].

ACE overexpression led to a marked up-regulation of ICAM-1 and VCAM-1 in monocytes. Expression and induction of these molecules has been consistently observed in the initial steps of atherosclerosis and in atherosclerotic plaques [50], [51]. Disruption or antibody-mediated blockage of these molecular targets proved to exert beneficial effects on atherogenesis [52], [53].

It is well documented that ACE-inhibition and/or anti-AngII-receptor treatment has anti-atherosclerotic effects in experimental models as well as patients with cardiovascular disease [54], [55], [56]. We found in our study that introduction of ACE into monocytes led to dramatically increased expression of AngII-receptors, AT1R and AT2R. ACE-inhibition or AngII-receptor blockage significantly decreased the adhesion of these monocytes to endothelial cells. These novel findings suggest that inhibition of local, monocyte-derived AngII-generation might exert anti-atherogenic actions.

Da Cunha et al. reported that subcutaneous infusions of AngII led to accelerated carotid atherosclerosis in apolipoprotein E-deficient mice. Additionally increased expression of adhesion molecules such as E-selectin, ICAM-1, VCAM-1, chemokine MCP-1, and MCSF was demonstrated. Enalapril, an ACE-inhibitor, reduced these expressions and the number of adhered macrophages and foam cells in the arterial wall [57].

We found that uremic serum on the one hand induces ACE overexpression, thus creating pro-atherogenic monocytes. In addition, uremic serum serves as an additional amplifier of monocyte-endothelial adhesion even for the cells already overexpressing ACE. This suggests that ACE induction is an important but most likely not the only mechanism by which uremia enhances monocyte endothelium interactions.

In summary we demonstrate uremia-induced elevation of ACE expression paralleled by a pro-atherogenic nature of ACE-overexpressing monocytes, partially mediated by enhancement of migratory and adhesion potential to endothelial monolayers. Inhibition of local, monocyte-derived AngII-generation exerts anti-atherosclerotic actions in vitro. These findings justify further investigation and verification in animal models.

Acknowledgments

We are very grateful to Mrs Manuela Hajri and Mrs Beate Heinze for their excellent technical assistance.

Author Contributions

Conceived and designed the experiments: BT CU MG. Performed the experiments: BT CU. Analyzed the data: BT CU. Contributed reagents/materials/analysis tools: ES RF. Contributed to the writing of the manuscript: BT MG.

References

1. Foley RN, Parfrey PS, Sarnak MJ (1998). Clinical epidemiology of cardiovascular disease in chronic renal disease. Am J Kidney 32: 112–119.
2. Cheung AK, Sarnak MJ, Yan G, Dwyer JT, Heyka RJ, et al. (2000) Atherosclerotic cardiovascular disease risks in chronic hemodialysis patients. Kidney Int 58: 353–362.
3. Vanholder R, Massy Z, Argiles A, Spasovski G, Verbeke F, et al. (2005) Chronic kidney disease as cause of cardiovascular morbidity and mortality. Nephrol Dial Transplant 20:1048–1056.
4. Chronic Kidney Disease Prognosis Consortium, Matsushita K, van der Velde M, Astor BC, Woodward M, et al. (2010) Association of estimated glomerular filtration rate and albuminuria with all-cause and cardiovascular mortality in general population cohorts: a collaborative meta-analysis. Lancet 12: 2073–2081.
5. Tyralla K, Amann K (2003) Morphology of the heart and arteries in renal failure. Kidney Int Suppl 84: 80–83.
6. Guerin AP, Blacher J, Pannier B, Marchais SJ, Safar ME, et al. (2001) Impact of aortic stiffness attenuation on survival of patients in end-stage renal failure. Circulation 103: 987–992.
7. Ulrich C, Seibert E, Heine GH, Fliser D, Girndt M (2011) Monocyte angiotensin converting enzyme expression may be associated with atherosclerosis rather than arteriosclerosis in hemodialysis patients. Clin J Am Soc Nephrol 6: 505–511.
8. Ross R (1993) The pathogenesis of atherosclerosis: a perspective for the 1990s. Nature 362: 801–809.
9. Steinberg D (2002) Atherogenesis in perspective: hypercholesterolemia and inflammation as partners in crime. Nature Med 8: 1211–1217.
10. Moore KJ, Tabas I (2011) Macrophages in the pathogenesis of atherosclerosis. Cell 145: 341–355.
11. Khallou-Laschet J, Varthaman A, Fornasa G, Compain C, Gaston AT, et al. (2010) Macrophage plasticity in experimental atherosclerosis. PLoS One 5: e8852.
12. Pello OM, Silvestre C, De Pizzol M, Andres V (2012) A glimpse on the phenomenon of macrophage polarization during atherosclerosis. Immunobiology 216: 1172–1176.
13. Martinez FO, Helming L, Gordon S (2009) Alternative activation of macrophages: an immunologic functional perspective. Annu Rev Immunol 27: 451–483.
14. Gratchev A, Kzhyshkowska J, Utikal J, Goerdt S (2005) Interleukin-4 and dexamethasone counterregulate extracellular matrix remodelling and phagocytosis in type-2 macrophages. Scand J Immunol 61: 10–17.
15. Xu W, Roos A, Schlagwein N, Woltman AM, Daha MR, et al. (2006) IL-10-producing macrophages preferentially clear early apoptotic cells. Blood 107: 4930–4937.
16. Kohlstedt K, Trouvain C, Namgaladze D, Fleming I (2011) Adipocyte-derived lipids increase angiotensin-converting enzyme (ACE) expression and modulate macrophage phenotype. Basic Res Cardiol 106: 205–215.
17. Chen X, Lu H, Zhao M, Tashiro K, Cassis LA, et al. (2013) Contributions of leukocyte angiotensin-converting enzyme to development of atherosclerosis. Arterioscler Thromb Vasc Biol 33: 2075–2080.
18. Schieffer B, Schieffer E, Hilfiker-Kleiner D, Hilfiker A, Kovanen PT, et al. (2000) Expression of angiotensin II and interleukin 6 in human coronary atherosclerotic plaques: potential implications for inflammation and plaque instability. Circulation 101: 1372–1378.
19. O'Brien KD, Shavelle DM, Caulfield MT, McDonald TO, Olin-Lewis K, et al. (2002) Association of angiotensin-converting enzyme with low-density lipoprotein in aortic valvular lesions and in human plasma. Circulation 106: 2224–2230.
20. Ouimet T, Lancelot E, Hyafil F, Rienzo M, Deux F, et al. (2012) Molecular and cellular targets of the MRI contrast agent P947 for atherosclerosis imaging. Mol Pharm 9: 850–861.
21. Shen XZ, Billet S, Lin C, Okwan-Duodu D, Chen X, et al. (2011) The carboxypeptidase ACE shapes the MHC class I peptide repertoire. Nat Immunol 12: 1078–1085.
22. Kitazono T, Padgett RC, Armstrong ML, Tompkins PK, Heistad DD (1995) Evidence that angiotensin II is present in human monocytes. Circulation 91: 1129–1134.
23. Yusuf S, Sleight P, Pogue J, Bosch J, Davies R, et al. (2000) Effects of an angiotensin-converting-enzyme inhibitor, ramipril, on cardiovascular events in high-risk patients. The Heart Outcomes Prevention Evaluation Study Investigators. N Engl J Med 342: 145–153.
24. Ulrich C, Heine GH, Seibert E, Fliser D, Girndt M (2010) Circulating monocyte subpopulations with high expression of angiotensin-converting enzyme predict mortality in patients with end-stage renal disease. Nephrol Dial Transplant 25: 2265–2272.
25. Ulrich C, Heine GH, Garcia P, Reichart B, Georg T, et al. (2006) Increased expression of monocytic angiotensin-converting enzyme in dialysis patients with cardiovascular disease. Nephrol Dial Transplant 21: 1596–1602.
26. Simolin MA, Pedersen TX, Bro S, Mäyränpää MI, Helske S, et al. (2009) ACE inhibition attenuates uremia-induced aortic valve thickening in a novel mouse model. BMC Cardiovasc Disord 9: 10.
27. Petrov MN, Shilo VY, Tarasov AV, Schwartz DE, Garcia JG, et al. (2012) Conformational changes of blood ACE in chronic uremia. PLoS One 7: e49290.
28. Finch JL, Suarez EB, Husain K, Ferder L, Cardema MC, et al. (2012) Effect of combining an ACE inhibitor and a VDR activator on glomerulosclerosis, proteinuria, and renal oxidative stress in uremic rats. Am J Physiol Renal Physiol 302: 141–149.
29. Mizobuchi M, Ogata H, Hosaka N, Kumata C, Nakazawa A, et al. (2011) Effects of calcimimetic combined with an angiotensin-converting enzyme inhibitor on uremic cardiomyopathy progression. Am J Nephrol 34: 256–260.
30. Schepers E, Meert N, Glorieux G, Goeman J, Van der Eycken J, et al. (2007) P-cresylsulphate, the main in vivo metabolite of p-cresol, activates leucocyte free radical production. Nephrol Dial Transplant 22: 592–596.
31. Shimizu H, Saito S, Higashiyama Y, Nishijima F, Niwa T (2013) CREB, NF-κB, and NADPH oxidase coordinately upregulate indoxyl sulfate-induced angiotensinogen expression in proximal tubular cells. Am J Physiol Cell Physiol 304: 685–692.
32. Sun CY, Chang SC, Wu MS (2012) Uremic toxins induce kidney fibrosis by activating intrarenal renin-angiotensin-aldosterone system associated epithelial-to-mesenchymal transition. PLoS One. 2012;7: e34026.
33. Ito S, Osaka M, Higuchi Y, Nishijima F, Ishii H, et al. (2010) Indoxyl sulfate induces leukocyte-endothelial interactions through up-regulation of E-selectin. J Biol Chem 285: 38869-38875.
34. Vanholder R, Schepers E, Pletinck A, Nagler EV, Glorieux G. (2014) The Uremic Toxicity of Indoxyl Sulfate and p-Cresyl Sulfate: A Systematic Review. J Am Soc Nephrol.
35. Pletinck A, Glorieux G, Schepers E, Cohen G, Gondouin B, et al. (2013) Protein-bound uremic toxins stimulate crosstalk between leukocytes and vessel wall. J Am Soc Nephrol 24: 1981–1994.
36. Metzger R, Franke FE, Bohle RM, Alhenc-Gelas F, Danilov SM (2011) Heterogeneous distribution of angiotensin I-converting enzyme (CD143) in the human and rat vascular systems: vessel, organ and species specificity. Microvasc Res 81: 206–215.
37. Diet F, Pratt RE, Berry GJ, Momose N, Gibbons GH, et al. (1996) Increased accumulation of tissue ACE in human atherosclerotic coronary artery disease. Circulation 94: 2756–2767.
38. Rafatian N, Milne RW, Leenen FH, Whitman SC (2013) Role of Renin Angiotensin System in Activation of Macrophages by modified Lipoproteins. Am J Physiol Heart Circ Physiol 305: 1309–1320.
39. Okumoto S, Taniguchi Y, Nakashima A, Masaki T, Ito T, et al. (2009) C–C chemokine receptor 2 expression by circulating monocytes influences atherosclerosis in patients on chronic hemodialysis. Ther Apher Dial 13: 205–212.
40. Stöger JL, Gijbels MJ, van der Velden S, Manca M, van der Loos CM, et al. (2012) Distribution of macrophage polarization markers in human atherosclerosis. Atherosclerosis 2012;225:461–468.
41. van Tits LJ, Stienstra R, van Lent PL, Netea MG, Joosten LA, et al. (2011) Oxidized LDL enhances pro-inflammatory responses of alternatively activated M2 macrophages: a crucial role for Krüppel-like factor 2. Atherosclerosis 214: 345–349.
42. Pourcet B, Pineda-Torra I (2013) Transcriptional regulation of macrophage arginase 1 expression and its role in atherosclerosis. Trends Cardiovasc Med 23: 143–152.
43. Libby P, Geng YJ, Aikawa M, Schoenbeck U, Mach F, et al. (1996) Macrophages and atherosclerotic plaque stability. Curr Opin Lipidol 7: 330–335.
44. Nelken NA, Coughlin SR, Gordon D, Wilcox JN (1991) Monocyte chemoattractant protein-1 in human atheromatous plaques. J Clin Invest 88: 1121–1127.
45. Wiesner P, Tafelmeier M, Chittka D, Choi SH, Zhang L, et al. (2013) MCP-1 binds to oxidized LDL and is carried by lipoprotein(a) in human plasma. J Lipid Res 54: 1877–1883.
46. Boring L, Gosling J, Cleary M, Charo IF (1998) Decreased lesion formation in CCR2-/- mice reveals a role for chemokines in the initiation of atherosclerosis. Nature 394: 894–897.
47. Dawson TC, Kuziel WA, Osahar TA, Maeda N (1999) Absence of CC chemokine receptor-2 reduces atherosclerosis in apolipoprotein E-deficient mice. Atherosclerosis 143:205–211.
48. Ni W, Kitamoto S, Ishibashi M, Usui M, Inoue S, et al. (2004) Monocyte chemoattractant protein-1 is an essential inflammatory mediator in angiotensin II-induced progression of established atherosclerosis in hypercholesterolemic mice. Arterioscler Thromb Vasc Biol 24: 534–539.
49. Ishibashi M, Hiasa K, Zhao Q, Inoue S, Ohtani K, et al. (2004) Critical role of monocyte chemoattractant protein-1 receptor CCR2 on monocytes in hypertension-induced vascular inflammation and remodeling. Circ Res 94: 1203–1210.
50. Blankenberg S, Barbaux S, Tiret L (2003) Adhesion molecules and atherosclerosis. Atherosclerosis 170: 191–203.
51. Tuttolomondo A, Di Raimondo D, Pecoraro R, Arnao V, Pinto A, et al. (2012) Atherosclerosis as an inflammatory disease: Curr Pharm Des 18: 4266–4288.
52. De Meyer I, Martinet W, De Meyer GR (2012) Therapeutic strategies to deplete macrophages in atherosclerotic plaques. Br J Clin Pharmacol 74: 246–263.

53. Lal H, Guleria RS, Foster DM, Lu G, Watson LE, et al. (2007) Integrins: novel therapeutic targets for cardiovascular diseases. Cardiovasc Hematol Agents Med Chem 5: 109–132.

54. Kojima C, Kawakami A, Takei T, Nitta K, Yoshida M (2007) Angiotensin-converting enzyme inhibitor attenuates monocyte adhesion to vascular endothelium through modulation of intracellular zinc. J Pharmacol Exp Ther 323: 855–860.

55. Bernardi S, Candido R, Toffoli B, Carretta R, Fabris B (2011) Prevention of accelerated atherosclerosis by AT1 receptor blockade in experimental renal failure. Nephrol Dial Transplant 26: 832–838.

56. Koga J, Egashira K, Matoba T, Kubo M, Ihara Y, et al (2008) Essential role of angiotensin II type 1a receptors in the host vascular wall, but not the bone marrow, in the pathogenesis of angiotensin II-induced atherosclerosis. Hypertens Res 31: 1791–1800.

57. da Cunha V, Tham DM, Martin-McNulty B, Deng G, Ho JJ, et al (2005) Enalapril attenuates angiotensin II-induced atherosclerosis and vascular inflammation. Atherosclerosis 178: 9–17.

Permissions

All chapters in this book were first published in PLOS ONE, by The Public Library of Science; hereby published with permission under the Creative Commons Attribution License or equivalent. Every chapter published in this book has been scrutinized by our experts. Their significance has been extensively debated. The topics covered herein carry significant findings which will fuel the growth of the discipline. They may even be implemented as practical applications or may be referred to as a beginning point for another development.

The contributors of this book come from diverse backgrounds, making this book a truly international effort. This book will bring forth new frontiers with its revolutionizing research information and detailed analysis of the nascent developments around the world.

We would like to thank all the contributing authors for lending their expertise to make the book truly unique. They have played a crucial role in the development of this book. Without their invaluable contributions this book wouldn't have been possible. They have made vital efforts to compile up to date information on the varied aspects of this subject to make this book a valuable addition to the collection of many professionals and students.

This book was conceptualized with the vision of imparting up-to-date information and advanced data in this field. To ensure the same, a matchless editorial board was set up. Every individual on the board went through rigorous rounds of assessment to prove their worth. After which they invested a large part of their time researching and compiling the most relevant data for our readers.

The editorial board has been involved in producing this book since its inception. They have spent rigorous hours researching and exploring the diverse topics which have resulted in the successful publishing of this book. They have passed on their knowledge of decades through this book. To expedite this challenging task, the publisher supported the team at every step. A small team of assistant editors was also appointed to further simplify the editing procedure and attain best results for the readers.

Apart from the editorial board, the designing team has also invested a significant amount of their time in understanding the subject and creating the most relevant covers. They scrutinized every image to scout for the most suitable representation of the subject and create an appropriate cover for the book.

The publishing team has been an ardent support to the editorial, designing and production team. Their endless efforts to recruit the best for this project, has resulted in the accomplishment of this book. They are a veteran in the field of academics and their pool of knowledge is as vast as their experience in printing. Their expertise and guidance has proved useful at every step. Their uncompromising quality standards have made this book an exceptional effort. Their encouragement from time to time has been an inspiration for everyone.

The publisher and the editorial board hope that this book will prove to be a valuable piece of knowledge for researchers, students, practitioners and scholars across the globe.

List of Contributors

Zaida Noemy Cabrera Jimenez, Benedito Jorge Pereira, João Egidio Romão Jr, Sonia Cristina da Silva Makida, Hugo Abensur, Rosa Maria Affonso Moyses, Rosilene Motta Elias
Renal Division, Internal Medicine, Hospital das Clínicas, University of São Paulo School of Medicine, São Paulo, Brazil

Dvora Rubinger, Rebecca Backenroth, Dan Sapoznikov
Nephrology and Hypertension Services, Department of Medicine, Hadassah University Medical Center, Jerusalem, Israel

Carlo A. Gaillard
Department of Nephrology, VU Medical Center, Amsterdam, The Netherlands

Neelke C. van der Weerd
Department of Nephrology, VU Medical Center, Amsterdam, The Netherlands
Department of Nephrology, Academic Medical Center, University of Amsterdam, Amsterdam, The Netherlands

Muriel P. C. Grooteman, Menso J. Nubé, Piet M. ter Wee
Department of Nephrology, VU Medical Center, Amsterdam, The Netherlands
Institute for Cardiovascular Research VU Medical Center (ICaR-VU), VU Medical Center, Amsterdam, The Netherlands

E. Lars Penne
Department of Nephrology, VU Medical Center, Amsterdam, The Netherlands
Department of Nephrology, University Medical Center Utrecht, Utrecht, The Netherlands

Michiel L. Bots
Julius Center for Health Sciences and Primary Care, University Medical Center Utrecht, Utrecht, The Netherlands

Marinus A. van den Dorpel
Department of Internal Medicine, Maasstad Hospital, Rotterdam, The Netherlands

Claire H. den Hoedt
Department of Internal Medicine, Maasstad Hospital, Rotterdam, The Netherlands
Department of Nephrology, University Medical Center Utrecht, Utrecht, The Netherlands

Albert H. A. Mazairac, Peter J. Blankestijn
Department of Nephrology, University Medical Center Utrecht, Utrecht, The Netherlands

Jack F. M. Wetzels
Department of Nephrology, Radboud University Nijmegen Medical Center, Nijmegen, The Netherlands

Erwin T. Wiegerinck, Dorine W. Swinkels
Department of Laboratory Medicine, Laboratory of Genetic, Endocrine and Metabolic Diseases, Radboud University Nijmegen Medical Center, Nijmegen, The Netherlands
Radboud University Nijmegen Medical Center, Nijmegen, The Netherlands

Yao-Ping Lin, Chih-Yu Yang
Institute of Clinical Medicine, School of Medicine, National Yang-Ming University, Taipei, Taiwan

Wen-Chung Yu
Department of Medicine, Taipei Veterans General Hospital, Taipei, Taiwan

Chen-Chung Liao
Proteomics Research Center, National Yang-Ming University, Taipei, Taiwan

Chin-Wen Chi
Department of Medical Research and Education, Taipei Veterans General Hospital, Taipei, Taiwan

Chao- Hsiung Lin
Proteomics Research Center, National Yang-Ming University, Taipei, Taiwan
Department of Medical Research and Education, Taipei Veterans General Hospital, Taipei, Taiwan
Department of Life Sciences and Institute of Genomic Sciences, National Yang-Ming University, Taipei, Taiwan
Department of Education and Research, Taipei City Hospital, Taipei, Taiwan

Vassilios Liakopoulos
Department of Nephrology, University of Thessaly, Larissa, Thessaly, Greece

Ioannis Stefanidis, Giorgos K. Sakkas
Department of Nephrology, University of Thessaly, Larissa, Thessaly, Greece
Centre for Research and Technology – Thessaly, Volos, Thessaly, Greece

Christoforos D. Giannaki
Department of Nephrology, University of Thessaly, Larissa, Thessaly, Greece
Centre for Research and Technology - Thessaly, Volos, Thessaly, Greece
Department of Life and Health Sciences, University of Nicosia, Nicosia, Cyprus

Georgios M. Hadjigeorgiou
Department of Neurology, University of Thessaly, Larissa, Thessaly, Greece
Centre for Research and Technology - Thessaly, Volos, Thessaly, Greece

Georgios N. Koukoulis
Department of Endocrinology, School of Medicine, University of Thessaly, Larissa, Thessaly, Greece

Eleftherios Lavdas
Department of Medical Radiological Technologists, Technological Educational Institute of Athens, Athens, Attika, Greece

Christina Karatzaferi, Yiannis Koutedakis
Department of Sport Science, University of Thessaly, Trikala, Thessaly, Greece
Centre for Research and Technology - Thessaly, Volos, Thessaly, Greece

Nikolaos Tsianas
Department of Nephrology, General Hospital of Trikala, Trikala, Thessaly Greece

Ferruh Artunc, Andreas Peter, Claus Thamer, Peter Weyrich, Hans-Ulrich Haering
Department of Internal Medicine, Division of Endocrinology, Diabetology, Vascular Disease, Nephrology and Clinical Chemistry, University of Tuebingen, Germany

Bjoern Friedrich
Department of Internal Medicine, Division of Endocrinology, Diabetology, Vascular Disease, Nephrology and Clinical Chemistry, University of Tuebingen, Germany
Dialysis Center, Leonberg, Germany

Christian Mueller, Tobias Breidthardt, Raphael Twerenbold
Department of Internal Medicine, Division of Cardiology, University of Basel, Basel, Switzerland

Laura E. A. Harrison, James O. Burton
Department of Renal Medicine, Royal Derby Hospital, Derby, United Kingdom

Christopher W. McIntyre
Department of Renal Medicine, Royal Derby Hospital, Derby, United Kingdom
School of Graduate Entry Medicine and Health, University of Nottingham, Derby, United Kingdom

Cheuk-Chun Szeto, Philip K. T. Li
Department of Medicine and Therapeutics, Chinese University of Hong Kong, Hong Kong, China

Tzong-Shyuan Lee
Department and Institute of Physiology, National Yang-Ming University, Taipei, Taiwan

Der-Cherng Tarng
Department and Institute of Physiology, National Yang-Ming University, Taipei, Taiwan
Institute of Clinical Medicine, National Yang-Ming University, Taipei, Taiwan
Division of Nephrology, Department of Medicine and Immunology Centre, Taipei Veterans General Hospital, Taipei, Taiwan

Ko-Lin Kuo
Department and Institute of Physiology, National Yang-Ming University, Taipei, Taiwan
School of Medicine, Tzu Chi University, Hualien, Taiwan
Division of Nephrology, Buddhist Tzu Chi General Hospital, Taipei Branch, Taipei, Taiwan

Chih-Pei Lin
Department of Biotechnology and Laboratory Science in Medicine and Institute of Biotechnology in Medicine, National Yang-Ming University, Taipei, Taiwan
Division of General Laboratory, Department of Pathology and Laboratory Medicine, Taipei Veterans General Hospital, Taipei, Taiwan

Szu-Chun Hung
School of Medicine, Tzu Chi University, Hualien, Taiwan
Division of Nephrology, Buddhist Tzu Chi General Hospital, Taipei Branch, Taipei, Taiwan

Yao-Ping Lin, Ching-Fang Tang
Division of Nephrology, Department of Medicine and Immunology Centre, Taipei Veterans General Hospital, Taipei, Taiwan
Filippo Martino, Mascha Schmidt, Yvonne Görzig
Institute for Molecular and Translational Treatment Strategies (IMTTS), Hannover Medical School, Hannover, Germany

Johan Lorenzen
Institute for Molecular and Translational Treatment Strategies (IMTTS), Hannover Medical School, Hannover, Germany
Department of Medicine, Division of Nephrology and Hypertension, Hannover Medical School, Hannover, Germany

Thomas Thum
Institute for Molecular and Translational Treatment Strategies (IMTTS), Hannover Medical School, Hannover, Germany
Centre of Clinical and Basic Research, IRCCS San Raffaele, Rome, Italy

Jan T. Kielstein, Julius Schmidt, Michael Broll
Department of Medicine, Division of Nephrology and Hypertension, Hannover Medical School, Hannover, Germany

Jie Cao, Qiuli Chen, Huaqun Zhang, Peipei Qi, Chao Liu, Xufang Yang, Jinhong Wang, Wei Pan
Department of Microbiology, Shanghai Key Laboratory of Medical Biodefense, Second Military Medical University, Shanghai, China

Shaohua Jiang
Department of Microbiology, Shanghai Key Laboratory of Medical Biodefense, Second Military Medical University, Shanghai, China,
Department of Cardiothoracic Surgery, The Military General Hospital of Tibet PLA, Lasa, China,

Hua Yang
Department of Microbiology, Shanghai Key Laboratory of Medical Biodefense, Second Military Medical University, Shanghai, China
Shanghai Key Laboratory of Tuberculosis, Shanghai Pulmonary Hospital, Tongji University School of Medicine, Shanghai, China

Niansong Wang
Department of Nephrology, Zhongshan Hospital, Fudan University, Shanghai, China
Department of Nephrology, Shanghai Sixth People's Hospital, Shanghai Jiao Tong University, Shanghai, China

Baohua Qian
Department of Blood Transfusion, Changhai Hospital, Second Military Medical University, Shanghai, China

Shuhan Sun
Department of Medical Genetics, Second Military Medical University, Shanghai, China

Meiliang Wang
Center for Experimental Medicine, Lanzhou General Hospital, Lanzhou Military Command, Lanzhou, Gansu, China

Ling Hui, Xiaoqin Ha
Center for Experimental Medicine, Lanzhou General Hospital, Lanzhou Military Command, Lanzhou, Gansu, China
Gansu Key Laboratory of Stem Cell and Gene Therapy, Lanzhou, Gansu, China

Jiuping Wang, Tianping Wang, Jing Li
Department of Infectious Diseases, Tangdu Hospital, the Fourth Military Medical University, Xi'an, Shaanxi, China

Hung-Yuan Chen, Yen-Lin Chiu, Shih-Ping Hsu, Mei-Fen Pai, Ju-Yeh Yang, Yu-Sen Peng
Division of Nephrology, Department of Internal Medicine, Far Eastern Memorial Hospital, New Taipei City, Taiwan
Division of Nephrology, Department of Internal Medicine, National Taiwan University Hospital and National Taiwan University College of Medicine, Taipei, Taiwan

Chien-Chu Lin
Division of Gastroenterology and Hepatology, Department of Internal Medicine, Far Eastern Memorial Hospital, New Taipei City, Taiwan

Ganpat J. Dahe, Sachin S. Kadam, Jayesh R. Bellare
Department of Chemical Engineering, Indian Institute of Technology Bombay, Powai, Mumbai, India

Siddharth S. Sabale, Dattatray P. Kadam
Department of Veterinary Pathology, Bombay Veterinary College, Parel, Mumbai, India

Laxman B. Sarkate
Department of Surgery & Radiology, Bombay Veterinary College, Parel, Mumbai, India

Yoke Mun Chan
Institute of Gerontology, University Putra Malaysia, Serdang, Malaysia
Department of Nutrition and Dietetics, Faculty of Medicine and Health Sciences, University Putra Malaysia, Serdang, Malaysia

Mohd Shariff Zalilah
Department of Nutrition and Dietetics, Faculty of Medicine and Health Sciences, University Putra Malaysia, Serdang, Malaysia

Sing Ziunn Hii
Viva Life Science Private Limited, Petaling Jaya, Malaysia

Seung Jun Kim, Hyung Jung Oh, Dong Eun Yoo, Dong Ho Shin, Mi Jung Lee, Hyoung Rae Kim, Jung Tak Park, Seung Hyeok Han, Tae-Hyun Yoo, Kyu Hun Choi
Department of Internal Medicine, College of Medicine, Yonsei University, Seoul, Korea

Shin-Wook Kang
Department of Internal Medicine, College of Medicine, Yonsei University, Seoul, Korea
Severance Biomedical Science Institute, Brain Korea 21, Yonsei University, Seoul, Korea

Ansgar Reising, Saskia Sambale, Julius J. Schmidt, Carsten Hafer, Bernhard M. W. Schmidt, Jan T. Kielstein
Department of Nephrology and Hypertension, Medical School Hannover, Hannover, Germany

Frank Donnerstag
Institute of Diagnostic and Interventional Neuroradiology, Medical School Hannover, Hannover, Germany

Cheng Li, Sheng Shen
Department of Renal Transplantation, Guangdong No.2 Provincial People's Hospital, Guangzhou, People's Republic of China

Huan-Huan Su, Ying-Wei Qiu, Wen-Feng Zhan, Jun-Zhang Tian, Gui-Hua Jiang
Department of Medical Imaging, Guangdong No.2 Provincial People's Hospital, Guangzhou, People's Republic of China,

Xiao-Fei Lv
State Key Laboratory of Oncology in South China and Department of Medical Imaging and Interventional Radiology, Sun Yat-Sen University Cancer Center, Guangzhou, People's Republic of China

Ria Arnold, Cindy S-Y. Lin, Arun V. Krishnan
Translational Neuroscience Facility, University of New South Wales, Sydney, New South Wales, Australia

Virginija Grinius
Department of Nephrology Prince of Wales Hospital, Sydney, New South Wales, Australia

Bruce A. Pussell, Timothy J. Pianta
Department of Nephrology Prince of Wales Hospital, Sydney, New South Wales, Australia
Prince of Wales Clinical School, University of New South Wales, Sydney, New South Wales, Australia

Matthew C. Kiernan
Prince of Wales Clinical School, University of New South Wales, Sydney, New South Wales, Australia
Neuroscience Research Australia, Sydney, New South Wales, Australia

James Howells
The University of Sydney and Institute of Clinical Neurosciences, Royal Prince Alfred Hospital, Sydney, New South Wales, Australia

Meg J. Jardine
Department of Nephrology Concord Repatriation General Hospital and The George Institute for Global Health, Sydney, New South Wales, Australia

Seung Joo Nam, Eui-Cheol Shin
Laboratory of Immunology and Infectious Diseases, Graduate School of Medical Science and Engineering, KAIST, Daejeon, Republic of Korea,

Yoon Seok Choi
Laboratory of Immunology and Infectious Diseases, Graduate School of Medical Science and Engineering, KAIST, Daejeon, Republic of Korea
Department of Internal Medicine, Chungnam National University College of Medicine, Daejeon, Republic of Korea

Jung Eun Lee, Jung Tak Park, Kyu Hun Choi, Beom Seok Kim
Department of Internal Medicine, Yonsei University College of Medicine, Seoul, Republic of Korea,

Hyon-Suk Kim
Department of Laboratory Medicine, Yonsei University College of Medicine, Seoul, Republic of Korea

Viknesh Selvarajah
Clinical Pharmacology Unit, Department of Medicine, University of Cambridge, Cambridge, United Kingdom
Department of Nephrology, Cambridge University Hospitals NHS Foundation Trust, Cambridge, United Kingdom

Sanjay Ojha
Department of Nephrology, Cambridge University Hospitals NHS Foundation Trust, Cambridge, United Kingdom

Laura Pasea
Centre for Applied Medical Statistics, Department of Public Health and Primary Care, Institute of Public Health, University of Cambridge, Cambridge, United Kingdom

Ian B. Wilkinson, Laurie A. Tomlinson
Cambridge Clinical Trials Unit, University of Cambridge, Cambridge, United Kingdom

I-Kuan Wang
Graduate Institute of Clinical Medical Science, China Medical University College of Medicine, Taichung, Taiwan
Division of Nephrology, China Medical University Hospital, Taichung, Taiwan
Department of Internal Medicine, China Medical University College of Medicine, Taichung, Taiwan

Chih-Chia Liang, Yao-Lung Liu, Chiz-Tzung Chang, Chiu-Ching Huang
Division of Nephrology, China Medical University Hospital, Taichung, Taiwan

Fung-Chang Sung, Cheng-Li Lin
Management Office for Health Data, China Medical University Hospital, Taichung, Taiwan,
Department of Public Health, China Medical University, Taichung, Taiwan

Po-Chang Lin
Division of Infection, China Medical University Hospital, Taichung, Taiwan

Tzung-Hai Yen
Division of Nephrology, Chang Gung Memorial Hospital, Taipei and Chang Gung Univeristy College of Medicine, Taoyuan, Taiwan

Donald E. Morisky
UCLA Fielding School of Public Health, Los Angeles, California, United States of America

Alexandre Granger Vallée
Nephrology, Dialysis and Intensive Care Unit, CHRU, Montpellier, France

Bernard Canaud, Leila Chenine, Hélène Leray-Moragues
Nephrology, Dialysis and Intensive Care Unit, CHRU, Montpellier, France
Dialysis Research and Training Institute, Montpellier, France

Annie Rodriguez
Dialysis Research and Training Institute, Montpellier, France

Marion Morena, Jean-Paul Cristol
Dialysis Research and Training Institute, Montpellier, France
Biochemistry Laboratory, CHRU, Montpellier, France
UMR 204, University of Montpellier I, Montpellier, France

Nicolas Molinari
UMR 729 MISTEA, DIM, CHRU, Montpellier, France

Lotfi Chalabi
AIDER, Montpellier, France

Ferruh Artunc, Robert Wagner, Andreas Peter, Hans-Ulrich Haering
Department of Internal Medicine, Division of Endocrinology, Diabetology, Vascular Disease, Nephrology and Clinical Chemistry, University of Tuebingen, Tuebingen, Germany

Bjoern Friedrich
Department of Internal Medicine, Division of Endocrinology, Diabetology, Vascular Disease, Nephrology and Clinical Chemistry, University of Tuebingen, Tuebingen, Germany Dialysis Center, Leonberg, Germany

Albina Nowak
Division of Internal Medicine, Division of Nephrology, University of Zurich, Zurich, Switzerland

Christian Mueller, Tobias Breidthardt, Raphael Twerenbold
Department of Internal Medicine, Division of Cardiology, University of Basel, Basel, Switzerland,

Stefan Ebmeyer
Fisher Scientific, Schwerte, Germany

Mengjing Wang, Haiming Li, Li You, Xiaoling Yu, Min Zhang, Chuanming Hao, Jing Chen
Division of Nephrology, Huashan Hospital, Shanghai Medical College, Fudan University, Shanghai, China

Ruijiang Zhu
Division of Radiology, Huashan Hospital, Shanghai Medical College, Fudan University, Shanghai, China

Zhijie Zhang
Department of Epidemiology and Biostatistics, School of Public Health, Fudan University, Shanghai, China
Biomedical statistical Center, Fudan University, Shanghai, China

Delong Zhao, Xuefeng Sun, Qi Huang, Yang Yang, Shimin Jiang, Yong Wang, Hanyu Zhu, Xiangmei Chen
Department of Nephrology, Chinese PLA General Hospital, State Key Laboratory of Kidney Disease (2011DAV00088), Beijing, China

Li Yao
Department of Nephrology, The First Affiliated Hospital, Chinese Medical University, Shenyang, China

Hongli Lin
Department of Nephrology, The First Affiliated Hospital, Dalian Medical College, Dalian, China,

Jijun Li
Department of Nephrology, The First Affiliated Hospital, General Hospital of PLA, Beijing, China,

Jiuyang Zhao
Department of Nephrology, The Second Affiliated Hospital, Dalian Medical College, Dalian, China,

Zhimin Zhang
Department of Nephrology, General Hospital of the General Headquarters, Beijing, China

Lide Lun
Department of Nephrology, General Hospital of the Air Force, Beijing, China

Jianrong Zhang
Department of Nephrology, General Hospital of the Force, Beijing, China

Mingxu Li
Department of Nephrology, General Hospital of the Navy, Beijing, China

Szu-Chun Hung
Division of Nephrology, Buddhist Tzu Chi General Hospital, Taipei Branch, Taipei, Taiwan

Yao-Ping Lin
Division of Nephrology, Department of Medicine, and Immunology Research Center, Taipei Veterans General Hospital, Taipei, Taiwan

Der-Cherng Tarng
Division of Nephrology, Department of Medicine, and Immunology Research Center, Taipei Veterans General Hospital, Taipei, Taiwan
Department and Institute of Physiology, School of Medicine, National Yang-Ming University, Taipei, Taiwan

Hsin-Lei Huang, Hsiao-Fung Pu
Department and Institute of Physiology, School of Medicine, National Yang-Ming University, Taipei, Taiwan

Eleonora Riccio, Maristella Minco, Gennaro Argentino, Roberta Russo, Stefania Brancaccio, Andrea Memoli, Bruno Memoli
Department of Public Health, Section of Nephrology, Federico II University of Naples, Naples, Italy

Mauro Cataldi
Department of Neuroscience, Reproductive and Odontostomatologic Sciences, Section of Pharmacology, Federico II University of Naples, Naples, Italy

Lucia Grumetto
Department of Pharmaceutical and Toxicological Chemistry, Federico II University of Naples, Naples, Italy

Loredana Postiglione
Department of Cellular and Molecular Biology and Pathology, Federico II University of Naples, Naples, Italy

Bruna Guida
Department of Clinical Medicine and Surgery, Federico II University of Naples, Naples, Italy

Bogusz Trojanowicz, Christof Ulrich, Eric Seibert, Roman Fiedler, Matthias Girndt
Department of Internal Medicine II, Martin-Luther-University Halle-Wittenberg, Germany

Index

www.ingramcontent.com/pod-product-compliance
Lightning Source LLC
LaVergne TN
LVHW081013210926
848485LV00004B/849